Rehabilitation for Persistent Pain across the Lifespan

Rehabilitation for Persistent Pain across the Lifespan

Editors

**Jo Nijs
Kelly Ickmans**

MDPI • Basel • Beijing • Wuhan • Barcelona • Belgrade • Manchester • Tokyo • Cluj • Tianjin

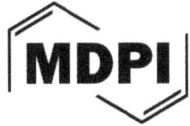

Editors
Jo Nijs
Department of Physiotherapy,
Human Physiology and
Anatomy, Faculty of Physical
Education and Physiotherapy,
Vrije Universiteit Brussel
Belgium

Kelly Ickmans
Department of Physiotherapy,
Human Physiology and Anatomy,
Faculty of Physical Education
and Physiotherapy,
Vrije Universiteit Brussel
Belgium

Editorial Office
MDPI
St. Alban-Anlage 66
4052 Basel, Switzerland

This is a reprint of articles from the Special Issue published online in the open access journal *Journal of Clinical Medicine* (ISSN 2077-0383) (available at: https://www.mdpi.com/journal/jcm/special_issues/Rehab_Pain).

For citation purposes, cite each article independently as indicated on the article page online and as indicated below:

LastName, A.A.; LastName, B.B.; LastName, C.C. Article Title. *Journal Name* **Year**, *Volume Number*, Page Range.

ISBN 978-3-03943-843-3 (Hbk)
ISBN 978-3-03943-844-0 (PDF)

© 2020 by the authors. Articles in this book are Open Access and distributed under the Creative Commons Attribution (CC BY) license, which allows users to download, copy and build upon published articles, as long as the author and publisher are properly credited, which ensures maximum dissemination and a wider impact of our publications.

The book as a whole is distributed by MDPI under the terms and conditions of the Creative Commons license CC BY-NC-ND.

Contents

About the Editors vii

Kelly Ickmans, Lennard Voogt and Jo Nijs
Rehabilitation Succeeds Where Technology and Pharmacology Failed: Effective Treatment of Persistent Pain across the Lifespan
Reprinted from: *J. Clin. Med.* **2019**, *8*, 2042, doi:10.3390/jcm8122042 1

Jo Nijs, Kelly Ickmans, David Beckwée and Laurence Leysen
Behavioral Graded Activity+ (BGA+) for Osteoarthritis: A Paradigm Shift from Disease-Based Treatment to Personalized Activity Self-Management
Reprinted from: *J. Clin. Med.* **2020**, *9*, 1793, doi:10.3390/jcm9061793 5

Lauren E. Harrison, Joshua W. Pate, Patricia A. Richardson, Kelly Ickmans, Rikard K. Wicksell and Laura E. Simons
Best-Evidence for the Rehabilitation of Chronic Pain Part 1: Pediatric Pain
Reprinted from: *J. Clin. Med.* **2019**, *8*, 1267, doi:10.3390/jcm8091267 11

An De Groef, Frauke Penen, Lore Dams, Elien Van der Gucht, Jo Nijs and Mira Meeus
Best-Evidence Rehabilitation for Chronic Pain Part 2: Pain during and after Cancer Treatment
Reprinted from: *J. Clin. Med.* **2019**, *8*, 979, doi:10.3390/jcm8070979 31

Anneleen Malfliet, Kelly Ickmans, Eva Huysmans, Iris Coppieters, Ward Willaert, Wouter Van Bogaert, Emma Rheel, Thomas Bilterys, Paul Van Wilgen and Jo Nijs
Best Evidence Rehabilitation for Chronic Pain Part 3: Low Back Pain
Reprinted from: *J. Clin. Med.* **2019**, *8*, 1063, doi:10.3390/jcm8071063 51

Michele Sterling, Rutger M. J. de Zoete, Iris Coppieters and Scott F. Farrell
Best Evidence Rehabilitation for Chronic Pain Part 4: Neck Pain
Reprinted from: *J. Clin. Med.* **2019**, *8*, 1219, doi:10.3390/jcm8081219 75

David Rice, Peter McNair, Eva Huysmans, Janelle Letzen and Patrick Finan
Best Evidence Rehabilitation for Chronic Pain Part 5: Osteoarthritis
Reprinted from: *J. Clin. Med.* **2019**, *8*, 1769, doi:10.3390/jcm8111769 95

Thomas Probst, Robert Jank, Nele Dreyer, Stefanie Seel, Ruth Wagner, Klaus Hanshans, Renate Reyersbach, Andreas Mühlberger, Claas Lahmann and Christoph Pieh
Early Changes in Pain Acceptance Predict Pain Outcomes in Interdisciplinary Treatment for Chronic Pain
Reprinted from: *J. Clin. Med.* **2019**, *8*, 1373, doi:10.3390/jcm8091373 127

Adrián Pérez-Aranda, Francesco D'Amico, Albert Feliu-Soler, Lance M. McCracken, María T. Peñarrubia-María, Laura Andrés-Rodríguez, Natalia Angarita-Osorio, Martin Knapp, Javier García-Campayo and Juan V. Luciano
Cost–Utility of Mindfulness-Based Stress Reduction for Fibromyalgia versus a Multicomponent Intervention and Usual Care: A 12-Month Randomized Controlled Trial (EUDAIMON Study)
Reprinted from: *J. Clin. Med.* **2019**, *8*, 1068, doi:10.3390/jcm8071068 137

Luis Suso-Martí, Jose Vicente León-Hernández, Roy La Touche, Alba Paris-Alemany and Ferran Cuenca-Martínez
Motor Imagery and Action Observation of Specific Neck Therapeutic Exercises Induced Hypoalgesia in Patients with Chronic Neck Pain: A Randomized Single-Blind Placebo Trial
Reprinted from: *J. Clin. Med.* **2019**, *8*, 1019, doi:10.3390/jcm8071019 157

Åsa Ringqvist, Elena Dragioti, Mathilda Björk, Britt Larsson and Björn Gerdle
Moderate and Stable Pain Reductions as a Result of Interdisciplinary Pain Rehabilitation—A Cohort Study from the Swedish Quality Registry for Pain Rehabilitation (SQRP)
Reprinted from: *J. Clin. Med.* **2019**, *8*, 905, doi:10.3390/jcm8060905 . . . . **175**

Matthias Vogel, Martin Krippl, Lydia Frenzel, Christian Riediger, Jörg Frommer, Christoph Lohmann and Sebastian Illiger
Dissociation and Pain-Catastrophizing: Absorptive Detachment as a Higher-Order Factor in Control of Pain-Related Fearful Anticipations Prior to Total Knee Arthroplasty (TKA)
Reprinted from: *J. Clin. Med.* **2019**, *8*, 697, doi:10.3390/jcm8050697 . . . . **203**

Ann-Christin Pfeifer, Pamela Meredith, Paul Schröder-Pfeifer, Juan Martin Gomez Penedo, Johannes C. Ehrenthal, Corinna Schroeter, Eva Neubauer and Marcus Schiltenwolf
Effectiveness of an Attachment-Informed Working Alliance in Interdisciplinary Pain Therapy
Reprinted from: *J. Clin. Med.* **2019**, *8*, 364, doi:10.3390/jcm8030364 . . . . **219**

Manuel Albornoz-Cabello, Jose Antonio Sanchez-Santos, Rocio Melero-Suarez, Alberto Marcos Heredia-Rizo and Luis Espejo-Antunez
Effects of Adding Interferential Therapy Electro-Massage to Usual Care after Surgery in Subacromial Pain Syndrome: A Randomized Clinical Trial
Reprinted from: *J. Clin. Med.* **2019**, *8*, 175, doi:10.3390/jcm8020175 . . . . **237**

Zoë C. Franklin, Paul S. Holmes and Neil E. Fowler
Eye Gaze Markers Indicate Visual Attention to Threatening Images in Individuals with Chronic Back Pain
Reprinted from: *J. Clin. Med.* **2019**, *8*, 31, doi:10.3390/jcm8010031 . . . . **251**

Elena Dragioti, Mathilda Björk, Britt Larsson and Björn Gerdle
A Meta-Epidemiological Appraisal of the Effects of Interdisciplinary Multimodal Pain Therapy Dosing for Chronic Low Back Pain
Reprinted from: *J. Clin. Med.* **2019**, *8*, 871, doi:10.3390/jcm8060871 . . . . **265**

Jon Ford, Andrew Hahne, Luke Surkitt, Alexander Chan and Matthew Richards
The Evolving Case Supporting Individualised Physiotherapy for Low Back Pain
Reprinted from: *J. Clin. Med.* **2019**, *8*, 1334, doi:10.3390/jcm8091334 . . . . **283**

Liye Zou, Yanjie Zhang, Lin Yang, Paul D. Loprinzi, Albert S. Yeung, Jian Kong, Kevin W Chen, Wook Song, Tao Xiao and Hong Li
Are Mindful Exercises Safe and Beneficial for Treating Chronic Lower Back Pain? A Systematic Review and Meta-Analysis of Randomized Controlled Trials
Reprinted from: *J. Clin. Med.* **2019**, *8*, 628, doi:10.3390/jcm8050628 . . . . **307**

About the Editors

Jo Nijs holds a PhD in rehabilitation science and physiotherapy. He is Professor at the Vrije Universiteit Brussel (Brussels, Belgium), physiotherapist/manual therapist at the University Hospital Brussels, Chair of oncological physiotherapy funded by the Berekuyl Academy, the Netherlands, and part of the Visiting Professor program of the University of Gothenburg (Sweden). Jo runs the Pain in Motion international research group (www.paininmotion.be). His research and clinical interests are patients with chronic pain and pain–movement interactions, with special emphasis on the central nervous system. The primary aim of his research is improving care for patients with chronic pain. At the age of 44, he has (co-)authored >260 peer reviewed publications (including papers in high impact journals such as *The Lancet* and *JAMA Neurology*), obtained €9.5 million grant income, supervised 18 PhD projects to completion and served on more than 290 occasions as an invited speaker at national and international meetings in 25 different countries (including 33 keynotes). He has trained around 3000 clinicians in 92 courses held in 12 different countries spread over 4 continents. His work has been cited over 7000 times (h-index: 47), with 26 citations per article (ISI Web of Knowledge). Jo is ranked 2nd in the world among chronic pain researchers (1st in Europe; expertscape.com), received the 2017 Excellence in Research Award from the JOSPT (USA), and the 2020 Francqui Collen Chair awarded by the University of Hasselt, Belgium.

Kelly Ickmans is part time Postdoctoral Research Fellow at the Research Foundation Flanders (FWO), Vrije Universiteit Brussel (Brussels, Belgium), where she is also part time Assistant Professor (ZAP). She is also an attending physiotherapist at the University Hospital Brussels (Brussels, Belgium) where she treats adults and children with chronic pain. In 2014, Kelly obtained her PhD in Rehabilitation Sciences and Physiotherapy. Within the international Pain in Motion research group (www.paininmotion.be), she leads the line of research on pediatric pain. Since the start of her research career in 2011, Kelly has (co-)authored over 80 peer-reviewed publications in international journals, including several papers in high impact journals. Her work has been cited over 1000 times in the scientific literature (h-index 18) with an average of 13 citations per article. She has furthermore published 4 chapters in (inter)national handbooks, served dozens of times as an invited speaker at national and international meetings in 8 different countries, delivered over 30 post-academic and refresher courses in different countries over the world, supervised 3 PhD projects to completion, and is currently (co-)supervisor of 8 PhD projects.

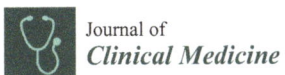

Editorial

Rehabilitation Succeeds Where Technology and Pharmacology Failed: Effective Treatment of Persistent Pain across the Lifespan

Kelly Ickmans [1,2,3,*], Lennard Voogt [1,4,5] and Jo Nijs [1,2]

1. Pain in Motion International Research Group, Department of Physiotherapy, Human Physiology and Anatomy, Faculty of Physical Education & Physiotherapy, Vrije Universiteit Brussel, Laarbeeklaan 103, 1090 Brussels, Belgium; l.p.voogt@hr.nl (L.V.); jo.nijs@vub.be (J.N.)
2. Department of Physical Medicine and Physiotherapy, Universitair Ziekenhuis Brussel, Laarbeeklaan 101, 1090 Brussels, Belgium
3. Research Foundation-Flanders (FWO), 1000 Brussels, Belgium
4. Research Centre for Health Care Innovations, Rotterdam University of Applied Sciences, 3015 EK Rotterdam, The Netherlands
5. Department of Physical Therapy Studies, Rotterdam University of Applied Sciences, 3015 EK Rotterdam, The Netherlands
* Correspondence: Kelly.Ickmans@vub.be; Tel.: +32-(0)24774503

Received: 14 November 2019; Accepted: 18 November 2019; Published: 21 November 2019

Chronic pain affects up to 30% of the adult population [1] and 11% to 38% of the childhood and adolescent population [2,3]. Its tremendous personal and socioeconomic impact is reflected by its cause of the highest number of years lived with disability [4] and being the most expensive cause of work-related disability in adults [5,6]. In children and adolescents, chronic pain causes decreased participation in recreational activities, difficulty maintaining social contacts, school absence and academic impairment, decreased health related quality of life, and increased health care utilization [3,7].

The area of rehabilitation research for patients having persistent pain is on the move with a substantial increase in the scientific understanding of persistent pain over the past decades. This rapid growth in pain science has inspired rehabilitation clinicians and researchers around the globe, leading to breakthrough research and the implementation of contemporary pain science in rehabilitation settings. Still, our understanding of persistent pain continues to grow, not in the least because of fascinating discoveries from areas such as psychoneuroimmunology, epigenetics, exercise physiology, clinical psychology, and nutritional (neuro)biology. This offers unique opportunities to further improve rehabilitation for patients with chronic pain. As age is a determining factor in the uniqueness of the bio-, psycho-, and social factors of persistent pain, this also implies that rehabilitation interventions should be tailored across the lifespan. Also, the diversity of health care disciplines involved in the rehabilitation of chronic pain (e.g., physicians, psychologists, physiotherapists, occupational therapists, nurses, coaches) provides a framework for upgrading rehabilitation for chronic pain towards comprehensive lifestyle approaches.

A number of articles published in this Special Issue draw specific attention to interdisciplinary multimodal rehabilitation programs for chronic pain. Ringqvist et al. [8] provide evidence that such programs delivered to adults in specialist care show moderate long-term effect sizes for pain, pain interference in daily life, and perceived health. Interestingly, Pfeifer et al. [9] provide preliminary support for the utility of incorporating an attachment-informed approach within these existing multimodal pain therapies, thereby aiming at advancing the working alliance between patient and therapist. In the realm of pediatric chronic pain rehabilitation, Harrison et al. [10] state that preliminary evidence on interdisciplinary outpatient treatments is promising with regard to improvements in pain intensity, pain-related disability, school attendance, catastrophizing, and symptoms of depression.

In addition, addressing multiple unfavorable lifestyle factors, such as physical inactivity, sedentary behavior, stress, smoking, unhealthy diet, and poor sleep concomitantly, seems to be a challenge for which such interdisciplinary pain rehabilitation programs may offer a comprehensive framework. Indeed, unfavorable lifestyle factors and pain have been shown to be interconnected [11]. This suggests that multimodal lifestyle-centered approaches may be effective for chronic pain. Actually, this matter is touched on in each of the five invited contributions on the best evidence rehabilitation for chronic pain [10,12–15], thus underscoring its topicality for persistent pain rehabilitation and providing important avenues for future research.

The invited contributions in this Special Issue are part of a "Best Evidence Rehabilitation for Chronic Pain" Series comprising five state-of-the-art papers from world leading experts regarding persistent pain. Part 1, by Harrison et al. [10], covers the current state-of-the-art rehabilitation approaches to treat persistent pain in children and adolescents. In addition, several emerging areas of interventions are highlighted to guide future research and clinical practice. Part 2, the article by De Groef et al. [12], provides the reader with a state-of-the-art overview of the best evidence rehabilitation modalities for patients having (persistent) pain during and following cancer treatment. This paper is of particular importance to the field of oncology, especially now that common practices to manage cancer pain are being challenged due to a lack of supporting evidence [16,17]. In parts 3 and 4, Malfliet et al. [13] and Sterling et al. [14] present an overview of the best evidence non-invasive rehabilitation for people having chronic low back pain and neck pain, respectively. Finally, in part 5, a state-of-the-art review of rehabilitation for osteoarthritis pain is provided by Rice et al. [15]. For each of these domains, the best evidence rehabilitation is reviewed in a way that clinicians can integrate it into their daily clinical routine. The "Best Evidence Tables", "Future Directions for Clinical Practice" sections, and key references to treatment manuals included in each of these papers serve to meet that aim. In addition, these overview articles also help clinical researchers to build upon the best evidence for designing future trials, implementation studies, and new innovative studies.

In summary, the collection of high-quality work presented in this Special Issue provides important new evidence from experimental lab-based as well as clinical studies, all focusing on rehabilitation for people with persistent pain. The review articles included in the "Best Evidence Rehabilitation for Chronic Pain" Series together delineate an important trend of continuously growing evidence supporting rehabilitation approaches for people with chronic pain. The more rehabilitation programs for people with chronic pain develop into multimodal lifestyle approaches, the stronger the evidence supporting them as key elements in the treatment for chronic pain. This is in sharp contrast with medical interventions for chronic pain such as (spinal) surgery, interventional treatments such as radiofrequency denervation, and analgesics that struggle following rigorous scientific evaluation [18–20], especially when side effects and cost-effectiveness are taken into account. Rehabilitation is succeeding where technology and pharmacology failed: providing effective treatment for people suffering from chronic pain. Still, much work needs to be done regarding implementation as well as scientific research. Therefore, we believe that the original and novel information along with the overview papers within the "Best Evidence Rehabilitation for Chronic Pain" Series in this Special Issue will serve as an important resource for researchers and an aid for clinicians to facilitate integration from research into daily clinical practice. Thereby, we hope to serve as a guiding light for future research in this area and to aid in further improvements in the quality of care for people with persistent pain across the lifespan.

Acknowledgments: No funding nor sponsorship was received for the present paper. Kelly Ickmans is a postdoctoral research fellow funded by the Research Foundation – Flanders (FWO). Jo Nijs is holder of a Chair entitled "Exercise immunology and chronic fatigue in health and disease" funded by the Berekuyl Academy, The Netherlands.

Conflicts of Interest: The authors declare no conflict of interest.

References

1. Mills, S.E.E.; Nicolson, K.P.; Smith, B.H. Chronic pain: A review of its epidemiology and associated factors in population-based studies. *Br. J. Anaesth.* **2019**, *123*, e273–e283. [CrossRef] [PubMed]
2. King, S.; Chambers, C.T.; Huguet, A.; MacNevin, R.C.; McGrath, P.J.; Parker, L.; MacDonald, A.J. The epidemiology of chronic pain in children and adolescents revisited: A systematic review. *Pain* **2011**, *152*, 2729–2738. [CrossRef] [PubMed]
3. Roth-Isigkeit, A.; Thyen, U.; Stoven, H.; Schwarzenberger, J.; Schmucker, P. Pain among children and adolescents: Restrictions in daily living and triggering factors. *Pediatrics* **2005**, *115*, e152–e162. [CrossRef] [PubMed]
4. Global Burden of Disease Study 2013 Collaborators. Global, regional, and national incidence, prevalence, and years lived with disability for 301 acute and chronic diseases and injuries in 188 countries, 1990–2013: A systematic analysis for the Global Burden of Disease Study 2013. *Lancet (Lond. Engl.)* **2015**, *386*, 743–800. [CrossRef]
5. Andersson, G.B. Epidemiological features of chronic low-back pain. *Lancet (Lond. Engl.)* **1999**, *354*, 581–585. [CrossRef]
6. Waddell, G.; Burton, A.K. Occupational health guidelines for the management of low back pain at work: Evidence review. *Occup. Med. (Oxf. Engl.)* **2001**, *51*, 124–135. [CrossRef] [PubMed]
7. Vervoort, T.; Logan, D.E.; Goubert, L.; De Clercq, B.; Hublet, A. Severity of pediatric pain in relation to school-related functioning and teacher support: An epidemiological study among school-aged children and adolescents. *Pain* **2014**, *155*, 1118–1127. [CrossRef] [PubMed]
8. Ringqvist, A.; Dragioti, E.; Bjork, M.; Larsson, B.; Gerdle, B. Moderate and stable pain reductions as a result of interdisciplinary pain rehabilitation-A cohort study from the Swedish quality registry for pain rehabilitation (SQRP). *J. Clin. Med.* **2019**, *8*, 905. [CrossRef] [PubMed]
9. Pfeifer, A.C.; Meredith, P.; Schroder-Pfeifer, P.; Gomez Penedo, J.M.; Ehrenthal, J.C.; Schroeter, C.; Neubauer, E.; Schiltenwolf, M. Effectiveness of an attachment-informed working alliance in interdisciplinary pain therapy. *J. Clin. Med.* **2019**, *8*, 364. [CrossRef] [PubMed]
10. Harrison, L.E.; Pate, J.W.; Richardson, P.A.; Ickmans, K.; Wicksell, R.K.; Simons, L.E. Best-evidence for the rehabilitation of chronic pain part 1: Pediatric pain. *J. Clin. Med.* **2019**, *8*, 1267. [CrossRef] [PubMed]
11. Nijs, J.; D'Hondt, E.; Clarys, P.; Deliens, T.; Polli, A.; Malfliet, A.; Coppieters, I.; Willaert, W.; Tumkaya Yilmaz, S.; Elma, O.; et al. Lifestyle and chronic pain across the lifespan: An inconvenient truth? *PM R J. Inj. Funct. Rehabil.* **2019**. [CrossRef] [PubMed]
12. De Groef, A.; Penen, F.; Dams, L.; Van der Gucht, E.; Nijs, J.; Meeus, M. Best-evidence rehabilitation for chronic pain part 2: Pain during and after cancer treatment. *J. Clin. Med.* **2019**, *8*, 979. [CrossRef] [PubMed]
13. Malfliet, A.; Ickmans, K.; Huysmans, E.; Coppieters, I.; Willaert, W.; Bogaert, W.V.; Rheel, E.; Bilterys, T.; Wilgen, P.V.; Nijs, J. Best evidence rehabilitation for chronic pain part 3: Low back pain. *J. Clin. Med.* **2019**, *8*, 1063. [CrossRef] [PubMed]
14. Sterling, M.; de Zoete, R.M.J.; Coppieters, I.; Farrell, S.F. Best evidence rehabilitation for chronic pain part 4: Neck pain. *J. Clin. Med.* **2019**, *8*, 1219. [CrossRef] [PubMed]
15. Rice, D.; McNair, P.; Huysmans, E.; Letzen, J.; Finan, P. Best evidence rehabilitation for chronic pain part 5: Osteoarthritis. *J. Clin. Med.* **2019**, *8*, 1769. [CrossRef] [PubMed]
16. Smith, E.M.L. Pharmacologic treatments for chronic cancer-related pain: Does anything work? *J. Clin. Oncol. Off. J. Am. Soc. Clin. Oncol.* **2019**, *37*, 1686–1689. [CrossRef] [PubMed]
17. Huang, R.; Jiang, L.; Cao, Y.; Liu, H.; Ping, M.; Li, W.; Xu, Y.; Ning, J.; Chen, Y.; Wang, X. Comparative efficacy of therapeutics for chronic cancer pain: A Bayesian network meta-analysis. *J. Clin. Oncol. Off. J. Am. Soc. Clin. Oncol.* **2019**, *37*, 1742–1752. [CrossRef] [PubMed]
18. Louw, A.; Diener, I.; Fernandez-de-Las-Penas, C.; Puentedura, E.J. Sham surgery in orthopedics: A systematic review of the literature. *Pain Med. (Malden Mass.)* **2017**, *18*, 736–750. [CrossRef] [PubMed]

19. Juch, J.N.S.; Maas, E.T.; Ostelo, R.; Groeneweg, J.G.; Kallewaard, J.W.; Koes, B.W.; Verhagen, A.P.; van Dongen, J.M.; Huygen, F.; van Tulder, M.W. Effect of radiofrequency denervation on pain intensity among patients with chronic low back pain: The mint randomized clinical trials. *JAMA* **2017**, *318*, 68–81. [CrossRef] [PubMed]
20. Nijs, J.; Leysen, L.; Vanlauwe, J.; Logghe, T.; Ickmans, K.; Polli, A.; Malfliet, A.; Coppieters, I.; Huysmans, E. Treatment of central sensitization in patients with chronic pain: Time for change? *Expert Opin. Pharmacother.* **2019**, *20*, 1961–1970. [CrossRef] [PubMed]

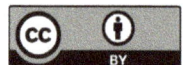

© 2019 by the authors. Licensee MDPI, Basel, Switzerland. This article is an open access article distributed under the terms and conditions of the Creative Commons Attribution (CC BY) license (http://creativecommons.org/licenses/by/4.0/).

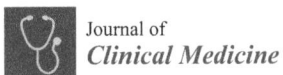

Editorial

Behavioral Graded Activity+ (BGA+) for Osteoarthritis: A Paradigm Shift from Disease-Based Treatment to Personalized Activity Self-Management

Jo Nijs [1,2,3,*], Kelly Ickmans [1,2,4], David Beckwée [5] and Laurence Leysen [1,5]

1. Pain in Motion International Research Group, Department of Physiotherapy, Human Physiology and Anatomy, Faculty of Physical Education & Physiotherapy, Vrije Universiteit Brussel, BE-1090 Brussels, Belgium; kelly.ickmans@vub.be (K.I.); Laurence.Leysen@vub.be (L.L.)
2. Chronic Pain Rehabilitation, Department of Physical Medicine and Physiotherapy, University Hospital Brussels, BE1090 Brussels, Belgium
3. Institute of Neuroscience and Physiology, University of Gothenburg, Box 430, SE-405 30 Göteborg, Sweden
4. Flemish Research Foundation (FWO), BE1050 Brussels, Belgium
5. Rehabilitation Research Group, Department of Physiotherapy, Human Physiology and Anatomy, Faculty of Physical Education & Physiotherapy, Vrije Universiteit Brussel, BE-1090 Brussels, Belgium; david.beckwee@vub.be
* Correspondence: Jo.Nijs@vub.be; Tel.: +32-2477-4489

Received: 3 June 2020; Accepted: 4 June 2020; Published: 9 June 2020

Abstract: Three promising directions for improving care for osteoarthritis (OA) include novel education strategies to target unhelpful illness and treatment beliefs; methods to enhance the efficacy of exercise interventions; and innovative, brain-directed treatments. Here we explain that each of those three promising directions can be combined through a paradigm-shift from disease-based treatments to personalized activity self-management for patients with OA. Behavioral graded activity (BGA) accounts for the current understanding of OA and OA pain and allows a paradigm shift from a disease-based treatment to personalized activity self-management for patients with OA. To account for the implementation barriers of BGA, we propose adding pain neuroscience education to BGA (referred to as BGA+). Rather than focusing on the biomedical (and biomechanical) disease characteristics of OA, pain neuroscience education implies teaching people about the underlying biopsychosocial mechanisms of pain. To account for the lack of studies showing that BGA is "safe" with respect to disease activity and the inflammatory nature of OA patients, a trial exploring the effects of BGA+ on the markers of inflammation is needed. Such a trial could clear the path for the required paradigm shift in the management of OA (pain) and would allow workforce capacity building that de-emphasizes biomedical management for OA.

Keywords: rehabilitation; chronic pain; inflammation

1. Introduction

Given the high number of treatment guidelines available, clinicians might be overwhelmed by the evidence on osteoarthritis (OA) management. Taking into account the socio-economic impact and high prevalence of OA, it is imperative that healthcare professionals have free access to up-to-date, evidence-based information to assist them in treatment decision-making. Therefore, in the *Journal of Clinical Medicine*'s Special Issue on "Rehabilitation for Persistent Pain Across the Lifespan", Rice et al. provide a state-of-the-art review of rehabilitation for OA pain [1]. In addition to providing a comprehensive and easily consumable overview of the best evidence on rehabilitation for OA pain, they also explore promising directions for clinical practice and discuss potential future research avenues. The promising directions for clinical practice include novel education strategies to target unhelpful illness and treatment beliefs; methods to enhance the efficacy of exercise interventions; and innovative, brain-directed treatments [1]. Here we explain that each of those three promising directions can be combined through a paradigm-shift from disease-based treatments to personalized activity self-management for patients with OA.

2. Disease-Based Osteoarthritis Treatment Offers Modest Effect Sizes

Current OA treatment guidelines have a disease-based, biomedical focus (e.g., joint replacement surgery). Even education and exercise therapy, cornerstones of international OA treatment guidelines [2–5], have a disease-based focus; education typically consists of accurate information to enhance the understanding of the condition (hip or knee OA) and its consequences, while the progression of exercises is typically guided by tolerable levels of pain and the patient's ability to perform a given exercise. Such a disease-based, biomedical focus is offline with our current understanding of OA pain [6], including its biopsychosocial nature and the role of central sensitization in amplifying the OA pain experience [7]. The effect sizes of disease-based education and exercise therapy for OA are moderate at best [5], allowing room for improvement. Such improvement might come from modifying existing disease-based educational and exercise therapy interventions to our current understanding of OA pain [6,8].

3. Personalized Activity Self-Management for Patients with Osteoarthritis

High all-cause mortality from knee OA is mediated mainly through walking disability [9], and encouraging people to walk and "get out and about" in addition to targeting OA can be protective against excessive mortality [10]. However, to people with OA, pain represents a major barrier to walking or any other physical activity [11–13]. An innovative and effective way of accounting for the current biopsychosocial understanding of OA pain and encouraging people to walk and "get out and about" and addressing pain as a barrier to physical activity, is through using behavioral-graded activity (BGA). BGA is a behavioral treatment integrating the concept of operant conditioning to increase the level of physical activity in the patient's daily life [14]. It is a highly personalized approach, targeting the patients' activity limitations and self-defined treatment goals (goal setting), and individually tailoring the baseline and grading levels for performing these daily activities. BGA allows OA patients to shift from having priority in pain control to priority in valued life goals.

The use of BGA for patients with OA pain is supported by a cluster-randomized clinical trial [14,15], suggesting that BGA is an effective treatment for relieving pain, improving physical functioning and physical performance, and preventing joint replacement surgery in patients with OA [14,15]. Compared to usual care, BGA resulted in superior exercise adherence and more physical activity in people with hip or knee OA [16]. Such increased physical activity levels not only result in less pain [17] but also hold the potential to decrease the low-grade inflammation that is characteristic of OA. Indeed, OA is characterized by a chronic low-grade inflammatory profile [18–20], and physical activity has strong anti-inflammatory effects [21–26], but studies in OA remain scarce. With its anti-inflammatory action, physical activity might even contribute to decreasing the mortality risk in patients with OA [27–29].

4. Implementation Barriers for a Personalized Activity Self-Management Approach

BGA accounts for the current understanding of OA and OA pain and allows a paradigm shift from a disease-based treatment to personalized activity self-management for patients with OA (Table 1). However, more than 10 years after the initial trial findings were published, BGA is not recommended by the European [30], American [4], or international [3] guidelines for OA management, preventing its implementation in clinical practice. Another implementation barrier relates to the common belief among both patients and therapists that OA pain is a "warning sign" of disease severity. Up to 89% of future therapists consider severe pain a reason for not using exercise in the treatment of OA, while 87% believe that increasing overall activity levels cannot stop the knee problem getting worse [31]. A multinational study concluded that workforce capacity building that de-emphasizes biomedical management for OA is urgently needed [32]. Beliefs about the consequences of exercise account for general practitioners' use of exercise in knee pain [33] (with 29% believing that rest was the optimum management approach for knee OA [34]). To account for these implementation barriers, we propose adding pain neuroscience education to BGA (referred to as BGA$^+$).

Table 1. Proposed paradigm shift from disease-based treatment to personalized activity self-management for osteoarthritis.

Current Best-Evidence: Disease-Based Treatment	Personalized Activity Self-Management
Disease-based, biomedically focussed eduation	Biopsychosocial education
Exercises target muscle strength, endurance, motor control, etc.	Physical activities targeting self-defined functional and/or social activities and life goals
Pain = sign of tissue damage, including inflammation	Pain = sign of nervous system sensitivity
Pain contingent approach to grading exercises	Operant conditioning and time contingent approach to grading daily activities

5. Pain Neuroscience Education + Behavioral Graded Activity = BGA$^+$

Indeed, patients with OA are confused about the cause of their pain and bewildered by its variability and randomness [35]. Without adequate information and advice from healthcare professionals, people do not know what they should and should not do, and, as a consequence, avoid activity for fear of causing harm. A Cochrane review concluded that providing reassurance and clear advice about the value of exercise in OA and opportunities to participate in exercise programs that people regard as enjoyable and relevant to their personal life may encourage greater exercise participation, which brings a range of health benefits to patients with OA [36]. Therefore, the addition of pain neuroscience education to BGA entails a dramatic shift in educating OA patients prior to exercise/activity interventions.

As explained by Rice et al. [1], rather than focusing on the biomedical (and biomechanical) disease characteristics of OA, pain neuroscience education implies teaching people about the underlying biopsychosocial mechanisms of pain. Pain neuroscience education is a remarkable example of how patients who receive proper guidance can really help themselves. Pain neuroscience education prepares patients for a time-contingent ("Perform the activity/exercise for five minutes, regardless of the pain."), cognition-targeted approach to daily (physical) activity and exercise therapy, as typically applied during BGA. Such a time-contingent approach replaces the classical symptom-contingent ("Stop the activity/exercise once it hurts") approach. A time-contingent approach to activities is often difficult for patients to comprehend and comply with and for therapists to implement. Indeed, a time-contingent approach to activities/exercises contradicts with the disease-based, biomedical focus on exercise and activity interventions with which therapists are often more comfortable with [37]. Pain neuroscience education specifically addresses this barrier for making a the paradigm shift to personalized activity self-management for patients with OA, both at the patient and the therapist level.

In a recent proof-of-concept study, we reported that pain neuroscience education, compared to biomedical-focused education, generates favorable effects on decreasing pain catastrophizing, excessive attention to pain, and activity-related fear at short and long-term follow-ups in people with knee OA [38]. In addition, a case series of 12 OA patients receiving pain neuroscience education prior to joint replacement surgery revealed that the fear of movement and sensitivity to pain decreased [39].

6. Conclusions

Taken together, BGA$^+$ addresses all three promising directions for clinical practice highlighted by Rice et al. [1]. BGA$^+$ includes a novel education strategy to target unhelpful illness and treatment beliefs; applies evidence-based methods to enhance the efficacy of physical activity/exercise interventions;

and can be considered an innovative, brain-directed treatment. Hence, BGA⁺ allows a paradigm-shift from disease-based treatments to personalized activity self-management for patients with OA. Still, to account for the implementation barrier, where OA patients fear that moving despite pain might aggravate disease activity, as well as the lack of studies showing that BGA is "safe" with respect to disease activity and the inflammatory nature of OA patients (therapist barrier), a trial exploring the effects of BGA⁺ on the markers of inflammation in patients with OA is urgently needed. Such a trial could clear the path for the required paradigm shift in the management of OA (pain) and would allow workforce capacity building that de-emphasizes biomedical management for OA [32].

Author Contributions: Conceptualization, J.N.; writing—original draft preparation, J.N.; writing—review and editing, J.N., K.I., D.B., L.L.; supervision, L.L. All authors have read and agreed to the published version of the manuscript

Funding: This research received no external funding.

Conflicts of Interest: J.N. coauthored a Dutch book on pain neuroscience education, but the royalties are collected by the Vrije Universiteit Brussel and not him personally. Besides that, the authors declare no conflict of interest.

References

1. Rice, D.; McNair, P.; Huysmans, E.; Letzen, J.; Finan, P. Best Evidence Rehabilitation for Chronic Pain Part 5: Osteoarthritis. *J. Clin. Med.* **2019**, *8*, 1769. [CrossRef]
2. Zhang, W.; Moskowitz, R.W.; Nuki, G.; Abramson, S.; Altman, R.D.; Arden, N.; Bierma-Zeinstra, S.; Brandt, K.D.; Croft, P.; Doherty, M.; et al. OARSI recommendations for the management of hip and knee osteoarthritis, Part II: OARSI evidence-based, expert consensus guidelines. *Osteoarthr. Cartil.* **2008**, *16*, 137–162. [CrossRef] [PubMed]
3. McAlindon, T.E.; Bannuru, R.R.; Sullivan, M.C.; Arden, N.K.; Berenbaum, F.; Bierma-Zeinstra, S.M.; Hawker, G.A.; Henrotin, Y.; Hunter, D.J.; Kawaguchi, H.; et al. OARSI guidelines for the non-surgical management of knee osteoarthritis. *Osteoarthr. Cartil.* **2014**, *22*, 363–388. [CrossRef]
4. Hochberg, M.C.; Altman, R.D.; April, K.T.; Benkhalti, M.; Guyatt, G.; McGowan, J.; Towheed, T.; Welch, V.; Wells, G.; Tugwell, P. American College of Rheumatology 2012 recommendations for the use of nonpharmacologic and pharmacologic therapies in osteoarthritis of the hand, hip, and knee. *Arthritis Care Res.* **2012**, *64*, 465–474. [CrossRef] [PubMed]
5. Fransen, M.; McConnell, S.; Harmer, A.R.; Van der Esch, M.; Simic, M.; Bennell, K.L. Exercise for osteoarthritis of the knee. *Cochrane Database Syst. Rev.* **2015**, *1*, Cd004376. [CrossRef]
6. Lluch Girbes, E.; Meeus, M.; Baert, I.; Nijs, J. Balancing "hands-on" with "hands-off" physical therapy interventions for the treatment of central sensitization pain in osteoarthritis. *Man. Ther.* **2014**, *20*, 349–352. [CrossRef] [PubMed]
7. Lluch, E.; Torres, R.; Nijs, J.; Van Oosterwijck, J. Evidence for central sensitization in patients with osteoarthritis pain: A systematic literature review. *Eur. J. Pain* **2014**, *18*, 1367–1375. [CrossRef] [PubMed]
8. Lluch Girbes, E.; Nijs, J.; Torres-Cueco, R.; Lopez, C. Pain treatment for patients with osteoarthritis and central sensitization. *Phys. Ther.* **2013**, *93*, 842–851. [CrossRef] [PubMed]
9. Liu, Q.; Niu, J.; Li, H.; Ke, Y.; Li, R.; Zhang, Y.; Lin, J. Knee Symptomatic Osteoarthritis, Walking Disability, NSAIDs Use and All-cause Mortality: Population-based Wuchuan Osteoarthritis Study. *Sci. Rep.* **2017**, *7*, 3309. [CrossRef]
10. Wilkie, R.; Parmar, S.S.; Blagojevic-Bucknall, M.; Smith, D.; Thomas, M.J.; Seale, B.J.; Mansell, G.; Peat, G. Reasons why osteoarthritis predicts mortality: Path analysis within a Cox proportional hazards model. *RMD Open* **2019**, *5*, e001048. [CrossRef]
11. Dobson, F.; Hinman, R.S.; Roos, E.M.; Abbott, J.H.; Stratford, P.; Davis, A.M.; Buchbinder, R.; Snyder-Mackler, L.; Henrotin, Y.; Thumboo, J.; et al. OARSI recommended performance-based tests to assess physical function in people diagnosed with hip or knee osteoarthritis. *Osteoarthr. Cartil.* **2013**, *21*, 1042–1052. [CrossRef] [PubMed]
12. Davis, M.A.; Ettinger, W.H.; Neuhaus, J.M.; Mallon, K.P. Knee osteoarthritis and physical functioning: Evidence from the NHANES I Epidemiologic Followup Study. *J. Rheumatol.* **1991**, *18*, 591–598. [PubMed]

13. Collins, J.E.; Katz, J.N.; Dervan, E.E.; Losina, E. Trajectories and risk profiles of pain in persons with radiographic, symptomatic knee osteoarthritis: Data from the osteoarthritis initiative. *Osteoarthr. Cartil.* **2014**, *22*, 622–630. [CrossRef] [PubMed]
14. Veenhof, C.; Koke, A.J.; Dekker, J.; Oostendorp, R.A.; Bijlsma, J.W.; van Tulder, M.W.; van den Ende, C.H. Effectiveness of behavioral graded activity in patients with osteoarthritis of the hip and/or knee: A randomized clinical trial. *Arthritis Rheum.* **2006**, *55*, 925–934. [CrossRef] [PubMed]
15. Pisters, M.F.; Veenhof, C.; Schellevis, F.G.; De Bakker, D.H.; Dekker, J. Long-term effectiveness of exercise therapy in patients with osteoarthritis of the hip or knee: A randomized controlled trial comparing two different physical therapy interventions. *Osteoarthr. Cartil.* **2010**, *18*, 1019–1026. [CrossRef]
16. Pisters, M.F.; Veenhof, C.; de Bakker, D.H.; Schellevis, F.G.; Dekker, J. Behavioural graded activity results in better exercise adherence and more physical activity than usual care in people with osteoarthritis: A cluster-randomised trial. *J. Physiother.* **2010**, *56*, 41–47. [CrossRef]
17. van Baar, M.E.; Assendelft, W.J.; Dekker, J.; Oostendorp, R.A.; Bijlsma, J.W. Effectiveness of exercise therapy in patients with osteoarthritis of the hip or knee: A systematic review of randomized clinical trials. *Arthritis Rheum.* **1999**, *42*, 1361–1369. [CrossRef]
18. Daghestani, H.N.; Kraus, V.B. Inflammatory biomarkers in osteoarthritis. *Osteoarthr. Cartil.* **2015**, *23*, 1890–1896. [CrossRef]
19. Greene, M.A.; Loeser, R.F. Aging-related inflammation in osteoarthritis. *Osteoarthr. Cartil.* **2015**, *23*, 1966–1971. [CrossRef]
20. Runhaar, J.; Bierma-Zeinstra, S.M.A. Should exercise therapy for chronic musculoskeletal conditions focus on the anti-inflammatory effects of exercise? *Br. J. Sports Med.* **2017**, *51*, 762–763. [CrossRef] [PubMed]
21. Petersen, A.M.; Pedersen, B.K. The anti-inflammatory effect of exercise. *J. Appl. Physiol.* **2005**, *98*, 1154–1162. [CrossRef]
22. Forti, L.N.; Van Roie, E.; Njemini, R.; Coudyzer, W.; Beyer, I.; Delecluse, C.; Bautmans, I. Effects of resistance training at different loads on inflammatory markers in young adults. *Eur. J. Appl. Physiol.* **2017**, *117*, 511–519. [CrossRef] [PubMed]
23. Liberman, K.; Forti, L.N.; Beyer, I.; Bautmans, I. The effects of exercise on muscle strength, body composition, physical functioning and the inflammatory profile of older adults: A systematic review. *Curr. Opin. Clin. Nutr. Metab. Care* **2017**, *20*, 30–53. [CrossRef] [PubMed]
24. Bautmans, I.; Njemini, R.; Vasseur, S.; Chabert, H.; Moens, L.; Demanet, C.; Mets, T. Biochemical changes in response to intensive resistance exercise training in the elderly. *Gerontology* **2005**, *51*, 253–265. [CrossRef] [PubMed]
25. Forti, L.N.; Van Roie, E.; Njemini, R.; Coudyzer, W.; Beyer, I.; Delecluse, C.; Bautmans, I. Load-Specific Inflammation Mediating Effects of Resistance Training in Older Persons. *J. Am. Med. Dir. Assoc.* **2016**, *17*, 547–552. [CrossRef] [PubMed]
26. Beyer, I.; Mets, T.; Bautmans, I. Chronic low-grade inflammation and age-related sarcopenia. *Curr. Opin. Clin. Nutr. Metab. Care* **2012**, *15*, 12–22. [CrossRef] [PubMed]
27. Wang, Y.; Nguyen, U.D.T.; Lane, N.E.; Lu, N.; Wei, J.; Lei, G.; Zeng, C.; Zhang, Y. Knee osteoarthritis, potential mediators, and risk of all-cause mortality: Data from the Osteoarthritis Initiative. *Arthritis Care Res.* **2020**. [CrossRef] [PubMed]
28. Hawker, G.A.; Croxford, R.; Bierman, A.S.; Harvey, P.J.; Ravi, B.; Stanaitis, I.; Lipscombe, L.L. All-cause mortality and serious cardiovascular events in people with hip and knee osteoarthritis: A population based cohort study. *PLoS ONE* **2014**, *9*, e91286. [CrossRef]
29. Veronese, N.; Cereda, E.; Maggi, S.; Luchini, C.; Solmi, M.; Smith, T.; Denkinger, M.; Hurley, M.; Thompson, T.; Manzato, E.; et al. Osteoarthritis and mortality: A prospective cohort study and systematic review with meta-analysis. *Semin. Arthritis Rheum.* **2016**, *46*, 160–167. [CrossRef]
30. Fernandes, L.; Hagen, K.B.; Bijlsma, J.W.; Andreassen, O.; Christensen, P.; Conaghan, P.G.; Doherty, M.; Geenen, R.; Hammond, A.; Kjeken, I.; et al. EULAR recommendations for the non-pharmacological core management of hip and knee osteoarthritis. *Ann. Rheum. Dis.* **2013**, *72*, 1125–1135. [CrossRef]
31. Vertommen, B. *Pain Attitudes and Beliefs of Physiotherapy Students Concerning the Management of Osteoarthritis*; Faculty of Medicine and Health Care, Antwerp University: Antwerp, Belgium, 2014; p. 38.

32. Briggs, A.M.; Hinman, R.S.; Darlow, B.; Bennell, K.L.; Leech, M.; Pizzari, T.; Greig, A.M.; MacKay, C.; Bendrups, A.; Larmer, P.J.; et al. Confidence and Attitudes Toward Osteoarthritis Care Among the Current and Emerging Health Workforce: A Multinational Interprofessional Study. *ACR Open Rheumatol.* **2019**, *1*, 219–235. [CrossRef] [PubMed]
33. Cottrell, E.; Roddy, E.; Rathod, T.; Porcheret, M.; Foster, N.E. What influences general practitioners' use of exercise for patients with chronic knee pain? Results from a national survey. *BMC Fam. Pract.* **2016**, *17*, 172. [CrossRef] [PubMed]
34. Cottrell, E.; Roddy, E.; Foster, N.E. The attitudes, beliefs and behaviours of GPs regarding exercise for chronic knee pain: A systematic review. *BMC Fam. Pract.* **2010**, *11*, 4. [CrossRef] [PubMed]
35. Selten, E.M.H.; Geenen, R.; Schers, H.J.; van den Hoogen, F.H.J.; van der Meulen-Dilling, R.G.; van der Laan, W.H.; Nijhof, M.W.; van den Ende, C.H.M.; Vriezekolk, J.E. Treatment Beliefs Underlying Intended Treatment Choices in Knee and Hip Osteoarthritis. *Int. J. Behav. Med.* **2018**, *25*, 198–206. [CrossRef] [PubMed]
36. Hurley, M.; Dickson, K.; Hallett, R.; Grant, R.; Hauari, H.; Walsh, N.; Stansfield, C.; Oliver, S. Exercise interventions and patient beliefs for people with hip, knee or hip and knee osteoarthritis: A mixed methods review. *Cochrane Database Syst. Rev.* **2018**, *4*, Cd010842. [CrossRef] [PubMed]
37. Nijs, J.; Roussel, N.; Paul van Wilgen, C.; Koke, A.; Smeets, R. Thinking beyond muscles and joints: Therapists' and patients' attitudes and beliefs regarding chronic musculoskeletal pain are key to applying effective treatment. *Man. Ther.* **2013**, *18*, 96–102. [CrossRef] [PubMed]
38. Lluch, E.; Duenas, L.; Falla, D.; Baert, I.; Meeus, M.; Sanchez-Frutos, J.; Nijs, J. Preoperative Pain Neuroscience Education Combined With Knee Joint Mobilization for Knee Osteoarthritis: A Randomized Controlled Trial. *Clin. J. Pain.* **2018**, *34*, 44–52. [CrossRef]
39. Louw, A.; Zimney, K.; Reed, J.; Landers, M.; Puentedura, E. Immediate preoperative outcomes of pain neuroscience education for patients undergoing total knee arthroplasty: A case series. *Physiother. Theory Pract.* **2019**, *35*, 543–553. [CrossRef]

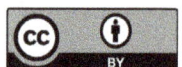

© 2020 by the authors. Licensee MDPI, Basel, Switzerland. This article is an open access article distributed under the terms and conditions of the Creative Commons Attribution (CC BY) license (http://creativecommons.org/licenses/by/4.0/).

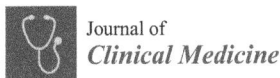

Review

Best-Evidence for the Rehabilitation of Chronic Pain Part 1: Pediatric Pain

Lauren E. Harrison [1], Joshua W. Pate [2], Patricia A. Richardson [1], Kelly Ickmans [3,4,5,6], Rikard K. Wicksell [7] and Laura E. Simons [1,*]

1. Department of Anesthesiology, Perioperative, and Pain Medicine, Stanford University School of Medicine, Stanford, CA 94304, USA
2. Faculty of Medicine and Health Sciences, Macquarie University, Sydney, NSW 2109, Australia
3. Research Foundation-Flanders (FWO), 1000 Brussels, Belgium
4. Department of Physiotherapy, Human Physiology and Anatomy (KIMA), Faculty of Physical Education & Physiotherapy, Vrije Universiteit Brussel, 1090 Brussels, Belgium
5. Pain in Motion International Research Group, 1090 Brussels, Belgium
6. Department of Physical Medicine and Physiotherapy, University Hospital Brussels, 1090 Brussels, Belgium
7. Department of Clinical Neuroscience, Psychology division, Karolinska Institutet, 171 65 Stockholm, Sweden
* Correspondence: lesimons@stanford.edu; Tel.: +32-650-736-0838

Received: 15 July 2019; Accepted: 16 August 2019; Published: 21 August 2019

Abstract: Chronic pain is a prevalent and persistent problem in middle childhood and adolescence. The biopsychosocial model of pain, which accounts for the complex interplay of the biological, psychological, social, and environmental factors that contribute to and maintain pain symptoms and related disability has guided our understanding and treatment of pediatric pain. Consequently, many interventions for chronic pain are within the realm of rehabilitation, based on the premise that behavior has a broad and central role in pain management. These treatments are typically delivered by one or more providers in medicine, nursing, psychology, physical therapy, and/or occupational therapy. Current data suggest that multidisciplinary treatment is important, with intensive interdisciplinary pain rehabilitation (IIPT) being effective at reducing disability for patients with high levels of functional disability. The following review describes the current state of the art of rehabilitation approaches to treat persistent pain in children and adolescents. Several emerging areas of interventions are also highlighted to guide future research and clinical practice.

Keywords: chronic pain; children pain rehabilitation; best evidence

1. Introduction

Chronic pain is a prevalent problem among children and adolescents, with epidemiological data indicating approximately 30% of children experience pain persisting for 3 months or longer [1,2]. The most common pain complaints in children include migraine, abdominal pain, and musculoskeletal pain [1]. The presence of chronic pain has a significant negative impact on functioning, with impairments across academic, social, and recreational domains, as well as family functioning [3]. Given this broad impact, treatment for chronic pain typically focuses on functional improvements across domains.

Rehabilitation for chronic pain applies the biopsychosocial model [4], which accounts for the complex interplay of the biological, psychological, social, and environmental factors that contribute to and maintain pain symptoms and related disability. Most interventions for chronic pain are within the realm of rehabilitation, based on the premise that behavior has a broad and central role in pain management. These treatments are typically delivered by one or more providers in medicine, nursing, psychology, physical therapy, and/or occupational therapy. In chronic pain management, as contrasted with acute pain treatment, the emphasis shifts from immediate analgesia to functional improvements in the presence of pain [5,6]. Given this, this review will focus solely on rehabilitation interventions, including psychological, behavioral, and physiological interventions.

Given all of the domains involved and impacted by chronic pain, treatment typically requires a comprehensive and multidisciplinary approach, most often achieved through psychological interventions, as well as physical and occupational therapies [7]. Multidisciplinary teams often consist of providers from several specialties who work together to develop a treatment plan for the patient and family [8]. An interdisciplinary model, comprised of the same specialists, differs slightly from a multidisciplinary team as the team members work together in a more fluid way (often housed within the same institution or clinic), with more extensive collaboration and shared treatment goals [8].

Rehabilitative treatments are also delivered across several levels of care, including outpatient, intensive outpatient (i.e., day treatment), and inpatient. Often thought of as the first level of care, outpatient interventions can be collaborative and multidisciplinary (e.g., if a psychologist and physical therapist were housed within the same medical system and corresponded regarding patient progress). However, outpatient interventions are typically delivered independent of each other. Unfortunately, adherence to treatment recommendations in outpatient pain clinics is often suboptimal [9], which underscores the importance of thorough assessment and delivery of tailored treatment approaches that best meet the individual needs of the child and family. Furthermore, patients with more severe pain-related disability or who have been unsuccessful in outpatient therapies may require more comprehensive and intensive interventions [8].

This review has several aims. First, we present an overview of the state-of-the-art of rehabilitative interventions for children and adolescents with chronic pain. In order to present the best evidence in rehabilitation for pediatric chronic pain, this review primarily relies on systematic reviews and meta-analyses. However, to incorporate the most recent evidence, methodologically sound clinical trials (e.g., randomized controlled trials, sample size > 20, clearly described interventions) that have not yet been integrated into the available reviews are included as well. For this review, a non-systematic search of the literature was performed in PubMed and Google Scholar using the following search strategy: ((child OR pediatric) OR adolescent AND (chronic pain (Text Word)) AND rehabilitation (Text Word)). The inclusion of chronic pain and rehabilitation terms resulted in a search that pulled for the primary rehabilitative interventions used to treat pediatric chronic pain. All titles and abstracts (total of 399) of articles were then separately screened by two authors (L.E.H., J.W.P.) for inclusion. Our second aim is to inform clinicians of innovative and emerging treatments that can potentially enhance treatment delivery and patient outcomes. Lastly, this review intends to identify evidence gaps among interventions that warrant further study, and to serve clinical researchers to build upon the best evidence for designing future trials, implementing studies, and developing innovative future studies.

2. State of the Art of Rehabilitation for Pediatric Chronic Pain

There is strong evidence to support early, targeted psychological and physiological intervention for pediatric chronic pain, with most approaches sharing common features: Pain education, psychological interventions, and physical and occupational therapies [7]. Psychological interventions for pediatric chronic pain focus on the self-management of pain and disability, with the ultimate goal of a return to baseline functioning [10,11]. Components of psychological interventions for chronic pain include, but are not limited to, psychoeducation, relaxation training, identifying and addressing negative cognitions, acceptance and values-based exercises, behavioral exposures, and parent coaching [12]. There is substantial evidence suggesting these interventions are effective at reducing pain severity, disability, and psychological distress (e.g., anxiety) in children with chronic pain [13–15]. Within pain conditions, psychological interventions have been found to effectively reduce pain in headache, abdominal pain, and musculoskeletal conditions, and functional disability in abdominal and musculoskeletal pain [14].

Physiological and rehabilitative interventions for pediatric chronic pain, including physical and occupational therapy, focus on improving physical functioning by progressively engaging children in previously avoided activities and taking a self-management approach to pain [16,17]. The goal of these interventions is to improve strength, flexibility, endurance, joint stability, tolerance for weight-bearing, coordination, balance, and proprioception [5,18–20]. Because the goal of these therapies is to promote independence (i.e., ability to manage daily life without excessive support from parents and caregivers) and a return to functioning (e.g., return to school and sport), active interventions (e.g., exercise) have a more significant role than passive interventions (e.g., massage or transcutaneous electrical nerve stimulation (TENS)) [21]. The goals of physical and occupational therapeutic interventions are often focused on independent functioning, as well as improved coping and increased self-efficacy, as opposed to pain reduction [22,23]. Following a thorough assessment within a biopsychosocial framework, including an assessment of functional goals, a developmentally-appropriate and individualized therapeutic treatment plan is developed and implemented [24]. The following section thoroughly reviews the evidence of effectiveness of the aforementioned rehabilitative treatments across outpatient, as well as intensive outpatient and inpatient treatment programs (see Table 1).

Table 1. Best Evidence for Rehabilitation in Pediatric Chronic Pain.

	Evidence Supporting Interventions	Examples of Resources
Individual Outpatient Interventions		
Pain Science Education	Heathcote et al., 2019 ** [25]; Moseley & Butler [26], 2015; Pas et al., 2018 [27] *	Tame the Beast What is Pain? The Mysterious Science of Pain PNE4Kids A Journey to Learn About Pain
Physiological Self-Regulation Training	Eccleston et al., 2002 [28] **	
Biofeedback	Benore and Banez, 2013 [29]; McKenna et al., 2015 [30] *	Breathe2Relax BellyBio
Progressive Muscle Relaxation	Palermo, 2012 [10]	Progressive Muscle Relaxation Script
Self-Hypnosis	Liossi et al., 2003 [31]; Tome-Pires & Miro, 2012 [32];	
Guided Imagery	Van Tilburg et al., 2009 [33] *	
Mindfulness-based Stress Reduction (MBSR) and Yoga	Evans et al., 2010 [34]; Jastrowski Mano et al., 2013 [35] *	
Cognitive Skills Training	Eccleston et al., 2015 [36] **; Fisher et al., 2014 [14] **; Palermo et al., 2010 [15] **	
Behavioral Exposure	Kanstrup et al., 2017 [37]; Kemani et al., 2018 [24]; Wicksell et al., 2007 [38] *; Wicksell et al., 2009 [39]	
Cognitive Behavioral Therapy for Insomnia (CBT-I)	Palermo et al., 2017 [40] *	iSleep App CBT-I App
Parent Coaching	Eccleston et al., 2014 [36] **; Palermo, 2012 [10]	Conquering Your Child's Chronic Pain Managing Your Child's Chronic Pain When Your Child Hurts Pain in Children and Young Adults: The Journey Back to Normal
Problem-Solving Skills Training	Law et al., 2017 [41]; Palermo et al., 2016 [42] *	
Multi-component Treatment Packages		
Cognitive-Behavioral Therapy	Eccleston et al., 2014 [36] **; Fisher et al., 2014 [14] **; Palermo et al., 2010 [15] **	Cognitive-Behavioral Therapy for Chronic Pain in Children and Adolescents
Acceptance and Commitment Therapy	Pielech et al., 2017 [43]; Wicksell et al., 2009 [39]	Acceptance and Mindfulness Treatments for Children and Adolescents
Physical Therapy Strength and Endurance Training Gait and Posture Training	Eccleston and Eccleston, 2004 [44]; Kempert et al., 2017b [45]; Mirek et al., 2019 [46]	
Occupational Therapy Independence with Activities of Daily Living Desensitization	Kempert et al., 2017a [47]; Kempert et al., 2017b [45] Sherry et al., 1999 [48]	

Table 1. Cont.

	Evidence Supporting Interventions	Examples of Resources
Interdisciplinary Outpatient Pain Treatment		
FIT Teens	Kashikar-Zuck et al., 2018 [49] *; Tran et al., 2016 [50] *	
2B Active	Dekker et al., 2016 [51]	
GET Living	GET Living, NCT: 03699007	
Intensive Interdisciplinary Pain Treatment (IIPT)	Hechler et al., 2015 [19] **	
Emerging Pain Treatment Intervention Formats		
One-day workshops	Coakley et al., 2018 [52]	The Comfort Ability
Internet and mobile applications	Bonnert et al., 2019 [53]; Palermo et al., 2018 [54]; Stinson et al., 2014 [55]	
Virtual Reality	Won et al., 2015 [56] *; Won et al., 2017 [57]	

Note: Tame the Beast and What is Pain? The Mysterious Science of Pain videos were not specifically developed for children. * denotes pilot studies; ** denotes systematic review and/or meta-analysis. All other studies listed are individual clinical trials or topical reviews.

2.1. Pain Related Education

The goal of psychoeducation is to provide the child and family with an explanation of the differences between acute and chronic pain and to emphasize the non-protective nature of chronic pain [12]. Psychoeducation is typically guided by the biopsychosocial model [4] and is an important component of treatment as it provides the family with a rationale as to how psychological interventions can be effective in addressing pain and associated disability [12]. Although psychoeducation is typically embedded in any comprehensive cognitive-behavioral treatment package, the clinicians and researchers in the field of physiotherapy have delved deeper into educating patients about pain science as a therapeutic tool and have worked to test the efficacy of pain science education both as a specific treatment component [26,58], as well as in combination with other biopsychosocially-oriented treatment components [59–61] Indeed, adding a cognition-targeted active approach to pain science (e.g., progression to the next phase of education is preceded by an intermediate phase of imagery or work on cognitions that might hinder progression) is considered critical in achieving larger long-term therapy effects, given that pain science as a stand-alone treatment only demonstrates small to medium effect sizes [62,63]. Although already used in clinical practice worldwide, research on pain science education in the pediatric pain field is just beginning.

Pain Science Education

"Pain science education", also called "pain neuroscience education" [63,64], "therapeutic neuroscience education" [65,66], or "explaining pain" [26], aims to change one's conceptual understanding of pain [67]. To enhance rehabilitation treatments, pain science education provides a foundation for understanding principles that guide biopsychosocial interventions for persistent pain [35]. Pain science education teaches people about the underlying biopsychosocial mechanisms of pain, including how the brain produces pain and that pain is often present without, or disproportionate to, tissue damage. In more complex and persistent pain states, this also includes peripheral and central sensitization, facilitation and inhibition, neuroplasticity, immune and endocrine changes [58]. Evidence shows that understanding pain decreases its threat value which, in turn, leads to more effective pain coping strategies [61,68]. Given that children with chronic pain often have significant problems with functioning (e.g., more school absenteeism and lower participation in daily, after-school, and family activities) contributing to lower quality of life, less physical fitness, and eventually more pain [69], pain science education may prepare and prime children with chronic pain for biopsychosocial treatments.

Pain science education is commonly part of multidisciplinary pain treatment [70] and can utilize freely available online resources [25] that complement pain science education/communication which is typically individually-tailored and thereby primarily delivered by a therapist. Additionally, PNE4Kids, a pain science curriculum for children (6–12 years old), has recently been developed [27] and is freely available for clinicians at http://www.paininmotion.be/pne4kids. Although there is meta-analytic evidence for adults suggesting that pain science education improves outcomes [71], evidence in pediatric chronic pain is scarce but promising with Andias et al. [72] providing support of a combined approach (pain science education + exercise therapy) in adolescents with chronic idiopathic neck pain, with data showing that this type of intervention is feasible and beneficial in pediatric patients with chronic pain. Yet, some methodological shortcomings were present in this study, such as the rather small sample size ($n = 43$) and the control group who did not receive any treatment (nor attention from the therapists). Therefore, further methodologically sound research is needed to assess both conceptual and behavioral change in relation to pain science education.

2.2. Physiological Self-Regulation Training

An often recommended intervention for children with chronic pain is training in self-regulation of physiological responses to pain (e.g., heart rate, breathing rate, skin temperature, and muscle tension). Relaxation-based strategies typically include deep-breathing exercises, progressive muscle relaxation, and imagery [10]. Studies have shown the direct benefits of relaxation techniques for children with persistent pain including slowing of heart rate and breathing, increased blood flow to the muscles, and decreased muscle tension e.g., [73]. These bodily changes have also been found to reduce the experience of stress and anxiety [74]. Often used in conjunction with relaxation training, biofeedback provides real-time feedback to the child related to the physiological processes and changes (e.g., changes in heart rate or skin temperature) that occur in the body when engaging in aforementioned relaxation techniques [29]. There is also some evidence for self-hypnosis. Several studies highlight the utility of self-hypnosis with pediatric procedural pain [30,31] and there is some evidence that it may be helpful with chronic conditions as well [32]. Examining a sample of 300 children with functional abdominal pain, Anbar [75] found that 80% of patients demonstrated improvement in pain following a course of self-hypnosis. Another study examined the efficacy of self-hypnosis in 26 children with chronic pain. Results demonstrated that self-hypnosis was significantly associated with decreased pain intensity, as well as improvements in functioning across academic and social domains and sleep [76].

Mindfulness-Based Stress Reduction and Yoga

Mindfulness-based stress reduction (MBSR) involves teaching patients mindfulness and focuses on bringing attention to the present moment, with the thought that shifting attention to the present allows for the use of positive coping strategies [77]. Data from pilot trials demonstrates evidence for the efficacy of MBSR for reduction of pain and stress, with improvements maintained at 6-month follow-up [35,78]. Additionally, there is some evidence for the role of yoga [34] and massage [79,80] in treating pediatric chronic pain. Integrating aspects of MBSR and yoga might help enhance interventions delivered within this population.

2.3. Cognitive Skills Training

Cognitive skills training focuses on the identification of negative and maladaptive thoughts/cognitions with the goal of systematically reframing and changing these thoughts [81]. Several clinical trials have demonstrated that children with chronic pain benefit from cognitive skills training [15]. Cognitive techniques such as cognitive restructuring, problem-solving, and positive self-talk, have been shown to be effective techniques for reducing negative thoughts associated with pain and related disability [10,13,14].

Incorporating components of Acceptance and Commitment Therapy (ACT) [82,83] into treatment may be beneficial, and there is evidence to suggest that ACT can be effective for children with chronic pain [39,84]. ACT focuses on increasing psychological flexibility and engagement in valued activities (e.g., willingness to go to school or to a friend's house even if pain is present) [82,85]. ACT differs from traditional cognitive therapy in that it focuses on changing the relationship the child has with distressing and negative thoughts as opposed to changing the thoughts themselves. This is done through exercises focused on cognitive defusion, which aims to increase the child's ability to notice the thought and how it influences behavior, rather than changing the content of the thought [86]. One study examining acceptance and values-based treatment for adolescents with chronic pain found that adolescents improved in self-reported functioning, as well as on objective measures of physical performance and reported a decrease in anxiety and catastrophizing [84] following intervention. Additionally, Wicksell and colleagues [85] examined mediators of change in ACT and found that ACT worked through improvements in processes related to psychological flexibility rather than through changes in traditional CBT constructs, providing additional evidence that ACT may be functionally different from traditional cognitive-behavioral treatments.

2.4. Behavioral Exposure

Operant-behavioral theories have long been applied to chronic pain populations to understand the association between pain severity and pain-related disability [87,88]. The Fear Avoidance Model [89,90] describes how heightened fear of pain and continued avoidance of activities that might exacerbate pain leads to prolonged disability, and recent work has focused on pain-related fear in children and adolescents and the application of the Fear Avoidance Model of Chronic Pain within pediatric patients [91,92]. Exposure-based treatments for pediatric chronic pain aim to improve functioning by exposing patients to activities they are currently avoiding due to fear of pain. In a study examining the efficacy of behavioral exposure within an ACT framework for children and adolescents with chronic pain, results demonstrated greater reductions in pain severity, functional disability, and fear of pain for patients who received the exposure treatment compared to those who received standard multidisciplinary treatment [39].

Graded in-vivo exposure, a treatment typically delivered by a psychologist and physio or occupational therapist [93,94], thus considered an interdisciplinary outpatient treatment, is now being evaluated in children and adolescents with chronic pain (described further in the Interdisciplinary Outpatient Pain Treatment section) [51]. The first single case experimental design (SCED) trial of graded in-vivo exposure in youth demonstrated robust improvements in pain-related avoidance and pain intensity with increased activity engagement at the end of treatment with decreases in pain-related fear and catastrophizing observed at 3-month follow-up with improvements across outcomes maintained at 6-month follow-up (Simons et al., [95]). Additionally, work has been done to incorporate interoceptive components, which involve having the child imagine increases in pain severity, into exposure treatments for children with chronic pain [96,97]. Use of interoceptive exposure techniques have been associated with decreased pain intensity and school avoidance, and data suggest that using these techniques are beneficial at reducing pain severity and altering relevant emotions related to pain [96].

2.5. Parent Coaching

While the aforementioned interventions often consider the child to be the primary treatment target, parents play a critical role in managing pain and maintaining or improving functioning [10]. At the very basic level, parents are often taught the relaxation and cognitive skills along with the child so that they are better able to help their child carry out the interventions at home [10]. Treatment with parents also focuses on shifting parent attention and behavioral responding toward encouraging function in the presence of persistent pain, while coaching the child to use coping skills to support functioning (i.e., contingency management). Findings from a systematic review of parent–child interventions, including cognitive-behavioral and family-focused treatments, found that these interventions could be beneficial in improving parent behaviors, e.g., reducing attention to pain symptoms, encourage functioning despite pain [36].

There is also evidence to suggest that parents of children with chronic pain experience significant emotional distress related to their child's pain (e.g., [98]). Recent work has been done to adapt problem-solving skills training (PSST), which teaches parents structured approaches to solving problems and targets parent distress, with results demonstrating that psychological interventions focused on reducing parent distress were effective [41,42]. Furthermore, a recent review [99] found that psychological interventions also improved parent mental health across a chronic illness sample, including parents of children with chronic pain. These findings support the notion that parent distress impacts child functioning [100]. Therefore, it is critical to consider parent distress when working with this population, as accurate assessment and treatment of parent distress, in addition to behavioral functioning, may have important implications for child outcomes. Additionally, there are several books written for parents that provide support and instruction on how to implement the aforementioned strategies and support coping and functioning in their children [44,101–103].

2.6. Physical Therapy

When working with children and adolescents with chronic pain, the key objectives of a physical therapist include encouraging the adoption of regular exercise, facilitating repeated exposure to movement in the presence of pain, and educating families regarding misconceptions about anatomy, physiology, pain, exercise and activity [48]. To assist the child in achieving functional goals, physical therapy works to improve strength, flexibility, endurance, joint stability, tolerance for weight-bearing, coordination, balance, and proprioception [5,18–20].

Exercise is a crucial component of rehabilitation for children and adolescents with chronic pain [7] and there are data to suggest that earlier experience with exercise is associated with better adherence [9]. Exercise activities for pain in the lower extremities may focus on jumping, fast-paced walking and/or running, climbing stairs, balance and coordination activities, and age-appropriate physical education activities and sport drills, whereas upper extremity exercises typically focus on strengthening and coordination drills [104]. It is important that exercises occur in a variety of settings, such as in the gym with equipment, at home without equipment, in a pool, or out in public settings, to assist with generalization of skills and reduce site-specific exercise behavior [105]. It is also important to take a behavioral management approach when increasing physical activity, most often achieved through gradual exposure to activities and pacing, which involves increasing intensity gradually as tolerance builds [19,48].

2.7. Occupational Therapy

Another vital component of rehabilitation for chronic pain is occupational therapy [8]. Occupational therapy differs from physical therapy in that the focus of interventions are on maximizing independence in age-appropriate activities of daily living and self-care (e.g., bathing, dressing, grooming), as well as academic (e.g., handwriting) and family activities (e.g., participation in chores) [17,19,48]. These goals are often achieved through individualized strategies such as psychoeducation, participation in games (e.g., standing up while playing a board game, or participating in games that requiring reaching or bending-designed based on patients functional goals), sensory discrimination, and developing a daily schedule to support engagement in meaningful activities throughout the day [5,8,106]. Desensitization, a technique used to reduce physical sensitivity to certain stimuli, is another important intervention provided though occupational therapy, particularly for patients with central pain sensitization (e.g., Complex Regional Pain Syndrome; CRPS) who experience difficulties tolerating physical stimulations and sensations on affected areas of the body. These patients may guard or protect the sensitive area in an attempt to avoid it being touched. In severe cases, patients may be unable to tolerate pressure from clothing items, such as socks, shoes, and tighter pants. To address this, the occupational therapist engages the patient in desensitization exercises, which may include rubbing the sensitive area with various textures including tissue, feather, textured fabrics, and towels, to gradually expose the nervous system to different sensations with the goal of retraining the brain to process these stimulations more typically [104].

An early meta-analytic review [107] found that conventional (i.e., monodisciplinary) physical and occupational therapy are better than no treatment or only medical treatment. There are also data to suggest that for specific conditions, such as CRPS, early individualized intensive physical therapy is considered best [108,109]. However, monodisciplinary rehabilitation treatments have been found to be inferior to multidisciplinary and interdisciplinary treatment approaches, where physical and occupation therapy are combined with psychological intervention [19,107].

2.8. Addressing Comorbidities

Sleep is an important aspect of health and development in childhood and adolescence. Unfortunately, disturbances to sleep, including insomnia and delayed sleep phase, are prevalent in children with chronic pain [110] and are associated with negative emotional, cognitive, and behavioral consequences [111]. Thus, thorough assessment of sleep and sleep hygiene (i.e., habits that might affect sleep onset or maintenance throughout the night, such as consumption of caffeine, spending too much time during the day in bed, use of electronics at bedtime) is warranted [10]. There is evidence to suggest psychological interventions are effective at addressing sleep problems. Specifically, cognitive behavioral therapy for insomnia (CBT-I) has been found to be effective for adolescents with co-occurring physical and psychological conditions, including adolescents with chronic pain [40]. Outcomes from the pilot trial demonstrated improvements in insomnia, as well as improvements in sleep quality and sleep hygiene, psychological symptoms, and overall health-related quality of life [40].

Additionally, chronic pain is often associated with comorbid psychiatric concerns including depression, anxiety disorders, and post-traumatic stress disorder (PTSD) [112] and the co-occurrence is likely bidirectional in nature. In other words, psychological symptoms could potentially be a contributing factor and an outcome of having chronic pain [33,113]. Additionally, there are data to suggest that chronic pain is a risk factor for suicidal ideation in adolescents, and clinicians should be alert to suicidal ideation and/or attempt within the population [114]. Consultation with and involvement of psychiatric care should be incorporated into treatment when appropriate. Further, assessing for adverse childhood events, trauma, or maltreatment may also be important and exposure to early childhood adversity may hinder the ability to effectively implement interventions. In addition to depression and anxiety, the presence of neurological and/or neuropsychiatric symptoms (e.g., conversion disorder) co-occur in pediatric pain populations [115]. Effective interventions need to target co-morbid mental health disorders and identify underlying mechanisms that serve to maintain mental health and pain conditions.

2.9. Interdisciplinary Outpatient Pain Treatment

Over the last several years, effort has been made to examination the efficacy of interdisciplinary interventions delivered at the outpatient level. Fibromyalgia Integrative Training for Teens (FIT Teens) combines cognitive-behavioral interventions with neuromuscular exercise training [49]. Results from the pilot randomized controlled trial (RCT) comparing FIT Teens to CBT-only demonstrated that adolescents who participated in FIT Teens experienced significant improvements in disability and greater decreases in pain intensity compared to the CBT-only condition, suggesting that FIT Teens provides additional benefits above and beyond CBT for children and adolescents with fibromyalgia. Additionally, there are several emerging interventions focusing on graded in-vivo exposure therapy (GET) for children and adolescents with chronic pain [51]; (GET Living, NCT: 03699007). One ongoing randomized controlled trial (RCT) in the Netherlands, "2B Active", combines GET and physical therapy to increase functioning by having patients complete activity exposures [51]. Additionally, there is an ongoing RCT in the United States comparing GET Living to multidisciplinary pain management in children with chronic pain (GET Living, NCT: 03699007). Similar to 2B Active, GET Living utilizes a psychologist and a physical therapist to deliver exposure interventions. However, different from 2B Active, GET Living specifically targets pain-related fear and avoidance.

2.10. Intensive Interdisciplinary Pain Treatment

Often when patients are unsuccessful at outpatient treatments, a more intensive, interdisciplinary pain treatment (IIPT) is required [19]. There is evidence from a systematic review and meta-analysis to suggest that IIPT may be effective at reducing disability and maintaining this reduction after treatment for a subgroup of patients [19]. Specifically, children and adolescents have demonstrated improvements in pain intensity, pain-related disability, and symptoms of depression post-treatment, with improvements maintained at 3-month follow-up. To be considered an IIPT program, the program includes three or more disciplines housed within the same facility (e.g., pain specialist, psychologist, and physical therapist) who work in an integrated manner to provide treatment in a day hospital or an inpatient setting. IIPT programs can be day treatment or inpatient and typically require the patient to participate in exercise-based therapies (PT and OT) as well as psychological interventions, for a total of eight hours per day [19].

Eccleston and colleagues [116] were the first to examine the effectiveness of intensive interdisciplinary pain treatment. The program examined was a 3-week multidisciplinary treatment for patients and parents, with results demonstrating immediate improvements in functioning. After a 3-month follow-up, data showed a significant decrease in anxiety, pain catastrophizing, disability, and improvements in school attendance. Another study compared a 3–4 week intensive day hospital rehabilitation program with standard outpatient treatments, which included various combinations of medical treatment, psychological, and physical therapies [117]. While there were improvements noted across both treatment groups, patients enrolled in the intensive day rehabilitation program had significantly larger improvements in functional disability, pain-related fear, and willingness to adopt a self-management approach to treating pain [117]. A recent study [5] examined the effects of an intensive day treatment program in which patients completed 1–2 half day sessions per week (lasting approximately 4 h each) for 4–8 weeks. Results indicated improvements in pain severity, as well as physical and psychological functioning [5]. To date, there has only been one randomized control trial (RCT) comparing intensive interdisciplinary pain treatment (IIPT) to a waitlist control group [106]. The IIPT utilized in this trial was a manualized program consisting of 6 treatment modules including pain psychoeducation, pain coping skills, cognitive intervention to target emotional distress, family therapy, physiotherapy, and parent sessions. Immediate effects were achieved for pain-related disability, school attendance, depression, and catastrophizing, with pain intensity and anxiety decreasing at 6-month follow up [106]. These results are consistent with outcomes from other intensive interdisciplinary pain rehabilitation treatment centers [108,118].

While all IIPT programs share the primary goal of improved functioning across domains, there is variability across programs with regard to structure, organization, and frequency of treatment delivery across disciplines [8]. One major distinction is that of intensive outpatient and inpatient treatment models. In comparing outcomes reported from intensive outpatient [108] and inpatient programs [118,119], patients in each program demonstrate significant functional improvements. Of note, several intensive pain rehabilitation programs offer both inpatient and day hospital programs, with patients triaged to level of care based on individual needs [17]. To our knowledge, outcomes between levels of care within the same facility have yet to be published. Another difference between intensive pain programs includes length of stay. For example, some programs have a fixed, 3-week length of stay, while others have a more flexible length of stay which is often established based on individual patient needs. Despite these differences, significant functional improvements are reported for these treatment programs. Continued examination of outcomes within and between treatment programs is warranted, as is further examination of mechanisms of change for patients undergoing IIPT treatment.

A recent study conducted a cost-analysis of an interdisciplinary pediatric pain clinic by retrospectively reviewing billing data for inpatient admissions, emergency department, and outpatient visits and associated costs and reimbursements [120]. Data examined included healthcare costs for patients 1 year prior to initiating interdisciplinary services with costs 1 year after initiating services.

Cost-analyses of pre-pain clinic costs found cost reductions 1 year post clinic participation (up to $36,228 to the hospital and $11,482 to insurance, per patient, per year), providing economic support for interdisciplinary intervention for children with chronic pain [120].

2.11. Emerging Pain Treatment Intervention Formats

One-day workshops. One day group-based psychological interventions for children with chronic pain have inherent benefits as it allows children and adolescents to meet peers with similar struggles and allows them to receive social support and benefit from shared experiences. These workshop programs can also be cost and time effective. One such program, The Comfort Ability [52] in an intensive one-day intervention, delivered concurrently to children and their parents, that introduces cognitive-behavioral skills of pain management and helps families develop a plan to support functional improvement. The workshop is currently available across 15 children's hospitals in the United States and Canada. Preliminary evaluation of this workshop demonstrates improvements in child functioning, depressive symptoms, and pain catastrophizing, which persist at 1-month follow-up. Additionally, parents report improvements in responses to their child's pain and beliefs regarding their child's ability to manage pain [52].

Internet and mobile applications. Recently, effort has been made to address access barriers for pediatric pain management services. Palermo and colleagues developed an 8-week online psychological intervention for children and their parents (WebMAP). Online modules included relaxation training, cognitive strategies, parent operant techniques, communication strategies, and interventions focused on sleep and activity engagement. Pilot data demonstrated that internet-delivered pain management reduced barriers of access to care and was effective at reducing pain-related disability [121]. The program was further developed into a mobile app version with data also indicating greater reduction in pain intensity and functional disability post treatment compared to waitlist control [54]. Other mobile-based technologies have been developed to assist patients in remotely self-monitoring symptoms and deliver interventions involving goal-setting for improving functioning, coping skills training and practice, and social support via discussion boards, goal sharing, and group-based challenges [55]. Additionally, an ACT based digital intervention for individuals with chronic pain has recently been developed in a series of studies with desktop as well as mobile use [122]. Results from an RCT with adults (n = 113) showed moderate to large effects in primary and secondary outcomes, with effects remaining 12 months following the end of treatment. Additionally, a review examining remotely delivered psychological therapies found that they were beneficial at reducing pain intensity across pain groups [123]. While these programs allow for patients to have access to treatment, remotely-delivered interventions may not be appropriate for all patients, and more complex patients would likely benefit from more intensive treatments.

Augmented reality and virtual reality. Augmented reality and virtual reality (VR) have been found to be an effective tool for reducing pain sensations in patients with acute pain [56,57,124]. One recent study examined the effects of VR in patients with chronic right arm pain secondary to a diagnosis of complex regional pain syndrome (CRPS), type 1. Similar to results found within acute and procedural pain samples, Matamala-Gomez and colleagues [125] found that multisensory interventions that manipulated body from VR modulated pain perceptions. Continued research on the effectiveness of VR within the pain rehabilitation setting is needed and should be a focus of future research within this population.

2.12. Summary of Rehabilitative Treatments for Pediatric Chronic Pain

In sum, rehabilitation for pediatric chronic pain applies the biopsychosocial model, which takes into account the complex interplay of biological, psychological, social, and environmental factors that contribute to and maintain pain and related disability. Given all of the domains impacted by pain, rehabilitation typically require a comprehensive and multidisciplinary approach. Currently, there is strong evidence to support early, targeted, treatments, with most rehabilitative interventions including pain education, psychological interventions, and physical and occupational therapies. Promising directions for clinical practice and research are discussed below.

3. Promising Directions for Clinical Practice

Given the expansive growth of rehabilitation interventions for youth with chronic pain, it is imperative to match individual patients with the appropriate treatment modality and level of intensity. The use of a screening tool, such as the Pediatric Pain Screening Tool (PPST) [126] could potentially be used to facilitate efficient treatment allocation. PPST is a 9-item screening tool used to identify prognostic factors (e.g., sleep disturbance, depression, anxiety) associated with adverse outcomes, with allocation to the high-risk group based upon responses to psychosocial items. The PPST can be easily delivered within a busy clinical setting and allows providers to quickly and effectively identify medium to high risk youth who may benefit from access to more comprehensive, multidisciplinary treatments [126]. Administering the PPST would allow patients to be triaged to the appropriate level of care, without having to trial treatments that might not be appropriate given their level of risk. For example, a patient who screens medium to high risk could be triaged to initiate both psychology and physical therapy, whereas a low-risk patient might benefit from physical therapy alone. Efforts to better match individual patients with specific treatments might help to reduce "treatment failure" that some patients experience when they engage in treatments that poorly match their current symptoms and functioning (e.g., the need for CBT-I for sleep difficulties).

Further, attempts to tailor the interventions delivered within each discipline might also be beneficial. For example, when a patient is triaged to psychology for pain management, extra effort should be made by the provider to assess what specific treatment modality might be most beneficial. For example, a patient with musculoskeletal pain who is experiencing high pain-related fear and avoidance may benefit from including a more targeted graded exposure treatment approach, as opposed to solely focusing on historically popular components of cognitive-behavioral interventions for chronic pain (e.g., relaxation skills training). Lastly, continued effort should be made address barriers to access of care and continued effort should be made to integrate one-day workshops that can be delivered on the weekends e.g., the Comfort Ability [52], as well as internet-based and mobile application treatments [54,55]. See Figure 1 for visual overview.

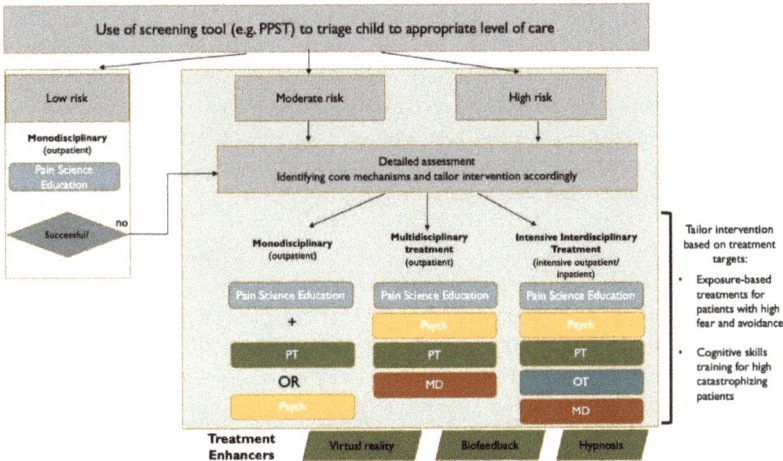

Figure 1. Schematic overview of Potential Future Directions for Clinical Practice. PPST = Pediatric Pain Screening Tool; PT = Physical Therapy; Psych = Psychology; MD = Medical Doctor; OT = Occupational Therapist.

4. Promising Directions for Research

Future research should focus on establishing clinical cut-off's for measures assessing core outcome domains, as this will allow for better evaluation of clinically significant change post-treatment. Along these lines, it will be important to explore emerging treatment targets (e.g., assessing pain-related fear and avoidance vs. pain catastrophizing vs. functional disability, pre/post treatment). It will also be important to continue to examine innovative and targeted multidisciplinary treatments. Over the last several years, effort has been made to develop interdisciplinary outpatient treatments, such as FIT Teens [49], 2B Active [51], and GET Living (NCT: 03699007), and preliminary outcomes are promising [51].

There is also a need to explore the processes and mechanisms of change within pain rehabilitation programs. In doing this, effort should be made to support collaboration between multiple disciplines involved in pediatric pain rehabilitation (e.g., psychology, physical therapy, occupation therapy, pain medicine). It may be also beneficial to establish standard pain program protocols, such as the one presented by Maynard, Amari, Wieczorek, Christensen and Slifer [118]. The use of a uniform protocol across IIPT programs would also allow for further examination of the mechanisms within these programs that account for the significant functional improvements these patients experience.

Examining outcomes across levels of care will also be important. Future randomized controlled trials should focus on examining outcomes between intensive day treatment and inpatient treatment. Such a trial might allow researchers to better understand what treatment works for whom, and why. Examination of outcomes across treatment settings would allow for further examination of the most efficient and cost-effective way to deliver empirically supported treatment to children and their families. Lastly, continued examination of outcomes for e-Health is also warranted. In addition to providing services to patients in low-resource areas, mobile- and internet-delivered programs for pain management could be used to supplement in person treatments as patients complete more intensive rehabilitation services and transition back into social and academic environments.

5. Conclusions

In conclusion, chronic pain is a prevalent and persistent problem in childhood and adolescence. Rehabilitation for pediatric chronic pain is typically based on learning theory and on the biopsychosocial model of pain, which accounts for the complex interplay of the biological, psychological, social, and environmental factors that contribute to and maintain pain symptoms and related disability. Given all of the systems involved and effected by chronic pain, the treatment of chronic pain requires comprehensive treatment approaches, including psychological intervention, physical therapy, and occupational therapy. With the emergence of several targeted interventions to address the individual challenges each patient with chronic pain faces coupled with new means of overcoming barriers to access, the field is well-positioned to alleviate the suffering of youth with chronic pain and reduce their risk of transitioning to adults with chronic pain.

Key Messages

1. Comprehensive multidisciplinary and interdisciplinary treatment based on behavioral medicine approaches are needed for children and adolescents with persistent pain.
2. Pain Science Education is commonly implemented with several resources currently available, yet evidence for its use is scarce.
3. Unique to pediatric rehabilitative approaches is the emphasis on including parents to optimize treatment outcomes.
4. Innovative pain treatment intervention formats such as mobile applications and virtual reality enhance the delivery and reach of evidence-based tools.
5. Comprehensive multidisciplinary/interdisciplinary treatment based on contemporary understanding of pain (neuro) science are needed for children and adolescents with persistent pain.

Author Contributions: Conceptualization, L.E.S., R.K.W., L.E.H., J.W.P., and K.I.; methodology, L.E.S., L.E.H., J.W.P., and K.I.; investigation, L.E.H. and J.W.P.; data curation, L.E.H. and J.W.P.; writing—original draft preparation, L.E.H., J.W.P., R.K.W., P.A.R., and K.I.; writing—review and editing, L.E.H., J.W.P., L.E.S., R.K.W., P.A.R., and K.I.; supervision, L.E.S. and R.K.W.; funding acquisition, L.E.S.

Funding: This research was funded by NIAMS/R21AR072921.

Conflicts of Interest: The authors declare no conflict of interest.

References

1. Huguet, A.; Miro, J. The severity of chronic pediatric pain: An epidemiological study. *J. Pain* **2008**, *9*, 226–236. [CrossRef]
2. King, S.; Chambers, C.T.; Huguet, A.; MacNevin, R.C.; McGrath, P.J.; Parker, L.; MacDonald, A.J. The epidemiology of chronic pain in children and adolescents revisited: A systematic review. *Pain* **2011**, *152*, 2729–2738. [CrossRef] [PubMed]
3. Palermo, T.M. Impact of recurrent and chronic pain on child and family daily functioning: A critical review of the literature. *J. Dev. Behav. Pediatr.* **2000**, *21*, 58–69. [CrossRef] [PubMed]
4. Engel, G.L. The biopsychosocial model and the education of health professionals. *Ann. N. Y. Acad. Sci.* **1978**, *310*, 169–181. [CrossRef] [PubMed]
5. Revivo, G.; Amstutz, D.K.; Gagnon, C.M.; McCormick, Z.L. Interdisciplinary Pain Management Improves Pain and Function in Pediatric Patients with Chronic Pain Associated with Joint Hypermobility Syndrome. *PM R* **2019**, *11*, 150–157. [CrossRef] [PubMed]
6. Wren, A.A.; Ross, A.C.; D'Souza, G.; Almgren, C.; Feinstein, A.; Marshall, A.; Golianu, B. Multidisciplinary Pain Management for Pediatric Patients with Acute and Chronic Pain: A Foundational Treatment Approach When Prescribing Opioids. *Children (Basel)* **2019**, *6*, 33. [CrossRef] [PubMed]
7. Clinch, J.; Eccleston, C. Chronic musculoskeletal pain in children: Assessment and management. *Rheumatology (Oxford)* **2009**, *48*, 466–474. [CrossRef]
8. Odell, S.; Logan, D.E. Pediatric pain management: The multidisciplinary approach. *J. Pain Res.* **2013**, *6*, 785–790. [CrossRef]
9. Simons, L.E.; Logan, D.E.; Chastain, L.; Cerullo, M. Engagement in multidisciplinary interventions for pediatric chronic pain: Parental expectations, barriers, and child outcomes. *Clin. J. Pain* **2010**, *26*, 291–299. [CrossRef]
10. Palermo, T.M. *Cognitive Behaioral Therapy for Chronic Pain in Children and Adolescents*; Oxford Press: New York, NY, USA, 2012.
11. Williams, A.C.; Eccleston, C.; Morley, S. Psychological therapies for the management of chronic pain (excluding headache) in adults. *Cochrane Database Syst. Rev.* **2012**, *11*, CD007407. [CrossRef]
12. Simons, L.E.; Basch, M.C. State of the art in biobehavioral approaches to the management of chronic pain in childhood. *Pain Manag.* **2016**, *6*, 49–61. [CrossRef] [PubMed]
13. Eccleston, C.; Palermo, T.M.; Williams, A.C.; Lewandowski Holley, A.; Morley, S.; Fisher, E.; Law, E. Psychological therapies for the management of chronic and recurrent pain in children and adolescents. *Cochrane Database Syst. Rev.* **2014**. [CrossRef]
14. Fisher, E.; Heathcote, L.C.; Palermo, T.M.; Williams, A.C.; Lau, J.; Eccleston, C. Systematic review and meta-analysis of psychological therapies for children with chronic pain. *J. Pediatr. Psychol.* **2014**, *39*, 763–782. [CrossRef] [PubMed]
15. Palermo, T.M.; Eccleston, C.; Lewandowski, A.S.; Williams, A.C.; Morley, S. Randomized controlled trials of psychological therapies for management of chronic pain in children and adolescents: An updated meta-analytic review. *Pain* **2010**, *148*, 387–397. [CrossRef] [PubMed]
16. Sieberg, C.B.; Smith, A.; White, M.; Manganella, J.; Sethna, N.; Logan, D.E. Changes in Maternal and Paternal Pain-Related Attitudes, Behaviors, and Perceptions across Pediatric Pain Rehabilitation Treatment: A Multilevel Modeling Approach. *J. Pediatr. Psychol.* **2017**, *42*, 52–64. [CrossRef] [PubMed]
17. Celedon, X.; Amari, A.; Ward, C.; Prestwich, S.; Slifer, K.J. Children and adolescents with chronic pain and functional disability: Use of a behavioral rehabilitation approach. *Curr. Phys. Med. Rehabil. Rep.* **2014**, *2*, 86–92. [CrossRef]

18. De Blecourt, A.C.; Schiphorst Preuper, H.R.; Van Der Schans, C.P.; Groothoff, J.W.; Reneman, M.F. Preliminary evaluation of a multidisciplinary pain management program for children and adolescents with chronic musculoskeletal pain. *Disabil. Rehabil.* **2008**, *30*, 13–20. [CrossRef]
19. Hechler, T.; Kanstrup, M.; Holley, A.L.; Simons, L.E.; Wicksell, R.; Hirschfeld, G.; Zernikow, B. Systematic Review on Intensive Interdisciplinary Pain Treatment of Children With Chronic Pain. *Pediatrics* **2015**, *136*, 115–127. [CrossRef]
20. Simons, L.E.; Sieberg, C.B.; Conroy, C.; Randall, E.T.; Shulman, J.; Borsook, D.; Berde, C.; Sethna, N.F.; Logan, D.E. Children with Chronic Pain: Response Trajectories after Intensive Pain Rehabilitation Treatment. *J. Pain* **2018**, *19*, 207–218. [CrossRef]
21. Landry, B.W.; Fischer, P.R.; Driscoll, S.W.; Koch, K.M.; Harbeck-Weber, C.; Mack, K.J.; Wilder, R.T.; Bauer, B.A.; Brandenburg, J.E. Managing Chronic Pain in Children and Adolescents: A Clinical Review. *PM R* **2015**, *7*, S295–S315. [CrossRef]
22. Banez, G.A. Chronic abdominal pain in children: What to do following the medical evaluation. *Curr. Opin. Pediatr.* **2008**, *20*, 571–575. [CrossRef] [PubMed]
23. Lynch-Jordan, A.M.; Sil, S.; Cunningham, N.; Kashikar-Zuck, S.; Goldschneider, K.R. Differential changes in functional disability and pain intensity over the course of psychological treatment for children with chronic pain. *Pain* **2014**, *155*, 1955–1961. [CrossRef] [PubMed]
24. Kemani, M.K.; Kanstrup, M.; Jordan, A.; Caes, L.; Gauntlett-Gilbert, J. Evaluation of an intensive interdisciplinary pain treatment based on acceptance and commitment therapy for adolescents with chronic pain and their parents: A nonrandomized clinical trial. *J. Pediatr. Psychol.* **2018**, *43*, 981–994. [CrossRef] [PubMed]
25. Heathcote, L.C.; Pate, J.W.; Park, A.L.; Leake, H.B.; Moseley, G.L.; Kronman, C.A.; Fischer, M.; Timmers, I.; Simons, L.E. Pain neuroscience education on YouTube. *PeerJ* **2019**, *7*, e6603. [CrossRef] [PubMed]
26. Moseley, G.L.; Butler, D.S. Fifteen Years of Explaining Pain: The Past, Present, and Future. *J. Pain* **2015**, *16*, 807–813. [CrossRef]
27. Pas, R.; Meeus, M.; Malfliet, A.; Baert, I.; Van Oosterwijck, S.; Leysen, L.; Nijs, J.; Ickmans, K. Development and feasibility testing of a Pain Neuroscience Education program for children with chronic pain: Treatment protocol. *Braz. J. Phys. Ther.* **2018**, *22*, 248–253. [CrossRef]
28. Eccleston, C.; Morley, S.; Williams, A.; Yorke, L.; Mastroyannopoulou, K. Systematic review of randomised controlled trials of psychological therapy for chronic pain in children and adolescents, with a subset meta-analysis of pain relief. *Pain* **2002**, *99*, 157–165. [CrossRef]
29. Scharff, L.; Marcus, D.A.; Masek, B.J. A controlled study of minimal-contact thermal biofeedback treatment in children with migraine. *J. Pediatr. Psychol.* **2002**, *27*, 109–119. [CrossRef] [PubMed]
30. Hawkins, P.J.; Liossi, C.; Ewart, B.; Hatira, P.; Kosmidis, V. Hypnosis in the alleviation of procedure related pain and distress in paediatric oncology patients. *Contemp. Hypn.* **1998**, *15*, 199–207. [CrossRef]
31. Liossi, C.; Hatira, P. Clinical hypnosis in the alleviation of procedure-related pain in pediatric oncology patients. *Int. J. Clin. Exp. Hypn.* **2003**, *51*, 4–28. [CrossRef] [PubMed]
32. Smith, J.T.; Barabasz, A.; Barabasz, M. Comparison of hypnosis and distraction in severely ill children undergoing painful medical procedures. *J. Couns. Psychol.* **1996**, *43*, 187. [CrossRef]
33. Cunningham, N.R.; Lynch-Jordan, A.; Mezoff, A.G.; Farrell, M.K.; Cohen, M.B.; Kashikar-Zuck, S. Importance of addressing anxiety in youth with functional abdominal pain: Suggested guidelines for physicians. *J. Pediatr. Gastroenterol. Nutr.* **2013**, *56*, 469. [CrossRef]
34. Evans, S.; Moieni, M.; Taub, R.; Subramanian, S.K.; Tsao, J.C.; Sternlieb, B.; Zeltzer, L.K. Iyengar yoga for young adults with rheumatoid arthritis: Results from a mixed-methods pilot study. *J. Pain Symptom. Manag.* **2010**, *39*, 904–913. [CrossRef] [PubMed]
35. Jastrowski Mano, K.E.; Salamon, K.S.; Hainsworth, K.R.; Anderson Khan, K.J.; Ladwig, R.J.; Davies, W.H.; Weisman, S.J. A randomized, controlled pilot study of mindfulness-based stress reduction for pediatric chronic pain. *Altern. Ther. Health Med.* **2013**, *19*, 8–14.
36. Eccleston, C.; Fisher, E.; Law, E.; Bartlett, J.; Palermo, T.M. Psychological interventions for parents of children and adolescents with chronic pain. *Cochrane Database Syst. Rev.* **2015**, *4*. [CrossRef]
37. Kanstrup, M.; Wicksell, R.; Kemani, M.; Wiwe Lipsker, C.; Lekander, M.; Holmström, L. A clinical pilot study of individual and group treatment for adolescents with chronic pain and their parents: Effects of acceptance and commitment therapy on functioning. *Children* **2016**, *3*, 30. [CrossRef] [PubMed]

38. Wicksell, R.K.; Melin, L.; Olsson, G.L. Exposure and acceptance in the rehabilitation of adolescents with idiopathic chronic pain—A pilot study. *Eur. J. Pain* **2007**, *11*, 267–274. [CrossRef] [PubMed]
39. Wicksell, R.K.; Melin, L.; Lekander, M.; Olsson, G.L. Evaluating the effectiveness of exposure and acceptance strategies to improve functioning and quailty of life in longstanding pediatric pain—A randomized controlled trial. *Pain* **2009**, *141*, 248–257. [CrossRef] [PubMed]
40. Palermo, T.M.; Beals-Erickson, S.; Bromberg, M.; Law, E.; Chen, M. A single arm pilot trial of brief cognitive behavioral therapy for insomnia in adolescents with physical and psychiatric comorbidities. *J. Clin. Sleep Med.* **2017**, *13*, 401–410. [CrossRef]
41. Law, E.F.; Fales, J.L.; Beals-Erickson, S.E.; Failo, A.; Logan, D.; Randall, E.; Weiss, K.; Durkin, L.; Palermo, T.M. A Single-Arm Feasibility Trial of Problem-Solving Skills Training for Parents of Children with Idiopathic Chronic Pain Conditions Receiving Intensive Pain Rehabilitation. *J. Pediatr. Psychol.* **2017**, *42*, 422–433. [CrossRef]
42. Palermo, T.M.; Law, E.; Bromberg, M.; Fales, J.L.; Eccleston, C.; Wilson, A.C. Problem solving skills training for parents of children with chronic pain: A pilot randomized controlled trial. *Pain* **2016**, *157*, 1213–1223. [CrossRef] [PubMed]
43. Pielech, M.; Vowles, K.; Wicksell, R.K. Acceptance and commitment therapy for pediatric chronic pain: Theory and application. *Children* **2017**, *4*, 10. [CrossRef]
44. Zeltzer, L.K.; Zeltzer, P. *Pain in Children and Young Adults: The Journey Back to Normal. Two Pediatricians' Mind-Body Guide for Parents*; Shilysca Press: Encino, CA, USA, 2016.
45. Kempert, H.; Benore, E.; Heines, R. Easily Administered Patient-Reported Outcome Measures: Adolescents' Perceived Functional Changes After Completing an Intensive Chronic Pain Rehabilitation Program. *Arch. Phys. Med. Rehabil.* **2017**, *98*, 58–63. [CrossRef]
46. Mirek, E.; Logan, D.; Boullard, K.; Hall, A.M.; Staffa, S.J.; Sethna, N. Physical Therapy Outcome Measures for Assessment of Lower Extremity Chronic Pain-Related Function in Pediatrics. *Pediatr. Phys. Ther.* **2019**, *31*, 200–207. [CrossRef] [PubMed]
47. Kempert, H.; Benore, E.; Heines, R. Physical and occupational therapy outcomes: Adolescents' change in functional abilities using objective measures and self-report. *Scand. J. Pain* **2017**, *14*, 60–66. [CrossRef]
48. Eccleston, Z.; Eccleston, C. Interdisciplinary management of adolescent chronic pain: Developing the role of physiotherapy. *Physiotherapy* **2004**, *90*, 77–81. [CrossRef]
49. Kashikar-Zuck, S.; Black, W.R.; Pfeiffer, M.; Peugh, J.; Williams, S.E.; Ting, T.V.; Thomas, S.; Kitchen, K.; Myer, G.D. Pilot randomized trial of integrated cognitive-behavioral therapy and neuromuscular training for juvenile fibromyalgia: The FIT Teens Program. *J. Pain* **2018**, *19*, 1049–1062. [CrossRef] [PubMed]
50. Tran, S.T.; Thomas, S.; DiCesare, C.; Pfeiffer, M.; Sil, S.; Ting, T.V.; Williams, S.E.; Myer, G.D.; Kashikar-Zuck, S. A pilot study of biomechanical assessment before and after an integrative training program for adolescents with juvenile fibromyalgia. *Pediatr. Rheumatol. Online J.* **2016**, *14*, 43. [CrossRef]
51. Dekker, C.; Goossens, M.E.; Bastiaenen, C.H.; Verbunt, J.A. Study protocol for a multicentre randomized controlled trial on effectiveness of an outpatient multimodal rehabilitation program for adolescents with chronic musculoskeletal pain (2B Active). *BMC Musculoskelet. Disord.* **2016**, *17*, 317. [CrossRef]
52. Coakley, R.M.; Wihak, T.; Kossowsky, J.; Iversen, C.; Donado, C. The Comfort Ability Pain Management Workshop: A Preliminary, Nonrandomized Investigation of a Brief, Cognitive, Biobehavioral, and Parent Training Intervention for Pediatric Chronic Pain. *J. Pediatr. Psychol.* **2018**, *43*, 252–265. [CrossRef]
53. Bonnert, M.; Olén, O.; Lalouni, M.; Hedman-Lagerlöf, E.; Särnholm, J.; Serlachius, E.; Ljótsson, B. Internet-Delivered Exposure-Based Cognitive-Behavioral Therapy for Adolescents With Functional Abdominal Pain or Functional Dyspepsia: A Feasibility Study. *Behav. Ther.* **2019**, *50*, 177–188. [CrossRef] [PubMed]
54. Palermo, T.M.; de la Vega, R.; Dudeney, J.; Murray, C.; Law, E. Mobile health intervention for self-management of adolescent chronic pain (WebMAP mobile): Protocol for a hybrid effectiveness-implementation cluster randomized controlled trial. *Contemp. Clin. Trials* **2018**, *74*, 55–60. [CrossRef] [PubMed]
55. Stinson, J.N.; Lalloo, C.; Harris, L.; Isaac, L.; Campbell, F.; Brown, S.; Ruskin, D.; Gordon, A.; Galonski, M.; Pink, L.R. iCanCope with Pain™: User-centred design of a web-and mobile-based self-management program for youth with chronic pain based on identified health care needs. *Pain Res. Manag.* **2014**, *19*, 257–265. [CrossRef]

56. Won, A.S.; Tataru, C.A.; Cojocaru, C.M.; Krane, E.J.; Bailenson, J.N.; Niswonger, S.; Golianu, B. Two virtual reality pilot studies for the treatment of pediatric CRPS. *Pain Med.* **2015**, *16*, 1644–1647. [CrossRef] [PubMed]
57. Won, A.S.; Bailey, J.; Bailenson, J.; Tataru, C.; Yoon, I.A.; Golianu, B. Immersive Virtual Reality for Pediatric Pain. *Children (Basel)* **2017**, *4*, 52. [CrossRef]
58. Louw, A.; Zimney, K.; Puentedura, E.J.; Diener, I. The efficacy of pain neuroscience education on musculoskeletal pain: A systematic review of the literature. *Physiother. Theory Pract.* **2016**, *32*, 332–355. [CrossRef]
59. Malfliet, A.; Kregel, J.; Coppieters, I.; De Pauw, R.; Meeus, M.; Roussel, N.; Cagnie, B.; Danneels, L.; Nijs, J. Effect of pain neuroscience education combined with cognition-targeted motor control training on chronic spinal pain: A randomized clinical trial. *JAMA Neurol.* **2018**, *75*, 808–817. [CrossRef] [PubMed]
60. Moseley, G.L. Joining forces-combining cognition-targeted motor control training with group or individual pain physiology education: A successful treatment for chronic low back pain. *J. Man. Manip. Ther.* **2003**, *11*, 88–94. [CrossRef]
61. Moseley, G.L. Combined physiotherapy and education is efficacious for chronic low back pain. *Aust. J. Physiother.* **2002**, *48*, 297–302. [CrossRef]
62. Malfliet, A.; Kregel, J.; Meeus, M.; Roussel, N.; Danneels, L.; Cagnie, B.; Dolphens, M.; Nijs, J. Blended-learning pain neuroscience education for people with chronic spinal pain: Randomized controlled multicenter trial. *Phys. Ther.* **2017**, *98*, 357–368. [CrossRef]
63. Nijs, J.; Van Wilgen, C.P.; Van Oosterwijck, J.; van Ittersum, M.; Meeus, M. How to explain central sensitization to patients with 'unexplained' chronic musculoskeletal pain: Practice guidelines. *Man. Ther.* **2011**, *16*, 413–418. [CrossRef] [PubMed]
64. Nijs, J.; Malfliet, A.; Ickmans, K.; Baert, I.; Meeus, M. Treatment of central sensitization in patients with 'unexplained' chronic pain: An update. *Expert Opin. Pharmacother.* **2014**, *15*, 1671–1683. [CrossRef] [PubMed]
65. Louw, A.; Puentedura, E.J.; Diener, I.; Peoples, R.R. Preoperative therapeutic neuroscience education for lumbar radiculopathy: A single-case fMRI report. *Physiother. Theory Pract.* **2015**, *31*, 496–508. [CrossRef] [PubMed]
66. Zimney, K.; Louw, A.; Puentedura, E.J. Use of Therapeutic Neuroscience Education to address psychosocial factors associated with acute low back pain: A case report. *Physiother. Theory Pract.* **2014**, *30*, 202–209. [CrossRef] [PubMed]
67. Pate, J.W.; Hush, J.M.; Hancock, M.J.; Moseley, G.L.; Butler, D.S.; Simons, L.E.; Pacey, V. A child's concept of pain: An international survey of pediatric pain experts. *Children* **2018**, *5*, 12. [CrossRef] [PubMed]
68. Moseley, G.L. A pain neuromatrix approach to patients with chronic pain. *Man. Ther.* **2003**, *8*, 130–140. [CrossRef]
69. Gold, J.I.; Yetwin, A.K.; Mahrer, N.E.; Carson, M.C.; Griffin, A.T.; Palmer, S.N.; Joseph, M.H. Pediatric chronic pain and health-related quality of life. *J. Pediatr. Nurs.* **2009**, *24*, 141–150. [CrossRef] [PubMed]
70. Robins, H.; Perron, V.; Heathcote, L.C.; Simons, L.E. Pain neuroscience education: State of the art and application in pediatrics. *Children (Basel)* **2016**, *4*, 43. [CrossRef]
71. Watson, J.A.; Ryan, C.G.; Cooper, L.; Ellington, D.; Whittle, R.; Lavender, M.; Dixon, J.; Atkinson, G.; Cooper, K.; Martin, D.J. Pain Neuroscience Education for Adults With Chronic Musculoskeletal Pain: A Mixed-Methods Systematic Review and Meta-Analysis. *J. Pain* **2019**. [CrossRef] [PubMed]
72. Andias, R.; Neto, M.; Silva, A.G. The effects of pain neuroscience education and exercise on pain, muscle endurance, catastrophizing and anxiety in adolescents with chronic idiopathic neck pain: A school-based pilot, randomized and controlled study. *Physiother. Theory Pract.* **2018**, *34*, 682–691. [CrossRef]
73. Kashikar-Zuck, S.; Vaught, M.H.; Goldschneider, K.R.; Graham, T.B.; Miller, J.C. Depression, coping, and functional disability in juvenile primary fibromyalgia syndrome. *J. Pain* **2002**, *3*, 412–419. [CrossRef] [PubMed]
74. Hicks, C.L.; Von Baeyer, C.L.; McGrath, P.J. Online psychological treatment for pediatric recurrent pain: A randomized evaluation. *J. Pediatr. Psychol.* **2006**, *31*, 724–736. [CrossRef] [PubMed]
75. Anbar, R.D. Hypnosis in pediatrics: Applications at a pediatric pulmonary center. *BMC Pediatr.* **2002**, *2*, 11. [CrossRef]
76. Delivet, H.; Dugue, S.; Ferrari, A.; Postone, S.; Dahmani, S. Efficacy of Self-hypnosis on Quality of Life For Children with Chronic Pain Syndrome. *Int. J. Clin. Exp. Hypn.* **2018**, *66*, 43–55. [CrossRef] [PubMed]

77. Shigaki, C.L.; Glass, B.; Schopp, L.H. Mindfulness-based stress reduction in medical settings. *J. Clin. Psychol. Med. Settings* **2006**, *13*, 209–216. [CrossRef]
78. Zernicke, K.A.; Campbell, T.S.; Blustein, P.K.; Fung, T.S.; Johnson, J.A.; Bacon, S.L.; Carlson, L.E. Mindfulness-based stress reduction for the treatment of irritable bowel syndrome symptoms: A randomized wait-list controlled trial. *Int. J. Behav. Med.* **2013**, *20*, 385–396. [CrossRef]
79. Field, T.; Hernandez-Reif, M.; Seligmen, S.; Krasnegor, J.; Sunshine, W.; Rivas-Chacon, R.; Schanberg, S.; Kuhn, C. Juvenile rheumatoid arthritis: Benefits from massage theraphy. *J. Pediatr. Psychol.* **1997**, *22*, 607–617. [CrossRef] [PubMed]
80. Suresh, S.; Wang, S.; Porfyris, S.; Kamasinski-sol, R.; Steinhorn, D.M. Massage therapy in outpatient pediatric chronic pain patients: Do they facilitate significant reductions in levels of distress, pain, tension, discomfort, and mood alterations? *Paediatr. Anaesth.* **2008**, *18*, 884–887. [CrossRef]
81. Beck, J.S. *Cognitive Behavior Therapy: Basics and Beyond*; Guilford Press: New York, NY, USA, 2011.
82. Hayes, S.C.; Strosahl, K.D.; Wilson, K.G. *Acceptance and Commitment Therapy: An Experiential Approach to Behavior Change*; Guilford Press: New York, NY, USA, 1999.
83. Coyne, L.W.; McHugh, L.; Martinez, E.R. Acceptance and commitment therapy (ACT): Advances and applications with children, adolescents, and families. *Child Adolesc. Psychiatr. Clin. N. Am.* **2011**, *20*, 379–399. [CrossRef]
84. Gauntlett-Gilbert, J.; Connell, H.; Clinch, J.; McCracken, L.M. Acceptance and values-based treatment of adolescents with chronic pain: Outcomes and their relationship to acceptance. *J. Pediatr. Psychol.* **2013**, *38*, 72–81. [CrossRef]
85. Wicksell, R.K.; Olsson, G.L.; Hayes, S.C. Mediators of change in acceptance and commitment therapy for pediatric chronic pain. *Pain* **2011**, *152*, 2792–2801. [CrossRef] [PubMed]
86. Masuda, A.; Feinstein, A.; Wendell, J.W.; Sheehan, S.T. Cognitive defusion versus thought distraction: A clinical rationale, training, and experiential exercise in altering psychological impacts of negative self-referential thoughts. *Behav. Modif.* **2010**, *34*, 520–538. [CrossRef] [PubMed]
87. Fordyce, W.E.; Folwer, R.S.; Lehmann, J.F.; D'elateur, B.J. Some implications of learning in problems of chronic pain. *J. Chronic Dis.* **1968**, *21*, 179–190. [CrossRef]
88. Walker, L.S. The evolution of research on recurrent abdominal pain: History, assumptions, and a conceptual model. *Prog. Pain Res. Manag.* **1999**, *13*, 141–172.
89. Simons, L.E.; Kaczynski, K.J. The Fear Avoidance model of chronic pain: Examination for pediatric application. *J. Pain* **2012**, *13*, 827–835. [CrossRef] [PubMed]
90. Vlaeyen, J.W.; Linton, S.J. Fear-avoidance model of chronic musculoskeletal pain: 12 years on. *Pain* **2012**, *153*, 1144–1147. [CrossRef] [PubMed]
91. Simons, L.E.; Sieberg, C.B.; Carpino, E.; Logan, D.; Berde, C. The Fear of Pain Questionnaire (FOPQ): Assessment of pain-related fear among children and adolescents with chronic pain. *J. Pain* **2011**, *12*, 677–686. [CrossRef] [PubMed]
92. Goubert, L.; Simons, L.E. Cognitive styles and processes in paediatric pain. In *Oxford Textbook of Pediatric Pain*; Oxford University Press: Oxford, UK, 2013; pp. 95–101.
93. Vlaeyen, J.W.S.; Morley, S.J.; Linton, S.J.; Boersma, K.; de Jong, J. *Pain-Related Fear: Exposure-Based Treatment of Chronic Pain*; IASP Press: Washington, DC, USA, 2012.
94. Vlaeyen, J.W.; de Jong, J.; Geilen, M.; Heuts, P.H.T.G.; van Breukelen, G. Graded exposure in vivo in the treatment of pain-related fear: A replicated single-case experimental design in four patients with chronic low back pain. *Behav. Res. Ther.* **2001**, *39*, 151–166. [CrossRef]
95. Simons, L.E.; Vlaeyen, J.W.S.; Declercq, L.; Smith, A.L.; Beebe, J.; Hogan, M.; Li, E.; Kronman, C.; Mahmud, F.; Corey, J.; et al. Avoid or engage? Outcomes of graded exposure in youth with chronic pain utilizing multi-level modeling of a single-case randomized design. *Pain* **2019**. submitted.
96. Hechler, T.; Dobe, M.; Damschen, U.; Blankenburg, M.; Schroeder, S.; Kosfelder, J.; Zernikow, B. The pain provocation technique for adolescents with chronic pain: Preliminary evidence for its effectiveness. *Pain Med.* **2010**, *11*, 897–910. [CrossRef]
97. Gruszka, P.; Schaan, L.; Adolph, D.; Pane-Farre, C.A.; Benke, C.; Schneider, S.; Hechler, T. Defence reponse mobilization in response to provocation or imagery of interoceptive sensations in adolescents with chronic pain: A study protocol. *Pain Rep.* **2018**, *3*. [CrossRef]

98. Palermo, T.M.; Eccleston, C. Parents of children and adolescents with chronic pain. *Pain* **2009**, *146*, 15. [CrossRef]
99. Law, E.F.; Fisher, E.; Eccleston, C.; Palermo, T.M. Psychological interventions for parents of children and adolescents with chronic illness. *Cochrane Database Syst. Rev.* **2019**. [CrossRef]
100. Simons, L.E.; Smith, A.; Kaczynski, K.; Basch, M. Living in fear of your child's pain: The Parent Fear of Pain Questionnaire. *Pain* **2015**, *156*, 694–702. [CrossRef]
101. Coakley, R.M. *When Your Child Hurts: Effective Stratgies to Increase Comfort, Reduce Stress, and Break the Cycle of Chronic Pain*; Yale University Press: New Haven, CT, USA, 2016.
102. Zeltzer, L.K.; Blackett Schlank, C. *Conquering Your Child's Chronic Pain*; HarperCollins: New York, NY, USA, 2005.
103. Palermo, T.M.; Law, E. *Managing Your Child's Chronic Pain*; Oxford University Press: Oxford, UK, 2015.
104. Sherry, D.D.; Wallace, C.A.; Kelley, C.; Kidder, M.; Sapp, L. Short-and long-term outcomes of children with complex regional pain syndrome type I treated with exercise therapy. *Clin. J. Pain* **1999**, *15*, 218–223. [CrossRef]
105. Eccleston, C.; Connell, H.; Carmichael, N. *Residential Treatment Settings for Adolescent Chronic Pain Management*; Humana Press: Totowa, NJ, USA, 2006.
106. Hechler, T.; Ruhe, A.-K.; Schmidt, P.; Hirsch, J.; Wager, J.; Dobe, M.; Krummenauer, F.; Zernikow, B. Inpatient-based intensive interdisciplinary pain treatment for highly impaired children with severe chronic pain: Randomized controlled trial of efficacy and economic effects. *Pain* **2014**, *155*, 118–128. [CrossRef]
107. Flor, H.; Fydrich, T.; Turk, D.C. Efficacy of multidisciplinary pain treatment centers: A meta-analytic review. *Pain* **1992**, *49*, 221–230. [CrossRef]
108. Logan, D.E.; Carpino, E.A.; Chiang, G.; Condon, M.; Firn, E.; Gaughan, V.J. A day-hospital approach to treatment of pediatric complex regional pain syndrome: Initial functional outcomes. *Clin. J. Pain* **2012**, *28*. [CrossRef]
109. Lee, B.H.; Scharff, L.; Sethna, N.; McCarthy, C.F.; Scott-Sutherland, J.; Shea, A.M.; Sullivan, P.; Meier, P.; Zurakowski, D.; Masek, B.J.; et al. Physical therapy and cognitive-behavioral treatment for complex regional pain syndromes. *J. Pediatr.* **2002**, *141*, 135–140. [CrossRef]
110. Valrie, C.R.; Bromberg, M.H.; Palermo, T.; Schanberg, L.E. A systematic review of sleep in pediatric pain populations. *J. Dev. Behav. Pediatr.* **2013**, *34*, 120–128. [CrossRef]
111. Palermo, T.M.; Kiska, R. Subjective sleep disturbances in adolescents with chronic pain: Relationship to daily functioning and quality of life. *J. Pain* **2005**, *6*, 201–207. [CrossRef]
112. McGrath, P.J.; Frager, G. Psychological barriers to optimal pain management in infants and children. *Clin. J. Pain* **1996**, *12*, 135–141. [CrossRef]
113. Cunningham, N.R.; Jagpal, A.; Tran, S.T.; Kashikar-Zuck, S.; Goldschneider, K.R.; Coghill, R.C.; Lynch-Jordan, A.M. Anxiety adversely impacts response to cognitive behavioral therapy in children with chronic pain. *J. Pediatr.* **2016**, *171*, 227–233. [CrossRef]
114. Van Tilburg, M.A.; Spence, N.J.; Whitehead, W.E.; Bangdiwala, S.; Goldston, D.B. Chronic pain in adolescents is associated with suicidal thoughts and behaviors. *J. Pain* **2011**, *12*, 1032–1039. [CrossRef]
115. Evans, J.R.; Benore, E.; Banez, G.A. Conversion disorder and pediatric chronic pain—Talking through the challenges. *Pediatr. Pain Lett.* **2015**, *17*, 16–20.
116. Eccleston, C.; Malleson, P.N.; Clinch, J.; Connell, H.; Sourbut, C. Chronic pain in adolescents: Evaluation of a programme of interdisciplinary cognitive behaviour therapy. *Arch. Dis. Child* **2003**, *88*, 881–885. [CrossRef]
117. Simons, L.E.; Sieberg, C.B.; Pielech, M.; Conroy, C.; Logan, D.E. What does it take? Comparing intensive rehabilitation to outpatient treatment for children with significant pain-related disability. *J. Pediatr. Psychol.* **2012**, *38*, 213–223. [CrossRef]
118. Maynard, C.S.; Amari, A.; Wieczorek, B.; Christensen, J.R.; Slifer, K.J. Interdisciplinary behavioral rehabilitation of pediatric pain-associated disability: Retrospective review of an inpatient treatment protocol. *J. Pediatr. Psychol.* **2009**, *35*, 128–137. [CrossRef]
119. Hechler, T.; Blankenburg, M.; Dobe, M.; Kosfelder, J.; Hübner, B.; Zernikow, B. Effectiveness of a multimodal inpatient treatment for pediatric chronic pain: A comparison between children and adolescents. *Eur. J. Pain* **2010**, *14*, 91–97. [CrossRef]
120. Mahrer, N.E.; Gold, J.I.; Luu, M.; Herman, P.M. A cost-analysis of an interdisciplinary pediatric chronic pain clinic. *J. Pain* **2018**, *19*, 158–165. [CrossRef]

121. Palermo, T.M.; Wilson, A.C.; Peters, M.; Lewandowski, A.S.; Somhegyi, H. Randomized controlled trial of an Internet-delivered family cognitive-behavioral therapy intervention for children and adolescents with chronic pain. *Pain* **2009**, *146*, 205–213. [CrossRef]
122. Lin, J.; Klatt, L.-I.; McCracken, L.M.; Baumeister, H. Psychological flexibility mediates the effect of an online-based acceptance and commitment therapy for chronic pain: An investigation of change processes. *Pain* **2018**, *159*, 663–672. [CrossRef]
123. Fisher, E.; Law, E.F.; Palermo, T.M.; Eccleston, C. Psychological therapies (remotely delivered) for the management of chronic and recurrent pain in children and adolescents. *Cochrane Database Syst. Rev.* **2014**, *2014*, CD011118.
124. Riva, G.; Baños, R.M.; Botella, C.; Mantovani, F.; Gaggioli, A. Transforming experience: The potential of augmented reality and virtual reality for enhancing personal and clinical change. *Front. Psychiatry* **2016**, *7*, 164. [CrossRef]
125. Matamala-Gomez, M.; Diaz Gonzalez, A.M.; Slater, M.; Sanchez-Vives, M.V. Decreasing Pain Ratings in Chronic Arm Pain Through Changing a Virtual Body: Different Strategies for Different Pain Types. *J. Pain* **2019**. [CrossRef]
126. Simons, L.E.; Smith, A.; Ibagon, C.; Coakley, R.M.; Logan, D.E.; Schecter, N.; Borsook, D.; Hill, J.C. Pediatric Pain Screen Tool (PPST): Rapid identification of risk in youth with pain complaints. *Pain* **2015**, *156*, 1511–1518. [CrossRef]

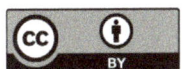

© 2019 by the authors. Licensee MDPI, Basel, Switzerland. This article is an open access article distributed under the terms and conditions of the Creative Commons Attribution (CC BY) license (http://creativecommons.org/licenses/by/4.0/).

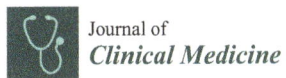 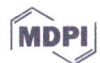

Review

Best-Evidence Rehabilitation for Chronic Pain Part 2: Pain during and after Cancer Treatment

An De Groef [1,2,*,†], Frauke Penen [1,2], Lore Dams [1,2], Elien Van der Gucht [1,2], Jo Nijs [3,4] and Mira Meeus [2,5]

1. Department of Rehabilitation Sciences, KU Leuven, University of Leuven, Herestraat 49, 3000 Leuven, Belgium
2. Department of Rehabilitation Sciences and Physiotherapy, MOVANT, University of Antwerp, Universiteitsplein 1, 2610 Antwerp, Belgium
3. Pain in Motion International Research Group, Department of Physiotherapy, Human Physiology and Anatomy (KIMA), Faculty of Physical Education & Physiotherapy, Vrije Universiteit Brussel (VUB), Laarbeeklaan 103, 1090 Brussels, Belgium
4. Department of Physical Medicine and Physiotherapy, University Hospital Brussels, Laarbeeklaan 101, 1090 Brussels, Belgium
5. Pain in Motion International Research Group, Department of Rehabilitation Sciences, Faculty of Medicine and Health Sciences, Ghent University, De Pintelaan 185, 9000 Ghent, Belgium
* Correspondence: an.degroef@kuleuven.be; Tel.: +32-16-342-171
† Support statement: ADG is a post-doctoral research fellow of the FWO-Flanders.

Received: 5 June 2019; Accepted: 4 July 2019; Published: 5 July 2019

Abstract: Pain during, and especially after, cancer remains underestimated and undertreated. Moreover, both patients and health care providers are not aware of potential benefits of rehabilitation strategies for the management of pain during and following cancer treatment. In this paper, we firstly provided a state-of-the-art overview of the best evidence rehabilitation modalities for patients having (persistent) pain during and following cancer treatment, including educational interventions, specific exercise therapies, manual therapies, general exercise therapies and mind-body exercise therapies. Secondly, the findings were summarized from a clinical perspective and discussed from a scientific perspective. In conclusion, best evidence suggests that general exercise therapy has small pain-relieving effects. Supporting evidence for mind-body exercise therapy is available only in breast cancer patients. At this moment, there is a lack of high-quality evidence to support the use of specific exercises and manual therapy at the affected region for pain relief during and after cancer treatment. No clinically relevant results were found in favor of educational interventions restricted to a biomedical approach of pain. To increase available evidence these rehabilitation modalities should be applied according to, and within, a multidisciplinary biopsychosocial pain management approach. Larger, well-designed clinical trials tailored to the origin of pain and with proper evaluation of pain-related functioning and the patient's pain experience are needed.

Keywords: cancer; pain; rehabilitation; exercise

1. Introduction

Since both prevalence and survival rates of cancer continue to rise, an increasing number of people have to cope with the debilitating effects of this disease and its treatment. Pain is one of the most prevalent and persistent problems reported by cancer patients and survivors [1,2]. A recent meta-analysis reported prevalence rates of 55% during cancer treatment and 40% after curative treatment [3]. Pain can interfere with activities of daily life, quality of life and fulfillment of a person's role in society. Yet, pain during, and especially after, cancer remains underestimated and undertreated [4].

Nowadays, pharmacological treatment is considered the standard approach for treating pain related to cancer (treatment) [5,6]. However, both patients and health care providers are often not aware of other possible rehabilitation strategies and their potential benefits in the management of pain during and after cancer treatment [5,7]. Cancer rehabilitation includes a multidisciplinary and biopsychosocial approach which aims to optimize functioning, well-being and participation of cancer survivors in general, as well as pain relief specifically [7,8]. An important role in the multidisciplinary team is reserved for the physical therapist, at all levels of cancer care (inpatient versus outpatient) and across the whole continuum of complexity of a patient's pain complaint [8]. Traditional rehabilitation modalities for pain during and following cancer treatment consist of both general (including mind-body exercises) and specific exercises as well as manual techniques to restore physical functioning. Additionally, awareness of the added value of educational interventions in a rehabilitation session has increased substantially and these interventions can no longer be ignored [9,10]. While literature on the beneficial effects of rehabilitation on physical symptoms (such as fatigue, exercise capacity) and general quality of life in cancer patients or survivors is overwhelming, evidence for pain relief in particular is rather scarce in this population.

In this paper, we firstly provided a state-of-the-art overview of the best evidence rehabilitation modalities for patients having (persistent) pain during and following cancer treatment. Secondly, the findings were summarized from a clinical perspective to facilitate integration from research into daily clinical practice. At last, the state-of-the-art overview was discussed from a scientific perspective. This way, future clinical researchers can build upon this best evidence when designing future trials, implementation studies or new innovative therapies.

2. State-of-the-Art

For this paper, we have identified scientific studies using broad search terms including 'pain', 'cancer' and 'rehabilitation' in MEDLINE (PubMed), SCOPUS and Pedro. To minimize selection bias and ensure the selection of high-quality evidence, systematic reviews and meta-analyses were preferred when possible. For the scope of this paper, evidence on rehabilitation modalities for pain during and following cancer was summarized in five categories, being educational interventions, specific exercise therapies, manual therapies, general exercise therapies and mind-body exercise therapies. The focus was limited to cancer patients and survivors with a primary cancer diagnosis and pain during and/or after active cancer treatment. Rehabilitation of advanced and metastatic cancers did not belong to the scope of this paper. Details on the target population, rehabilitation modality, comparator, pain-related outcomes, rehabilitation setting, rehabilitation providers and conclusions regarding the pain-related outcomes can be found in Table 1.

2.1. Education

In general, patient education interventions can be defined as "the process by which health professionals and others impart information to patients that will alter their health behaviors or improve their health status" [11].

Table 1. Detailed best evidence table.

Author, Year (Design)	Target Population	Rehabilitation Modality	Comparator	Pain-Related Outcomes	Rehabilitation Setting	Rehabilitation Providers	Conclusion
1. Education							
Oldenmenger et al. 2018 (Systematic review of RCTs)	- adults - solid malignancies - cancer-related pain	Educational intervention: information, behavioural instructions + advice (by verbal, written, audio- or videotaped or computer-aided modalities)	Usual care or active control intervention	- pain intensity (NRS or VAS) - pain interference (Brief Pain Inventory or an equivalent) - knowledge about cancer-related pain, pain barriers (Barriers Questionnaire) - medication adherence (Medication Adherence Scale, Medication Event Monitoring System or self-report)	Outpatient and inpatient	(Oncology) nurse, research assistant/nurse	stat. sign. differences in favour of education were found for: - pain intensity in 31% of studies *(only evaluated in 40% of included RCTs)* - pain interference in 33% of studies *(only evaluated in 68% of studies)* - pain knowledge or barriers in 84% of studies *(only evaluated in 84% of included RCTs)* - medication adherence in 50% of studies *(only evaluated in 23% of included RCTs)*
Prevost et al. 2016 (systematic review of (non-) RCTs)	- adults - cancer patients with pain	Patient educational programs (PEP): information, behavioural instructions + advice (by verbal, written, audio- or videotaped, telecare, or computer-aided modalities)	Usual care, general patient education, nutrition education	- pain intensity (NRS) - pain interference (Brief Pain Inventory or an equivalent) - knowledge about cancer-related pain, pain barriers (Barriers Questionnaire) - medication adherence (questionnaires or self-reported)	Ambulatory, home care, and hospital settings	(Oncology) nurse	stat. sign. differences in favour of education were found for: - pain intensity in 52% of studies - pain interference in 12% of studies *(only evaluated in 37% of included RCTs)* - pain knowledge and barriers in 81% of studies *(only evaluated in 70% of included RCTs)* - medication adherence in 45% of studies *(only evaluated in 25% of included RCTs)*
Ling et al. 2012 (review of RCTs)	- adults - cancer-related pain	Educational intervention: information, behavioural instructions and advice by means of verbal, written or audio/video-tape messages	Non-educational treatment, no treatment or usual care	- pain intensity (Brief Pain Inventory, Total Pain Quality Management) - pain interference (Brief Pain Inventory, Total Pain Quality Management)	Outpatient	Healthcare staff	- 50% of studies reported stat. sign. decrease in pain intensity - no stat. sign. results for pain interference

Table 1. *Cont.*

Author, Year (Design)	Target Population	Rehabilitation Modality	Comparator	Pain-Related Outcomes	Rehabilitation Setting	Rehabilitation Providers	Conclusion
2. Specific exercise therapy							
McNeely et al. 2010 (review + meta-analysis of RCTs)	- female adults - breast cancer patients who had surgical removal of breast tumour, axillary lymph node dissection or sentinel node biopsy - during and after cancer treatment	1) Active or active-assisted ROM exercises; 2) Passive ROM/manual stretching exercises; 3) Stretching exercises (including formal exercise interventions such as yoga and Tai Chi Chuan); 4) Strengthening or resistance exercises. Carried out following surgery, during adjuvant treatment and following cancer treatment	1) Early (day 1–3 post-surgery) vs. delayed (day 4 or later post-surgery) 2) usual care/comparison 3) supervised vs. unsupervised	- pain incidence - pain intensity (VAS)	Outpatient and inpatient	Physical therapist, manual therapist, occupational therapist or exercise specialist	1) *Early vs. delayed post-operative exercises:* - no stat. sign. difference in pain incidence at 2w, 1Mo, 6Mo and 2y FU (Bendz et al 2002) and 3Mo FU (Le Vu 1997) 2) *Specific exercises vs. usual care/comparison* - no stat. sign. difference in pain incidence post-intervention (OR: 1.65; 95% CI: 2.50 to 0.81) or at 6Mo FU (OR: 1.51; 95% CI: 2.35 to 0.67) (Beurskens et al 2007) - stat. sign. different decrease in pain intensity: −3.4 vs. −0.5 ($p < 0.01$) at 3Mo; −3.8 vs. −1.0 ($p > 0.05$) at 6Mo (Beurskens et al 2007) 3) *Supervised vs. unsupervised* - no stat. sign. difference in pain intensity post-intervention (MD: −5.40 points; CI: −19.16 to 8.36) (Hwang et al 2008)
De Groef et al. 2015 (review of (pseudo-) RCTs)	- female adults- breast cancer - maximum of 6 weeks postoperative	Active exercises	1) Early (day 1–3 post-surgery) vs. delayed (day 4 or later post-surgery) 2) usual care/comparison/no exercise program	- pain incidence - pain intensity (NRS or VAS)	Outpatient	NS	1) *Early vs. delayed post-operative exercises:* - no stat. sign. differences for pain intensity (reported in only one study, Bendz et al 2002) 2) *Specific exercises vs. usual care* - no stat. sign. difference in pain incidence post-intervention (OR: 1.65; 95% CI: 2.50 to 0.81) or at 6Mo FU (OR: 1.51; 95% CI: 2.35 to 0.67) (Beurskens et al 2007) - stat. sign. different decrease in pain intensity: −3.4 vs. −0.5 ($p < 0.01$) at 3Mo; −3.8 vs. −1.0 ($p > 0.05$) at 6Mo (Beurskens et al 2007)

Table 1. Cont.

Author, Year (Design)	Target Population	Rehabilitation Modality	Comparator	Pain-Related Outcomes	Rehabilitation Setting	Rehabilitation Providers	Conclusion
Carvalho et al. 2012 (review + meta-analyses of RCTs)	- adults - head and neck cancer - during and after cancer treatment - with dysfunction of the shoulder due to having received any type of cancer treatment	1) Active or active-assisted range of motion exercises 2) Passive range of motion exercises 3) Stretching exercises 4) Resistance exercises 5) Proprioceptive neuromuscular facilitation 6) Any other exercise with a focus on shoulder dysfunction treatment or prevention, whether combined or not with pharmacological intervention.	No treatment, usual care, placebo, sham exercises or pharmacological interventions	- pain subscale of the Shoulder Pain and Disability Index (SPADI) (0-100)	Inpatient: Cross Cancer Institute and University of Alberta in Edmonton, Canada (McNeely et al 2004 and 2008)	NS	- stat. sign. beneficial effects for Progressive Strengthening Training (12 weeks) compared to standard care for pain subscale of the SPADI; MD −6.26 95% CI (12.20 to −0.31)

3. Manual therapy

Author, Year (Design)	Target Population	Rehabilitation Modality	Comparator	Pain-Related Outcomes	Rehabilitation Setting	Rehabilitation Providers	Conclusion
De Groef et al. 2015 (review of (pseudo-) RCTs)	- female adults: breast cancer - max 6 weeks postoperative.	Passive mobilizations	1) Early (day 1–3 post-surgery) vs. delayed (day 4 or later post-surgery) 2) Usual care/comparison/no exercise program	- pain incidence - pain intensity (NRS or VAS)	Outpatient	NS	- pain or sensitivity problems: 74% in no physical therapy vs. 70% mobilisation group vs. 72% massage groups vs. 68% mobilisation and massage group at 3 Mo ($p > 0.05$) - locoregional pain: 5% in mobilization group vs. 13% in no mobilization group ($p = 0.03$) at 8-24 Mo Follow-Up (Le Vu et al., 1997)
Shin et al. 2016 (review + meta-analyses of RCTs)	- adults and children - metastatic, colorectal, advanced, breast, lung, paediatric and non-specified cancer	Massage therapy: tissue manipulation using a carrier oil or blended carrier oil with essential oils (i.e., aromatherapy); excluding touch therapies such as therapeutic touch, acupressure, and reflexology.	No massage	- pain intensity (NRS, VRS or VAS)	Outpatient and inpatient	Trained therapists or not mentioned	- massage significant effect in 1/5 studies on present pain intensity (NRS 0-10): MD −1.60, 95% CI (−2.67 to −0.53)
Boyd et al. 2016 (review + meta-analyses of RCTs)	- adults - metastatic, colorectal, advanced, breast, paediatric and non-specified cancer - with pain	Massage therapy: the systematic manipulation of soft tissue with the hands that positively affects and promotes healing, reduces stress, enhances muscle relaxation, improves local circulation, and creates a sense of well-being.	Sham, no treatment, or active comparator (i.e, participants are actively receiving any type of intervention)	- pain intensity/severity (VAS)	Inpatient, at patient's or therapist's home or a hospice	Massage therapist, unspecified therapist, nurse, healing-arts specialist, caregiver, or a researcher trained in massage	- 79% (11/14) of studies showed significant beneficial effects of massage therapy on pain intensity - meta-analysis massage vs. no treatment including 3 studies: SMD—0.20, 95% CI (−0.99 to 0.59); reduction in pain intensity = −5.075, 95% CI (−24.80 to 14.63) - meta-analysis massage vs. active comparator including 6 studies: SMD = −0.55, 95% CI (−1.23 to 0.14); reduction in pain intensity = −13.63, 95% CI (−30.78 to 3.5)

Table 1. Cont.

4. General exercise therapy

Author, Year (Design)	Target Population	Rehabilitation Modality	Comparator	Pain-Related Outcomes	Rehabilitation Setting	Rehabilitation Providers	Conclusion
Nakano et al. 2018 (SR and meta-analyses of RCTs)	- adults - during and after cancer treatment	1) Aerobic exercise program 2) Resistance exercise program 3) Mixed exercise program	Not receiving any (major) exercise intervention or other interventions (e.g., cognitive behavioural therapy); groups with only attention, relaxation, or education	- EORTC-QLQ-C30 – pain symptom subscale	NS	NS	- overall effect of exercise on EORTC-QLQ-C30 – pain symptom subscale: SMD −0.17, 95% CI (−0.32 to −0.03); p = .02; - no stat. sign. difference among 3 subgroups: 1) aerobic exercise program (4 studies): NS 2) resistance exercise program (3 studies): NS 3) mixed exercise program (4 studies): SMD −0.28; 95% CI (−0.47 to −0.09); p = .005
Mishra et al. 2012 (SR and meta-analyses of RCTs and CCTs)	- adults - after cancer treatment (i.e., survivors) - excluding those who are terminally ill and receiving hospice care	Exercise interventions and any physical activity causing an increase in energy expenditure, and involving a planned or structured movement of the body performed in a systematic manner in terms of frequency, intensity, and duration and is designed to maintain or enhance health-related outcomes	No exercise, another intervention, or usual care (e.g., with no specific exercise program prescribed)	- pain intensity (EORTC-QLQ-C30 – pain symptom subscale or Shoulder Pain and Disability Index (SPADI))	NS	NS	- pain intensity: −0.29 95% CI (−0.55 to −0.04) standard deviation units after 12 weeks follow-up; (4 studies) A standard deviation unit is equivalent to about a 28-point change on the QLQ-C30 pain sub-scale
Mishra et al. 2012 (SR and meta-analyses of RCTs and CCTs)	- adults - during active cancer treatment - excluding those who are terminally ill and receiving hospice care	Exercise interventions and any physical activity causing an increase in energy expenditure, and involving a planned or structured movement of the body performed in a systematic manner in terms of frequency, intensity, and duration and is designed to maintain or enhance health-related outcomes	No exercise, another intervention, or usual care (e.g., with no specific exercise program prescribed)	- Pain intensity (MOS SF-36 – pain subscale, EORTC QLQ-C30 – pain symptom subscale, VAS, MD Anderson Symptom Inventory – pain subscale)	Individual or group, home or facility based	Professionally led or not	- no significant effect was obtained when pooling trials that reported change in pain from baseline to follow-up nor overall pain for follow-up values

Table 1. Cont.

Author, Year (Design)	Target Population	Rehabilitation Modality	Comparator	Pain-Related Outcomes	Rehabilitation Setting	Rehabilitation Providers	Conclusion
5. Mind-body therapy							
Pinto-Carral et al. 2018 (SR and meta-analyses of RCTs and CCTs)	- adults - breast cancer - during and after cancer treatment	Pilates exercises: focused on core muscle strengthening, spine flexibility and shoulder girdle range of motion	Other exercise interventions	- Pain intensity (Brief Pain Inventory, VAS)	NS	Specialized pilates centres (outpatient) or at home	- stat. sign effect for pain intensity: SMD −0.48; 95% CI (−0.88 to −0.07)
Danhauer et al 2019 (SR of RCTs)	- adults - breast, prostate, lymphoma colorectal or mixed cancer groups - during and after cancer treatment	Yoga: multicomponent protocols, (i.e., movement/postures, breathing and mediation) based on several different yoga types (Anusara, Eischens, Iyengar, Tibetan, Bali, Vivekananda Yoga Anusandhana Samsthana)	Waitlist, usual care or active comparator	- Pain (not further specified)	NS	NS	- 1/1 study stat. sign. improvement of pain *during cancer treatment* - 2/3 studies stat. sign. improvement of pain *after cancer treatment*
Pan et al. 2015 (SR and MA of RCT)	- adults - breast cancer - after active cancer treatment	Tai Chi Chuan (NS)	Psychosocial therapy intervention, standard care, health education	- pain (not specified health-related quality of life questionnaire or SF-36)	NS	NS	- no stat. sign. effect for pain: SMD 0.11; 95% CI (−0.41 to 0.18)

Stat. sign. = Statistically Significant; RCT = Randomized Controlled Trial; SR = Systematic Review; NRS = Numeric Rating Scale; VAS = Visual Analogue Scale; VRS = Verbal Rating Scale; SMD = Standardized Mean Difference; MD = Mean Difference; CI = Confidence Interval; Mo = Months; w = weeks; y = years; EORTC-QLQ-C30 = European Organization for Research and Treatment of Cancer Quality of Life Questionnaire-C30; MOS SF-36 = Medical Outcome Study 36-Item Short From Survey; NS = Not specified.

In the broad field of rehabilitation, the importance of education has increased tremendously over the past years, especially in patients with musculoskeletal pain [12]. In the oncological field, several reviews have summarized the effectiveness of educational interventions on pain intensity, the use of analgesics, side effects and misconceptions on opioids, in patients with pain from active cancer [13–17]. Within the rehabilitation scope of this paper, we found three systematic reviews that had summarized the effectiveness of an educational intervention in the form of individual information, behavioral instructions and advice in relation to management of pain related to cancer (treatment) [16–18] (Table 1, Section 1. Education). Comparing educational interventions with usual care, they had found a statistically significant difference in pain intensity in 31% [17], 50% [18] and 52% [16] of the included studies, respectively. Up to 33% [17] and 12% [16] of included studies also showed significant beneficial effects on pain interference with daily activities. Interestingly, Prevost et al. (2016) found that 81% of the studies had significantly improved knowledge and beliefs regarding pain and 45% of studies had improvement in adherence with prescribed analgesics in the education group [16]. In the review of Oldenmenger et al., 68% of the studies showed a significant difference in pain knowledge or barriers, including poor knowledge and misconceptions about pain medication and their side-effects. This last one also evaluated medication adherence and found a statistically significant increase in the education group in 50% of studies [17].

However, these studies could neither find a relation between pain knowledge/barriers and pain intensity, nor medication adherence among the included trials reporting both outcomes [17]. Few studies reported effect sizes and despite their significance, these effect sizes were small and of limited clinical relevance in all included studies [18]. Also, response rates are low with only an improvement in pain in 20% of all included patients in the review of Oldenmenger et al [17].

A possible explanation for these rather limited beneficial effects may be the narrow scope of the educational interventions. Indeed, the content of the educational interventions can vary widely among studies and can have different scopes. The emphasis of the educational interventions in these reviews was restricted to a biomedical approach of pain. This is illustrated by the fact that most education was given by (oncology) nurses and medical doctors and mainly covered the consequences of cancer treatment and the pharmacological and medical management of these sequellae. However, considering the increased knowledge of pain pathophysiology, education should additionally incorporate a more biopsychosocial explanation of pain [10], as this has been supported by research in various other chronic musculoskeletal pain populations. This modern educational approach has a broader scope and aims at removing barriers for all aspects of pain management (including self-management and rehabilitation). It targets the patient's cognitions and knowledge of pain as well as his/her pain-related behavior and thereby aims for a shift from a passive therapy-receiver to an active self-manager [9,10,16,17]. Additionally, education may vary in type (face-to-face, leaflet, video), provider and duration. Furthermore, populations and mechanisms of pain in the included studies were quite heterogeneous, making it unclear whether pain was related to active cancer and/or a consequence of cancer treatment modalities [14,16].

All things concerned, although the effect of educational interventions in a rehabilitation setting seems promising, the ambiguity of its essential components when applied in a cancer population still remains to be further unraveled.

2.2. Specific Exercise Therapy

Specific exercise therapy typically includes active and/or active-assisted strengthening, mobilizing and stretching exercises to restore function of the affected region [19]. The literature on the effectiveness of specific exercise for pain in cancer survivors is scarce [20]. A tremendous amount of research has been done on the effect of specific exercises for other upper limb dysfunctions during and after head, neck and breast cancer. Range of motion, upper limb strength and upper limb function in general may be affected after surgery and radiotherapy due to formation of fibrosis and scar tissue, nerve damage, muscle tightness, lymphedema (including axillary cording) and pain [20–22]. Specific exercises are indeed prescribed to optimize and/or restore joint and muscle function of the affected region. Reduction in pain is often presumed to occur subsequently. However, pain might be a primary indication for specific exercises as well. In particular, for nociceptive and neuropathic pain at the affected region, specific exercises may aid in increased blood flow, as well as a reduced hyperesthesia, inflammation, biomechanical deficits and muscle spasms [5,23,24]. To our knowledge, only four systematic reviews have summarized randomized controlled trials on the effectiveness of specific exercises in an oncological population that included pain outcome measures [19–21,25] (Table 1, Section 2. Specific exercise therapy).

First, in breast cancer patients, three reviews have summarized the effectiveness of different exercise programs compared to usual care or no exercises [19,20,25]. The exercise programs varied in content (mobilization, stretching, strengthening and stabilization exercises) and in duration (timing, frequency and intensity). For (shoulder) pain, with the exception of one study, no differences between two groups were found. This study compared active exercises with a leaflet and showed beneficial effects on pain intensity on a visual analogue scale (0–10) three months (−2.7 95% CI (−3.6 to −1.9)) and six months (−2.5 95% CI (−3.5 to −1.6)) following surgery [26]. Remarkably, almost all studies reported beneficial effects of exercises on shoulder range of motion and/or shoulder function in general.

Additionally, several studies showed no difference in an early or delayed start of specific exercises after surgery for pain incidence and pain intensity up to two years follow-up [19,20]. Comparing a supervised versus non-supervised program [27], differences in neither pain incidence nor intensity were found [19].

Another Cochrane review and meta-analysis (including two studies) in patients treated for head and neck cancer pain showed significant beneficial effects of a progressive strengthening training program on pain [21]. However, results were not clinically relevant.

In conclusion, there is currently no evidence available that supports the use of specific exercise therapy for relieving pain in cancer patients or cancer survivors. Several reasons for this can be postulated. First, these exercise programs were designed to increase physical impairments, including impaired range of motion and strength, and pain was only considered as a secondary outcome. The latter implies that the available trials were not designed to examine the potential for specific exercises on pain relief (i.e., the trials might have been underpowered to detect clinically important changes in pain; the trials included all cancer patients or cancer survivors, while not all patients suffer from clinically relevant levels of pain, in turn decreasing the ability of a treatment to generate important changes). Moreover, most studies only evaluated pain intensity. Other dimensions of pain, or rather pain-related disability, are outcomes of higher clinical relevance and may reflect true effects of specific exercise interventions. Lastly, the underlying mechanism of the patients' pain complaint was not taken into account when providing the exercise therapy to the patients suffering from cancer or post-cancer pain. Pain during and after cancer treatment can have many origins with different associated indications for exercise therapy. Therefore, prescription guidelines on specific exercises for pain after cancer treatment are not available and it remains to be established which type(s) of exercise therapy (strengthening, mobilizing and stretching exercises) is indicated depending on the predominant pain mechanism at different time points throughout cancer treatment and thereafter.

The most important message from the limited amount of research is that specific exercises are safe. However, evidence on the best type of exercise, the exact modalities and timing is inconclusive [19–21,25].

2.3. Manual Therapy

Within the cancer field, studies of manual therapy address passive joint mobilizations and massage therapy. First, manual passive mobilizations primarily aim at restoring joint range of motion trough alleviating capsular restrictions, distracting (soft) tissues and providing movement and lubrication for normal articular cartilage. Additionally, pain relief may be achieved through the activation of mechanoreceptors and stimulation of fast-conducting fibers [28]. The review of De Groef et al. included one RCT on the effectiveness of passive mobilizations after breast cancer surgery [20] (Table 1, Section 3. Manual Therapy). This study indicated beneficial effects of passive mobilizations during the first week post-surgery on long-term prevalence of locoregional pain. However, this one study shows high risk of bias, so results are inconclusive [29].

Second, research on massage therapy in cancer population on the other hand is overwhelming. Massage can be defined as the manipulation of the soft tissues of the body, performed by the hands, for the purpose of producing effects on the vascular, muscular, and nervous systems [30]. Two most recent systematic reviews of RCTs are discussed here (Table 1, Section 3. Manual Therapy). A Cochrane review on massage, including 19 studies of which 5 reported the effects on pain, showed beneficial effects of massage therapy in only one study [31]. Another review found beneficial effects of massage in 79% of the included studies [32]. However, beneficial effects on pain intensity were very small and of limited clinical relevance as illustrated by the meta-analyses: Standardized Mean Difference (SMD) of −0.20 (95% CI, −0.99 to 0.59) for massage versus no treatment and SMD of −0.55 (95% CI, −1.23 to 0.14) for massage versus an active comparator (including attention, usual care, standard treatment, a reading group comparator, and caring presence) [32]. The review indeed concluded in the evidence synthesis that only weak recommendations can be made for massage therapy and that effects are clinically irrelevant [32]. As suggested by the definition of massage therapy, other effects aimed at with massage therapy may be a reduction in anxiety and stress and an enhancement of personal sense of well-being through the effect on body and mind [32]. However, the studies in both reviews were of very low quality and included a mix of primary, advanced, and metastatic cancers; concluding that there is a lack of clear evidence to support the use of massage for pain relief in people with cancer at this moment [31,32].

2.4. General Exercise Therapy

Exercise can be defined as "any physical activity causing an increase in energy expenditure, and involving a planned or structured movement of the body performed in a systematic manner in terms of frequency, intensity, and duration and is designed to maintain or enhance health-related outcomes" (American College of Sports Medicine). Typically, aerobic and resistance training are considered when discussing general exercise therapy [33,34]. A systematic review of systematic reviews by Stout et al. summarized results of 53 reviews on exercise in cancer populations [35]. They concluded that exercise was beneficial before, during, and after cancer treatment, across all cancer types, and for a wide range of physical outcome parameters. Moreover, exercise was found to be safe during all cancer stages. Several reviews in different cancer populations indeed confirmed the beneficial effect of exercise on quality of life [36–38]. Despite this large amount of studies and clear guidelines, no recommendations for using general exercise therapy for the treatment of pain in cancer populations were extracted.

Frist, Nakano et al. published the most recent meta-analysis limited to RCTs using the European Organization for Research and Treatment of Cancer Quality of Life Questionnaire-C30 (EORTC-QLQ-C30) [39] (Table 1, Section 4. General exercise therapy). They summarized the effect of aerobic and/or general resistance exercises on physical symptoms, including pain, for cancer patients and survivors in any setting. The meta-analysis showed that pain in the intervention group (receiving aerobic and/or resistance exercises) was significantly lower compared to no intervention. However, the effect size was only small (SMD of −0.17 (95%CI, −0.32 to 0.03)) and no differences among the 3 types of exercises interventions could be extracted [39]. Second, two Cochrane reviews of Mishra et al. summarized the effectiveness of exercise interventions on health-related quality of life, including pain, during active cancer treatment [34] and in cancer survivors [33], respectively (Table 1, Section 4. General exercise therapy). During active cancer treatment, no significant effects for pain relief in favor of general exercises were described. In cancer survivors, pooled data of four studies showed beneficial effects of exercise for pain with a small effect size (SMD of −0.29 (95% CI, −0. 55 to −0.04)). Another noteworthy Cochrane review summarized the beneficial effects of general physical activity, including activities as part of occupation, active transportation, household and gardening chores, and recreational activities [40]. Exercise was considered as a subcategory of physical activity. This review showed beneficial effects for a wide range of health-related outcome parameters. For pain however, 9 out of the 63 included trials that reported a pain outcome measurement showed no beneficial effects [40].

These reviews summarized the effectiveness of aerobic and/or resistance exercise therapy as an intervention [33,34,39,40]. The type of exercise therapy and specific modality most efficient for pain relief was not clear. In the general population, exercise is considered very important in pain management because of its possible beneficial effect on central pain (inhibitory) mechanisms, the autonomic nervous system, the immune system (anti-inflammatory effect) and subsequent hypoalgesic effect [41–43]. However, the response to exercise is more variable in chronic musculoskeletal pain populations and may even result in hyperalgesia [41–43]. For cancer populations, even less is known about pain processing during and after exercise therapy, and a possible impaired analgesic response to exercise (therapy) and physical activity. Remarkably, in particular for hormone therapy related arthralgia, which is experienced by up to 50% breast cancer survivors treated with aromatase inhibitors, general exercise therapy holds high value [44–46]. Findings from a high-quality randomized controlled trial indicated that 150 minutes per week of aerobic exercise and supervised strength training twice per week can lead to clinically relevant improvements in pain [46].

In conclusion, general exercise therapy is safe and well tolerated, both during and after cancer treatment. However, only limited evidence is available on the beneficial effects for pain relief during and after cancer treatment in general. The exact exercise modalities to ensure this pain relief are not described [33,34,39]. However, a combination of aerobic training and strengthening exercises is recommended for pain relief in patients with hormone therapy related arthralgia [46].

2.5. Mind-Body Exercise Therapy

Mind-body exercises intend to enhance the mind's capacity to positively affect bodily functions and symptoms, including pain, by combining exercises with mental focus [47]. They have gained interest in many fields of rehabilitation, including cancer.

First, pilates has found its way into many rehabilitation practices. One review showed that pilates was statistically more effective than the interventions in the control groups for reducing pain among women with breast cancer, showing a moderate effect (SMD of −0.48 (95%CI, −0.88 to −0.07)) [48] (Table 1, Section 5. Mind-body therapy). However, only women with breast cancer were included. Yoga is becoming very popular in cancer rehabilitation as well, as reflected by the 29 RCTs summarized in the review of Danhauer et al. [49] (Table 1, Section 5. Mind-body therapy). They reported improvements in general quality of life, fatigue, and perceived stress. Pain was investigated only in a very small number of studies showing inconclusive results [49]. Another popular type of mind-body exercises is Tai Chi Chuan. However, for pain in breast cancer survivors, pooled results of three RCTs could not demonstrate beneficial effects (SMD of 0.11 (95%CI, −0.41 to 0.18)) [50] (Table 1, Section 5. Mind-body therapy).

The positive effect of mind-body therapies, in particular yoga in e.g., breast cancer patients, seems more obvious for psychological wellbeing, including stress, anxiety and depression [47,49]. Similarly, for massage therapy, through a reduction in anxiety and stress and enhancement of personal sense of well-being a relief in physical symptoms, including pain, may be achieved [32,47].

Mind-body exercise therapy are often considered as complementary therapeutic interventions and may play an important role in cancer rehabilitation. While pilates seems to have clinically important pain-relieving effects in women with breast cancer, evidence for yoga as a pain-relieving intervention in cancer populations is inconclusive.

3. Promising Directions for Clinical Practice

Both clinicians and researchers highlight and emphasize the tremendous need of a systematic follow-up of side-effects related to cancer and its treatment(s), including pain, in order to improve quality of life of cancer survivors. Indeed, besides treatment of cancer itself and follow-up of relapses, a systematic prospective care pathway is minimally required for each cancer patient [51–55]. The key elements of such a care model are (1) a proactive approach to regularly examine and question patients on pain and pain-related disability; (2) providing ongoing assessment during all stages of cancer treatment (often in absence of problems) and (3) uniform efforts to enable early interventions for pain management, including mono- and complex multidisciplinary interventions, both in inpatient and outpatient settings [51–55].

A first step in improving clinical practice through clinical care pathways would be early detection and proper diagnosis of pain in cancer. A clear diagnosis of a patient's pain complaint is a critical step in clinical decision-making. Over the past decades, knowledge on the origin of pain during and after cancer treatment has increased [5,7]. From a tumor-related and a treatment-related classification of pain, there was a major shift to a mechanism-based classification of cancer pain [56,57]. During adjuvant treatment of a primary cancer, the tumour is removed, so it is expected that pain is no more related to cancer, per se. In the early stage of cancer treatment, nociceptive and/or neuropathic pain caused by surgery, radiotherapy and/or chemotherapy is present in most cases [24,58]. At this stage, pain is related to tissue damage and if adequately managed, can be considered as a short-term side effect. In a later stage, when these local effects of the different cancer treatment modalities should have been healed, the initial causes of pain may be overshadowed by sensitization of the central nervous system in a subgroup of cancer survivors [58–60]. In this case, pain is no longer related to tissue damage and can be explained by enhanced processing of sensory input (sensitization) within the peripheral and/or central nervous system and by altered pain modulation, leading to so called central sensitization pain or nociplastic pain [61]. Specifically for the cancer population, it is important to recognize that local tissue damage or peripheral mechanisms can continue to contribute to their pain complaint for a long time after completion of acute treatment, together with other sustaining psychosocial factors e.g., postmastectomy pain syndrome and chemotherapy-induced peripheral neuropathy [5] or related to ongoing treatment modalities for several years such as arthralgia related to hormonal therapy [62]. For effective pain management, identification of the predominant pain mechanism is warranted. Clinical guidelines for the identification of the predominant pain mechanism in cancer survivors are available, however not validated [58].

Secondly, through the clinical care pathway, referral for adequate pain management is facilitated [51]. As summarized above, a tremendous amount of research is available on rehabilitation modalities for a wide range of physical symptoms during and after cancer treatment. Despite its high prevalence rates and high disabling impact, in many studies "pain" was not used as outcome measure. Too often pain is considered as "being part of" cancer survivorship, resulting in minimal effort to detect pain and referral for adequate treatment. Although research is limited, the reviews described above point towards promising pain-relieving effects of rehabilitation modalities for pain management during and after cancer treatment. However, effect sizes are only small to moderate and research is limited to mostly breast cancer populations. Based on this, the following modalities can be carefully recommended in general. Firstly, both at the start and during a rehabilitation program, the added value of an educational intervention based on modern pain (neuro)science—including a biopsychosocial explanation of pain—should be considered to remove barriers for rehabilitation and promote adequate pain behavior and cognitions [10]. In particular, in patients with maladaptive pain beliefs and behavior, an educational intervention is warranted to explain pain and how different therapy modalities can potentially influence this. Correct interpretation of symptoms during treatment will facilitate shared decision-making and further therapy adherence. Secondly, currently no evidence supports the pain-relieving effect of specific exercises and mobilizations during and after cancer treatment. Whether these rehabilitation modalities have a role in particular for acute nociceptive and neuropathic pain related to joint and muscle dysfunctions at the affected region should be further investigated [20–22,24]. Thirdly, general exercise therapy may result in pain relief. However, more research is needed on the modalities (type, frequency, intensity and duration) to increase effect sizes and ensure reduction in pain and/or pain-related disability and avoid pain flares after exercise [33,34,39]. Indeed, in a subgroup of cancer survivors with predominant nociplastic pain, endogenous pain modulation may be impaired and alter the response to both specific and general exercise therapy. However, it is important to note and explain that rehabilitation interventions, including exercise therapy, are still safe both during and after cancer treatment. In particular, for cancer survivors with hormone therapy related arthralgia, general exercise therapy is recommended [46]. At last, mind-body interventions, including general exercises such as yoga and pilates, might have a complementary role. However, besides the pain-relieving effects of pilates in women with breast cancer, study results are inconclusive. It has been argued that the pain-relieving effect occurs through a reduction in anxiety and stress and enhancement of personal sense of well-being [32]. The evidence on the influence of various psychosocial and emotional factors on the (persistence of) pain has increased past decades [9,63]. Especially in cancer populations, the cancer diagnosis, treatment but also the fear of cancer reoccurrence can induce stress, depression and anxiety among others [64]. As proposed for the educational interventions, a biopsychosocial explanation of pain is necessary. Therefore, mind-body therapies fit within this approach and may be valuable modalities to address pain and its psychosocial sustaining factors. The remark has to be made to what extent these mind-body therapies belong to the rehabilitation domain. Other interventions, e.g., mindfulness, mediation, acupuncture, ... are often considered as complementary mind-body interventions as well. However, since the element of bodily movement in these interventions is not apparent, they are beyond the scope of this paper. Given the multiple cancer treatment modalities, pain is often not the only side effect during and after cancer treatment. When initiating rehabilitation modalities for pain, in particular exercise therapy, other comorbidities should be taken into account when developing a treatment plan. Fatigue is often associated with pain and vice versa, and may hamper regular performance of general exercise. Several cancer treatments have a toxic effect on the cardiovascular system among others, leading to decreased exercise tolerance. When establishing an exercise program, this has to be taken into account [65].

Pain management during and after cancer treatment is not restricted to pharmacological therapy and rehabilitation interventions. Other disciplines should be part of the rehabilitation team and multidisciplinary treatment should be provided if necessary. Increased stress, anxiety and sleep disturbances have been described to interfere with pain and/or pain-related disability and therefore should be addressed if necessary [9,66]. Social workers may be important to address problems with participation in society [67]. Other lifestyle interventions, including nutrition, smoking and excess alcohol consumption, have been proposed to improve cancer survivorship and quality of life and therefore their role in pain relief should be considered as well [68].

Additionally, pioneering studies are emerging on the use of eHealth in the cancer population. Applications for symptom monitoring, including cancer pain, are already available and show promising results [17,69]. These applications may also increase the accessibility to educational resources and self-management strategies [69]. A recent review confirmed that applications supporting self-management improve pain and fatigue outcomes in cancer survivors [70]. In line with this, telecoaching interventions may be of value to increase adherence to specific exercise programs [71] and/or physical activity in general in cancer patients [72]. These technological highlights keep manifesting, but researchers warn that high-quality studies are currently still ongoing and these interventions should be developed and tested properly before being recommended [69].

4. Promising Directions for Research

Current state-of-the art rehabilitation for pain during and after cancer treatment is limited. When positive pain-relieving effects for rehabilitation interventions are found, effect sizes are most often small to moderate. Different explanations can be given for this. In clinical practice different interventions are combined, which is an important strength of rehabilitation for pain, but unfortunately hard to translate into research. Additionally, pain relief from a comparative intervention, standard intervention or even no intervention may occur and result in small effect sizes as well. Typically, responders and non-responders can be identified in clinical trials, especially when the intervention is not tailored to e.g., the predominant pain mechanism. This may result in overall small effect sizes at group level. Therefore, a balance between a pragmatic approach and highly standardized conditions is needed in research. In the following paragraph, items that should be considered in further research are discussed.

Firstly, both from a clinical and scientific perspective, it is highly important to correctly diagnose pain and identify the predominant pain mechanism of a patient's pain complaint. Clinical guidelines for this purpose are described, however not validated [58,73]. Several studies did not clearly describe whether pain was related to cancer itself or whether it was a side effect of the different treatment modalities. Pain can be a symptom of cancer. However, pain due to cancer often means it has already metastasized. For this paper, the focus was limited to cancer patients and survivors with a primary cancer diagnosis and pain during and/or after active cancer treatment, so it is expected that pain is no more related to the cancer itself. In future studies, this should be specified when diagnosing pain in cancer patients and survivors. Associated with this, due to the prolonged side effects of certain treatment modalities, e.g., radiotherapy and hormone therapy, it is in many cases difficult to distinguish whether a patient's pain complaint is still related to local tissue damage (nociceptive and/or neuropathic pain) or rather to altered pain processing in nociplastic pain without dominant peripheral input. Studies on the effectiveness of rehabilitation modalities tailored to the predominant pain mechanism might result in larger effect sizes [58,74].

Secondly, besides a proper diagnosis of a patient's pain complaint in order to tailor rehabilitation modalities, a comprehensive pain assessment is warranted. The Initiative on Methods, Measurement, and Pain Assessment in Clinical Trials (IMMPACT) recommends six core outcome domains that should be considered when designing clinical trials on pain management. These domains include: (1) different dimensions of pain; (2) physical functioning; (3) emotional functioning; (4) participant ratings of improvement and satisfaction with treatment; (5) symptoms and adverse events; and (6) participant disposition [75]. Indeed, in order to unravel the concept of pain, outcomes should not be limited to the impairment itself, but also include pain-related functioning. Moreover, it is argued that rehabilitation modalities and other interventions should focus on improvement of daily functioning and pain-related disability, which will ultimately lead to reductions in patient's pain intensity (or at least the debilitating nature of pain). On the other hand, generic outcome measures such as general quality of life may lack responsiveness to detect (more subtle) changes in pain [16,75]. Additionally, various psychosocial factors play an essential part in the pain experience and the degree to which someone perceives their pain as disabling. The effect of rehabilitation interventions on psychosocial outcomes and possible moderating and mediating role of these factors in response to treatment for pain during and after cancer treatment should be explored in future studies. At last, to explore the duration of response and sustainability of rehabilitation interventions for pain relief, an adequate follow-up period should be provided.

Thirdly, besides the high burden for the patient in the first place, the socio-economic impact of pain during and after cancer treatment should be investigated. The number of people with long-term sick leave or reduced working hours after cancer continues to rise. Pain, low (perceived) physical functioning and low self-efficacy are factors associated with delayed return to work [76,77]. Additionally, rehabilitation entails a substantial financial cost for the health care system. Increasing the effectiveness of rehabilitation for pain may decrease the number of rehabilitation and costs associated with other more expensive pain management strategies. Therefore, proper health- and socio-economic analyses are needed to change practice.

Fourthly, technological developments in rehabilitation should not be ignored, as they may lead to innovative treatment avenues for cancer survivors as well. For example, preliminary study results show that effects of virtual and augmented reality for rehabilitation of phantom limb pain [78], (neuropathic) pain related to multiple sclerosis [79] and spinal cord injury [80] and pain in children [81] are promising. In cancer patients, it may be valuable to distract patients from pain, to increase motivation and participation with a better response to treatment as a result. This may be an interesting research topic in the future.

At last, an overwhelming amount of evidence is available in certain cancer populations, e.g., breast cancer. More trials in other cancer populations, such as colon and gynecological cancers are needed before any general recommendations can be given. Additionally, rehabilitation for pain in advanced cancers, palliative settings and populations with social disparities may warrant a different approach and thus needs further investigation.

5. Conclusions

While literature on the beneficial effects of rehabilitation modalities for symptoms such as fatigue, exercise tolerance and general quality of life is overwhelming, evidence for pain relief during and after cancer treatment is rather scarce. In conclusion, best evidence suggests that general exercise therapy has small pain-relieving effects. Evidence for mind-body exercise therapy in breast cancer is promising given the moderate effect size. At this moment, there is a lack of high-quality evidence to support the use of specific exercises and manual therapy at the affected region for pain relief during and after cancer treatment. No clinically relevant results were found for educational interventions restricted to a biomedical approach of pain. To increase available evidence, these rehabilitation modalities should be applied according to and within a multidisciplinary biopsychosocial pain management approach. Larger, well-designed clinical trials tailored to the origin of pain and with proper evaluation including pain-related functioning and other outcomes related the patient's pain experience are needed.

6. Clinical Implications

- Rehabilitation modalities, including manual therapy, specific and general exercise therapy, are safe and well tolerated during and after cancer.
- Evidence for pain relief is scarce but promising.
- Despite the unclarity of essential components of education to improve pain, its role in rehabilitation during and after cancer may be crucial for pain relief.
- Mind-body interventions including e.g., pilates may be complementary.

7. Research Agenda

- Distinct prescription guidelines for specific and general exercise therapy according to the FITT principles should be explored.
- Validated guidelines for the accurate identification of the predominant pain mechanism in cancer are warranted.
- The effectiveness of rehabilitation tailored to the predominant pain mechanism should be investigated.

Author Contributions: Conceptualization, A.D.G., M.M. and J.N.; Literature search and data extraction, A.D.G., F.P., L.D. and E.V.d.G.; Writing, Original Draft Preparation, A.D.G., F.P., L.D and E.V.d.G.; Writing, Review & Editing, J.N. and M.M.; Supervision, J.N. and M.M.

Funding: This work is partially funded by the Berekuyl Academy Chair, funded by the European College for Lymphatic Therapy, the Netherlands, and awarded to Jo Nijs, Vrije Universiteit Brussel, Belgium.

Conflicts of Interest: The authors declare no conflict of interest.

References

1. Torre, L.A.; Bray, F.; Siegel, R.L.; Ferlay, J.; Lortet-Tieulent, J.; Jemal, A. Global cancer statistics, 2012. *CA Cancer J. Clin.* **2015**, *65*, 87–108. [CrossRef] [PubMed]
2. Ferlay, J.; Colombet, M.; Soerjomataram, I.; Dyba, T.; Randi, G.; Bettio, M.; Gavin, A.; Visser, O.; Bray, F. Cancer incidence and mortality patterns in Europe: Estimates for 40 countries and 25 major cancers in 2018. *Eur. J. Cancer* **2018**, *103*, 356–387. [CrossRef] [PubMed]

3. Van den Beuken-van Everdingen, M.H.; Hochstenbach, L.M.; Joosten, E.A.; Tjan-Heijnen, V.C.; Janssen, D.J. Update on Prevalence of Pain in Patients With Cancer: Systematic Review and Meta-Analysis. *J. Pain Symptom Manag.* **2016**, *51*, 1070–1090.e1079. [CrossRef] [PubMed]
4. Pachman, D.R.; Barton, D.L.; Swetz, K.M.; Loprinzi, C.L. Troublesome symptoms in cancer survivors: Fatigue, insomnia, neuropathy, and pain. *J. Clin. Oncol.* **2012**, *30*, 3687–3696. [CrossRef] [PubMed]
5. Glare, P.A.; Davies, P.S.; Finlay, E.; Gulati, A.; Lemanne, D.; Moryl, N.; Oeffinger, K.C.; Paice, J.A.; Stubblefield, M.D.; Syrjala, K.L. Pain in cancer survivors. *J. Clin. Oncol.* **2014**, *32*, 1739–1747. [CrossRef] [PubMed]
6. Bennett, M.I.; Kaasa, S.; Barke, A.; Korwisi, B.; Rief, W.; Treede, R.D. The IASP classification of chronic pain for ICD-11: Chronic cancer-related pain. *Pain* **2019**, *160*, 38–44. [CrossRef] [PubMed]
7. Egan, M.Y.; McEwen, S.; Sikora, L.; Chasen, M.; Fitch, M.; Eldred, S. Rehabilitation following cancer treatment. *Disabil. Rehabil.* **2013**, *35*, 2245–2258. [CrossRef]
8. Cheville, A.L.; Mustian, K.; Winters-Stone, K.; Zucker, D.S.; Gamble, G.L.; Alfano, C.M. Cancer Rehabilitation: An Overview of Current Need, Delivery Models, and Levels of Care. *Phys. Med. Rehabil. Clin. N. Am.* **2017**, *28*, 1–17. [CrossRef]
9. Nijs, J.; Leysen, L.; Pas, R.; Adriaenssens, N.; Meeus, M.; Hoelen, W.; Ickmans, K.; Moloney, N. Treatment of pain following cancer: Applying neuro-immunology in rehabilitation practice. *Disabil. Rehabil.* **2016**. [CrossRef]
10. Nijs, J.; Wijma, A.J.; Leysen, L.; Pas, R.; Willaert, W.; Hoelen, W.; Ickmans, K.; Wilgen, C.P.V. Explaining pain following cancer: A practical guide for clinicians. *Braz. J. Phys. Ther.* **2018**. [CrossRef]
11. Koongstvedt, P. *The Managed Health Care Handbook*; Aspen Publishers: Gaithersburg, MD, USA, 2001.
12. Louw, A.; Zimney, K.; Puentedura, E.J.; Diener, I. The efficacy of pain neuroscience education on musculoskeletal pain: A systematic review of the literature. *Physiother. Theory Pract.* **2016**, *32*, 332–355. [CrossRef] [PubMed]
13. Lee, Y.J.; Hyun, M.K.; Jung, Y.J.; Kang, M.J.; Keam, B.; Go, S.J. Effectiveness of education interventions for the management of cancer pain: A systematic review. *Asian Pac. J. Cancer Prev.* **2014**, *15*, 4787–4793. [CrossRef] [PubMed]
14. Bennett, M.I.; Bagnall, A.M.; Jose Closs, S. How effective are patient-based educational interventions in the management of cancer pain? Systematic review and meta-analysis. *Pain* **2009**, *143*, 192–199. [CrossRef] [PubMed]
15. Koller, A.; Miaskowski, C.; De Geest, S.; Opitz, O.; Spichiger, E. A systematic evaluation of content, structure, and efficacy of interventions to improve patients' self-management of cancer pain. *J. Pain Symptom Manag.* **2012**, *44*, 264–284. [CrossRef] [PubMed]
16. Prevost, V.; Delorme, C.; Grach, M.C.; Chvetzoff, G.; Hureau, M. Therapeutic Education in Improving Cancer Pain Management: A Synthesis of Available Studies. *Am. J. Hosp. Palliat. Care* **2016**, *33*, 599–612. [CrossRef] [PubMed]
17. Oldenmenger, W.H.; Geerling, J.I.; Mostovaya, I.; Vissers, K.C.P.; de Graeff, A.; Reyners, A.K.L.; van der Linden, Y.M. A systematic review of the effectiveness of patient-based educational interventions to improve cancer-related pain. *Cancer Treat. Rev.* **2018**, *63*, 96–103. [CrossRef] [PubMed]
18. Ling, C.C.; Lui, L.Y.; So, W.K. Do educational interventions improve cancer patients' quality of life and reduce pain intensity? Quantitative systematic review. *J. Adv. Nurs.* **2012**, *68*, 511–520. [CrossRef] [PubMed]
19. McNeely, M.L.; Campbell, K.; Ospina, M.; Rowe, B.H.; Dabbs, K.; Klassen, T.P.; Mackey, J.; Courneya, K. Exercise interventions for upper-limb dysfunction due to breast cancer treatment. *Cochrane Database Syst. Rev.* **2010**. [CrossRef]
20. De Groef, A.; Van Kampen, M.; Dieltjens, E.; Christiaens, M.R.; Neven, P.; Geraerts, I.; Devoogdt, N. Effectiveness of postoperative physical therapy for upper-limb impairments after breast cancer treatment: A systematic review. *Arch. Phys. Med. Rehabil.* **2015**, *96*, 1140–1153. [CrossRef]
21. Carvalho, A.P.; Vital, F.M.; Soares, B.G. Exercise interventions for shoulder dysfunction in patients treated for head and neck cancer. *Cochrane Database Syst. Rev.* **2012**. [CrossRef]
22. Sierla, R.; Mun Lee, T.S.; Black, D.; Kilbreath, S.L. Lymphedema following breast cancer: Regions affected, severity of symptoms, and benefits of treatment from the patients' perspective. *Clin. J. Oncol. Nurs.* **2013**, *17*, 325–331. [CrossRef] [PubMed]

23. Andersen, L.L.; Kjaer, M.; Sogaard, K.; Hansen, L.; Kryger, A.I.; Sjogaard, G. Effect of two contrasting types of physical exercise on chronic neck muscle pain. *Arthritis Rheum.* **2008**, *59*, 84–91. [CrossRef] [PubMed]
24. Stubblefield, M.D.; Keole, N. Upper Body Pain and Functional Disorders in Patients With Breast Cancer. *PM & R* **2013**, *6*, 170–183. [CrossRef]
25. Tatham, B.; Smith, J.; Cheifetz, O.; Gillespie, J.; Snowden, K.; Temesy, J.; Vandenberk, L. The efficacy of exercise therapy in reducing shoulder pain related to breast cancer: A systematic review. *Physiother. Can.* **2013**, *65*, 321–330. [CrossRef] [PubMed]
26. Beurskens, C.H.; van Uden, C.J.; Strobbe, L.J.; Oostendorp, R.A.; Wobbes, T. The efficacy of physiotherapy upon shoulder function following axillary dissection in breast cancer, a randomized controlled study. *BMC Cancer* **2007**, *7*, 166. [CrossRef] [PubMed]
27. Hwang, J.H.; Chang, H.J.; Shim, Y.H.; Park, W.H.; Park, W.; Huh, S.J.; Yang, J.H. Effects of supervised exercise therapy in patients receiving radiotherapy for breast cancer. *Yonsei Med. J.* **2008**, *49*, 443–450. [CrossRef]
28. Egmond, D.L.; Mink, A.J.F.; Vorselaars, B.V.; Schuitemaker, R. *Extermiteiten, Manuele Therapie in Enge en Ruime Zin*; Bohn Stafleu van Loghum: Houten, The Netherlands, 2014.
29. Le Vu, B.; Dumortier, A.; Guillaume, M.V.; Mouriesse, H.; Barreau-Pouhaer, L. Efficacy of massage and mobilization of the upper limb after surgical treatment of breast cancer. *Bull. Du Cancer* **1997**, *84*, 957–961.
30. Fellowes, D.; Barnes, K.; Wilkinson, S. Aromatherapy and massage for symptom relief in patients with cancer. *Cochrane Database Syst. Rev.* **2004**. [CrossRef]
31. Shin, E.S.; Seo, K.H.; Lee, S.H.; Jang, J.E.; Jung, Y.M.; Kim, M.J.; Yeon, J.Y. Massage with or without aromatherapy for symptom relief in people with cancer. *Cochrane Database Syst. Rev.* **2016**. [CrossRef]
32. Boyd, C.; Crawford, C.; Paat, C.F.; Price, A.; Xenakis, L.; Zhang, W.; Evidence for Massage Therapy Working Group. The Impact of Massage Therapy on Function in Pain Populations—A Systematic Review and Meta-Analysis of Randomized Controlled Trials: Part II, Cancer Pain Populations. *Pain Med.* **2016**, *17*, 1553–1568. [CrossRef]
33. Mishra, S.I.; Scherer, R.W.; Geigle, P.M.; Berlanstein, D.R.; Topaloglu, O.; Gotay, C.C.; Snyder, C. Exercise interventions on health-related quality of life for cancer survivors. *Cochrane Database Syst. Rev.* **2012**, *8*. [CrossRef] [PubMed]
34. Mishra, S.I.; Scherer, R.W.; Snyder, C.; Geigle, P.M.; Berlanstein, D.R.; Topaloglu, O. Exercise interventions on health-related quality of life for people with cancer during active treatment. *Cochrane Database Syst. Rev.* **2012**. [CrossRef]
35. Stout, N.L.; Baima, J.; Swisher, A.K.; Winters-Stone, K.M.; Welsh, J. A Systematic Review of Exercise Systematic Reviews in the Cancer Literature (2005–2017). *PM & R* **2017**, *9*, S347–S384. [CrossRef]
36. Bourke, L.; Boorjian, S.A.; Briganti, A.; Klotz, L.; Mucci, L.; Resnick, M.J.; Rosario, D.J.; Skolarus, T.A.; Penson, D.F. Survivorship and improving quality of life in men with prostate cancer. *Eur. Urol.* **2015**, *68*, 374–383. [CrossRef] [PubMed]
37. Zeng, Y.; Huang, M.; Cheng, A.S.; Zhou, Y.; So, W.K. Meta-analysis of the effects of exercise intervention on quality of life in breast cancer survivors. *Breast Cancer* **2014**. [CrossRef] [PubMed]
38. Furmaniak, A.C.; Menig, M.; Markes, M.H. Exercise for women receiving adjuvant therapy for breast cancer. *Cochrane Database Syst. Rev.* **2016**. [CrossRef]
39. Nakano, J.; Hashizume, K.; Fukushima, T.; Ueno, K.; Matsuura, E.; Ikio, Y.; Ishii, S.; Morishita, S.; Tanaka, K.; Kusuba, Y. Effects of Aerobic and Resistance Exercises on Physical Symptoms in Cancer Patients: A Meta-analysis. *Integr. Cancer Ther.* **2018**, *17*, 1048–1058. [CrossRef]
40. Lahart, I.M.; Metsios, G.S.; Nevill, A.M.; Carmichael, A.R. Physical activity for women with breast cancer after adjuvant therapy. *Cochrane Database Syst. Rev.* **2018**. [CrossRef]
41. Lima, L.V.; Abner, T.S.; Sluka, K.A. Does exercise increase or decrease pain? Central mechanisms underlying these two phenomena. *J. Physiol.* **2017**. [CrossRef]
42. Naugle, K.M.; Fillingim, R.B.; Riley, J.L., III. A meta-analytic review of the hypoalgesic effects of exercise. *J. Pain* **2012**, *13*, 1139–1150. [CrossRef]
43. Rice, D.; Nijs, J.; Kosek, E.; Wideman, T.; Hasenbring, M.I.; Koltyn, K.; Graven-Nielsen, T.; Polli, A. Exercise induced hypoalgesia in pain-free and chronic pain populations: State of the art and future directions. *J. Pain* **2019**. [CrossRef] [PubMed]
44. Nahm, N.; Mee, S.; Marx, G. Efficacy of management strategies for aromatase inhibitor-induced arthralgia in breast cancer patients: A systematic review. *Asian Pac. J. Clin. Oncol.* **2018**. [CrossRef] [PubMed]

45. Yang, G.S.; Kim, H.J.; Griffith, K.A.; Zhu, S.; Dorsey, S.G.; Renn, C.L. Interventions for the Treatment of Aromatase Inhibitor-Associated Arthralgia in Breast Cancer Survivors: A Systematic Review and Meta-analysis. *Cancer Nurs.* **2017**, *40*, E26–E41. [CrossRef] [PubMed]
46. Irwin, M.L.; Cartmel, B.; Gross, C.P.; Ercolano, E.; Li, F.; Yao, X.; Fiellin, M.; Capozza, S.; Rothbard, M.; Zhou, Y.; et al. Randomized exercise trial of aromatase inhibitor-induced arthralgia in breast cancer survivors. *J. Clin. Oncol.* **2015**, *33*, 1104–1111. [CrossRef] [PubMed]
47. Husebø, A.M.L.; Husebø, T.L. Quality of Life and Breast Cancer: How Can Mind–Body Exercise Therapies Help? An Overview Study. *Sports* **2017**, *5*, 79. [CrossRef] [PubMed]
48. Pinto-Carral, A.; Molina, A.J.; de Pedro, A.; Ayan, C. Pilates for women with breast cancer: A systematic review and meta-analysis. *Complementary Ther. Med.* **2018**, *41*, 130–140. [CrossRef] [PubMed]
49. Danhauer, S.C.; Addington, E.L.; Cohen, L.; Sohl, S.J.; Van Puymbroeck, M.; Albinati, N.K.; Culos-Reed, S.N. Yoga for symptom management in oncology: A review of the evidence base and future directions for research. *Cancer* **2019**. [CrossRef] [PubMed]
50. Pan, Y.; Yang, K.; Shi, X.; Liang, H.; Zhang, F.; Lv, Q. Tai chi chuan exercise for patients with breast cancer: A systematic review and meta-analysis. *Evid. Based Complementary Altern. Med.* **2015**, *2015*, 535237. [CrossRef]
51. Stout, N.L.; Binkley, J.M.; Schmitz, K.H.; Andrews, K.; Hayes, S.C.; Campbell, K.L.; McNeely, M.L.; Soballe, P.W.; Berger, A.M.; Cheville, A.L.; et al. A prospective surveillance model for rehabilitation for women with breast cancer. *Cancer* **2012**, *118*, 2191–2200. [CrossRef]
52. Holland, J.C.; Reznik, I. Pathways for psychosocial care of cancer survivors. *Cancer* **2005**, *104*, 2624–2637. [CrossRef]
53. Coccia, P.F.; Pappo, A.S.; Beaupin, L.; Borges, V.F.; Borinstein, S.C.; Chugh, R.; Dinner, S.; Folbrecht, J.; Frazier, A.L.; Goldsby, R.; et al. Adolescent and Young Adult Oncology, Version 2.2018, NCCN Clinical Practice Guidelines in Oncology. *J. Natl. Compr. Cancer Netw.* **2018**, *16*, 66–97. [CrossRef] [PubMed]
54. Kvale, E.; Urba, S.G. NCCN guidelines for survivorship expanded to address two common conditions. *J. Natl. Compr. Cancer Netw.* **2014**, *12*, 825–827. [CrossRef]
55. Alfano, C.M.; Kent, E.E.; Padgett, L.S.; Grimes, M.; de Moor, J.S. Making Cancer Rehabilitation Services Work for Cancer Patients: Recommendations for Research and Practice to Improve Employment Outcomes. *PM & R* **2017**, *9*, S398–S406. [CrossRef]
56. Smart, K.M.; Blake, C.; Staines, A.; Doody, C. The Discriminative validity of "nociceptive," "peripheral neuropathic," and "central sensitization" as mechanisms-based classifications of musculoskeletal pain. *Clin. J. Pain* **2011**, *27*, 655–663. [CrossRef] [PubMed]
57. Chimenti, R.L.; Frey-Law, L.A.; Sluka, K.A. A Mechanism-Based Approach to Physical Therapist Management of Pain. *Phys. Ther.* **2018**, *98*, 302–314. [CrossRef] [PubMed]
58. Nijs, J.; Leysen, L.; Adriaenssens, N.; Aguilar Ferrandiz, M.E.; Devoogdt, N.; Tassenoy, A.; Ickmans, K.; Goubert, D.; van Wilgen, C.P.; Wijma, A.J.; et al. Pain following cancer treatment: Guidelines for the clinical classification of predominant neuropathic, nociceptive and central sensitization pain. *Acta Oncol.* **2016**, *55*, 659–663. [CrossRef] [PubMed]
59. Fernandez-Lao, C.; Cantarero-Villanueva, I.; Fernandez-de-las-Penas, C.; Del-Moral-Avila, R.; Menjon-Beltran, S.; Arroyo-Morales, M. Widespread mechanical pain hypersensitivity as a sign of central sensitization after breast cancer surgery: Comparison between mastectomy and lumpectomy. *Pain Med.* **2011**, *12*, 72–78. [CrossRef]
60. Andrykowski, M.A.; Curran, S.L.; Carpenter, J.S.; Studts, J.L.; Cunningham, L.; McGrath, P.C.; Sloan, D.A.; Kenady, D.E. Rheumatoid symptoms following breast cancer treatment: A controlled comparison. *J. Pain Symptom Manag.* **1999**, *18*, 85–94. [CrossRef]
61. Kosek, E.; Cohen, M.; Baron, R.; Gebhart, G.F.; Mico, J.A.; Rice, A.S.; Rief, W.; Sluka, A.K. Do we need a third mechanistic descriptor for chronic pain states? *Pain* **2016**, *157*, 1382–1386. [CrossRef]
62. Niravath, P. Aromatase inhibitor-induced arthralgia: A review. *Ann. Oncol.* **2013**, *24*, 1443–1449. [CrossRef]
63. Edwards, R.R.; Dworkin, R.H.; Sullivan, M.D.; Turk, D.C.; Wasan, A.D. The Role of Psychosocial Processes in the Development and Maintenance of Chronic Pain. *J. Pain* **2016**, *17*, T70–T92. [CrossRef] [PubMed]
64. Heathcote, L.C.; Eccleston, C. Pain and cancer survival: A cognitive-affective model of symptom appraisal and the uncertain threat of disease recurrence. *Pain* **2017**, *158*, 1187–1191. [CrossRef] [PubMed]
65. Jones, L.W.; Eves, N.D.; Haykowsky, M.; Freedland, S.J.; Mackey, J.R. Exercise intolerance in cancer and the role of exercise therapy to reverse dysfunction. *Lancet Oncol.* **2009**, *10*, 598–605. [CrossRef]

66. Ciuca, A.; Baban, A. Psychological factors and psychosocial interventions for cancer related pain. *Rom. J. Intern. Med.* **2017**, *55*, 63–68. [CrossRef] [PubMed]
67. Kiasuwa Mbengi, R.; Otter, R.; Mortelmans, K.; Arbyn, M.; Van Oyen, H.; Bouland, C.; de Brouwer, C. Barriers and opportunities for return-to-work of cancer survivors: Time for action—rapid review and expert consultation. *Syst. Rev.* **2016**, *5*, 35. [CrossRef]
68. Rock, C.L.; Doyle, C.; Demark-Wahnefried, W.; Meyerhardt, J.; Courneya, K.S.; Schwartz, A.L.; Bandera, E.V.; Hamilton, K.K.; Grant, B.; McCullough, M.; et al. Nutrition and physical activity guidelines for cancer survivors. *CA Cancer J. Clin.* **2012**, *62*, 243–274. [CrossRef]
69. Davis, S.W.; Oakley-Girvan, I. Achieving value in mobile health applications for cancer survivors. *J. Cancer Surviv.* **2017**, *11*, 498–504. [CrossRef]
70. Hernandez Silva, E.; Lawler, S.; Langbecker, D. The effectiveness of mHealth for self-management in improving pain, psychological distress, fatigue, and sleep in cancer survivors: A systematic review. *J. Cancer Surviv.* **2019**, *13*, 97–107. [CrossRef]
71. Harder, H.; Holroyd, P.; Burkinshaw, L.; Watten, P.; Zammit, C.; Harris, P.R.; Good, A.; Jenkins, V. A user-centred approach to developing bWell, a mobile app for arm and shoulder exercises after breast cancer treatment. *J. Cancer Surviv.* **2017**, *11*, 732–742. [CrossRef]
72. Kuijpers, W.; Groen, W.G.; Aaronson, N.K.; van Harten, W.H. A systematic review of web-based interventions for patient empowerment and physical activity in chronic diseases: Relevance for cancer survivors. *J. Med. Internet Res.* **2013**, *15*, e37. [CrossRef]
73. Leysen, L.; Adriaenssens, N.; Nijs, J.; Pas, R.; Bilterys, T.; Vermeir, S.; Lahousse, A.; Beckwee, D. Chronic pain in breast cancer survivors: Nociceptive, neuropathic or central sensitization pain? *Pain Pract.* **2018**. [CrossRef] [PubMed]
74. Kumar, S.P.; Prasad, K.; Kumar, V.K.; Shenoy, K.; Sisodia, V. Mechanism-based Classification and Physical Therapy Management of Persons with Cancer Pain: A Prospective Case Series. *Indian J. Palliat. Care* **2013**, *19*, 27–33. [CrossRef] [PubMed]
75. Dworkin, R.H.; Turk, D.C.; Farrar, J.T.; Haythornthwaite, J.A.; Jensen, M.P.; Katz, N.P.; Kerns, R.D.; Stucki, G.; Allen, R.R.; Bellamy, N.; et al. Core outcome measures for chronic pain clinical trials: IMMPACT recommendations. *Pain* **2005**, *113*, 9–19. [CrossRef] [PubMed]
76. Sun, Y.; Shigaki, C.L.; Armer, J.M. Return to work among breast cancer survivors: A literature review. *Support. Care Cancer* **2017**, *25*, 709–718. [CrossRef] [PubMed]
77. Mehnert, A. Employment and work-related issues in cancer survivors. *Crit. Rev. Oncol. Hematol.* **2011**, *77*, 109–130. [CrossRef] [PubMed]
78. Dunn, J.; Yeo, E.; Moghaddampour, P.; Chau, B.; Humbert, S. Virtual and augmented reality in the treatment of phantom limb pain: A literature review. *NeuroRehabilitation* **2017**, *40*, 595–601. [CrossRef] [PubMed]
79. Maggio, M.G.; Russo, M.; Cuzzola, M.F.; Destro, M.; La Rosa, G.; Molonia, F.; Bramanti, P.; Lombardo, G.; De Luca, R.; Calabro, R.S. Virtual reality in multiple sclerosis rehabilitation: A review on cognitive and motor outcomes. *J. Clin. Neurosci.* **2019**. [CrossRef] [PubMed]
80. Pozeg, P.; Palluel, E.; Ronchi, R.; Solca, M.; Al-Khodairy, A.W.; Jordan, X.; Kassouha, A.; Blanke, O. Virtual reality improves embodiment and neuropathic pain caused by spinal cord injury. *Neurology* **2017**, *89*, 1894–1903. [CrossRef] [PubMed]
81. Arane, K.; Behboudi, A.; Goldman, R.D. Virtual reality for pain and anxiety management in children. *Can. Fam. Phys.* **2017**, *63*, 932–934.

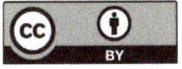

© 2019 by the authors. Licensee MDPI, Basel, Switzerland. This article is an open access article distributed under the terms and conditions of the Creative Commons Attribution (CC BY) license (http://creativecommons.org/licenses/by/4.0/).

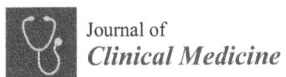

Article

Best Evidence Rehabilitation for Chronic Pain Part 3: Low Back Pain

Anneleen Malfliet [1,2,3,4,5,*], Kelly Ickmans [1,2,3,4], Eva Huysmans [1,2,3,4,6], Iris Coppieters [2,3,4,5], Ward Willaert [2,3,5], Wouter Van Bogaert [2,3], Emma Rheel [2,3,7], Thomas Bilterys [2,3], Paul Van Wilgen [2,3,8] and Jo Nijs [2,3,4,*]

1. Research Foundation–Flanders (FWO), 1090 Brussels, Belgium
2. Department of Physiotherapy, Human Physiology and Anatomy (KIMA), Faculty of Physical Education & Physiotherapy, Vrije Universiteit Brussel, 1090 Brussels, Belgium
3. Pain in Motion International Research Group, 1090 Brussels, Belgium
4. Department of Physical Medicine and Physiotherapy, University Hospital Brussels, Laarbeeklaan 101, 1090 Brussels, Belgium
5. Department of Rehabilitation Sciences and Physiotherapy, Faculty of Medicine and Health Sciences, Ghent University, 9000 Gent, Belgium
6. Department of Public Health (GEWE), Faculty of Medicine and Pharmacy, Vrije Universiteit Brussel, 1090 Brussels, Belgium
7. Department of Experimental-Clinical and Health Psychology, Ghent University, 9000 Ghent, Belgium
8. Transcare, Transdisciplinary Pain Management Centre, 9728 EE Groningen, The Netherlands
* Correspondence: anneleen.malfliet@vub.be (A.M.); Jo.Nijs@vub.be (J.N.)

Received: 6 June 2019; Accepted: 16 July 2019; Published: 19 July 2019

Abstract: Chronic Low Back Pain (CLBP) is a major and highly prevalent health problem. Given the high number of papers available, clinicians might be overwhelmed by the evidence on CLBP management. Taking into account the scale and costs of CLBP, it is imperative that healthcare professionals have access to up-to-date, evidence-based information to assist them in treatment decision-making. Therefore, this paper provides a state-of-the-art overview of the best evidence non-invasive rehabilitation for CLBP. Taking together up-to-date evidence from systematic reviews, meta-analysis and available treatment guidelines, most physically inactive therapies should not be considered for CLBP management, except for pain neuroscience education and spinal manipulative therapy if combined with exercise therapy, with or without psychological therapy. Regarding active therapy, back schools, sensory discrimination training, proprioceptive exercises, and sling exercises should not be considered due to low-quality and/or conflicting evidence. Exercise interventions on the other hand are recommended, but while all exercise modalities appear effective compared to minimal/passive/conservative/no intervention, there is no evidence that some specific types of exercises are superior to others. Therefore, we recommend choosing exercises in line with the patient's preferences and abilities. When exercise interventions are combined with a psychological component, effects are better and maintain longer over time.

Keywords: pain neuroscience; musculoskeletal pain; rehabilitation medicine; physiotherapy; lifestyle

1. Introduction

Chronic Low Back Pain (CLBP) is a major health problem worldwide and prevalence numbers have increased substantially in the past decades [1]. A global systematic review reports a linear correlation between age and CLBP prevalence, more specifically, individuals aged between 20 and 59 have a CLBP prevalence of 19.6%, while the prevalence in older people is 25.4% [2]. Besides pain, disability is reported very frequently. CLBP is a major contributor to the global disability burden, and continues to be the leading cause of years lived with disability [3,4]. About half of the people who experience LBP will seek care [5]. Given the high prevalence numbers of CLBP [2], this relates to excessive direct and indirect health care costs as well as a major social and economic impact [6,7].

Current guidelines recommend non-pharmacological and non-invasive management, including the advice to stay active, the use of patient education and exercise therapy [8]. Yet, given the high number of treatment guidelines, systematic reviews and randomized controlled trials on CLBP management, clinicians might be overwhelmed by the evidence available. Taking into account the scale and costs of the CLBP problem, it is imperative that healthcare professionals involved in CLBP management should have access to up-to-date, evidence-based information to assist them in treatment decision-making. Therefore, this paper aims to endorse consistent best practice, to reduce unwarranted variation and to diminish the use of low-value interventions in CLBP care.

Here, a state-of-the-art overview of the best evidence non-invasive rehabilitation for people having CLBP is provided. The best evidence non-invasive rehabilitation is reviewed in a way that clinicians can integrate the evidence into their daily clinical routine. In addition, the state-of-the-art overview also serves clinical researchers to build upon the best evidence for designing future trials and implementation studies, and to develop new innovative studies.

2. State of the Art

To cover the best evidence non-invasive rehabilitation, this section relies on systematic reviews and meta-analyses primarily. A non-systematic search of the literature was performed in PubMed, Web of Science and Google Scholar using the following search terms: rehabilitation, chronic low back pain, chronic back pain, chronic lumbar pain, chronic lower back pain. When possible, we used 'systematic review', and 'meta-analysis' filters. Additionally, information from several international clinical guidelines was retrieved and discussed.

Given the strong empirical support indicating that pain severity alone is not a robust predictor of function and improvement, we will focus both on pain and function as outcomes for chronic low back pain management [9,10].

2.1. Evidence from Systematic Reviews, and Meta-Analyses

A non-systematic search for evidence on non-invasive rehabilitation modalities for CLBP increases the understanding that CLBP is not only a common health problem but is also highly investigated. Unfortunately, many systematic reviews focus on LBP in general, and include both (sub)acute and chronic LBP. When the results of both populations were merged together in a review and specific conclusions for CLBP could not be identified, these papers were excluded from this overview. An outline of the available systematic reviews and meta-analyses that focused solely on CLBP, or in which CLBP results could be isolated, can be found in Table 1. If more than one systematic review was found regarding a specific topic, priority was given to including a meta-analysis (if available) and/or the most recent paper available.

The overview of evidence available from systematic review and meta-analyses is presented using the subdivision based on physically '*active*' and '*inactive*' interventions. Yet, this subdivision is chosen for practical reasons, and relies on whether an intervention requires the patient to be physically active or not. Therefore, pain neuroscience education will be discussed as part of the physically inactive interventions. Yet, we would like to stress that pain neuroscience education requires mental and cognitive activity of the patient given the required interaction between patient and therapist.

Table 1. Best evidence table for non-invasive rehabilitation in people with chronic low back pain: evidence from systematic reviews and meta-analyses.

Author, Year	LoE	Intervention and Sample	Main Outcomes and Results	Mono-/Multi-/Transdisciplinary [Involved Rehabilitation Professions]	Remarks	Recommended for Clinical Practice?
Physically inactive interventions						
Noori, 2019 [11]	1A	Therapeutic ultrasound ($n = 333$)	3 studies: ↓ pain after ultrasound compared to placebo or exercise. 3 studies: no effect	Not stated [Not stated]	Small samples, most studies lack follow-up period. No meta-analyses.	Lack of strong evidence for the use of ultrasound (LoC 1)
Li, 2019 [12]	1A	Kinesiotape ($n = 627$) *Meta-analysis*	Pain intensity: No significant effect. Disability: Significant ↓ in Oswestry Disability Index, but not in Roland Morris Disability Questionnaire	Monodisciplinary [Physiotherapist]	/	Lack of evidence for the use of kinesiotape (LoC 1)
Wood, 2019 [13]	1A	Pain Neuroscience Education (PNE) ($n = 615$) *Meta-analysis*	PNE alone: no significant change in pain, but significant ↓ in disability and kinesiophobia at short term compared to an alternative intervention. PNE combined with other PT interventions: significant ↓ in pain at short-term.	Monodisciplinary [Physiotherapist or general practitioners]	Heterogeneity in outcome measures.	Moderate quality evidence to use pain neuroscience education as adjunct to usual physiotherapy (LoC 1)
Resende, 2018 [14]	1A	Transcutaneous electrical nerve stimulation (TENS) ($n = 575$) *Meta-analysis*	Pain: Significant reduction during therapy, but not immediately after therapy or at 1 or 3mo follow-up. Disability: No effect during, or after therapy.	Not stated [Not stated]	Similar conclusion in other meta-analysis on effects of TENS on chronic back pain (Wu, 2018) [15]	Not recommended to use for CLBP (LoC 1)
Furlan, 2015 [16]	1A	Massage ($n = 2548$) *Meta-analysis*	Compared to inactive control: Massage may be more effective for pain and disability at short term. Conclusions at long term are unclear. Compared to active control: Results are unclear, no conclusions can be made at short- and long-term follow-up.	Not stated [Not stated]	Subacute and CLBP results are presented as one group. Very low quality of evidence.	Massage is not recommended to treat CLBP (LoC 1)
Orrock, 2013 [17]	1A	Osteopathic intervention ($n = 330$)	Similar effect of osteopathic intervention when compared to sham intervention or exercise and PT.	Monodisciplinary [Osteopath]	Only two studies available. No meta-analysis.	Not recommended due to lack of evidence (LoC 1)

Table 1. *Cont.*

Author, Year	LoE	Intervention and Sample	Main Outcomes and Results	Mono-/Multi-/Transdisciplinary [Involved Rehabilitation Professions]	Remarks	Recommended for Clinical Practice?
Rubinstein, 2019 [18]	1A	Spinal manipulative therapy (n = 9211) *Meta-analysis*	Pain: Moderate evidence that spinal manipulative therapy provides statistically better results than other interventions (exercise, PT, back school, medical care) at 6mo, but not at 1 and 12mo follow-up. Function: Moderate quality evidence that spinal manipulative therapy provides a small, statistically better result than other interventions at 1mo, but not at 6 or 12mo follow-up.	Monodisciplinary [Physiotherapist, chiropractor, manual therapist, osteopath]	Many studies with high risk of bias.	Possible adjunctive therapy. Produces similar effects to recommended therapies. Possibility of adverse events. (LoC 1)
Physically active interventions						
Hajihasani, 2019 [19]	1A	Adding Cognitive Behavioral Therapy (CBT) to PT (n = 965)	Compared to PT alone: Pain: mixed results, significant ↓ in 5 out of 10 studies; Disability: mixed results, significant ↓ in 4 out of 7 studies; Quality of Life: mixed results, significant ↓ in 2 out of 5 studies; Depression: mixed results, 2 studies show no changes, while one study shows exacerbation of depressive symptoms after adding CBT.	Mono- or multidisciplinary [Psychologist and physiotherapist]	No meta-analysis.	Mixed results, no clear indication for adding CBT to PT (LoC 1)
Zhang, 2019 [20]	1A	Group-based physiotherapist-led behavioral psychological interventions (n = 1927) *Meta-analysis*	Compared to waitlist or usual care: Significant pain reduction at short-, intermediate, and long-term follow-up. Compared to active treatment: No difference between groups at short- or intermediate, but significant lower pain after behavioral therapy at long-term follow-up.	Monodisciplinary [Physiotherapist]	Heterogeneity in methods.	Yes, while there is no difference with active treatments at short and intermediate follow-up, behavioral treatments appear more effective at long-term follow-up. There are indications that the addition of behavioral components can reduce sick leave.
Vanti, 2019 [21]	1A	Walking interventions (n = 510) *Meta-analysis*	Pain, disability, quality of life and fear-avoidance improve equally by walking or exercise.	Not stated [Physiotherapist]	Same conclusion in similar meta-analysis by Sitthiporn-vorakul, 2018 [22]	Walking is not more effective for reducing pain and disability compared to exercise or education, but can be used as a low-budget and easy accessible alternative (LoC 1)

Table 1. *Cont.*

Author, Year	LoE	Intervention and Sample	Main Outcomes and Results	Mono-/Multi-/Transdisciplinary [Involved Rehabilitation Professions]	Remarks	Recommended for Clinical Practice?
Van Erp, 2018 [23]	1A	Primary Care Interventions Using a Biopsychosocial Approach (n = 1426)	**Compared to education/advice:** Functional disability ↓ at short, mid and long term; Pain ↓ at short, mid and long term; Quality of life: No differences **Compared to physical activity therapy:** Functional disability: No differences; Pain: mixed results, 2 out of 4 studies report significant ↓ in pain in biopsychosocial approach	Mono- or multidisciplinary [Physiotherapist, combined with nurses, psychologist, or occupational therapist]	Heterogeneity in study and treatment designs. No meta-analysis.	Use of bio-psychosocial interventions in primary care is beneficial over education and advice (LoC 1)
Wewege, 2018 [24]	1A	Aerobic and resistance exercise interventions (n = 322) *Meta-analysis*	**Pooled results of aerobic and resistance training:** Small significant improvement in pain and a trend towards significance for decreased disability and improved mental health. No differences were found for physical health (SF36).	Monodisciplinary [Physiotherapist or exercise therapist]	/	Moderate quality evidence for the use of aerobic and resistance training (LoC 1)
Luomajoki, 2018 [25]	1A	Movement control exercise therapy (n = 781) *Meta-analysis*	**In global group:** Short-term ↓ in disability, but not in pain compared to active control treatment. No long-term effects. **In subgroup with movement control impairment:** Short- and long-term ↓ in pain and disability.	Monodisciplinary [Physiotherapist]	Small sample sized and heterogeneity of included studies.	Very low to moderate quality of evidence to use movement control exercises in CLBP AND movement control impairment (LoC 1)
Parreira, 2017 [26]	1A	Back School (n = 4105) *Meta-analysis*	Pain: Low quality of evidence for reduction at short term, but not at intermediate or long-term follow-up compared to no treatment. Disability: Low quality of evidence that back schools are not effective at intermediate or long-term follow-up compared to no treatment.	Monodisciplinary [Physiotherapist or medical specialist]	Low quality of evidence	Because of low quality of evidence, back schools are not recommended for CLBP (LoC 1)

Table 1. Cont.

Author, Year	LoE	Intervention and Sample	Main Outcomes and Results	Mono-/Multi-/Transdisciplinary [Involved Rehabilitation Professions]	Remarks	Recommended for Clinical Practice?
Du, 2017 [27]	1A	Self-management (n = 2188) Meta-analysis	Pain: Significant reduction using self-management at immediate, short-term, intermediate and long-term follow-up compared to a control intervention. Disability: Significant reduction using self-management at immediate, short-term, intermediate and long-term follow-up compared to a control intervention.	Mono- or multidisciplinary, and/or internet-based [Physiotherapist, psychologist, exercise therapist, and/or internet-based]	/	Yes, there is moderate-quality evidence that self-management has a moderate effect on pain intensity, and small to moderate effect on disability (LoC 1)
López-de-Uralde-Villanueva, 2016 [28]	1A	Graded Activity and Graded Exposure (n = 1486) Meta-analysis	Graded activity vs other forms of exercises: No difference for disability, quality of life or pain at any time-point. Graded activity vs waitlist or usual care: Graded activity is more effective to reduce disability, but not pain at short- and long-term follow-up. Graded activity vs graded exposure: Graded exposure was more effective to reduce disability and catastrophizing in the short term. There is no difference between both regarding the effect on pain.	Not stated [Not stated]	Poor methodological quality of many included studies. Possible publication bias could not be assessed.	There is limited evidence that graded activity significantly reduces disability in the short and long term compared to a control intervention, but not when compared to an active control intervention. There is strong evidence that graded activity cannot change pain in the short, intermediate, and long term compared to a control intervention. There are indicative findings that graded exposure is better than graded activity at decreasing disability and catastrophizing in the short term. (LoC 1)
Saragiotto, 2016 [29]	1A	Motor control exercise (n = 2431) Meta-analysis	Compared to other exercises: Small, but not clinically important effect on pain and disability at short term, but not at intermediate or long-term follow-up. Compared to manual therapy: No effect on pain and disability. Compared to minimal intervention: Clinical important effect on pain at short- and long-term. Small, but not clinically important effect on disability at short- intermediate and long-term.	Not stated [Not stated]	/	Motor control exercises are more effective than a minimal intervention, but is not more effective than other forms of exercise or manual therapy (LoC 1)

Table 1. Cont.

Author, Year	LoE	Intervention and Sample	Main Outcomes and Results	Mono-/Multi-/Transdisciplinary [Involved Rehabilitation Professions]	Remarks	Recommended for Clinical Practice?
Kälin, 2016 [30]	1A	Sensory discrimination training (n = 255)	Both sensory discrimination and control treatments (TENS, back school, sham treatment) led to a decrease in pain and an improvement in function.	Monodisciplinary [Physiotherapist]	Conflicting evidence, low quality of included studies. No meta-analysis.	Conflicting evidence, no clear conclusion or recommendation possible (LoC 1)
Yamato, 2015 [31]	1A	Pilates (n = 510) *Meta-analysis*	Pain: Pilates is more effective at short and intermediate term compared to minimal intervention, but not compared to other exercise interventions. Disability: Pilates is more effective at short and intermediate term compared to minimal intervention, but not compared to other exercise interventions.	Monodisciplinary [Pilates instructor]	Although the review focused on (sub)acute and chronic LBP, but all included studies dealt about CLBP.	Pilates is more effective than minimal intervention (low- to moderate quality of evidence), but there is no evidence for the superiority of Pilates to other forms of exercise (LoC 1)
Kamper, 2015 [32]	1A	Multidisciplinary biopsychosocial rehabilitation (n = 6858) *Meta-analysis*	**Compared to usual care:** Multidisciplinary biopsychosocial rehabilitation is more effective to reduce pain and disability, even at long-term. **Compared to physical treatment:** Multidisciplinary biopsychosocial rehabilitation is more effective to reduce pain and disability, even at long-term.	Multidisciplinary [Physical, psychological, educational, and/or work-related components delivered by expert healthcare providers]	Clinical heterogeneity among included studies.	Yes, multidisciplinary biopsychosocial rehabilitation is more effective than usual care or physical treatment (LoC 1)
Searle, 2015 [33]	1A	Exercise interventions (n = 4462) *Meta-analysis*	**General comparison:** Exercise has a small but significant benefit for the treatment of non-specific CLBP and is more effective than conservative therapies (wait list or usual activities, general practitioner care, electrotherapies and manipulative therapies). **Sub-analysis:** Strength/resistance, coordination/stabilization, and combined exercise is more effective than conservative therapies, but not cardiorespiratory exercise.	Not stated [Not stated]	Heterogeneity in application of exercise interventions.	Yes. Beneficial effect of strength/resistance and coordination/stabilization exercise programs over other interventions (LoC 1)

Table 1. *Cont.*

Author, Year	LoE	Intervention and Sample	Main Outcomes and Results	Mono-/Multi-/Transdisciplinary [Involved Rehabilitation Professions]	Remarks	Recommended for Clinical Practice?
McCaskey, 2014 [34]	1A	Proprioceptive exercises (n = 1380)	**Perceptual proprioceptive training:** More effective for pain reduction than back school. Two studies, very low quality of evidence. **Joint repositioning training:** More effective for short-term pain reduction than no intervention. No difference with other exercises. Low quality of evidence. **Multimodal proprioceptive training:** More effective for short-term pain reduction than no intervention. No difference with other exercises. Low quality of evidence.	Monodisciplinary [Physiotherapist]	Overall low quality of evidence. No meta-analysis.	No consistent benefit in adding proprioceptive exercises for CLPB rehabilitation (LoC 1)
Yue, 2014 [35]	1A	Sling exercise (n = 706) *Meta-analysis*	Sling exercises are not more effective for improving pain or function compared to other forms of exercise.	Not stated [Not stated]	Low quality of included studies.	Based on the available evidence, sling exercises are not recommended (LoC 1)
Holtzman, 2013 [36]	1A	Yoga (n = 851) *Meta-analysis*	Pain and disability improved directly post-treatment (moderate to large effect sizes) and remained at long-term follow-up (small to medium effect sizes). Effects were compared to no treatment/waitlist, stretching, usual care, education and exercise.	Monodisciplinary [Yoga therapist]	Heterogeneity in yoga interventions. High quality of included studies.	Yes, possible adjunctive to PT intervention (LoC 1)
Hoffman, 2007 [37]	1A	Psychological interventions (n = 1747) *Meta-analysis*	**Compared to waitlist:** Psychological interventions are superior to reduce pain intensity and health-related quality of life. **Compared to active control (e.g., treatment as usual) intervention:** Psychological interventions are not superior	Mono- or multidisciplinary [Not stated]	/	Psychological interventions are more effective than no intervention, but not compared to active interventions (LoC 1)

Level of Evidence (LoE): 1A: Systematic review of randomized controlled trials; 1B: Individual randomized controlled trials; 2A: Systematic review of cohort studies; 2B: Individual cohort study or low quality randomized controlled trials; 3A: Systematic review of case-control studies; 3B: individual case-control study; 4: Case-series; 5: Expert opinion. Level of Conclusion (LoC): LoC 1: Research of evidence level 1A or at least 2 independent conducted studies of evidence level 1B; LoC 2: 1 research of evidence level 1B or at least 2 independent conducted studies of evidence level 2B or 3B; LoC 3 1 research of evidence level 2B, 3B or 4; LoC 4: Opinion of experts or Inconclusive or inconsistent results between various studies. Abbreviations: LoE = Level of Evidence; LoC = Level of Conclusion; PT= physiotherapy; CLBP = Chronic Low Back Pain.

2.2. Physically Inactive Interventions

Investigated inactive techniques for CLBP include therapeutic ultrasound, kinesiotape, pain neuroscience education, transcutaneous electrical nerve stimulation, massage, osteopathic intervention, and spinal manipulative therapy (including high-velocity low-amplitude spinal manipulations as well as low-velocity low-amplitude mobilizations). Out of these therapies, only two are recommended, and only when implemented as adjunctive therapy: pain neuroscience education and spinal manipulative therapy. All other inactive interventions (i.e., therapeutic ultrasound, kinesiotape, transcutaneous electrical nerve stimulation, massage and osteopathic interventions) are not recommended for CLBP management based on available evidence.

Pain neuroscience education aims to decrease the threat value of pain by increasing the patient's knowledge about pain and by reconceptualizing pain [38]. As stand-alone intervention, this treatment modality can reduce disability and kinesiophobia short term, but is not able to change pain [13]. However, when combined with other physiotherapeutic interventions, pain neuroscience education can significantly reduce pain short term [13]. Therefore, pain neuroscience education can be considered as a first step before applying an active intervention for people with CLBP. Given that many people with CLBP display kinesiophobia (i.e., fear of movement and avoidance behavior, which is a barrier for positive treatment outcome) [39], and active interventions are recommended (see below: 'active interventions' and 'international guidelines') [40], pain neuroscience education can prime people for further treatment by adapting beliefs and expectations. We would like to emphasize that—although here discussed among physically inactive interventions—pain neuroscience education requires a certain degree of activity of the patient. Pain neuroscience education should be delivered using intense interaction between the patient and the therapist, and therefore requires mental and cognitive activity of the patient [41,42]. Additionally, pain neuroscience education appears to enhance physical activation and its effects on pain, given the evidence that combining pain neuroscience education with a (therapeutic) exercise intervention is more effective than an exercise intervention alone (large effect size for pain intensity) [13,43]. Manuals to implement pain neuroscience education are available in books [44,45], and tools for clinical practice can be found online [46].

Similarly, spinal manipulative therapy can be used in clinical practice for CLBP management, but only as part of a treatment package (i.e., adjunctive therapy) given the moderate quality evidence from improvements in pain and function at short-term follow-up (1 month) but not at long term (6 or 12 months follow-up) [18,40,47,48]. Importantly, evidence reports several possible adverse events related to spinal manipulative therapy, which should be taken into account by the clinician before using these techniques. Reported adverse events include severe back pain, acute flare-up of back pain, inability to sleep because of pain, muscle soreness and stiffness, exacerbation of symptoms, and tiredness [18]. Interestingly, a randomized controlled trial examined if the effects on pain differed between region-specific and non-region-specific spinal manipulations in people with CLBP (n = 148) [49]. While both groups showed a reduction in pain intensity after the manipulation, they did not find any differences between region-specific and non-region-specific techniques. This finding appears to refute any local, biomechanical mechanisms behind the effectiveness of these techniques [49]. Changes in pain in response to manipulative techniques in people with CLBP could therefore be more related to a cascade of neurophysiological responses from both the peripheral and central nervous system as well as nonspecific effects such as expectations and psychosocial factors, rather than local tissue changes [49].

As the effects of spinal manipulative techniques in CLBP might be explained by similar mechanisms contributing to the positive effects of pain neuroscience education, some researchers suggest to combine both recommended physically inactive adjunctive therapies discussed here [50,51]. Given their similar recommendation (i.e., as adjuvant therapy to active treatment modalities), discussing their simultaneous application in clinical practice becomes relevant. Because of the aim of pain neuroscience education to shift the patient's focus away from the tissues in the low back as the source of their pain, many could conclude that pain neuroscience education should be used solely within a hands-off treatment approach.

Yet, the meta-analysis of Wood et al. (2018) includes papers that combine pain neuroscience education with other physiotherapeutic interventions such as exercise/activity and/or manual therapy [13]. Outcomes appeared to favor the combination of pain neuroscience education with movement, either passive (manual therapy) and/or active. This suggests that combining pain neuroscience education with "hands-on" approaches results in more favorable responses than pain neuroscience education alone [51]. Yet, given the statement of The American Physical Therapy Association (APTA) that warns us for the negative effects of applying physically inactive treatments (i.e., they can delay recovery and lead to poor long-term outcomes by reinforcing a passive role, promoting inactivity and disability behavior, and 'medicalizing' the patient), combining pain neuroscience education with active exercise therapy might still be preferred over any physically inactive approach.

If a clinician were to combine pain neuroscience education with "hands-on" techniques, care should be taken that all communication to the patient fits within the biopsychosocial framework of PNE. Therefore, it should be avoided to present manual techniques within a biomedical pain model, in which the therapist is deemed to "fix" a structure [52,53]. Instead, communication can focus on the desensitizing effects of "hands-on" techniques and threatening words such as "pain" can be replaced by more neutral terms like "symptoms" [52,54].

2.3. Physically Active Interventions

Given the listed active interventions in Table 1 and their recommendations, physically active interventions appear to have more potential to alter symptoms in CLBP than physically inactive interventions. Yet, the following four treatment modalities are not recommended due to lack of qualitative evidence and/or conflicting evidence: back schools, sensory discrimination training, proprioceptive exercises, and sling exercises [26,30,34,35]. Therefore, based on current evidence, these types of therapy should not be considered for CLBP management.

The other active therapies for CLBP listed in Table 1 can be subdivided in physiotherapeutic treatment modalities that include a psychological component (i.e., multimodal), and treatment modalities that focus purely on physical exercises and movements. All included exercise modalities (aerobic exercise, strength/resistance exercise, coordination/stabilization exercise, motor control, and pilates) can effectively reduce pain and disability compared to minimal, passive/conservative, or no intervention [24,29,31,33]. However, when compared to each other (or to other active treatments), no differences can be found between different exercise modalities [24,29,31,33]. This is at odds with evidence in healthy people, where—for example—resistance training can reduce pain sensitivity to a greater extent than aerobic exercise [55].

Taken together, the information available regarding exercise interventions in CLBP and the wide variety in duration, intensity and methods of training, we cannot recommend which groups or types of exercise interventions are most effective [24,29,31,33]. From a motivational point of view, we recommend taking the patient's preferences and abilities into account when deciding upon exercise modalities to use. Interestingly, when exercise therapy reduces pain and disability in people with CLBP, the improvements are often unrelated to an improvement in physical function [56]. Therefore, it is suggested that other exercise-induced changes like improved psychological status and cognitions (e.g., reduced anxiety, catastrophizing, and fear) influence pain and disability more than changes in physical function. This might explain the difficulties currently encountered to identify the optimal exercise modality and dosage for CLBP management [24,57]. This statement is (partly) underscored by the evidence on treatment modalities that combine exercises with a psychological component (i.e., biopsychosocial approach) [20,23,32].

Three systematic reviews (two of which included a meta-analysis) focused on the effectiveness of a biopsychosocial treatment approach [20,23,32]. This approach involves a physical component combined with a psychological component and/or a social/work targeted component [32]. Results of this approach compared to other active treatments are promising. For example, while there was no difference at short- and intermediate-term follow-up, behavioral psychological interventions were more effective to reduce pain at short-term and long-term follow-up than active treatments without a psychological component [20,58,59]. Interestingly, the best results were found for multidisciplinary biopsychosocial rehabilitation [32]. Importantly, the systematic review and meta-analysis investigating this rehabilitation approach does not allow to differentiate whether the positive results emanate from the multidisciplinary approach, the biopsychosocial focus, or both, as comparator studies all involved a monodisciplinary biomedical approach (e.g., electrotherapy, aerobic, stretching and strengthening exercises, traction, TENS, manual therapy, back school, surgery, etc.) [32]. Yet, both compared to monodisciplinary usual care and to monodisciplinary physical treatment, multidisciplinary biopsychosocial rehabilitation was found to be more effective to reduce pain and disability, even at long-term follow-ups [60–67]. These results indicate that a multidisciplinary biopsychosocial approach can provide CLBP patients with relevant tools to maintain positive treatment effects long term. This is underscored by evidence that the effect on work equates to a person having roughly double the odds of being at work after 12 months if they received a multidisciplinary rehabilitation program rather than a physical treatment alone [32,68–71]. Interestingly, studies focusing on the costs-effectiveness of interdisciplinary rehabilitation programs for chronic (pediatric) pain in general found significant reductions in medical costs post-treatment compared to the pretreatment phase [72–74].

Yet, a multidisciplinary approach can be time-consuming, and resource intensive. As there is currently no evidence available that directly compares a biopsychosocial approach in a monodisciplinary versus a multidisciplinary setting, future researchers should focus on the question if it is the multidisciplinary or rather biopsychosocial focus that explains these positive results. Interestingly, a large randomized controlled trial recently conducted by our group has investigated the effectiveness of a biopsychosocial approach (i.e., combining pain neuroscience education and cognition-targeted exercise therapy) delivered monodisciplinary by a physiotherapist only [75]. This approach was able to reduce pain, symptoms of central sensitization, and to improve psychophysiological measures of central sensitization, disability, pain cognitions, mental health and physical functioning (medium to large effect sizes) compared to an active control treatment. Using this example, we want to underscore that even in a monodisciplinary setting a biopsychosocial approach can be effective and should be targeted by clinicians. A treatment manual of this approach is published and can be accessed freely online (https://bit.ly/2WcA1re) [76].

The added value of a combined, biopsychosocial approach (i.e., adding psychological components to active physiotherapy treatments) is further underscored by a systematic review and meta-analysis that focused on the effectiveness of stand-alone psychological interventions for CLBP [37]. This review concluded that, compared to a waitlist, psychological interventions were superior to reduce pain intensity and improve quality of life, but showed equal results when compared to an active (i.e., exercise) control intervention [37].

Additionally, we would like to highlight the possible advantage of incorporating graded exposure techniques into the management of chronic low back pain. Graded exposure is a treatment modality that identifies feared exercises or activities, and exposes the patient to these exercises or activities in a hierarchical fashion, starting with an exercise or activity that elicits minimal amounts of fear and progressing only when this fear reduces [28]. One systematic review and meta-analysis focusses both on graded activity and graded exposure in nonspecific CLBP [28]. While graded activity can only improve disability when compared to a waitlist or usual care control group and does not show superior to other forms of exercises, there is some indicative research showing that graded exposure is more effective than graded activity to improve disability and catastrophizing short term [28]. However, currently there are no systematic reviews or meta-analyses available to allow firm conclusions on the potential of graded exposure in chronic low back pain management. Therefore, we suggest that clinicians can screen for the possible presence of feared movements and activities, and to tackle them using graded exposure techniques upon occurrence [77,78].

Last, we would like to underline a recent meta-analysis on the effectiveness of walking interventions [21]. When compared to education or other active exercises, walking improves pain, disability, quality of life and fear-avoidance to a similar extent. Therefore, walking interventions are not recommended as sole use, but given the low-budget and easy, accessible characteristics of walking, it can be a valuable home-based addition to other therapy modalities as it can increase physical activity, overcome activity avoidance, and minimize barriers for other types of exercise [21,22]. Walking at a low to moderate intensity imposes low risk of (musculoskeletal) injury and can improve aerobic capacity, body mass index, systolic/diastolic blood pressure, triglyceride levels, and high-density lipoprotein cholesterol levels in both healthy and sedentary individuals [22,79,80]. Therefore, clinicians should consider implementing walking exercises for CLBP management, when combined with other types of recommended, active treatment.

2.4. International Guidelines

A critical review of LBP guidelines (2017) [81] used the Appraisal of Guidelines Research and Evaluation (AGREE) instrument to assess their quality and recommends four (out of 17 available) guidelines for LBP management [40,82–84]. Two of these guidelines (NICE guidelines and Dutch physiotherapy guidelines) focused on CLBP as a specific group apart from (sub)acute LBP [40,82] and will be discussed here. For the NICE guidelines, we refer to the updated version that was published in 2016. Additionally, the recommendations of two more recently published guidelines that were not yet included in the critical review will be discussed [85,86]. An overview of the recommendations included in these (clinical) guidelines can be found in Table 2. We will not discuss all recommendations in detail here but will rather highlight some striking features and parallels between guidelines.

Although several differences exist between the different guidelines, exercise is recommended in all of them [40,82,85,86]. Interestingly, all of them also recognize that none of the exercise modalities is superior to the others: health care providers can choose any type of exercise (general, aerobic, strengthening, yoga, group-based or individual, etc.), but should specifically consider the patient's preferences, needs and capabilities while choosing the exercise modality. The NICE guidelines even take it one step further and identify exercise as key treatment modality for LBP, given the recommendation to only consider manual therapy and/or psychological therapies if it is a part of a treatment package including exercise [40]. For multidisciplinary biopsychosocial rehabilitation—the intervention that shows high potential based on available systematic reviews and meta-analysis (see Table 1)—the NICE guidelines recommend considering this approach when significant psychosocial obstacles limit recovery, or when previous treatments have not been effective.

Importantly, these guidelines all agree not to recommend transcutaneous electrical nerve stimulation, interferential therapy (electrotherapy), or ultrasound for the treatment of CLBP. Other not-to-use modalities in CLBP management as identified in at least one of these guidelines are: traction, biofeedback, massage, laser therapy, taping, lumbar support, postural exercises, orthotics, and percutaneous electrical nerve stimulation. Interestingly, all modalities that are not recommended comprise physically inactive techniques, i.e., this implies lack of participation from the individual receiving the therapy intervention. This is in line with the conclusions made based on the systematic reviews (and meta-analysis) included in Table 1. The American Physical Therapy Association (APTA) even warns us of the negative effects of applying physically inactive treatments for any type of patient: these treatments can delay recovery and lead to poor long-term outcomes by reinforcing a passive role, promoting inactivity and disability behavior, and 'medicalizing' the patient [87]. Given the 'active' focus of recommended treatment modalities, this advice should also be taken into consideration when treating patients with CLBP. While physically inactive treatments (like manual therapy) appear to have potentially positive effects, they should not be used as sole treatment but rather in a multimodal approach focusing mainly on activating the patient [40].

Table 2. Overview of recommendations in (clinical) guidelines for chronic low back pain management.

Guideline		Recommendation for CLBP
Bekkering et al. Dutch Physiotherapy Guidelines for Low Back Pain (2003) [82]	Recommended	- **Exercise therapy (not clear which exercises are best):** Strong evidence that exercise therapy is equally effective compared to passive physiotherapy techniques. Strong evidence that exercise therapy is more effective than standard care by the general practitioner. - **Behavioral treatment: may be useful.** Strong evidence for a moderately positive effect on pain compared to no treatment, waitlist or placebo. Effectiveness compared to other treatments not clear.
	Not recommended	- Traction - Biofeedback - Massage - Transcutaneous electrical nerve stimulation - Ultrasound - Electrotherapy - Laser therapy
Wong et al. Clinical guidelines for the noninvasive management of low back pain (2016) [86]	Recommended	- **Education:** Advice and information promoting self-management, evidence-based information on expected course and effective self-care options, advice to stay active. - **Exercises:** No recommendations for or against any specific type of exercise, consider patient preferences. - **Manual therapy,** including spinal manipulation - **Multimodal rehabilitation:** including physical and psychological interventions (e.g., cognitive/behavioral approached and exercise). - Recommended by some guidelines: Massage, acupuncture, antidepressants.
	Not recommended	- Muscle relaxants - Gabapentin - **Passive modalities,** including transcutaneous electrical nerve stimulation, laser, interferential therapy and ultrasound.

Table 2. *Cont.*

Guideline		Recommendation for CLBP
Qaseem et al. Noninvasive treatments for acute, subacute and chronic low back pain (2017) [85]	Recommended	- **Exercise**: Moderate-quality evidence for small improvements in pain relief and function when compared to no exercise or usual care. No evidence on which exercise regimen is best. - **Motor control exercise**: Low-quality evidence for the effectiveness of motor control exercise (small improvements in pain and function) compared to minimal intervention, general exercise, and multimodal physical therapy. Low quality of evidence found no differences between motor control exercises plus exercise or exercise alone. - **Tai Chi**: Low-quality evidence showed that Tai Chi results in moderate pain reduction compared to waitlist or no intervention. - **Yoga**: Low-quality evidence showed that yoga results in a small pain reduction compared to exercise. - **Psychological therapies**: Low-quality evidence showed positive effects of progressive relaxation therapy, mindfulness relaxation, electromyography biofeedback training, operant therapy and cognitive behavioral therapy compared to waitlist. Low-quality evidence shows no difference between psychological therapies and exercise or physical therapy, and no difference between psychological therapies plus exercise and exercise alone. - **Multidisciplinary rehabilitation**: Moderate-quality evidence for effectiveness to improve pain and disability compared to usual care, no treatment, or physical therapy.
	Not Clear	- **Pilates** - **Acupuncture**: Low-to-moderate-quality evidence shows effectiveness of acupuncture but compared to no treatment or sham treatment. No improvement found in function. - **Spinal manipulation** - **Low-level laser therapy**
	Not recommended	- **TENS** - **Ultrasound** - **Lumbar support** - **Taping**

Table 2. Cont.

Guideline		Recommendation for CLBP
National Guideline Centre. NICE Guideline Low back pain and sciatica (2016) [40]	Recommended	- **Self-management**: Provide advice and information tailored to the patient's needs and capacities, including information on the nature of the pain, and encouragement to continue normal activities. - **Exercise**: Consider group exercise programs, take into account the patient's specific needs, preferences and capabilities when choosing the type of exercise. - **Manual therapy (spinal manipulation, mobilization or soft tissue techniques)**: Can be used, but only as part of a treatment package including exercise, with or without psychological therapy. - **Cognitive behavioral therapy**: As part of a treatment package, including exercise, with or without manual therapy. - **Multidisciplinary biopsychosocial rehabilitation**: Consider a combined physical and psychological intervention incorporating cognitive behavioral techniques when significant psychosocial obstacles limit recovery, or when previous treatments have not been effective. - **Return to work**: Promote and facilitate. - Normal activities of daily living: Promote and facilitate.
	Not recommended	- Opioids - Postural exercise or education - Orthotics, belt, corsets or rocker sole shoes - Traction - Acupuncture - Ultrasound - Percutaneous electrical nerve stimulation - Transcutaneous electrical nerve stimulation - Interferential therapy

3. Promising Directions for Clinical Practice

Over the past decades, scientific understanding of CLBP has increased substantially. This has shifted treatment approaches away from pure biomedical treatments to multimodal approaches that acknowledge the complex biopsychosocial nature of CLBP. The latter includes addressing lifestyle factors, like physical activity and sedentary behavior, exercise, stress, sleep, and nutritional aspects (Figure 1). In the general chronic pain population, the influence of lifestyle factors like (chronic) stress, insomnia and sleep problems, depression, smoking, alcohol, obesity and nutrition are already acknowledged [88–92]. Additionally, the overview of best evidence non-invasive rehabilitation for CLBP in this paper highlights the importance of physical activity and exercise therapy for CLBP management. Still, within CLBP management specifically, other lifestyle factors have received little attention in scientific literature so far. Yet, a multimodal lifestyle-centered approach (Figure 1) could lead to a long-term decrease of the psychological and socio-economic burden of chronic pain.

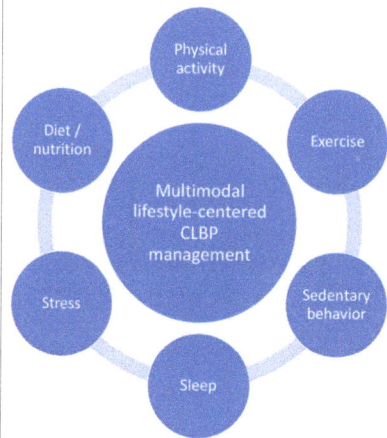

Figure 1. Promising direction for further research: a multimodal lifestyle-centered approach for people with chronic low back pain (CLBP).

Incorporating stress management in CLBP treatment could help patients to cope with everyday stressors, and leads to a clinically meaningful reduction in disability even at long-term (one year) follow-up [93]. Stress management can help to increase acceptance of physical discomfort and difficult emotions [93]. The advantage of a multimodal approach that addresses different lifestyle factors can be underscored by the interconnection between stress and sleep in people with CLBP [94]. Numerous studies report a strong association between anxiety levels and insomnia severity [95,96], and daily life stress can negatively impact sleep [97]. As poor sleep acts as a precipitating and perpetuating factor [98], and can represent a barrier for effective chronic pain management [99], its importance for CLBP management is evident. Additionally, people with chronic pain will spontaneously engage in more physical activity following a better night of sleep [100], again underscoring the importance of a multimodal lifestyle-centered approach.

Similar to sleep, overweightness and obesity are risk factors for developing LBP, and are associated with more severe and debilitating pain as pain intensity and disability show dose-responses to Body Mass Index, waist circumference, percent fat, and fat mass [101–107]. Unfortunately, overweight and obesity are an often overlooked lifestyle factor of importance in CLBP, while overweight/obese people with CLBP are likely to have more complex needs requiring a focus on lifestyle factors [108]. A recent study examining a nonsurgical weight loss program (i.e., physical exercise plus changes in dietary behavior) found that people with CLBP (n = 46) not only lost body weight, but also experienced less pain and disability [109]. Given the uncontrolled nature of this study, methodologically-sound randomized controlled trials examining the added value of such an approach are needed. Yet, if therapists were to implement a weight reduction program for CLBP management, this program should include changes in diet, behavior and physical activity [109], given the American College of Sports Medicine Position Stand that a moderate dietary restriction combined with a physical activity program (i.e., a deficit of 500 to 700 kcal on the energy balance) is effective and delivers long-term results [110].

Importantly, such multimodal lifestyle approach should primarily be implemented as a patient-centered approach, tailoring the included treatment aspects to the preferences and attitudes of the individual. This includes continuous (non-)verbal communication, education during all aspects of treatments, patient-defined goals, patient-empowerment, and a confident therapist who has sufficient social and interpersonal skills and shows specific knowledge [111]. To optimize the success rate of this approach, principles of self-monitoring, goal setting and feedback can also be integrated [112,113]. Given the need for behavioral changes in such a lifestyle approach, motivational interviewing techniques can help the therapist to overcome difficulties experienced by the patient to engage in this positive health behavior [114]. For example, consequences of an unhealthy lifestyle, as well as barriers for change, can be discussed, together with examples of how a better lifestyle can impact pain and quality of life, including a plan-of-action [115]. Motivational interviewing aims to develop autonomous motivation in the patient by increasing perceived competence, self-regulation and self-efficacy [115]. As higher self-efficacy is one of the key factors associated with better treatment outcome in chronic pain, motivational interviewing techniques are useful to consider even beyond CLBP management [116,117]. Clinicians and researchers should focus on this multimodal approach to CLBP to aim for long-term improvements in pain, disability and quality of life, rather than a short-term relief. As this approach could increase the empowerment of the patient and thus increase their personal control over the symptoms, the need for constant follow-up and supervision of a physiotherapist—and the related socio-economic costs—could be diminished.

4. Conclusions

Given the high prevalence of CLBP, and the overwhelming evidence available on its possible management, this paper aimed to give a clear overview of best evidence practice. To conclude, most physically inactive therapies should not be considered for CLBP management, except for pain neuroscience education and spinal manipulative therapy if combined with exercise therapy, with or without psychological therapy. Regarding active therapy, back schools, sensory discrimination training, proprioceptive exercises, and sling exercises should not be considered for CLBP management due to a lack of qualitative evidence and/or conflicting evidence. Exercise interventions, on the other hand, are recommended, but while all exercise modalities appear effective compared to minimal, passive/conservative or no intervention, there is no evidence that some specific types of exercises are superior to others. Therefore, we recommend choosing exercise modalities according with the patient's preferences and abilities. When combining exercise interventions with a psychological component, effects are better than an approach without psychological component and remain at long term.

Key messages for CLBP rehabilitation

- Do not consider the use of therapeutic ultrasound, kinesiotape, transcutaneous electrical nerve stimulation, massage and osteopathic interventions.
- Pain neuroscience education and spinal manipulative therapy can have positive effects but should not be used as stand-alone treatment. Consider these modalities only as part of a treatment package including exercise, with or without psychological therapy.
- Do not consider back school, sensory discrimination training, proprioceptive exercises, and sling exercises.
- Exercise therapy is highly recommended, but it is not clear which duration, intensity and methods of training are best.

- Consider a combined physical and psychological intervention incorporating cognitive behavioral techniques to maintain positive effects at long-term.

Author Contributions: Conceptualization, A.M, K.I. and J.N.; Literature search and data extraction, A.M.; Writing, Original Draft Preparation, A.M..; Writing, Review & Editing, all authors; Supervision, J.N.

Acknowledgments: Anneleen Malfliet, Kelly Ickmans, and Eva Huysmans funded by the Research Foundation Flanders (FWO), Belgium. This work is partially funded by the Berekuyl Academy Chair, funded by the European College for Lymphatic Therapy, The Netherlands, and awarded to Jo Nijs, Vrije Universiteit Brussel, Belgium. Iris Coppieters and Thomas Bilterys are both funded by the Applied Biomedical Research Program (TBM) of the Agency for Innovation by Science and Technology (IWT) and the Research Foundation Flanders (FWO), Belgium.

Conflicts of Interest: Jo Nijs has co-authored a Dutch book for clinicians on pain neuroscience education, but the royalties for that book are collected by the Vrije Universiteit Brussel and not him personally. Besides that, the authors have no conflict of interest to disclose.

References

1. Clark, S.; Horton, R. Low Back Pain: A Major Global Challenge. *Lancet* **2018**, *391*, 2302. [CrossRef]
2. Meucci, R.D.; Fassa, A.G.; Faria, N.M. Prevalence of Chronic Low Back Pain: Systematic Review. *Rev. Saude Publica* **2015**, *49*, 73. [CrossRef] [PubMed]
3. Hurwitz, E.L.; Randhawa, K.; Yu, H.; Cote, P.; Haldeman, S. The Global Spine Care Initiative: A Summary of the Global Burden of Low Back and Neck Pain Studies. *Eur. Spine J.* **2018**, *27*, 796–801. [CrossRef] [PubMed]
4. James, S.L.; Abate, D.; Abate, K.H.; Abay, S.M.; Abbafati, C.; Abbasi, N.; Abbastabar, H.; Abd-Allah, F.; Abdela, J.; Abdelalim, A.; et al. Global, Regional, and National Incidence, Prevalence, and Years Lived with Disability for 354 Diseases and Injuries for 195 Countries and Territories, 1990–2017: A Systematic Analysis for the Global Burden of Disease Study 2017. *Lancet* **2018**, *392*, 1789–1858. [CrossRef]
5. Ferreira, M.L.; Machado, G.; Latimer, J.; Maher, C.; Ferreira, P.H.; Smeets, R.J. Factors Defining Care-Seeking in Low Back Pain—A Meta-Analysis of Population Based Surveys. *Eur. J. Pain* **2010**, *14*, 747.e1–747.e7. [CrossRef] [PubMed]
6. Gore, M.; Sadosky, A.; Stacey, B.R.; Tai, K.; Leslie, D. The Burden of Chronic Low Back Pain: Clinical Comorbidities, Treatment Patterns, and Health Care Costs in Usual Care Settings. *Spine* **2012**, *37*, E668–E677. [CrossRef] [PubMed]
7. Balague, F.; Mannion, A.F.; Pellise, F.; Cedraschi, C. Non-Specific Low Back Pain. *Lancet* **2012**, *379*, 482–491. [CrossRef]
8. O'Connell, N.E.; Cook, C.E.; Wand, B.M.; Ward, S.P. Clinical Guidelines for Low Back Pain: A Critical Review of Consensus and Inconsistencies across three major guidelines. *Best Pract. Res. Clin. Rheumatol.* **2016**, *30*, 968–980. [CrossRef]
9. Fraenkel, L.; Falzer, P.; Fried, T.; Kohler, M.; Peters, E.; Kerns, R.; Leventhal, H. Measuring Pain Impact Versus Pain Severity Using a Numeric Rating Scale. *J. Gen. Intern. Med.* **2012**, *27*, 555–560. [CrossRef]
10. Turk, D.C.; Fillingim, R.B.; Ohrbach, R.; Patel, K.V. Assessment of Psychosocial and Functional Impact of Chronic Pain. *J. Pain* **2016**, *17*, T21–T49. [CrossRef]
11. Noori, S.A.; Rasheed, A.; Aiyer, R.; Jung, B.; Bansal, N.; Chang, K.; Ottestad, E.; Gulati, A. Therapeutic Ultrasound for Pain Management in Chronic Low Back Pain and Chronic Neck Pain: A Systematic Review. *Pain Med.* **2019**. [CrossRef] [PubMed]
12. Li, Y.; Yin, Y.; Jia, G.; Chen, H.; Yu, L.; Wu, D. Effects of Kinesiotape on Pain and Disability in Individuals with Chronic Low Back Pain: A Systematic Review and Meta-Analysis of Randomized Controlled Trials. *Clin. Rehabil.* **2018**, *33*, 596–606. [CrossRef] [PubMed]
13. Wood, L.; Hendrick, P.A. A Systematic Review and Meta-Analysis of Pain Neuroscience Education for Chronic Low Back Pain: Short-and Long-Term Outcomes of Pain and Disability. *Eur. J. Pain* **2019**, *23*, 234–249. [CrossRef] [PubMed]
14. Resende, L.; Merriwether, E.; Rampazo, E.P.; Dailey, D.; Embree, J.; Deberg, J.; Liebano, R.E.; Sluka, K.A. Meta-Analysis of Transcutaneous Electrical Nerve Stimulation for Relief of Spinal Pain. *Eur. J. Pain* **2018**, *22*, 663–678. [CrossRef] [PubMed]

15. Wu, L.C.; Weng, P.W.; Chen, C.H.; Huang, Y.Y.; Tsuang, Y.H.; Chiang, C.J. Literature Review and Meta-Analysis of Transcutaneous Electrical Nerve Stimulation in Treating Chronic Back Pain. *Reg. Anesth. Pain Med.* **2018**, *43*, 425–433. [CrossRef] [PubMed]
16. Furlan, A.D.; Giraldo, M.; Baskwill, A.; Irvin, E.; Imamura, M. Massage for Low-Back Pain. *Cochrane Database Syst. Rev.* **2015**, *9*, CD001929. [CrossRef] [PubMed]
17. Orrock, P.J.; Myers, S.P. Osteopathic Intervention in Chronic Non-Specific Low Back Pain: A Systematic Review. *BMC Musculoskelet. Disord.* **2013**, *14*, 129. [CrossRef]
18. Rubinstein, S.M.; de Zoete, A.; van Middelkoop, M.; Assendelft, W.J.J.; de Boer, M.R.; van Tulder, M.W. Benefits and Harms of Spinal Manipulative Therapy for the Treatment of Chronic Low Back Pain: Systematic Review and Meta-Analysis of Randomised Controlled Trials. *BMJ* **2019**, *364*, l689. [CrossRef]
19. Hajihasani, A.; Rouhani, M.; Salavati, M.; Hedayati, R.; Kahlaee, A.H. The Influence of Cognitive Behavioral Therapy on Pain, Quality of Life, and Depression in Patients Receiving Physical Therapy for Chronic Low Back Pain: A Systematic Review. *PMR* **2019**, *11*, 167–176. [CrossRef]
20. Zhang, Q.; Jiang, S.; Young, L.; Li, F. The Effectiveness of Group-Based Physiotherapy-Led Behavioral Psychological Interventions on Adults with Chronic Low Back Pain: A Systematic Review and Meta-Analysis. *Am. J. Phys. Med. Rehabil.* **2019**, *98*, 215–225. [CrossRef]
21. Vanti, C.; Andreatta, S.; Borghi, S.; Guccione, A.A.; Pillastrini, P.; Bertozzi, L. The Effectiveness of Walking Versus Exercise on Pain and Function in Chronic Low Back Pain: A Systematic Review and Meta-Analysis of Randomized Trials. *Disabil. Rehabil.* **2019**, *41*, 622–632. [CrossRef]
22. Sitthipornvorakul, E.; Klinsophon, T.; Sihawong, R.; Janwantanakul, P. The Effects of Walking Intervention in Patients with Chronic Low Back Pain: A Meta-Analysis of Randomized Controlled Trials. *Musculoskelet. Sci. Pract.* **2018**, *34*, 38–46. [CrossRef]
23. van Erp, R.M.A.; Huijnen, I.P.J.; Jakobs, M.L.G.; Kleijnen, J.; Smeets, R. Effectiveness of Primary Care Interventions Using a Biopsychosocial Approach in Chronic Low Back Pain: A Systematic Review. *Pain Pract.* **2019**, *19*, 224–241. [CrossRef]
24. Wewege, M.A.; Booth, J.; Parmenter, B.J. Aerobic Vs. Resistance Exercise for Chronic Non-Specific Low Back Pain: A Systematic Review and Meta-Analysis. *J. Back Musculoskelet. Rehabil.* **2018**, *31*, 889–899. [CrossRef]
25. Luomajoki, H.A.; Beltran, M.B.B.; Careddu, S.; Bauer, C.M. Effectiveness of Movement Control Exercise on Patients with Non-Specific Low Back Pain and Movement Control Impairment: A Systematic Review and Meta-Analysis. *Musculoskelet. Sci. Pract.* **2018**, *36*, 1–11. [CrossRef]
26. Parreira, P.; Heymans, M.W.; van Tulder, M.W.; Esmail, R.; Koes, B.W.; Poquet, N.; Lin, C.C.; Maher, C.G. Back Schools for Chronic Non-Specific Low Back Pain. *Cochrane Database Syst. Rev.* **2017**, *8*, CD011674. [CrossRef]
27. Du, S.; Hu, L.; Dong, J.; Xu, G.; Chen, X.; Jin, S.; Zhang, H.; Yin, H. Self-Management Program for Chronic Low Back Pain: A Systematic Review and Meta-Analysis. *Patient Educ. Couns.* **2017**, *100*, 37–49. [CrossRef]
28. López-de-Uralde-Villanueva, I.; Muñoz-García, D.; Gil-Martínez, A.; Pardo-Montero, J.; Muñoz-Plata, R.; Angulo-Díaz-Parreño, S.; Gómez-Martínez, M.; la Touche, R. A Systematic Review and Meta-Analysis on the Effectiveness of Graded Activity and Graded Exposure for Chronic Nonspecific Low Back Pain. *Pain Med.* **2016**, *17*, 172–188. [CrossRef]
29. Saragiotto, B.T.; Maher, C.G.; Yamato, T.P.; Costa, L.O.; Costa, L.C.; Ostelo, R.W.; Macedo, L.G. Motor Control Exercise for Nonspecific Low Back Pain: A Cochrane Review. *Spine* **2016**, *41*, 1284–1295. [CrossRef]
30. Kalin, S.; Rausch-Osthoff, A.K.; Bauer, C.M. What Is the Effect of Sensory Discrimination Training on Chronic Low Back Pain? A Systematic Review. *BMC Musculoskelet. Disord.* **2016**, *17*, 143. [CrossRef]
31. Yamato, T.P.; Maher, C.G.; Saragiotto, B.T.; Hancock, M.J.; Ostelo, R.W.; Cabral, C.M.; Costa, L.C.; Costa, L.O. Pilates for Low Back Pain: Complete Republication of a Cochrane Review. *Spine* **2016**, *41*, 1013–1021. [CrossRef] [PubMed]
32. Kamper, S.J.; Apeldoorn, A.T.; Chiarotto, A.; Smeets, R.J.; Ostelo, R.W.; Guzman, J.; van Tulder, M.W. Multidisciplinary Biopsychosocial Rehabilitation for Chronic Low Back Pain: Cochrane Systematic Review and Meta-Analysis. *BMJ* **2015**, *350*, h444. [CrossRef] [PubMed]
33. Searle, A.; Spink, M.; Ho, A.; Chuter, V. Exercise Interventions for the Treatment of Chronic Low Back Pain: A Systematic Review and Meta-Analysis of Randomised Controlled Trials. *Clin. Rehabil.* **2015**, *29*, 1155–1167. [CrossRef] [PubMed]

34. McCaskey, M.A.; Schuster-Amft, C.; Wirth, B.; Suica, Z.; de Bruin, E.D. Effects of Proprioceptive Exercises on Pain and Function in Chronic Neck- and Low Back Pain Rehabilitation: A Systematic Literature Review. *BMC Musculoskelet. Disord.* **2014**, *15*, 382. [CrossRef] [PubMed]
35. Yue, Y.S.; Wang, X.D.; Xie, B.; Li, Z.H.; Chen, B.L.; Wang, X.Q.; Zhu, Y. Sling Exercise for Chronic Low Back Pain: A Systematic Review and Meta-Analysis. *PLoS ONE* **2014**, *9*, e99307. [CrossRef]
36. Holtzman, S.; Beggs, R.T. Yoga for Chronic Low Back Pain: A Meta-Analysis of Randomized Controlled Trials. *Pain Res. Manag.* **2013**, *18*, 267–272. [CrossRef] [PubMed]
37. Hoffman, B.M.; Papas, R.K.; Chatkoff, D.K.; Kerns, R.D. Meta-Analysis of Psychological Interventions for Chronic Low Back Pain. *Health Psychol.* **2007**, *26*, 1–9. [CrossRef]
38. Malfliet, A.; Kregel, J.; Meeus, M.; Roussel, N.; Danneels, L.; Cagnie, B.; Dolphens, M.; Nijs, J. Blended Learning Pain Neuroscience Education for People with Chronic Spinal Pain: A Randomized-Controlled Multi-Centre Trial. *Phys. Ther.* **2017**, *98*, 357–358. [CrossRef]
39. Picavet, H.S.J.; Vlaeyen, J.W.S.; Schouten, J.S.A.G. Pain Catastrophizing and Kinesiophobia: Predictors of Chronic Low Back Pain. *Am. J. Epidemiol.* **2002**, *156*, 1028–1034. [CrossRef]
40. National Institute for Health and Care Excellence. *Nice Guidelines: Low Back Pain and Sciatica in over 16s: Assessment and Management*; National Institute for Health and Care Excellence: London, UK, 2016.
41. Van Ittersum, M.W.; Van Wilgen, C.P.; Van der Schans, C.P.; Lambrecht, L.; Groothoff, J.W.; Nijs, J. Written Pain Neuroscience Education in Fibromyalgia: A Multicenter Randomized Controlled Trial. *Pain Pract.* **2013**, *14*, 689–700. [CrossRef]
42. Nijs, J.; Meeus, M. Five Requirements for Effective Pain Neuroscience Education in Physiotherapy Practice. nuzzel.com. 2015. Available online: http://www.paininmotion.be/blog/detail/five-requirements-effective-pain-neuroscience-education-physiotherapy-practice (accessed on 5 May 2019).
43. Bodes Pardo, G.; Girbes, E.L.; Roussel, N.A.; Izquierdo, T.G.; Penick, V.J.; Martin, D.P. Pain Neurophysiology Education and Therapeutic Exercise for Patients with Chronic Low Back Pain: A Single-Blind Randomized Controlled Trial. *Arch. Phys. Med. Rehabil.* **2018**, *99*, 338–347. [CrossRef] [PubMed]
44. Butler, D.S.; Moseley, G.L. *Explain Pain*; Noigroup Publications: Adelaide, Australia, 2003.
45. Van Wilgen, C.P.; Nijs, J. *Pijneducatie—Een Praktische Handleiding Voor (Para)Medici*; Bohn Stafleu van Loghum: Houten, The Netherlands, 2010.
46. Pain in Motion. Tools for Clinical Practice. Available online: http://www.paininmotion.be/education/tools-for-clinical-practice (accessed on 5 May 2019).
47. Rubinstein, S.M.; van Middelkoop, M.; Assendelft, W.J.; de Boer, M.R.; van Tulder, M.W. Spinal Manipulative Therapy for Chronic Low-Back Pain. *Cochrane Database Syst. Rev.* **2011**, *16*, CD008112.
48. O'Keeffe, M.; O'Connell, N.E. Letter to the Editor. Response Letter To: Benefits and Harms of Spinal Manipulative Therapy for the Treatment of Chronic Low Back Pain: Systematic Review and Meta-Analysis of Randomised Controlled Trials. *BMJ* **2019**, *364*, l689.
49. de Oliveira, R.F.; Liebano, R.E.; Lda, C.C.; Rissato, L.L.; Costa, L.O. Immediate Effects of Region-Specific and Non-Region-Specific Spinal Manipulative Therapy in Patients with Chronic Low Back Pain: A Randomized Controlled Trial. *Phys. Ther.* **2013**, *93*, 748–756. [CrossRef] [PubMed]
50. Louw, A.; Nijs, J.; Puentedura, E.J. A Clinical Perspective on a Pain Neuroscience Education Approach to Manual Therapy. *J. Man. Manip. Ther.* **2017**, *25*, 160–168. [CrossRef] [PubMed]
51. Puentedura, E.J.; Flynn, T. Combining Manual Therapy with Pain Neuroscience Education in the Treatment of Chronic Low Back Pain: A Narrative Review of the Literature. *Physiother. Theory Pract.* **2016**, *32*, 408–414. [CrossRef] [PubMed]
52. Bialosky, J.E.; George, S.Z.; Bishop, M.D. How Spinal Manipulative Therapy Works: Why Ask Why? *J. Orthop. Sports Phys. Ther.* **2008**, *38*, 293–295. [CrossRef]
53. Nijs, J.; Roussel, N.; van Wilgen, C.P.; Koke, A.; Smeets, R. Thinking Beyond Muscles and Joints: Therapists' and Patients' Attitudes and Beliefs Regarding Chronic Musculoskeletal Pain Are Key to Applying Effective Treatment. *Man. Ther.* **2013**, *18*, 96–102. [CrossRef]
54. Lluch Girbes, E.; Meeus, M.; Baert, I.; Nijs, J. Balancing "Hands-on" with "Hands-Off" Physical Therapy Interventions for the Treatment of Central Sensitization Pain in Osteoarthritis. *Man. Ther.* **2015**, *20*, 349–352. [CrossRef]
55. Naugle, K.M.; Fillingim, R.B.; Riley, J.L., III. A Meta-Analytic Review of the Hypoalgesic Effects of Exercise. *J. Pain* **2012**, *13*, 1139–1150. [CrossRef]

56. Steiger, F.; Wirth, B.; de Bruin, E.D.; Mannion, A.F. Is a Positive Clinical Outcome after Exercise Therapy for Chronic Non-Specific Low Back Pain Contingent Upon a Corresponding Improvement in the Targeted Aspect(S) of Performance? A Systematic Review. *Eur. Spine J.* **2012**, *21*, 575–598. [CrossRef] [PubMed]
57. Booth, J.; Moseley, G.L.; Schiltenwolf, M.; Cashin, A.; Davies, M.; Hubscher, M. Exercise for Chronic Musculoskeletal Pain: A Biopsychosocial Approach. *Musculoskelet. Care* **2017**, *15*, 413–421. [CrossRef] [PubMed]
58. Walti, P.; Kool, J.; Luomajoki, H. Short-Term Effect on Pain and Function of Neurophysiological Education and Sensorimotor Retraining Compared to Usual Physiotherapy in Patients with Chronic or Recurrent Non-Specific Low Back Pain, a Pilot Randomized Controlled Trial. *BMC Musculoskelet. Disord.* **2015**, *16*, 83. [CrossRef] [PubMed]
59. Vibe Fersum, K.; O'Sullivan, P.; Skouen, J.S.; Smith, A.; Kvale, A. Efficacy of Classification-Based Cognitive Functional Therapy in Patients with Non-Specific Chronic Low Back Pain: A Randomized Controlled Trial. *Eur. J. Pain* **2013**, *17*, 916–928. [CrossRef] [PubMed]
60. Von Korff, M.; Balderson, B.H.; Saunders, K.; Miglioretti, D.L.; Lin, E.H.; Berry, S.; Moore, J.E.; Turner, J.A. A Trial of an Activating Intervention for Chronic Back Pain in Primary Care and Physical Therapy Settings. *Pain* **2005**, *113*, 323–330. [CrossRef] [PubMed]
61. Linton, S.J.; Boersma, K.; Jansson, M.; Svard, L.; Botvalde, M. The Effects of Cognitive-Behavioral and Physical Therapy Preventive Interventions on Pain-Related Sick Leave: A Randomized Controlled Trial. *Clin. J. Pain* **2005**, *21*, 109–119. [CrossRef] [PubMed]
62. Monticone, M.; Ferrante, S.; Rocca, B.; Baiardi, P.; Farra, F.D.; Foti, C. Effect of a Long-Lasting Multidisciplinary Program on Disability and Fear-Avoidance Behaviors in Patients with Chronic Low Back Pain: Results of a Randomized Controlled Trial. *Clin. J. Pain* **2013**, *29*, 929–938. [CrossRef]
63. Lambeek, L.C.; van Mechelen, W.; Knol, D.L.; Loisel, P.; Anema, J.R. Randomised Controlled Trial of Integrated Care to Reduce Disability from Chronic Low Back Pain in Working and Private Life. *BMJ* **2010**, *340*, c1035. [CrossRef]
64. Nicholas, M.K.; Wilson, P.H.; Goyen, J. Operant-Behavioural and Cognitive-Behavioural Treatment for Chronic Low Back Pain. *Behav. Res. Ther.* **1991**, *29*, 225–238. [CrossRef]
65. Strand, L.I.; Ljunggren, A.E.; Haldorsen, E.M.; Espehaug, B. The Impact of Physical Function and Pain on Work Status at 1-Year Follow-up in Patients with Back Pain. *Spine* **2001**, *26*, 800–808. [CrossRef]
66. Roche, G.; Ponthieux, A.; Parot-Shinkel, E.; Jousset, N.; Bontoux, L.; Dubus, V.; Penneau-Fontbonne, D.; Roquelaure, Y.; Legrand, E.; Colin, D.; et al. Comparison of a Functional Restoration Program with Active Individual Physical Therapy for Patients with Chronic Low Back Pain: A Randomized Controlled Trial. *Arch. Phys. Med. Rehabil.* **2007**, *88*, 1229–1235. [CrossRef]
67. Roche-Leboucher, G.; Petit-Lemanac'h, A.; Bontoux, L.; Dubus-Bausiere, V.; Parot-Shinkel, E.; Fanello, S.; Penneau-Fontbonne, D.; Fouquet, N.; Legrand, E.; Roquelaure, Y.; et al. Multidisciplinary Intensive Functional Restoration Versus Outpatient Active Physiotherapy in Chronic Low Back Pain: A Randomized Controlled Trial. *Spine* **2011**, *36*, 2235–2242. [CrossRef]
68. Bendix, A.F.; Bendix, T.; Hæstrup, C.; Busch, E. A Prospective, Randomized 5-Year Follow-up Study of Functional Restoration in Chronic Low Back Pain Patients. *Eur. Spine J.* **1998**, *7*, 111–119. [CrossRef]
69. Bendix, A.F.; Bendix, T.; Ostenfeld, S.; Bush, E.; Andersen, A. Active Treatment Programs for Patients with Chronic Low Back Pain: A Prospective, Randomized, Observer-Blinded Study. *Eur. Spine J.* **1995**, *4*, 148–152. [CrossRef]
70. Kool, J.; Bachmann, S.; Oesch, P.; Knuesel, O.; Ambergen, T.; de Bie, R.; van den Brandt, P. Function-Centered Rehabilitation Increases Work Days in Patients with Nonacute Nonspecific Low Back Pain: 1-Year Results from a Randomized Controlled Trial. *Arch. Phys. Med. Rehabil.* **2007**, *88*, 1089–1094. [CrossRef]
71. Streilbelt, M.; Thren, K.; Muller-Fahrnow, W. Effects of Fce-Based Multidisciplinary Rehabilitation in Patients with Chronic Musculoskeletal Disorders—Results of a Randomized Controlled Trial. *Physikalische Medizin Rehabilitationsmedizin Kurortmedizin* **2009**, *19*, 34–41.
72. Sletten, C.D.; Kurklinsky, S.; Chinburapa, V.; Ghazi, S. Economic Analysis of a Comprehensive Pain Rehabilitation Program: A Collaboration between Florida Blue and Mayo Clinic Florida. *Pain Med.* **2015**, *16*, 898–904. [CrossRef]
73. Evans, J.R.; Benore, E.; Banez, G.A. The Cost-Effectiveness of Intensive Interdisciplinary Pediatric Chronic Pain Rehabilitation. *J. Pediatr. Psychol.* **2015**, *41*, 849–856. [CrossRef]

74. Gatchel, R.J.; McGeary, D.D.; McGeary, C.A.; Lippe, B. Interdisciplinary Chronic Pain Management: Past, Present, and Future. *Am. Psychol.* **2014**, *69*, 119–130. [CrossRef]
75. Malfliet, A.; Kregel, J.; Coppieters, I.; de Pauw, R.; Meeus, M.; Roussel, N.; Cagnie, B.; Danneels, L.; Nijs, J. Effect of Pain Neuroscience Education Combined with Cognition-Targeted Motor Control Training on Chronic Spinal Pain: A Randomized Clinical Trial. *JAMA Neurol.* **2018**, *75*, 808–817. [CrossRef]
76. Malfliet, A.; Kregel, J.; Meeus, M.; Cagnie, B.; Roussel, N.; Dolphens, M.; Danneels, L.; Nijs, J. Applying Contemporary Neuroscience in Exercise Interventions for Chronic Spinal Pain: Treatment Protocol. *Braz. J. Phys. Ther.* **2017**, *21*, 378–387. [CrossRef]
77. Woods, M.P.; Asmundson, G.J. Evaluating the Efficacy of Graded in Vivo Exposure for the Treatment of Fear in Patients with Chronic Back Pain: A Randomized Controlled Clinical Trial. *Pain* **2008**, *136*, 271–280. [CrossRef]
78. Vlaeyen, J.W.; de Jong, J.; Geilen, M.; Heuts, P.H.; van Breukelen, G. The Treatment of Fear of Movement/(Re)Injury in Chronic Low Back Pain: Further Evidence on the Effectiveness of Exposure in Vivo. *Clin. J. Pain* **2002**, *18*, 251–261. [CrossRef]
79. Tully, M.A.; Cupples, M.E.; Hart, N.D.; McEneny, J.; McGlade, K.J.; Chan, W.S.; Young, I.S. Randomised Controlled Trial of Home-Based Walking Programmes at and Below Current Recommended Levels of Exercise in Sedentary Adults. *J. Epidemiol. Community Health* **2007**, *61*, 778–783. [CrossRef]
80. Tschentscher, M.; Niederseer, D.; Niebauer, J. Health Benefits of Nordic Walking: A Systematic Review. *Am. J. Prev. Med.* **2013**, *44*, 76–84. [CrossRef]
81. Chetty, L. A Critical Review of Low Back Pain Guidelines. *Workplace Health Saf.* **2017**, *65*, 388–394. [CrossRef]
82. Bekkering, G.E.; Hendriks, E.; Koes, B.; Oostendorp, R.A.B.; Rwjg, O.; Jmc, T.; Tulder, M. Dutch Physiotherapy Guidelines for Low Back Pain. *Physiotherapy* **2003**, *89*, 82–96. [CrossRef]
83. Australian Acute Musculoskeletal Pain Guidelines Group. *Evidencebased Management of Acute Musculoskeletal Pain*; Australian Academic Press: Brisbane, Australia, 2004.
84. van Tulder, M.; Becker, A.; Bekkering, T.; Breen, A.; del Real, M.T.; Hutchinson, A.; Koes, B.; Laerum, E.; Malmivaara, A. Chapter 3. European Guidelines for the Management of Acute Nonspecific Low Back Pain in Primary Care. *Eur. Spine J.* **2006**, *15*, S169–S191. [CrossRef]
85. Qaseem, A.; Wilt, T.J.; McLean, R.M.; Forciea, M.A. Noninvasive Treatments for Acute, Subacute, and Chronic Low Back Pain: A Clinical Practice Guideline from the American College of Physicians. *Ann. Intern. Med.* **2017**, *166*, 514–530. [CrossRef]
86. Wong, J.J.; Cote, P.; Sutton, D.A.; Randhawa, K.; Yu, H.; Varatharajan, S.; Goldgrub, R.; Nordin, M.; Gross, D.P.; Shearer, H.M.; et al. Clinical Practice Guidelines for the Noninvasive Management of Low Back Pain: A Systematic Review by the Ontario Protocol for Traffic Injury Management (Optima) Collaboration. *Eur. J. Pain* **2016**, *21*, 201–216. [CrossRef]
87. White, N.T.; Delitto, A.; Manal, T.J.; Miller, S. The American Physical Therapy Association's Top Five Choosing Wisely Recommendations. *Phys. Ther.* **2015**, *95*, 9–24. [CrossRef]
88. Morin, C.M.; Gibson, D.; Wade, J. Self-Reported Sleep and Mood Disturbance in Chronic Pain Patients. *Clin. J. Pain* **1998**, *14*, 311–314. [CrossRef]
89. Finan, P.H.; Goodin, B.R.; Smith, M.T. The Association of Sleep and Pain: An Update and a Path Forward. *J. Pain* **2013**, *14*, 1539–1552. [CrossRef]
90. Finan, P.H.; Smith, M.T. The Comorbidity of Insomnia, Chronic Pain, and Depression: Dopamine as a Putative Mechanism. *Sleep Med. Rev.* **2013**, *17*, 173–183. [CrossRef]
91. Van Hecke, O.; Torrance, N.; Smith, B.H. Chronic Pain Epidemiology—Where Do Lifestyle Factors Fit In? *Br. J. Pain* **2013**, *7*, 209–217. [CrossRef]
92. Abdallah, C.G.; Geha, P. Chronic Pain and Chronic Stress: Two Sides of the Same Coin? *Chronic Stress* **2017**, *1*. [CrossRef]
93. Cherkin, D.C.; Sherman, K.J.; Balderson, B.H.; Cook, A.J.; Anderson, M.L.; Hawkes, R.J.; Hansen, K.E.; Turner, J.A. Effect of Mindfulness-Based Stress Reduction Vs Cognitive Behavioral Therapy or Usual Care on Back Pain and Functional Limitations in Adults with Chronic Low Back Pain: A Randomized Clinical Trial. *JAMA* **2016**, *315*, 1240–1249. [CrossRef]
94. Tang, N.K.Y.; Wright, K.J.; Salkovskis, P.M. Prevalence and Correlates of Clinical Insomnia Co-Occurring with Chronic Back Pain. *J. Sleep Res.* **2007**, *16*, 85–95. [CrossRef]

95. Denis, D.; Akhtar, R.; Holding, B.C.; Murray, C.; Panatti, J.; Claridge, G.; Sadeh, A.; Barclay, N.L.; O'Leary, R.; Maughan, B.; et al. Externalizing Behaviors and Callous-Unemotional Traits: Different Associations with Sleep Quality. *Sleep* **2017**, *40*, zsx070. [CrossRef]
96. Nakamura, M.; Nagamine, T. Neuroendocrine, Autonomic, and Metabolic Responses to an Orexin Antagonist, Suvorexant, in Psychiatric Patients with Insomnia. *Innov. Clin. Neurosci.* **2017**, *14*, 30–37.
97. Kim, E.J.; Dimsdale, J.E. The Effect of Psychosocial Stress on Sleep: A Review of Polysomnographic Evidence. *Behav. Sleep Med.* **2007**, *5*, 256–278. [CrossRef]
98. Jungquist, C.R.; O'Brien, C.; Matteson-Rusby, S.; Smith, M.T.; Pigeon, W.R.; Xia, Y.; Lu, N.; Perlis, M.L. The Efficacy of Cognitive-Behavioral Therapy for Insomnia in Patients with Chronic Pain. *Sleep Med.* **2010**, *11*, 302–309. [CrossRef]
99. Pigeon, W.R.; Moynihan, J.; Matteson-Rusby, S.; Jungquist, C.R.; Xia, Y.; Tu, X.; Perlis, M.L. Comparative Effectiveness of Cbt Interventions for Co-Morbid Chronic Pain & Insomnia: A Pilot Study. *Behav. Res. Ther.* **2012**, *50*, 685–689.
100. Tang, N.K.Y.; Sanborn, A.N. Better Quality Sleep Promotes Daytime Physical Activity in Patients with Chronic Pain? A Multilevel Analysis of the within-Person Relationship. *PLoS ONE* **2014**, *9*, e92158. [CrossRef]
101. Vismara, L.; Menegoni, F.; Zaina, F.; Galli, M.; Negrini, S.; Capodaglio, P. Effect of Obesity and Low Back Pain on Spinal Mobility: A Cross Sectional Study in Women. *J. Neuroeng. Rehabil.* **2010**, *7*, 3. [CrossRef]
102. Shiri, R.; Karppinen, J.; Leino-Arjas, P.; Solovieva, S.; Viikari-Juntura, E. The Association between Obesity and Low Back Pain: A Meta-Analysis. *Am. J. Epidemiol.* **2010**, *171*, 135–154. [CrossRef]
103. Hershkovich, O.; Friedlander, A.; Gordon, B.; Arzi, H.; Derazne, E.; Tzur, D.; Shamis, A.; Afek, A. Associations of Body Mass Index and Body Height with Low Back Pain in 829,791 Adolescents. *Am. J. Epidemiol.* **2013**, *178*, 603–609. [CrossRef]
104. Paulis, W.D.; Silva, S.; Koes, B.W.; van Middelkoop, M. Overweight and Obesity Are Associated with Musculoskeletal Complaints as Early as Childhood: A Systematic Review. *Obes. Rev.* **2014**, *15*, 52–67. [CrossRef]
105. Zhang, T.T.; Liu, Z.; Liu, Y.L.; Zhao, J.J.; Liu, D.W.; Tian, Q.B. Obesity as a Risk Factor for Low Back Pain: A Meta-Analysis. *Clin. Spine Surg.* **2018**, *31*, 22–27. [CrossRef]
106. Hussain, S.M.; Urquhart, D.M.; Wang, Y.; Shaw, J.E.; Magliano, D.J.; Wluka, A.E.; Cicuttini, F.M. Fat Mass and Fat Distribution Are Associated with Low Back Pain Intensity and Disability: Results from a Cohort Study. *Arthritis Res. Ther.* **2017**, *19*, 26. [CrossRef]
107. Dario, A.B.; Ferreira, M.L.; Refshauge, K.; Sanchez-Romera, J.F.; Luque-Suarez, A.; Hopper, J.L.; Ordonana, J.R.; Ferreira, P.H. Are Obesity and Body Fat Distribution Associated with Low Back Pain in Women? A Population-Based Study of 1128 Spanish Twins. *Eur. Spine J.* **2016**, *25*, 1188–1195. [CrossRef]
108. Williams, A.; Wiggers, J.; O'Brien, K.M.; Wolfenden, L.; Yoong, S.; Campbell, E.; Robson, E.; McAuley, J.; Haskins, R.; Kamper, S.J.; et al. A Randomised Controlled Trial of a Lifestyle Behavioural Intervention for Patients with Low Back Pain, Who Are Overweight or Obese: Study Protocol. *BMC Musculoskelet. Disord.* **2016**, *17*, 70. [CrossRef]
109. Roffey, D.M.; Ashdown, L.C.; Dornan, H.D.; Creech, M.J.; Dagenais, S.; Dent, R.M.; Wai, E.K. Pilot Evaluation of a Multidisciplinary, Medically Supervised, Nonsurgical Weight Loss Program on the Severity of Low Back Pain in Obese Adults. *Spine J.* **2011**, *11*, 197–204. [CrossRef]
110. Donnelly, J.E.; Blair, S.N.; Jakicic, J.M.; Manore, M.M.; Rankin, J.W.; Smith, B.K. American College of Sports Medicine Position Stand. Appropriate Physical Activity Intervention Strategies for Weight Loss and Prevention of Weight Regain for Adults. *Med. Sci. Sports Exerc.* **2009**, *41*, 459–471. [CrossRef]
111. Wijma, A.J.; Bletterman, A.N.; Clark, J.R.; Vervoort, S.; Beetsma, A.; Keizer, D.; Nijs, J.; van Wilgen, C.P. Patient-Centeredness in Physiotherapy: What Does It Entail? A Systematic Review of Qualitative Studies. *Physiother Theory Pract.* **2017**, *33*, 825–840. [CrossRef]
112. Perez, R.B.; Dixon, S.; Culver, S.; Sletten, C.D. Intensive Interdisciplinary Treatment for a Patient with Coexisting Pain and Obesity: A Case Study. *Obes. Res. Clin. Pract.* **2018**, *12*, 397–400. [CrossRef]
113. Michie, S.; Richardson, M.; Johnston, M.; Abraham, C.; Francis, J.; Hardeman, W.; Eccles, M.P.; Cane, J.; Wood, C.E. The Behavior Change Technique Taxonomy (V1) of 93 Hierarchically Clustered Techniques: Building an International Consensus for the Reporting of Behavior Change Interventions. *Ann. Behav. Med.* **2013**, *46*, 81–95. [CrossRef]

114. Briggs, A.M.; Jordan, J.E.; O'Sullivan, P.B.; Buchbinder, R.; Burnett, A.F.; Osborne, R.H.; Straker, L.M. Individuals with Chronic Low Back Pain Have Greater Difficulty in Engaging in Positive Lifestyle Behaviours Than Those without Back Pain: An Assessment of Health Literacy. *BMC Musculoskelet. Disord.* **2011**, *12*, 161. [CrossRef]
115. Lee, H.; Wiggers, J.; Kamper, S.J.; Williams, A.; O'Brien, K.M.; Hodder, R.K.; Wolfenden, L.; Yoong, S.L.; Campbell, E.; Haskins, R.; et al. Mechanism Evaluation of a Lifestyle Intervention for Patients with Musculoskeletal Pain Who Are Overweight or Obese: Protocol for a Causal Mediation Analysis. *BMJ Open* **2017**, *7*, e014652. [CrossRef]
116. Miles, C.L.; Pincus, T.; Carnes, D.; Homer, K.E.; Taylor, S.J.; Bremner, S.A.; Rahman, A.; Underwood, M. Can We Identify How Programmes Aimed at Promoting Self-Management in Musculoskeletal Pain Work and Who Benefits? A Systematic Review of Sub-Group Analysis within Rcts. *Eur. J. Pain* **2011**, *15*, 775.e1–775.e11.
117. Kores, R.C.; Murphy, W.D.; Rosenthal, T.L.; Elias, D.B.; North, W.C. Predicting Outcome of Chronic Pain Treatment Via a Modified Self-Efficacy Scale. *Behav. Res. Ther.* **1990**, *28*, 165–169. [CrossRef]

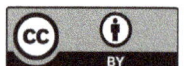

© 2019 by the authors. Licensee MDPI, Basel, Switzerland. This article is an open access article distributed under the terms and conditions of the Creative Commons Attribution (CC BY) license (http://creativecommons.org/licenses/by/4.0/).

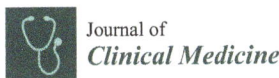

Review

Best Evidence Rehabilitation for Chronic Pain Part 4: Neck Pain

Michele Sterling [1,2,3,*], Rutger M. J. de Zoete [1,2], Iris Coppieters [4,5] and Scott F. Farrell [1,2,3]

1. RECOVER Injury Research Centre, The University of Queensland, 4006 Brisbane, Australia
2. NHMRC Centre of Research Excellence in Road Traffic Injury Recovery, The University of Queensland, 4006 Brisbane, Australia
3. Menzies Health Institute Queensland, Griffith University, 4222 Gold Coast, Australia
4. Pain in Motion International Research Group, Department of Physiotherapy, Human Physiology and Anatomy, Faculty of Physical Education & Physiotherapy, Vrije Universiteit Brussel, 1090 Brussels, Belgium
5. Department of Rehabilitation Sciences and Physiotherapy, Faculty of Medicine and Health Sciences, Ghent University, 9000 Ghent, Belgium
* Correspondence: m.sterling@uq.edu.au

Received: 16 July 2019; Accepted: 8 August 2019; Published: 15 August 2019

Abstract: Neck pain, whether from a traumatic event such as a motor vehicle crash or of a non-traumatic nature, is a leading cause of worldwide disability. This narrative review evaluated the evidence from systematic reviews, recent randomised controlled trials, clinical practice guidelines, and other relevant studies for the effects of rehabilitation approaches for chronic neck pain. Rehabilitation was defined as the aim to restore a person to health or normal life through training and therapy and as such, passive interventions applied in isolation were not considered. The results of this review found that the strongest treatment effects to date are those associated with exercise. Strengthening exercises of the neck and upper quadrant have a moderate effect on neck pain in the short-term. The evidence was of moderate quality at best, indicating that future research will likely change these conclusions. Lower quality evidence and smaller effects were found for other exercise approaches. Other treatments, including education/advice and psychological treatment, showed only very small to small effects, based on low to moderate quality evidence. The review also provided suggestions for promising future directions for clinical practice and research.

Keywords: neck pain; rehabilitation; exercise; psychology review

1. Introduction

The health and economic burdens due to neck and back pain are substantial, being the leading cause of years-lived-with-disability worldwide [1]. The societal burden of these conditions is driven by the fact that many cases do not recover from acute episodes but go on to develop persistent or recurrent pain [2,3]. Neck pain may arise as a consequence of traumatic injury, usually a motor vehicle crash (whiplash associated disorder—WAD) or be of a non-traumatic onset such as occurs in office workers (termed 'non-traumatic neck pain' in this review). Some argue that there is little difference between the two neck pain conditions and have developed classification systems that do not differentiate between them [4]. However, direct comparisons between WAD and non-traumatic neck pain have found the former group report higher levels of pain and disability [5], greater psychological distress [5], more marked hyperalgesia and hypoesthesia indicative of nociplastic pain [6,7], and have worse outcomes at follow-up [8]. These findings suggest that different mechanisms may underlie WAD and non-traumatic neck pain and subsequently different classification systems and treatments may be necessary depending on the patient presentation.

The aim of this review is a state-of-the-art overview of the best evidence rehabilitation for patients with neck pain. The best evidence rehabilitation is reviewed in a way that clinicians can integrate the evidence into their daily clinical routine. In addition, the state-of-the-art overview also serves clinical researchers to build upon the best evidence for designing future trials, implementation studies, and to develop new innovative studies.

2. State-of-the-Art

For this best evidence review, rehabilitation was defined as aiming to restore a person with neck pain to health or normal life through training and therapy (Oxford dictionary definition). It will include a review of active non-interventional treatments such as exercise, psychology, and multimodal approaches. Interventional procedures (e.g., radio-frequency neurotomy), pharmaceutical treatment, and passive treatments—such as acupuncture or manual therapy alone and not used in conjunction with more active treatments—will not be included. For this review, a non-systematic search of scientific studies was performed in MEDLINE (PubMed), Scopus, CINAHL, and Pedro using the following search terms: chronic neck pain, neck pain, whiplash associated disorders, rehabilitation, exercise. To minimize selection bias and to ensure high quality evidence was selected, systematic reviews and meta-analyses were preferred and sought where possible. Recent high quality randomised clinical trials (RCTs) not already included in systematic reviews were included as well as information from large population-based cohorts and international clinical guidelines. High quality trials were defined as those receiving a Pedro score of 6/10 or greater and Pedro scores are provided for each trial included in this review. Both WAD and non-traumatic neck pain were included with the aim of separating the results for both neck pain groups where possible. This review did not include cervical radiculopathy.

A summary of the results are provided in Table 1.

Table 1. Best evidence summary—systematic reviews and RCTs if conducted after publication of a relevant systematic review.

Intervention	Target Population	Level of Evidence	Quality of Evidence	Effect Size	Site of Care	Rehabilitation Professions	Key References and/or Treatment Manuals
Reassurance, advice, education							
Video in ED focussing on activation	WAD (n = 348)	Level I [9]	Moderate	Small effect compared to no treatment at intermediate follow-up, RR 0.79 (0.59 to 1.06), NNT:23	ED	All	See systematic review
WAD information pamphlet	WAD (n = 102)	Level I [9]	Low	No effect compared to generic advice	ED	All	See systematic review
Booklet or email	NTNP (n = 64)	Level 1 [10]	Moderate	No effect compared to massage or exercise	Primary	All	See systematic review
Booklet/neck school	NTNP (n = 411)	Level 1 [11]	Very low to low	No effect	Primary and secondary	All	
Exercise							
Strengthening (upper quarter)	WAD and NTNP (n = 241)	Level 1 [12]	Moderate	Moderate to large at short-term follow-up, SMD (pain) −0.71 (−1.33 to −0.10)	Primary and secondary	Exercise professionals	See systematic review
	Office workers with neck pain (n = 605)	Level 1 [13]	Moderate	Moderate effect vs. no intervention, SMD pain = 0.59 (0.29 to 0.89)	Workplace		
Endurance training (upper quarter)	WAD and NTNP (n = 198)	Level 1 [12]	Moderate	Small at short-term follow-up	Primary and secondary	Physiotherapists	See systematic review
Muscle control (stabilisation)	WAD and NTNP (n = 71)	Level 1 [12]	Moderate	Small at intermediate-term follow-up Small to moderate effect on pain in the short to intermediate term (SMD pain −0.59 (95% CI: −0.97 to −0.20))	Primary and secondary	Physiotherapists	See systematic review
	NTNP (n = 174)	Level 1 [14]	Low to moderate	Small effect on disability (SMD disability −0.44 (95% CI: −0.81 to −0.08) vs. other treatments	Primary and secondary	Physiotherapists	
Stretching (neck & shoulder)	Workers (n = 96)	Level II [15]	Pedro (8/10)	Small effect on pain & disability compared to ergonomic advice (−1.4; 95% CI −2.2 to −0.7 for pain; −4.8; 95% CI −9.3 to −0.4 for disability)	Work place	Exercise professionals	Exercise protocol available at [15]

Table 1. Cont.

Intervention	Target Population	Level of Evidence	Quality of Evidence	Effect Size	Site of Care	Rehabilitation Professions	Key References and/or Treatment Manuals
Eye-neck co-ordination/proprioception	WAD & NTNP (n = 103)	Level I [16]	Very low	Small effect on pain MD: −1.6 (−3.6 to 0.3) compared to no exercise Meta-analysis for other outcomes could not be conducted	Primary and Secondary	Physiotherapists	See systematic review
Qigong	WAD and NTNP (n = 191)	Level I [12]	Moderate	Small at intermediate-term follow-up	Primary and secondary	Exercise professionals	See systematic review
Yoga	NTNP (n = 686)	Level I * (high heterogeneity) [17]	Moderate	Moderate effect on pain and disability vs. various other treatments including exercise, SMD pain = −1.13 (−1.60 to −0.66), SMD disability −0.92 (−1.38 to 0.47)	Primary and secondary	Exercise professionals	See systematic review
General exercise	WAD, NTNP, workers (n = 386)	Level I [13,18]		No effect	Primary and secondary	Exercise professionals	See systematic review
Psychological treatments alone (CBT)	WAD and NTNP (n = 168)	Level I [19]	Very low to moderate	Small effect on pain and disability when compared to no treatment, SMD pain = −0.58 (−1.01 to −0.16), SMD disability = −0.61 (−1.21 to −0.01)	Primary and secondary	Psychology professionals	See systematic review
Combined psychological and physical treatments delivered by physiotherapists	WAD (n = 211)	Level I * (high heterogeneity) [20]	Moderate quality	No effect on pain and disability Medium effect on fear of avoidance	Primary	Physiotherapists	See systematic review
	Acute WAD (n = 108)	Level II [RCT] [21]	NA Pedro (8/10)	Medium to large effect on pain related disability compared to exercise only		Physiotherapists	Treatment protocols available at [21]
Physiotherapist manual therapy	WAD and NTNP (n = 345)	Level I [22]		No effect compared to exercise alone	Primary and secondary		

Levels of Evidence were defined as per the Oxford Centre for Evidence Based Medicine [23]. Quality of Evidence as per reported in Systematic reviews or per Pedro scale for RCTs. * Indicates systematic reviews with high heterogeneity indicating caution is required with interpretation of results. WAD: whiplash associated disorders; NTNP: non-traumatic neck pain; ED: emergency department; SMD: standardised mean difference; MD: mean difference; NNT: number needed to treat.

3. Reassurance, Advice, and Education

It is acknowledged that the provision of reassurance, advice, and education are subtly different paradigms, but as they are often difficult to study in isolation, they have been included together for the purposes of this review.

Providing advice and reassurance to the patient with neck pain is the first step in the rehabilitation process and is often the first-line treatment recommended by clinical practice guidelines [24,25]. Currently, there is no clear guidance on the recommended content of reassurance, beyond the message of a favourable prognosis and full recovery [24]. In a recent qualitative study, the views of both patients with WAD and non-traumatic neck pain were sought about the issues that concerned them most. We found that both groups of patients wanted similar kinds of information that were consistent with themes of worry about possible undetected structural damage; distress about difficulty undertaking usual activities; concerns about the future and hardships such as treatment costs and insurance claims [26]. These findings may provide some direction to the nature of reassurance required by patients with neck pain.

Various information and educational approaches including information booklets, websites, and videos have been investigated for their effectiveness in improving outcomes following whiplash injury [9]. This Cochrane review identified three overall themes for patient education: advice on increasing activity, advice focusing on pain and stress coping skills, and workplace ergonomics and advice on self-care strategies. The review found that an educational video of advice in the hospital Emergency Department that focussed on resuming activity was more beneficial in decreasing acute WAD symptoms than no treatment at 24 weeks follow-up (RR 0.79, 95% CI: 0.59 to 1.06) but not at 6 and 52 weeks. The number of patients who must receive this educational video intervention for one to benefit was 23. The results were based on one RCT only. No other educational intervention was found to be effective, including a WAD information pamphlet provided in ED [9]. Later systematic reviews have found that structured patient education alone did not yield large benefits in clinical effectiveness compared with other conservative interventions for patients with WAD or non-traumatic neck pain [10,11].

Recent RCTs not included in the above-mentioned reviews have found similar results. An educational treatment of pain management focusing on understanding/acceptance of pain, goal setting, and participation in social- and work-related contexts was less effective in improving a physical quality of life measure when compared to a multimodal treatment (the same education in addition to exercise) for a mixed traumatic/non-traumatic neck pain sample [27] (Pedro 6/10). A preliminary RCT in a small sample of women with mixed chronic neck pain also found that pain education was less effective when delivered alone than when delivered in conjunction with exercise [28] (Pedro 7/10).

Education directed toward increasing a patient's knowledge of pain neuroscience has gained traction in recent years, mostly in the field of low back pain. Systematic reviews have found that this approach has a small to moderate effect on pain and disability in the short-term immediately following the intervention for patients with low back pain [29]. There is also moderate level evidence that the use of pain neuroscience education alongside other physiotherapy interventions probably improves disability and pain in the short term in chronic low back pain [30]. Pain neuroscience has been less investigated in neck pain, with one preliminary RCT showing potential benefit when combined with exercise for adolescents with non-traumatic neck pain [31] (Pedro 7/10).

Clinical message: Tested educational/advice treatments alone show only small effects for patients with neck pain (WAD and non-traumatic neck pain). Better effects may be seen when educational approaches are used in conjunction with exercise. The optimal content to be included in educational approaches is not known.

4. Exercise

Various types of exercise have been evaluated for their effectiveness in neck pain, including general exercise and activity, neck specific strengthening or control exercises, and sensorimotor exercises. Systematic reviews generally include all exercise types together. A recent comprehensive Cochrane systematic review found no high quality evidence, indicating that there is still uncertainty about the effectiveness of exercise for neck pain [12]. In an attempt to gain clarity around the effectiveness of exercise alone, this review included only trials with single interventions that compared exercise with a control or comparative group. Additionally, the authors used an exercise classification system based on a clinical rationale for selecting studies with similar interventions to assist with interpretation and inclusion within the meta-analyses [12].

Moderate quality evidence supported the use of upper quarter (neck, scapula, and upper limb) strength training to improve pain immediately post treatment with a moderate to large effect (pooled SMD (pain) −0.71 (95% CI: −1.33 to −0.10)) at short-term follow-up. There was also moderate quality evidence to support: (i) upper-quarter endurance training for a small beneficial effect on pain immediately post treatment and short-term follow-up; (ii) neck and shoulder girdle muscle control (stabilisation) exercises to improve pain and function at intermediate term follow-up (MD pain (100 point scale) −14.90 (95% CI: −22.40 to −7.39)); and (iii) Qigong (mindfulness and slow movement exercise) to minimally improve function but not global patient perceived effect in the short term. Low quality evidence suggested that breathing exercises; general fitness training; stretching alone; and vestibular rehabilitation type exercises may not change pain or function at immediate post treatment to short-term follow-up. Very low quality evidence suggested that neuromuscular eye–neck co-ordination/proprioceptive exercises may improve pain and function at short-term follow-up, supporting findings of a previous systematic review [16].

From this review, it should be noted that the best available evidence is at a moderate quality level, meaning that further research is likely to have an important impact on the effect estimate. The review also did not differentiate between WAD and non-traumatic neck pain, but there may well be different responses to exercise (and other treatments) between the two neck pain groups as a consequence of their different clinical presentation and features outlined earlier in this review. A later review found similar results, concluding that supervised qigong, yoga, and combined programs including strengthening, range of motion, and flexibility are effective for the management of persistent neck pain, with no one program superior to another [32]. These authors also noted that effect sizes are small indicating a small clinical benefit of exercise for chronic neck pain [32].

Other systematic reviews have investigated the evidence for one specific exercise type. Exercises to improve control of the cranio-cervical flexion movement were found to have small to moderate effect on pain in the short to intermediate term (SMD pain −0.59 (95% CI: −0.97 to −0.20)) and a small effect on disability (SMD disability −0.44 (95% CI: −0.81 to −0.08)) when compared to other treatments (other exercise, manual therapy) in people with non-traumatic neck pain [14]. However, the meta-analysis revealed high heterogeneity indicating that results should be interpreted with caution. Another systematic review without meta-analysis found that motor control exercises may not be any more effective than a standard strengthening exercise program [33]. Yoga was found to have moderate positive effects on pain (SMD −1.13 (95% CI:−1.60 to −0.66)) and disability (SMD = −0.92 (95% CI: −1.38 to −0.47)) over other treatments (mostly other exercise) for people with chronic non-traumatic neck pain [17] but the results had high heterogeneity, indicating caution is required with interpretation.

Two systematic reviews have evaluated the effect of general exercise and activity for neck pain with both reviews acknowledging the limited number of trials available for inclusion. One review found that there were no clinically meaningful differences between comprehensive exercise programs, which included general exercise, and minimal intervention controls in the medium and long term [18]. A second review including studies of both non-traumatic neck pain and WAD found small effects on pain that were probably not clinically significant [34].

Clinicians may want to understand if one form of exercise is more effective than another. While all systematic reviews note small effects for most exercise types, it has been commonly assumed that there is no difference between them. However, few direct head-to-head comparisons of different exercise types have been undertaken and therefore firm conclusions cannot be drawn. Some data suggest differential effects of exercise type on pain sensitivity. For example, isometric exercise may exert greater hypoalgesic effects than aerobic exercise, at least in the short term [35], so it is possible that further research may show that exercise type has different influences on pain.

Clinical message: Exercise seems to have beneficial effects on neck pain (WAD and non-traumatic neck pain), although high quality evidence is lacking. There is moderate evidence indicating that strengthening exercises of the upper quarter may have a moderate effect on pain, but further research may change this result. At present, there is no data available to show that one form of exercise is more effective than another. There is also no data to indicate the optimal dose or intensity. Until further evidence becomes available, clinicians may want to take patient preference and their clinical expertise with exercise prescription into account when providing an exercise intervention. They should also consider the potential overall health benefits of exercise (particularly aerobic and strengthening exercises).

5. Work Place Neck Pain

Office workers have the highest annual prevalence of neck pain (up to 63% depending on neck pain definition) of all occupations [36]. Neck pain is a recurrent condition with 60–80% of workers reporting a recurrence one year after the initial episode [37]. Ergonomic interventions such as adjustments to the physical work space and equipment are commonly employed, with the aim of reducing physical strain to the musculoskeletal system, thus reducing risk of injury. A recent Cochrane review found inconsistent evidence that the use of an arm support or an alternative mouse may reduce the incidence of neck and should disorders (risk ratio (RR) 0.52 (95% CI: 0.27 to 0.99)). For other physical ergonomic interventions, they found no evidence of an effect and for organisational interventions, such as increased work breaks, very low-quality evidence was found for an effect on the incidence of upper limb pain [38]. Another recent systematic review found low quality evidence that ergonomic programs do not reduce the risk of a new episode of neck pain (OR 1.00 (95% CI: 0.74 to 1.35)) but moderate quality evidence that an exercise program substantially reduces the risk of a new episode of neck pain (OR 0.32 (95% CI: 0.12 to 0.86)) [39]. The latter finding was based on two RCTs, one included aerobic, strengthening, and stretching exercises and the other strengthening and stretching exercises [39].

For workers with neck and/or upper limb pain, another Cochrane review found very low quality evidence that exercise interventions were no more effective than no treatment on pain disability and sick leave [40]. This review also found that ergonomic interventions did not decrease pain in the short term but did decrease pain in the long term (low quality evidence) [40]. An earlier review found moderate quality evidence that a multiple-component intervention (including mental health education, physical health education, relaxation and breaks, activity modifications, and physical environmental modifications) reduced sickness absence in the intermediate-term (OR 0.56 (95% CI: 0.33 to 0.95)) which was not sustained over time but no intervention had an effect on pain [41]. However, a more recent review and meta-analysis concluded that workplace-based strengthening exercises were effective in reducing neck pain in office workers with a larger effect if the exercises were targeted to the neck/shoulder with moderate quality evidence (SMD pain = 0.59 (95% CI 0.29 to 0.89)) [13]. There was a dose–response relationship with greater participation in the exercise being associated with a larger effect [13]. These conclusions were supported by another review that concluded that there is level II evidence recommending that clinicians include strengthening exercise to improve neck pain and quality of life [42]. Recommendations arising from all reviews were that further large high quality clinical trials are needed.

Since the publication of these reviews, several RCTs have investigated various interventions for workplace related neck pain. Neck and shoulder stretching exercise and ergonomic advice improved neck pain and disability to a greater extent than ergonomic advice alone, with small effects (−1.4; 95% CI: −2.2 to −0.7 for visual analogue scale; −4.8; 95% CI: −9.3 to −0.4 for Northwick Park Neck Pain Questionnaire) in workers with at least moderate neck pain (Pedro 8/10) [15]. However, Caputo and colleagues found no difference between a twice-weekly 7-week group-based neck and shoulder resistance exercise programme compared to group-based stretching and postural exercise of the same duration [43] (Pedro 7/10).

Clinical message: Work-place strengthening programs may be effective for office workers with non-traumatic neck pain and for preventing neck pain in asymptomatic workers. Evidence for the effectiveness of ergonomic interventions is inconsistent.

6. Psychological Treatments

Similar to all chronic pain conditions, neck pain is associated with psychological factors such as cognitive distress, anxiety, depressed mood, fear of pain and/or movement [44,45] and in the case of WAD, posttraumatic stress symptoms [45]. Psychological factors likely play a role in the transition from acute to chronic pain [46] and contribute to the extent and severity of pain and disability reported [46]. Treatments directed at psychological factors can decrease pain and disability [47].

Cognitive behavioural therapy (CBT) is one of the most common psychological treatments used in the treatment of chronic pain conditions. CBT works by means of modifying maladaptive and dysfunctional thoughts (e.g., catastrophising, kinesiophobia) and improving mood (e.g., anxiety and depression), leading to gradual changes in cognition and illness behaviour. With respect to neck pain, a recent Cochrane review found the quality of the evidence to be very low to moderate with only six high quality RCTs being available for inclusion [19]. CBT was found to be more effective for short-term pain (SMD pain −0.58 (95% CI: −1.01 to −0.16)) and disability (SMD disability −0.61 (95% CI: −1.21 to −0.01)) reduction only when compared to no treatment. There was moderate quality evidence that CBT was better than other interventions for improving kinesiophobia at intermediate-term follow-up (SMD −0.39 (95% CI: −0.69 to −0.08)). For subacute neck pain, CBT was significantly better than other types of treatment at reducing pain in the short-term (SMD pain −0.24 (95% CI: −0.48 to 0.00)), but there were no effects on disability and kinesiophobia. Looking at psychological treatments more broadly, Shearer and colleagues found no evidence for or against the use of psychological interventions (including relaxation training and CBT) in patients with recent onset neck pain or WAD [48]. For chronic neck pain, they found evidence that a progressive goal attainment program may be helpful.

The results of both systematic reviews illustrate the dearth of clinical trials investigating psychological treatments for neck pain with only 10 RCTs eligible for inclusion. This is in comparison to say low back pain, where systematic reviews have included up to 30 RCTs [49,50].

Clinical message: There is little evidence available to determine if psychological treatments alone are effective for neck pain (WAD and non-traumatic neck pain).

7. Combined Treatments—Physical and Psychological Treatments

Many clinical trials have investigated interventions of mixed treatments and or disciplines. The most recognised of these approaches is multidisciplinary rehabilitation. No systematic reviews for multidisciplinary rehabilitation of chronic neck pain were located. A review of this approach for chronic low back pain found modest positive effects on pain and disability compared to usual care or physical rehabilitation [51].

A more common approach studied in patients with neck pain is to add a psychological treatment to a physiotherapy program with both components delivered by physiotherapists. A recent systematic review and meta-analysis of this combined approach found that, for neck pain and WAD, there was no effect on pain or disability but statistically and probably clinically relevant effects on fear of movement beliefs (SMD −0.5 (95% CI: −0.95 to −0.05)) and pain catastrophizing (SMD −0.31 (95% CI: −0.54 to −0.08)) [20]. However, the meta-analysis revealed high heterogeneity, potentially as the psychological interventions and usual physiotherapy/usual care were not uniform across the included

RCTs. The definition of psychological intervention in this review was kept broad. Studies with larger effects were more closely examined, revealing that these RCTs tended to use individually tailored interventions. In addition, these interventions addressed patients' maladaptive cognition through the use of various cognitive techniques (e.g., identifying and challenging negative thoughts) while aiming to modify patients' maladaptive behaviours and increasing level of activities using a range of behavioural strategies (e.g., breathing and relaxation techniques, goal setting, and graded activities). Furthermore, some of these studies also encouraged patients to participate in the decision making regarding goal settings and treatment. One of these studies included patients with WAD [52], with the other being of patients with low back pain [53].

Since this review, one additional RCT investigating effects of combined psychological/physiotherapy interventions has been published, all with slightly different approaches. A recent RCT (StressModex) showed that a physiotherapist delivered exercise program and a psychological treatment targeting initial stress related symptoms in patients with acute WAD and at high risk of poor recovery, was more effective than exercise alone on pain related disability (primary outcome) (Neck Disability Index at 6 weeks: −10.0 (−15.5 to −4.8); at 6 months: −7.8 (−13.8 to −1.8) and at 12 months: −10.1 (−16.3 to −4.0)) and stress, depression and self-efficacy (secondary outcomes) [21]. The effect size on the primary outcome was moderate to large. The psychological component of the combined intervention was consistent with that outlined in the above systematic review [20]—it was a targeted intervention using cognitive strategies and behavioural strategies. Whilst there has been no direct head to head comparison, the results of StressModex are superior to what has been found for both 'psychologically informed' physiotherapy (MINT trial) [54] and early multidisciplinary care [55] for acute WAD. In both these trials, there was no stratification of patients based on risk to recovery and treating all patients as a homogenous group may dilute any treatment effect. The former trial used less targeted strategies for dealing with psychological factors where the physiotherapists questioned patients to identify treatment targets, such as beliefs about pain and coping strategies. It is possible that the approach used in the MINT trial was too broad and although attempted to address psychosocial factors, lacked the specificity to be effective. StressModex specifically targeted one psychological risk factor and trained physiotherapists in its management as opposed to a more broad approach and this may be a reason for the stronger effects seen. In the latter multidisciplinary trial, patients were less compliant with psychology treatment compared to physiotherapy. Patients in the acute stage of a physical injury may not see the relevance of seeing a psychologist for what they perceive is a physical injury. This may be further justification for an enhanced role of physiotherapists in the management of acute WAD (and other musculoskeletal injuries), with that role including the management of psychological aspects of the condition in addition to physical ones.

With respect to non-traumatic neck pain, few trials have tested a combined physiotherapy/psychological intervention. One RCT of fair quality (Pedro 5/10) found no added benefit of a cognitive behavioural intervention to exercise on disability but clinically meaningful reductions in pain [56].

Taken together, the results of these studies suggest that psychological treatments delivered by physiotherapists may need to be individually targeted (personalized rehabilitation) as opposed to a broad psychologically-informed approach. Further research is required to determine the important and effective components of a physiotherapist-delivered psychological intervention.

Clinical message: Combined psychological and physiotherapy interventions delivered by physiotherapists may be more effective than physiotherapy alone for WAD but these results need further replication. The psychological component may be more effective if it specifically targets individual psychological factors.

8. Combined Treatments—Exercise and Passive Treatments

Manual therapy is a common treatment provided to patients with neck pain. It was not an aim of this review to synthesise evidence for passive treatments used in isolation. However, as manual therapy is often combined with exercise in clinical practice, it is worthwhile to consider if its addition has any greater effects than exercise alone. A systematic review of RCTs including both WAD and non-traumatic neck pain concluded that combined manual therapy and exercise was no more effective than exercise alone in reducing neck pain intensity, neck disability, or improving quality of life [22]. In contrast, Hildago et al. [57] found moderate evidence supporting combined manual therapy and exercise for acute to sub-acute neck pain and moderate to strong evidence for chronic neck pain. In their systematic review, Sutton and colleagues [58] found that multimodal care—including education, exercise, and manual therapy—can benefit patients with WAD and non-traumatic neck pain. They also concluded that there is no additional benefit to providing frequent sessions of multimodal care to patients with neck pain over an extended time period [58].

Clinical message: Adding manual therapy to exercise may be more beneficial than exercise alone, but the evidence is conflicting.

9. Lifestyle Interventions

In recent times, attention has been paid to the potential role of lifestyle factors in the development of chronic musculoskeletal pain. Epidemiological studies have found that higher levels of physical activity are associated with less neck and shoulder pain [59] and physical inactivity and high Body Mass Index are associated with an increased risk of chronic pain in the low back and neck/shoulders in the general adult population [60]. Sleep problems have also been shown to be associated with an increased risk of chronic pain in the low back and neck/shoulders [61]. These data suggest that interventions directed at improving lifestyle factors may be effective for musculoskeletal pain, including neck pain, but few trials have been conducted in this area. Williams and colleagues found that a 6-month telephone-based healthy lifestyle coaching service intervention provided no benefit (primary outcome was pain) over usual care for obese patients with low back pain [62] (Pedro 8/10). The intervention was not successful in changing the targeted lifestyle factors such as weight, physical activity, diet, and sleep and this may explain the lack of effect on pain [62]. No recent trials of lifestyle interventions for neck pain were found but this could be an area of future research.

Clinical message: The effect of lifestyle interventions on chronic neck pain is unknown as no studies have yet been conducted.

10. Patient Stratification and Sub-Grouping

The mostly small effects seen in clinical trials for musculoskeletal pain conditions have led to suggestions that the small effects are due to the heterogeneity of the conditions and their subsequent differential response. In response, there has been much debate about the merits or otherwise of sub-grouping patients which may in turn lead to the identification of the most effective treatment for each sub-group [63]. Some RCTs, using patient sub-grouping, have been conducted in low back pain with limited effects seen [64]. With respect to neck pain, few studies looking at the benefits and effects of patient sub-grouping have been conducted and all have been in WAD. In a preliminary RCT, a neck and shoulder girdle specific exercise program was found to be more effective in patients with chronic WAD and signs of central sensitisation (widespread mechanical and cold hyperalgesia) when compared to those without these features [65] (Pedro 7/10). However, in this trial, the sub-group analyses were not pre-defined and prior sample size calculations did not consider sub-group analyses, indicating that the results should be interpreted with a high degree of caution. In a later trial with a priori sample size calculations that included investigation of the moderating effects of several variables on the outcomes, the results were not replicated [66]. No evidence was found that measures of central sensitisation or psychological variables of posttraumatic stress symptoms moderated the effect of a 12-week exercise intervention in patients with chronic WAD [66]. Similarly, in patients with acute WAD (<4 weeks post injury) providing different treatments based on the individual patient's sensory and psychological presentation provided no better effect than usual care [55]. In this RCT, if patients presented with widespread hyperalgesia and significant psychological distress, they received physiotherapy exercise, medication, and psychological treatment, whereas those without these features received physiotherapy exercise alone. This pragmatic approach using patient sub-grouping was compared to usual care [55]. In summary, sub-grouping patients with WAD based on sensory and psychological measures has not yet been successful.

Another approach has been to stratify patients, usually those with an acute condition, based on their risk of recovery or non-recovery. Again, most research in this area has been in WAD. A clinical prediction rule to identify both chronic moderate/severe disability and full recovery at 12 months post-injury was recently developed [67,68]. The results indicated that an initial Neck Disability Index score of ≥40%, age ≥35 years, and a score of ≥6 on a hyperarousal symptom scale (symptoms of trouble falling asleep, irritability, difficulty concentrating, being overly alert, and easily startled) could accurately predict patients with moderate/severe disability at 12 months. It is also important to predict patients who will recover well as these patients will likely require less intensive intervention. Initial Neck Disability Index scores of ≤32% and age ≤35 years predicted full recovery at 12 months post-injury. Further evaluation of the clinical prediction rule has shown that it performs comparably to the more generic and commonly used Orebro Musculoskeletal Pain Questionnaire (short form) [69] and may have better specificity (unpublished data).

The aim of a prognostic clinical prediction rule is to target treatment toward the identified risk groups. For the whiplash clinical prediction rule, it is proposed that patients identified at low-risk of poor recovery require minimal treatment consisting of advice, reassurance and simple exercises [70]. In contrast, it is suggested that patients identified at high risk of poor recovery will require further assessment of potentially contributory factors including psychological distress, nociceptive processing, and neck movement and strength [70]. Whether or not this risk stratified targeted approach results in better patient outcomes is currently being evaluated with no data yet available.

Clinical message: Risk-stratification may be useful for patients with WAD but further research is required before treatment based on stratification can be recommended.

11. Promising Directions for Clinical Practice

Despite the existence of numerous clinical practice guidelines for non-traumatic neck pain and WAD, most recommendations are based on low to moderate quality evidence or on consensus. Clinicians need to be aware of this situation and while broadly following the clinical guideline recommendations, be astute to the individual patient presentation, and adapt their treatments as required. Nonetheless, it is clear that traditional rehabilitation approaches are not very effective and that a step-change is needed to improve this situation. It is difficult to nominate promising directions for clinical practice, as many areas require further research, so the following two sections overlap to some extent. However, some findings if widely adopted in the clinical arena have the potential for an immediate effect to improve health outcomes. Some of these are outlined.

Risk screening or stratification of patients early in development of their neck pain condition followed by provision of a clinical pathway of care based on the patient's risk of developing chronic/persistent pain. There are several tools available to achieve this—WhipPredict for patients with WAD, the short-form Orebro Musculoskeletal screen for WAD and non-traumatic neck pain, and StartMSK for non-traumatic neck pain (see Table 2 for availability). Research suggests that rehabilitation health care providers are not aware of prognostic indicators and do not use clinical risk screening tools for patients with neck pain [71,72]. The majority of patients will fall into the 'low risk' category; in other words, they should recover well with minimal treatment comprising a few sessions of advice, reassurance, and exercise. Those deemed at 'high risk' require further evaluation including assessment of psychological factors, nociplastic pain, and more complex movement problems that then could be specifically addressed. Whilst this stratified care model and subsequent care pathway is yet to be fully evaluated for neck pain, there has been substantial research of a similar approach for low back pain. Some trials in low back pain show good effect [73] but others have been more equivocal [74]. In this latter trial conducted in the USA, the intervention resulted in use of the STarT Back risk screening tool, but it did not change health care provider treatment decisions. Some reasons for this proposed by the researchers were unacceptability to clinicians, inadequate leadership and system support, ineffective implementation, and inadequate potency [74]. Neck pain researchers should take note of these issues and they could be addressed in risk-stratified neck pain trials.

Table 2. Promising directions for clinical practice.

Treatment Approach	Resources
Risk screening/stratification of patients to determine risk of poor or delayed recovery	• WhipPredict (Whiplash Clinical Prediction Tool) [67,68]. Electronic version available at https://recover.centre.uq.edu.au/research/clinician-resources • Hard copy available on author request • Orebro Musculoskeletal Screening Tool Short-Form [69] Available at https://www.cesphn.org.au/documents/filtered-document-list/204-oerebro-musculoskeletal-pain-screening-questionnaire/file • StartMSK [75]. Available at https://www.keele.ac.uk/startmsk/moreaboutthetool/
Clinical pathways of care based on risk stratification	• Under evaluation. Protocol available at [70]
Development of skills of rehabilitation professionals to integrate some psychological treatments into standard physical rehabilitation	• There are various protocols available but few that are specific to neck pain • The integration of a psychological treatment targeting stress related symptoms in people with acute WAD is available at the following reference [21]
Provide advice and reassurance to patients that is more targeted to their needs	• Preliminary findings of the needs of patients with WAD and neck pain [26,76,77]

The development of more horizontal across discipline (versus vertical siloed uni-discipline) skills for rehabilitation professionals. It is clear that, like all musculoskeletal conditions, neck pain is heterogeneous and the management of particularly the 'high risk' patient group requires skills that cut across various disciplines. An example of cross discipline skills is the utilisation of physiotherapists to deliver psychological type treatments. With respect to the targeting of psychosocial risk factors in high risk patients, it has been previously argued in this review that individual specificity will be required, with preliminary evidence showing a broader approach may not be as effective. If further research supports this tenet, then rehabilitation professionals will need to upskill in the identification and management of psychosocial risk factors. At least anecdotally, there seems to be some resistance to this but the evidence is strong that psychosocial factors pay a role in musculoskeletal outcomes and rehabilitation professionals including physiotherapists are well positioned to deliver care that may be considered outside their traditional realm. One cautionary note. It is not advocated that rehabilitation professionals deliver care to patients with a psychopathology such as severe depression or posttraumatic stress disorders and these patients will need referral to a mental health professional. Rehabilitation professionals will require skills in assessment of patient mental health so that appropriate referral can be initiated. The upskilling of the rehabilitation workforce should commence from early undergraduate training and this may be already happening in some locations but is lagging behind in others [78].

Provide advice and reassurance that is consistent with identified patient needs. Qualitative research has begun to identify the needs of people with neck pain with respect to the information they are seeking and these findings should lay the foundation for future trials. Some of the factors emerging when talking to people with neck pain may not be traditionally included in advice and reassurance delivered by rehabilitation health care providers. An example is concerns around treatment costs and insurance claims reported by patients with WAD [26]. Psychological distress associated with claims processes have been shown to interfere with recovery and quality of life [79]. Providing information to patients regarding these processes may assist recovery. Another example would be information about likely prognosis nominated as important by patients [76], but which health care providers may not usually provide or be uncomfortable with how to deliver this information to patients. We have consistently found that physiotherapists are not well aware of the consistent predictors of poor recovery after whiplash injury [71,80], so may not routinely assess for such factors with the view of gauging prognosis. There are clinical prediction rules available to identify patients both at risk of poor recovery and those that will recover well [67–69] but to date the clinical uptake of these has been slow. This may require more effective knowledge transfer and potentially a cultural change within the physiotherapy profession.

12. Promising Directions for Research

Exercise is the staple approach for most rehabilitation professionals, but further evidence is required to guide this key area of management. The role of exercise in managing neck pain should be clarified including the comparisons of different exercise modalities (strengthening, muscle control, aerobic, and so forth) and dosages. The rationale underpinning the use of exercise is to specifically target underlying physical impairments, which will then impact on pain and disability [81]. However, this assumption has been challenged. In a systematic review for low back pain, little correlation between improvements in clinical outcomes such as pain and disability and improvements in physical function with exercise were found [82]. Similar results were found in a review of neck pain [83] and in a RCT of hip pain [84]. The results of both reviews suggest that improvements in self-reported clinical measures with exercise may be more associated with other factors such as psychological and/or central nervous system responses than by the rectification of specific physical impairments. Certainly, it is clear that exercise exerts central inhibitory effects termed exercise induced hypoalgesia (EIH) [85] and that EIH is impaired in some people with chronic pain including neck pain [35,86]. Further research is required to understand central nervous system responses to exercise in chronic pain and how it may be possible to enhance the EIH response to improve patient outcomes [87].

Physical rehabilitation is not the only treatment approach to show mostly small to moderate effects on outcomes. Psychological treatments for chronic musculoskeletal pain show similar effect sizes despite a large number of clinical trials available [88]. Few trials have investigated psychological treatments for neck pain, but based on the chronic pain literature as a whole, it would be expected that similar small effects would also be found. Interestingly, recent calls have been made from the psychology field to consider the body as well as the brain when considering painful conditions. These authors call this 'embodied pain' defined by the premise that cognition extends beyond the brain so that an ever-changing body is at the core of how experiences are shaped such as by the unconscious workings of the immune system or the collaborative efforts made to avoid movement [89]. Whilst it is very early days, efforts to combine psychological treatment with physical exercise ("body") treatment for neck pain may show greater effects than either treatment alone [21], warranting further investigation.

Many reviews of musculoskeletal pain call for further research to identify who does or does not respond to treatment [90,91]. It would be fair to say that little progress has been made in this direction for any condition including neck pain. To date, clinical trials have not been able to identify factors associated with treatment response. An early under-powered RCT of exercise for chronic WAD reported that patients with cold and mechanical hyperalgesia were less likely to respond to exercise [65], but this result could not be replicated in a larger adequately powered study [66]. Similarly, no trials investigating moderating factors on treatment effect for non-traumatic neck pain were identified. Such knowledge would facilitate more individualized patient care.

The development and testing of innovative methods to include lifestyle interventions for neck pain is needed. It is known that many lifestyle factors are associated with chronic musculoskeletal pain including physical activity [60], sleep [92], smoking [93], stress [94,95], and possibly diet [96]. At the current time, it is not known if addressing these factors will prevent the development of neck pain or the transitions to recovery once an injury has occurred [97].

Other areas requiring research and clinical attention include the development and implementation of modern methods of treatment delivery, in order to enhance access to treatment. Technology assisted methods, such as telehealth, have been successfully used in the rehabilitation of conditions, such as stroke [98] and post orthopaedic surgery [99], and show promise for the delivery of psychological treatment. Such approaches have not been readily taken up in musculoskeletal pain practice, perhaps due to the perception that passive hands-on treatment is required. However, the evidence dictates that passive treatment is not essential for neck pain conditions. Rather, active treatment approaches that improve patient self-efficacy are preferable due the stronger evidence base and these could be delivered in more innovative ways than the traditional face-to-face sessions.

Key messages:

- Strengthening exercises of the neck and upper quadrant have a moderate effect on neck pain in the short-term. This conclusion is based on moderate quality evidence.
- Other exercise approaches demonstrate small effects based mostly on low quality evidence.
- Reassurance/advice/education generally show small effects based on low to moderate quality evidence.
- Psychological treatments alone have small effects based on very low to moderate quality evidence.
- Combined psychological and physical treatments delivered by physiotherapists may be more effective.
- Clinical guidelines are mostly based upon low to moderate quality evidence or consensus, so future research will likely change these conclusions.
- Clinicians should consider the limitations of the evidence regarding rehabilitation for chronic neck pain, and as such broadly follow clinical guidelines; however, adapt treatment to each patient as appropriate.

Finally, and by no means the least important, is that improved understanding of biological processes underlying neck pain is required as this will provide direction for new and innovative treatments. There is evidence available indicating impaired immune responses in WAD and neck arm pain [100], some evidence of quantitative imaging biomarkers [101] and emerging data of genetic variants of stress biomarkers associated with non-recovery after whiplash injury [102].

Author Contributions: M.S. conceived the content, wrote the paper and approved the final version. R.M.J.d.Z. and S.F.F. contributed and approved the final version of the paper. I.C. conceived the design of the paper and approved the final version of the manuscript.

Conflicts of Interest: The authors declare no conflict of interest.

References

1. Hurwitz, E.L.; Randhawa, K.; Yu, H.; Cote, P.; Haldeman, S. The Global Spine Care Initiative: A summary of the global burden of low back and neck pain studies. *Eur. Spine J.* **2018**, *27*, 796–801. [CrossRef] [PubMed]
2. Sterling, M.; Hendrikz, J.; Kenardy, J. Compensation claim lodgement and health outcome developmental trajectories following whiplash injury: A prospective study. *Pain* **2010**, *150*, 22–28. [CrossRef] [PubMed]

3. Carroll, L.J.; Hogg-Johnson, S.; Cote, P.; Van der Velde, G.; Holm, L.W.; Carragee, E.J.; Hurwitz, E.L.; Peloso, P.M.; Cassidy, J.D.; Guzman, J.; et al. Course and prognostic factors for neck pain in workers: Results of the Bone and Joint Decade 2000–2010 Task Force on Neck Pain and Its Associated Disorders. *Spine* **2008**, *33*, S93–S100. [CrossRef] [PubMed]
4. Haldeman, S.; Carroll, L.; Cassidy, D.; Schubert, J.; Nygren, A. The Bone and Joint Decade 2000–2010 Task Force on Neck Pain and Its Associated Disorders Executive Summary. *Spine* **2008**, *33*, S5–S7. [CrossRef] [PubMed]
5. Ris, I.; Juul-Kristensen, B.; Boyle, E.; Kongsted, A.; Manniche, C.; Sogaard, K. Chronic neck pain patients with traumatic or non-traumatic onset: Differences in characteristics. A cross-sectional study. *Scand. J. Pain* **2017**, *14*, 1–8. [CrossRef]
6. Scott, D.; Jull, G.; Sterling, M. Widespread sensory hypersensitivity is a feature of chronic whiplash-associated disorder but not chronic idiopathic neck pain. *Clin. J. Pain* **2005**, *21*, 175–181. [CrossRef]
7. Chien, A.; Eliav, E.; Sterling, M. Sensory hypoaesthesia is a feature of chronic whiplash but not chronic idiopathic neck pain. *Man. Ther.* **2010**, *15*, 48–53. [CrossRef]
8. Anstey, R.; Kongsted, A.; Kamper, S.; Hancock, M.J. Are people with whiplash-associated neck pain different from people with nonspecific neck pain? *J. Orthop. Sports Phys. Ther.* **2016**, *46*, 894–901. [CrossRef]
9. Gross, A.; Forget, M.; St George, K.; Fraser, M.; Graham, N.; Perry, L.; Burnie, S.; Goldsmith, C.; Haines, T.; Brunarski, D. Patient education for neck pain. *Cochrane Database Syst. Rev.* **2012**, CD005106. [CrossRef]
10. Yu, H.; Cote, P.; Southerst, D.; Wong, J.; Varatharajan, S.; Shearer, H.; Gross, D.; Van der Velde, G.; Carroll, L.; Mior, S.; et al. Does structured patient education improve the recovery and clinical outcomes of patients with neck pain? A systematic review from the Ontario Protocol for Traffic Injury Management (OPTIMa) Collaboration. *Spine J.* **2016**, *16*, 1524–1540. [CrossRef]
11. Ainpradub, K.; Sitthipornvorakul, E.; Janwantanakul, P.; Van der Beek, A.J. Effect of education on non-specific neck and low back pain: A meta-analysis of randomized controlled trials. *Man. Ther.* **2016**, *22*, 31–41. [CrossRef] [PubMed]
12. Gross, A.; Kay, T.M.; Paquin, J.P.; Blanchette, S.; Lalonde, P.; Christie, T.; Dupont, G.; Graham, N.; Burnie, S.J.; Gelley, G.; et al. Exercises for mechanical neck disorders. *Cochrane Database Syst. Rev.* **2015**, *1*, Cd004250. [CrossRef] [PubMed]
13. Chen, X.; Coombes, B.K.; Sjogaard, G.; Jun, D.; O'Leary, S.; Johnston, V. Workplace-based interventions for neck pain in office workers: systematic review and meta-analysis. *Phys. Ther.* **2018**, *98*, 40–62. [CrossRef] [PubMed]
14. Martin-Gomez, C.; Sestelo-Diaz, R.; Carrillo-Sanjuan, V.; Navarro-Santana, M.J.; Bardon-Romero, J.; Plaza-Manzano, G. Motor control using cranio-cervical flexion exercises versus other treatments for non-specific chronic neck pain: A systematic review and meta-analysis. *Musculoskelet. Sci. Pract.* **2019**, *42*, 52–59. [CrossRef] [PubMed]
15. Tunwattanapong, P.; Kongkasuwan, R.; Kuptniratsaikul, V. The effectiveness of a neck and shoulder stretching exercise program among office workers with neck pain: A randomized controlled trial. *Clin. Rehabil.* **2016**, *30*, 64–72. [CrossRef] [PubMed]
16. McCaskey, M.A.; Schuster-Amft, C.; Wirth, B.; Suica, Z.; de Bruin, E.D. Effects of proprioceptive exercises on pain and function in chronic neck-and low back pain rehabilitation: A systematic literature review. *BMC Musculoskelet. Disord.* **2014**, *15*, 382. [CrossRef] [PubMed]
17. Li, Y.; Li, S.; Jiang, J.; Yuan, S. Effects of yoga on patients with chronic nonspecific neck pain: A prisma systematic review and meta-analysis. *Medicine* **2019**, *98*, e14649. [CrossRef] [PubMed]
18. Griffin, A.; Leaver, A.; Moloney, N. General exercise does not improve long-term pain and disability in individuals with whiplash-associated disorders: A systematic review. *J. Orthop. Sports Phys. Ther.* **2017**, *47*, 472–480. [CrossRef]
19. Monticone, M.; Cedraschi, C.; Ambrosini, E.; Rocca, B.; Fiorentini, R.; Restelli, M.; Gianola, S.; Ferrante, S.; Zanoli, G.; Moja, L. Cognitive-behavioural treatment for subacute and chronic neck pain. *Cochrane Database Syst. Rev.* **2015**, Cd010664. [CrossRef]
20. Silva Guerrero, A.V.; Maujean, A.; Campbell, L.; Sterling, M. A systematic review and meta-analysis of the effectiveness of psychological interventions delivered by physiotherapists on pain, disability and psychological outcomes in musculoskeletal pain conditions. *Clin. J. Pain* **2018**, *34*, 838–857. [CrossRef]

21. Sterling, M.; Smeets, R.; Warren, J.; Kenardy, J. Physiotherapist-delivered stress inoculation training integrated with exercise versus physiotherapy exercise alone for acute whiplash-associated disorder (StressModex): A randomised controlled trial of a combined psychological/physical intervention. *Br. J. Sports Med.* **2019**. [CrossRef] [PubMed]
22. Fredin, K.; Loras, H. Manual therapy, exercise therapy or combined treatment in the management of adult neck pain—A systematic review and meta-analysis. *Musculoskelet. Sci. Pract.* **2017**, *31*, 62–71. [CrossRef] [PubMed]
23. Oxford Centre for Evidence Based Medicine. Levels of Evidence. Available online: https://www.cebm.net/2009/06/oxford-centre-evidence-based-medicine-levels-evidence-march-2009/ (accessed on 28 June 2019).
24. SIRA. *Guidelines for the Management of Acute Whiplash-Associated Disorders for Health Professionals*; State Insurance Regulatory Authority (NSW): Sydney, Australia, 2014; p. 16.
25. Blanpied, P.R.; Gross, A.R.; Elliott, J.M.; Devaney, L.L.; Clewley, D.; Walton, D.M.; Sparks, C.; Robertson, E.K. Neck pain: Revision 2017. *J. Orthop. Sports Phys. Ther.* **2017**, *47*, A1–A83. [CrossRef] [PubMed]
26. Silva Guerrero, A.V.; Maujean, A.; Setchell, J.; Sterling, M. A comparison of perceptions of reassurance in patients with non-traumatic neck pain and whiplash associated disorders (WAD) in consultations with primary care practitioners—An online Survey. In Proceedings of the WCPT Conference, Geneva, Switzerland, 10–13 May 2019.
27. Ris, I.; Sogaard, K.; Gram, B.; Agerbo, K.; Boyle, E.; Juul-Kristensen, B. Does a combination of physical training, specific exercises and pain education improve health-related quality of life in patients with chronic neck pain? A randomised control trial with a 4-month follow up. *Man. Ther.* **2016**, *26*, 132–140. [CrossRef] [PubMed]
28. Brage, K.; Ris, I.; Falla, D.; Sogaard, K.; Juul-Kristensen, B. Pain education combined with neck-and aerobic training is more effective at relieving chronic neck pain than pain education alone—A preliminary randomized controlled trial. *Man. Ther.* **2015**, *20*, 686–693. [CrossRef] [PubMed]
29. Tegner, H.; Frederiksen, P.; Esbensen, B.A.; Juhl, C. Neurophysiological pain education for patients with chronic low back pain: A systematic review and meta-analysis. *Clin. J. Pain* **2018**, *34*, 778–786. [CrossRef] [PubMed]
30. Wood, L.; Hendrick, P.A. A systematic review and meta-analysis of pain neuroscience education for chronic low back pain: Short-and long-term outcomes of pain and disability. *Eur. J. Pain* **2019**, *23*, 234–249. [CrossRef] [PubMed]
31. Andias, R.; Neto, M.; Silva, A.G. The effects of pain neuroscience education and exercise on pain, muscle endurance, catastrophizing and anxiety in adolescents with chronic idiopathic neck pain: A school-based pilot, randomized and controlled study. *Physiother. Theory Pract.* **2018**, *34*, 682–691. [CrossRef]
32. Southerst, D.; Nordin, M.C.; Cote, P.; Shearer, H.M.; Varatharajan, S.; Yu, H.; Wong, J.J.; Sutton, D.A.; Randhawa, K.A.; Van der Velde, G.M.; et al. Is exercise effective for the management of neck pain and associated disorders or whiplash-associated disorders? A systematic review by the Ontario Protocol for Traffic Injury Management (OPTIMa) Collaboration. *Spine J.* **2016**, *16*, 1503–1523. [CrossRef]
33. Hanney, W.J.; Kolber, M.J.; Cleland, J.A. Motor control exercise for persistent nonspecific neck pain. *Phys. Ther. Rev.* **2010**, *15*, 84–91. [CrossRef]
34. De Zoete, R.M.J.; Brown, L.; Oliveira, K.; Penglaze, L.; Rex, R.; Sawtell, B.; Sullivan, T. The effectiveness of general physical exercise for individuals with chronic neck pain: A systematic review of randomised controlled trials. *Eur. J. Physiother.* **2019**, 1–7. [CrossRef]
35. Smith, A.; Ritchie, C.; Pedler, A.; McCamley, K.; Roberts, K.; Sterling, M. Exercise induced hypoalgesia is elicited by isometric, but not aerobic exercise in individuals with chronic whiplash associated disorders. *Scand. J. Pain* **2017**, *15*, 14–21. [CrossRef] [PubMed]
36. Cote, P.; Van der Velde, G.; Cassidy, J.D.; Carroll, L.J.; Hogg-Johnson, S.; Holm, L.W.; Carragee, E.J.; Haldeman, S.; Nordin, M.; Hurwitz, E.L.; et al. The burden and determinants of neck pain in workers: Results of the bone and joint decade 2000-2010 task force on neck pain and its associated disorders. *Spine* **2008**, *33*, S60–S74. [CrossRef] [PubMed]
37. Carroll, L.; Hogg-Johnson, S.; Van der Velde, G.; Haldeman, S.; Holm, L.; Carragee, E.; Hurwitz, E.; Cote, P.; Nordin, M.; Peloso, P.; et al. Course and prognostic factors for neck pain in the general population. *Spine* **2008**, *33*, S75–S82. [CrossRef] [PubMed]

38. Hoe, V.C.; Urquhart, D.M.; Kelsall, H.L.; Zamri, E.N.; Sim, M.R. Ergonomic interventions for preventing work-related musculoskeletal disorders of the upper limb and neck among office workers. *Cochrane Database Syst. Rev.* **2018**, *10*, Cd008570. [CrossRef] [PubMed]
39. de Campos, T.F.; Maher, C.G.; Steffens, D.; Fuller, J.T.; Hancock, M.J. Exercise programs may be effective in preventing a new episode of neck pain: A systematic review and meta-analysis. *J. Physiother.* **2018**, *64*, 159–165. [CrossRef]
40. Verhagen, A.P.; Bierma-Zeinstra, S.M.; Burdorf, A.; Stynes, S.M.; de Vet, H.C.; Koes, B.W. Conservative interventions for treating work-related complaints of the arm, neck or shoulder in adults. *Cochrane Database Syst. Rev.* **2013**, *12*, Cd008742. [CrossRef]
41. Aas, R.W.; Tuntland, H.; Holte, K.A.; Roe, C.; Lund, T.; Marklund, S.; Moller, A. Workplace interventions for neck pain in workers. *Cochrane Database Syst. Rev.* **2011**, *13*, Cd008160. [CrossRef]
42. Louw, S.; Makwela, S.; Manas, L.; Meyer, L.; Terblaanche, D.; Brink, Y. Effectiveness of exercise in office workers with neck pain: A systematic review and meta-analysis. *S. Afr. J. Physiother.* **2017**, *73*, 392. [CrossRef]
43. Caputo, G.M.; Di Bari, M.; Naranjo Orellana, J. Group-based exercise at workplace: Short-term effects of neck and shoulder resistance training in video display unit workers with work-related chronic neck pain-a pilot randomized trial. *Clin. Rheumatol.* **2017**, *36*, 2325–2333. [CrossRef]
44. Hogg-Johnson, S.; Van der Velde, G.; Carroll, L.; Holm, L.; Cassidy, D.; Guzman, J.; Cote, P.; Haldeman, S.; Ammendolia, C.; Carragee, E.; et al. The burden and determinants of neck pain in the general population. *Spine* **2008**, *33*, S39–S51. [CrossRef] [PubMed]
45. Campbell, L.; Smith, A.; McGregor, L.; Sterling, M. psychological factors and the development of chronic whiplash associated disorder(s): A systematic review. *Clin. J. Pain* **2018**, *34*, 755–768. [CrossRef] [PubMed]
46. Borsook, D.; Youssef, A.M.; Simons, L.; Elman, I.; Eccleston, C. When pain gets stuck: The evolution of pain chronification and treatment resistance. *Pain* **2018**, *159*, 2421–2436. [CrossRef] [PubMed]
47. Williams, A.; Eccleston, C.; Morley, S. Psychological therapies for the management of chronic pain (excluding headache) in adults. *Cochrane Database Syst. Rev.* **2012**, *11*, CD007407. [CrossRef] [PubMed]
48. Shearer, H.M.; Carroll, L.J.; Wong, J.J.; Cote, P.; Varatharajan, S.; Southerst, D.; Sutton, D.A.; Randhawa, K.A.; Yu, H.; Mior, S.A.; et al. Are psychological interventions effective for the management of neck pain and whiplash-associated disorders? A systematic review by the ontario protocol for traffic injury management (optima) collaboration. *Spine J.* **2016**, *16*, 1566–1581. [CrossRef]
49. Richmond, H.; Hall, A.M.; Copsey, B.; Hansen, Z.; Williamson, E.; Hoxey-Thomas, N.; Cooper, Z.; Lamb, S.E. The effectiveness of cognitive behavioural treatment for non-specific low back pain: A systematic review and meta-analysis. *PLoS ONE* **2015**, *10*, e0134192. [CrossRef] [PubMed]
50. Henschke, N.; Ostelo, R.W.; Van Tulder, M.W.; Vlaeyen, J.W.; Morley, S.; Assendelft, W.J.; Main, C.J. Behavioural treatment for chronic low-back pain. *Cochrane Database Syst. Rev.* **2010**, Cd002014. [CrossRef] [PubMed]
51. Kamper, S.J.; Apeldoorn, A.T.; Chiarotto, A.; Smeets, R.J.E.M.; Ostelo, R.W.J.G.; Guzman, J.; Van Tulder, M.W. Multidisciplinary biopsychosocial rehabilitation for chronic low back pain. *Cochrane Database Syst. Rev.* **2014**, CD000963. [CrossRef]
52. Bring, A.; Asenlof, P.; Soderlund, A. What is the comparative effectiveness of current standard treatment, against an individually tailored behavioural programme delivered either on the Internet or face-to-face for people with acute whiplash associated disorder? A randomized controlled trial. *Clin. Rehabil.* **2016**, *30*, 441–453. [CrossRef]
53. Vibe Fersum, K.; O'Sullivan, P.; Skouen, J.S.; Smith, A.; Kvale, A. Efficacy of classification-based cognitive functional therapy in patients with non-specific chronic low back pain: A randomized controlled trial. *Eur. J. Pain* **2013**, *17*, 916–928. [CrossRef]
54. Lamb, S.E.; Gates, S.; Williams, M.A.; Williamson, E.M.; Mt-Isa, S.; Withers, E.J.; Castelnuovo, E.; Smith, J.; Ashby, D.; Cooke, M.; et al. Emergency department treatments and physiotherapy for acute whiplash: A pragmatic, two-step, randomised controlled trial. *Lancet* **2013**, *381*, 546–556. [CrossRef]
55. Jull, G.; Kenardy, J.; Hendrikz, J.; Cohen, M.; Sterling, M. Management of acute whiplash: A randomized controlled trial of multidisciplinary stratified treatments. *Pain* **2013**, *154*, 1798–1806. [CrossRef] [PubMed]
56. Thompson, D.P.; Oldham, J.A.; Woby, S.R. Does adding cognitive-behavioural physiotherapy to exercise improve outcome in patients with chronic neck pain? A randomised controlled trial. *Physiotherapy* **2016**, *102*, 170–177. [CrossRef] [PubMed]

57. Hidalgo, B.; Hall, T.; Bossert, J.; Dugeny, A.; Cagnie, B.; Pitance, L. The efficacy of manual therapy and exercise for treating non-specific neck pain: A systematic review. *J. Back Musculoskelet. Rehabil.* **2018**, *30*, 1149–1169. [CrossRef] [PubMed]
58. Sutton, D.A.; Cote, P.; Wong, J.J.; Varatharajan, S.; Randhawa, K.A.; Yu, H.; Southerst, D.; Shearer, H.M.; Van der Velde, G.M.; Nordin, M.C.; et al. Is multimodal care effective for the management of patients with whiplash-associated disorders or neck pain and associated disorders? A systematic review by the Ontario Protocol for Traffic Injury Management (OPTIMa) Collaboration. *Spine J.* **2016**, *16*, 1541–1565. [CrossRef] [PubMed]
59. Guddal, M.H.; Stensland, S.O.; Smastuen, M.C.; Johnsen, M.B.; Zwart, J.A.; Storheim, K. Physical activity level and sport participation in relation to musculoskeletal pain in a population-based study of adolescents: The Young-HUNT study. *Orthop. J. Sports Med.* **2017**, *5*, 2325967116685543. [CrossRef] [PubMed]
60. Nilsen, T.I.; Holtermann, A.; Mork, P.J. Physical exercise, body mass index, and risk of chronic pain in the low back and neck/shoulders: Longitudinal data from the Nord-Trondelag Health Study. *Am. J. Epidemiol.* **2011**, *174*, 267–273. [CrossRef]
61. Mork, P.J.; Vik, K.L.; Moe, B.; Lier, R.; Bardal, E.M.; Nilsen, T.I. Sleep problems, exercise and obesity and risk of chronic musculoskeletal pain: The Norwegian HUNT study. *Eur. J. Public Health* **2014**, *24*, 924–929. [CrossRef]
62. Williams, A.; Wiggers, J.; O'Brien, K.M.; Wolfenden, L.; Yoong, S.L.; Hodder, R.K.; Lee, H.; Robson, E.K.; McAuley, J.H.; Haskins, R.; et al. Effectiveness of a healthy lifestyle intervention for chronic low back pain: A randomised controlled trial. *Pain* **2018**, *159*, 1137–1146. [CrossRef]
63. Wand, B.M.; O'Connell, N.E. Chronic non-specific low back pain—sub-groups or a single mechanism? *BMC Musculoskelet. Disord.* **2008**, *9*, 11. [CrossRef]
64. Thackeray, A.; Fritz, J.M.; Childs, J.D.; Brennan, G.P. The effectiveness of mechanical traction among subgroups of patients with low back pain and leg pain: a randomized trial. *J. Orthop. Sports Phys. Ther.* **2016**, *46*, 144–154. [CrossRef] [PubMed]
65. Jull, G.; Sterling, M.; Kenardy, J.; Beller, E. Does the presence of sensory hypersensitivity influence outcomes of physical rehabilitation for chronic whiplash?—A preliminary RCT. *Pain* **2007**, *129*, 28–34. [CrossRef] [PubMed]
66. Michaleff, Z.; Maher, C.; Lin, C.; Rebbeck, T.; Connelly, L.; Jull, G.; Sterling, M. Comprehensive physiotherapy exercise program or advice alone for chronic whiplash (PROMISE): A pragmatic randomised controlled trial (ACTRN12609000825257). *Lancet* **2014**, *384*, 133–141. [CrossRef]
67. Ritchie, C.; Hendrikz, J.; Jull, G.; Elliott, J.; Sterling, M. External validation of a clinical prediction rule to predict full recovery and continued moderate/severe disability following acute whiplash injury. *J. Orthop. Sports Phys. Ther.* **2015**, *45*, 242–250. [CrossRef] [PubMed]
68. Ritchie, C.; Hendrikz, J.; Kenardy, J.; Sterling, M. Development and validation of a screening tool to identify both chronicity and recovery following whiplash injury. *Pain* **2013**, *154*, 2198–2206. [CrossRef] [PubMed]
69. Linton, S.J.; Nicholas, M.; MacDonald, S. Development of a short form of the orebro musculoskeletal pain screening questionnaire. *Spine* **2011**, *36*, 1891–1895. [CrossRef] [PubMed]
70. Rebbeck, T.; Leaver, A.; Bandong, A.N.; Kenardy, J.; Refshauge, K.; Connelly, L.; Cameron, I.; Mitchell, G.; Willcock, S.; Ritchie, C.; et al. Implementation of a guideline-based clinical pathway of care to improve health outcomes following whiplash injury (Whiplash ImPaCT): Protocol of a randomised, controlled trial. *J. Physiother.* **2016**, *62*, 111. [CrossRef] [PubMed]
71. Kelly, J.; Ritchie, C.; Sterling, M. Agreement is very low between a clinical prediction rule and physiotherapist assessment for classifying the risk of poor recovery of individuals with acute whiplash injury. *Musculoskelet. Sci. Pract.* **2018**, *39*, 73–79. [CrossRef]
72. Kelly, J.; Sterling, M.; Rebbeck, T.; Bandong, A.N.; Leaver, A.; Mackey, M.; Ritchie, C. Health practitioners' perceptions of adopting clinical prediction rules in the management of musculoskeletal pain: A qualitative study in Australia. *BMJ Open* **2017**, *7*, e015916. [CrossRef]
73. Hill, J.; Whitehurst, D.; Lewis, M.; Bryan, S.; Dunn, K.M.; Foster, N.; Konstantinou, K.; Main, C.; Sowden, G.; Somerville, S.; et al. Comparison of stratified primary care management for low back pain with current best practice (STarT Back): A randomised controlled trial. *Lancet* **2011**, *378*, 1560–1571. [CrossRef]

74. Cherkin, D.; Balderson, B.; Wellman, R.; Hsu, C.; Sherman, K.J.; Evers, S.C.; Hawkes, R.; Cook, A.; Levine, M.D.; Piekara, D.; et al. Effect of low back pain risk-stratification strategy on patient outcomes and care processes: The match randomized trial in primary care. *J. Gen. Intern. Med.* **2018**, *33*, 1324–1336. [CrossRef] [PubMed]
75. Campbell, P.; Hill, J.C.; Protheroe, J.; Afolabi, E.K.; Lewis, M.; Beardmore, R.; Hay, E.M.; Mallen, C.D.; Bartlam, B.; Saunders, B.; et al. Keele Aches and Pains Study protocol: Validity, acceptability, and feasibility of the Keele STarT MSK tool for subgrouping musculoskeletal patients in primary care. *J. Pain Res.* **2016**, *9*, 807–818. [CrossRef] [PubMed]
76. Sterling, J.; Maujean, A.; Sterling, M. Information needs of patients with whiplash associated disorders: A Delphi study of patient beliefs. *Musculoskelet. Sci. Pract.* **2018**, *33*, 29–34. [CrossRef] [PubMed]
77. Maujean, A.; Sterling, J.; Sterling, M. What information do patients need following a whiplash injury? The perspectives of patients and physiotherapists. *Disabil. Rehabil.* **2017**, *40*, 1135–1141. [CrossRef] [PubMed]
78. Hush, J.M.; Nicholas, M.; Dean, C.M. Embedding the IASP pain curriculum into a 3-year pre-licensure physical therapy program: redesigning pain education for future clinicians. *Pain Rep.* **2018**, *3*, e645. [CrossRef] [PubMed]
79. Grant, G.M.; O'Donnell, M.L.; Spittal, M.J.; Creamer, M.; Studdert, D.M. Relationship between stressfulness of claiming for injury compensation and long-term recovery: A prospective cohort study. *JAMA Psychiatry* **2014**, *71*, 446–453. [CrossRef] [PubMed]
80. Ng, T.; Pedler, A.; Vicenzino, B.; Sterling, M. Physiotherapists' beliefs about whiplash injury: A cross-cultural comparison between Singapore and Queensland. *Physiother. Res. Int.* **2015**, *20*, 77–86. [CrossRef] [PubMed]
81. Falla, D.; Hodges, P.W. Individualized Exercise Interventions for Spinal Pain. *Exerc. Sport Sci. Rev.* **2017**, *45*, 105–115. [CrossRef]
82. Steiger, F.; Wirth, B.; de Bruin, E.D.; Mannion, A.F. Is a positive clinical outcome after exercise therapy for chronic non-specific low back pain contingent upon a corresponding improvement in the targeted aspect(s) of performance? A systematic review. *Eur. Spine J.* **2012**, *21*, 575–598. [CrossRef]
83. Chen, K.; De Zoete, R.M.J.; Sterling, M. Relationships between Improvement in Patient-reported Outcomes and Physical Performance after Specific Exercise Intervention for Chronic Neck Pain: A Systematic Review. *Musc Sc and Prac.*. under review.
84. Bieler, T.; Siersma, V.; Magnusson, S.P.; Kjaer, M.; Beyer, N. Exercise induced effects on muscle function and range of motion in patients with hip osteoarthritis. *Physiother. Res. Int.* **2018**, *23*, e1697. [CrossRef] [PubMed]
85. Naugle, K.M.; Fillingim, R.B.; Riley, J.L., III. A meta-analytic review of the hypoalgesic effects of exercise. *J. Pain* **2012**, *13*, 1139–1150. [CrossRef] [PubMed]
86. Vaegter, H.B.; Handberg, G.; Graven-Nielsen, T. Hypoalgesia after exercise and the cold pressor test is reduced in chronic musculoskeletal pain patients with high pain sensitivity. *Clin. J. Pain* **2016**, *32*, 58–69. [CrossRef] [PubMed]
87. Rice, D.; Nijs, J.; Kosek, E.; Wideman, T.; Hasenbring, M.I.; Koltyn, K.; Graven-Nielsen, T.; Polli, A. Exercise-induced hypoalgesia in pain-free and chronic pain populations: state of the art and future directions. *J. Pain* **2019**. [CrossRef] [PubMed]
88. Eccleston, C.; Crombez, G. Advancing psychological therapies for chronic pain. *F1000 Res.* **2017**, *6*, 461. [CrossRef] [PubMed]
89. Tabor, A.; Keogh, E.; Eccleston, C. Embodied pain-negotiating the boundaries of possible action. *Pain* **2017**, *158*, 1007–1011. [CrossRef] [PubMed]
90. Bisset, L.M.; Vicenzino, B. Physiotherapy management of lateral epicondylalgia. *J. Physiother.* **2015**, *61*, 174–181. [CrossRef] [PubMed]
91. Bennell, K. Physiotherapy management of hip osteoarthritis. *J. Physiother.* **2013**, *59*, 145–157. [CrossRef]
92. Aili, K.; Nyman, T.; Svartengren, M.; Hillert, L. Sleep as a predictive factor for the onset and resolution of multi-site pain: A 5-year prospective study. *Eur. J. Pain* **2015**, *19*, 341–349. [CrossRef]
93. McLean, S.M.; May, S.; Klaber-Moffett, J.; Sharp, D.M.; Gardiner, E. Risk factors for the onset of non-specific neck pain: A systematic review. *J. Epidemiol. Community Health* **2010**, *64*, 565–572. [CrossRef]
94. Ortego, G.; Villafane, J.H.; Domenech-Garcia, V.; Berjano, P.; Bertozzi, L.; Herrero, P. Is there a relationship between psychological stress or anxiety and chronic nonspecific neck-arm pain in adults? A systematic review and meta-analysis. *J. Psychosom. Res.* **2016**, *90*, 70–81. [CrossRef] [PubMed]

95. Maujean, A.; Gullo, M.J.; Andersen, T.E.; Ravn, S.L.; Sterling, M. Post-traumatic stress symptom clusters in acute whiplash associated disorder and their prediction of chronic pain-related disability. *Pain Rep.* **2017**, *2*, e631. [CrossRef] [PubMed]
96. Skillgate, E.; Pico-Espinosa, O.J.; Hallqvist, J.; Bohman, T.; Holm, L.W. Healthy lifestyle behavior and risk of long duration troublesome neck pain or low back pain among men and women: Results from the Stockholm Public Health Cohort. *Clin. Epidemiol.* **2017**, *9*, 491–500. [CrossRef] [PubMed]
97. Malfliet, A.; Bilterys, T.; Van Looveren, E.; Meeus, M.; Danneels, L.; Ickmans, K.; Cagnie, B.; Mairesse, O.; Neu, D.; Moens, M.; et al. The added value of cognitive behavioral therapy for insomnia to current best evidence physical therapy for chronic spinal pain: Protocol of a randomized controlled clinical trial. *Braz. J. Phys. Ther.* **2019**, *23*, 62–70. [CrossRef] [PubMed]
98. Dodakian, L.; McKenzie, A.L.; Le, V.; See, J.; Pearson-Fuhrhop, K.; Burke Quinlan, E.; Zhou, R.J.; Augsberger, R.; Tran, X.A.; Friedman, N.; et al. A home-based telerehabilitation program for patients with stroke. *Neurorehabilitation Neural Repair* **2017**, *31*, 923–933. [CrossRef] [PubMed]
99. Shukla, H.; Nair, S.R.; Thakker, D. Role of telerehabilitation in patients following total knee arthroplasty: Evidence from a systematic literature review and meta-analysis. *J. Telemed. Telecare* **2017**, *23*, 339–346. [CrossRef] [PubMed]
100. Gold, J.E.; Hallman, D.M.; Hellstrom, F.; Bjorklund, M.; Crenshaw, A.G.; Djupsjobacka, M.; Heiden, M.; Mathiassen, S.E.; Piligian, G.; Barbe, M.F. Systematic review of biochemical biomarkers for neck and upper-extremity musculoskeletal disorders. *Scand. J. Work Environ. Health* **2016**, *42*, 103–124. [CrossRef] [PubMed]
101. Gold, J.E.; Hallman, D.M.; Hellstrom, F.; Bjorklund, M.; Crenshaw, A.G.; Mathiassen, S.E.; Barbe, M.F.; Ali, S. Systematic review of quantitative imaging biomarkers for neck and shoulder musculoskeletal disorders. *BMC Musculoskelet. Disord.* **2017**, *18*, 395. [CrossRef]
102. Borstov, A.; Smith, L.; Diatchenko, L.; Soward, J.; Ulirsch, C.; Rossi, R.; Swor, W.; Hauda, D.; Peak, J.; Jones, D.; et al. Polymorphisms in the glucocorticoid receptor co-chaperone FKBP5 predict persistent musculoskeletal pain after traumatic stress exposure. *Pain* **2013**, *154*, 1419–1426.

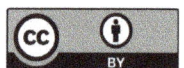

© 2019 by the authors. Licensee MDPI, Basel, Switzerland. This article is an open access article distributed under the terms and conditions of the Creative Commons Attribution (CC BY) license (http://creativecommons.org/licenses/by/4.0/).

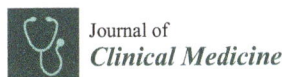

Review

Best Evidence Rehabilitation for Chronic Pain Part 5: Osteoarthritis

David Rice [1,2,*], Peter McNair [1], Eva Huysmans [3,4,5,6,7], Janelle Letzen [8] and Patrick Finan [8]

1. Health and Rehabilitation Research Institute, Auckland University of Technology, Auckland 1142, New Zealand; peter.mcnair@aut.ac.nz
2. Waitemata Pain Service, Department of Anaesthesiology and Perioperative Medicine, Waitemata District Health Board, Auckland 1142, New Zealand
3. Pain in Motion International Research Group; Eva.Huysmans@vub.be
4. Department of Physiotherapy, Human Physiology and Anatomy, Faculty of Physical Education & Physiotherapy, Vrije Universiteit Brussel, 1090 Brussel, Belgium
5. Department of Public Health (GEWE), Faculty of Medicine and Pharmacy, Vrije Universiteit Brussel, 1090 Brussels, Belgium
6. I-CHER, Interuniversity Center for Health Economics Research, 1090 Brussels, Belgium
7. Department of Physical Medicine and Physiotherapy, Universitair Ziekenhuis Brussel, 1090 Brussels, Belgium
8. Department of Psychiatry & Behavioral Sciences, Johns Hopkins University, Baltimore, MD 21287, USA; jletzen1@jhmi.edu (J.L.); pfinan1@jhu.edu (P.F.)
* Correspondence: david.rice@aut.ac.nz

Received: 14 September 2019; Accepted: 30 September 2019; Published: 24 October 2019

Abstract: Osteoarthritis (OA) is a leading cause of chronic pain and disability in older adults, which most commonly affects the joints of the knee, hip, and hand. To date, there are no established disease modifying interventions that can halt or reverse OA progression. Therefore, treatment is focused on alleviating pain and maintaining or improving physical and psychological function. Rehabilitation is widely recommended as first-line treatment for OA as, in many cases, it is safer and more effective than the best-established pharmacological interventions. In this article, we describe the presentation of OA pain and give an overview of its peripheral and central mechanisms. We then provide a state-of-the-art review of rehabilitation for OA pain—including self-management programs, exercise, weight loss, cognitive behavioral therapy, adjunct therapies, and the use of aids and devices. Next, we explore several promising directions for clinical practice, including novel education strategies to target unhelpful illness and treatment beliefs, methods to enhance the efficacy of exercise interventions, and innovative, brain-directed treatments. Finally, we discuss potential future research in areas, such as treatment adherence and personalized rehabilitation for OA pain.

Keywords: osteoarthritis; musculoskeletal pain; rehabilitation medicine; physiotherapy; psychology; non-pharmacological

1. Introduction

Osteoarthritis (OA) is the most common form of arthritis and a leading cause of chronic pain and disability, affecting ~250 million people worldwide [1]. OA can occur in any synovial joint, but the knee, hip, and joints of the hand are most commonly affected [2,3]. Important risk factors for the development of OA include increasing age, female gender, previous joint trauma, and (as yet largely unidentified) genetic factors [2,4]. In addition, increased mechanical stress on the joints caused by factors, such as malalignment [2], increased body weight [5,6], and manual work [7–9], also play an important role. While the signature characteristic of OA is a loss of articular cartilage, it is apparent that many other joint structures can become affected as the disease progresses, including the subchondral bone, fibrocartilage, capsule, ligaments, synovial membrane, and periarticular muscles [10].

1.1. OA Pain Presentation

Pain is the primary symptom that motivates people with OA to seek medical attention and it is associated with functional limitations [11–13], emotional distress [14,15], fear of movement [16–18], sleep problems [15,19], fatigue [15,20], and an overall marked reduction in quality of life [21,22]. Joint pain might also have direct neuromuscular consequences, including muscle weakness [23], impaired muscle force control [24], and gait adaptations [25], some of which may affect joint loading [26,27] and increase the risk of further pain and structural deterioration [28–30].

Individuals with symptomatic OA commonly report pain in response to activities of daily living that involve movement or mechanical loading of the affected joint, such as walking across the room, getting up from sitting, or opening a jar [31]. Pain at rest and night pain are also frequently reported [31]. The painful joint(s) is commonly described as more sensitive to touch and pressure [32] and in some cases, changes in temperature [33,34]. Two distinct types of joint pain are commonly reported—a dull background aching, throbbing pain, and a sharp, stabbing pain that is intermittent but more severe [31,35]. In knee OA, specifically, this intermittent, sharp pain often arises unpredictably and is associated with giving way or locking of the knee [31]. A minority of people with OA [36–38] describe pain qualities, such as burning, shooting, or electric shocks, and more recent evidence shows that some describe perceptual disturbances, including feeling as if their painful limb is altered in size [39–41], missing [32,42], or difficult to control [39,42].

OA pain is often described as highly variable, fluctuating in intensity both within and between days [43–45]. In the long-term, the natural course of OA pain also varies across individuals. When reassessed over several months or years, many people with OA (35–60%) report a more or less consistent joint pain that does not markedly change over time [46–48]. For others, pain is described as consistently worsening, progressing from a predominantly load-dependent intermittent pattern of pain, to a more constant, severe pain [35,49]. Conversely, ~12–30% of people report sustained lessening of pain intensity over several years [47,50,51]. Thus, although OA has traditionally been thought of as a progressive condition, the evidence suggests that long-term worsening of pain is far from inevitable.

1.2. Mechanisms of OA Pain

Historically, OA pain has been viewed as a symptom, being driven by the activation of articular nociceptors in response to structural damage of the joint [52,53]. While joint nociception is one important factor contributing to OA pain, interdisciplinary research has revealed that OA pain is better understood within a biopsychosocial framework [54–56]—being influenced by a complex array of interacting factors.

1.2.1. Peripheral Mechanisms of OA Pain

Notably, articular cartilage is aneural, and therefore cannot generate nociception [57]. In contrast, other joint structures, such as the subchondral bone, periosteum, ligaments, capsule, synovium, and parts of the meniscus are richly innervated by nociceptors [58,59]. Despite this, demonstrating a strong link between joint structural deterioration and OA pain has proven to be elusive. For the individual person with OA, there does not appear to be a meaningful relationship between the structural changes that were observed on x-ray and the intensity of the pain experience [60,61]. At a population level, the relationship is somewhat stronger, with those who have severe radiographic OA more likely to experience frequent pain [57,62,63]. However, as many as 75–80% of community dwelling adults with evidence of radiographic OA do not experience frequent joint pain [64,65], while, conversely, as few as 10–15% of people who experience frequent joint pain have definite radiographic evidence of OA [60,64,65]. Furthermore, the radiographic progression of OA can be discordant with changes in joint pain [48,66].

The relatively poor relationship between radiographic findings and OA pain can be partly explained by the lack of sensitivity of x-ray to joint structural changes, particularly in soft tissue and subchondral bone [56,67]. Thus, several studies have examined the relationship between joint MRI features and OA pain. In recent systematic reviews of studies involving people with radiographically established knee OA [68,69], two MRI findings have been consistently associated with both incident joint pain and worsening OA pain—bone marrow lesions (BMLs) and synovitis. BMLs are ill-defined, hyperintense marrow signals on fluid-sensitive, fat-suppressed MRI [70,71]. While still unclear, it is thought that BMLs may trigger nociception through microfracture of the subchondral bone, an increase in intraosseous pressure and/or neoinnervation accompanying vascular in growth [71–73]. With respect to synovitis, several inflammatory molecules directly activate chemosensitive nociceptors in the joint, while others also produce potent, long lasting decreases in the firing threshold of nociceptors and increase their spontaneous discharge, a process that is known as peripheral sensitization [58,59]. Thus, synovitis, and the accompanying peripheral sensitization, may substantially increase joint nociceptor discharge, both at rest and during movement. While once considered a non-inflammatory condition, there is now compelling evidence that synovitis is a common feature of OA [74].

1.2.2. Central Mechanisms of OA Pain

Despite advances in our understanding of important sources of joint nociception, it is evident that joint MRI features can also be discordant with pain. For example, at least one abnormal joint MRI feature can be found in >80% of pain-free community dwelling adults [67]. Notably, MRI identified synovitis might be present in ~30–35% of pain-free individuals [67,75], while BMLs may be observed in ~30–50% of people who are pain free [75–77] and, even in those with established OA, progression or resolution of synovitis [78] and BMLs [79] are not always related to changes in pain. These findings suggest that other factors also play an important role in determining individual differences in OA pain severity. In this regard, extensive preclinical evidence exists that, in the presence of ongoing joint nociception, a maladaptive gain of neural signaling in the central nociceptive pathways within the spinal cord and brain occurs in animal models of arthritis [80–83], a process that is known as central sensitization. Importantly, central sensitization results in sensory input being strongly amplified when it reaches nociceptive pathways at the level of the spinal cord and brain [84], thereby increasing the frequency, severity, and spread of pain [85–87]. In recent decades, mounting evidence from human studies suggests that central sensitization is evident in at least a subgroup of people with OA [88], is an important driver of pain severity [85,87], and at least partly explains the discordance between pain intensity and joint structural changes [89]. In addition, several neuroimaging studies have now demonstrated altered brain structure and brain activation patterns in people with symptomatic OA. Commonly, limbic areas of the brain are more active in people with OA than in controls [90–94], both at rest and in response to standardized painful stimuli. In addition, changes in gray matter volume [93,95,96] and white matter integrity [96] have been shown in several brain regions important to nociceptive processing.

It is now well established that psychosocial and lifestyle factors (e.g., sleep) play an important role in amplifying or attenuating the pain experience [97,98], and may be involved in the initiation and maintenance of central sensitization [98–102]. These factors can also have an important influence on disability, independent of their effect on pain [103–106]. For example, sleep problems are common in OA, with at least 50% of individuals reporting difficulties in initiating or maintaining sleep [19,107]. The interrelations between sleep and pain have been well characterized over the past two decades, with epidemiological, experimental, and clinical research providing broad support for a bidirectional relationship [98]. Consistent with these findings, a number of studies have linked sleep problems with increased pain and pain sensitivity among individuals with OA [108–112], which suggests that sleep could be an important treatment target for reducing OA pain—although clinical trials have not always supported that premise [113].

As many as 40% of people with OA have anxiety, depression, or both, as compared to 5–17% in the general population [114]. OA pain and depressive symptoms interact in a recursive cycle, with each contributing to increased fatigue and disability, which may lead to pain worsening over time [20]. Furthermore, in a large sample of pain-free adults, high anxiety was found to predict new onset joint pain over a 12-month follow up period [115] and it was associated with increased pain sensitivity in people with established knee OA [115]. Similarly, people with OA who had the highest levels of psychological distress and pain vigilance showed a generalized increase in pain sensitivity [116], while higher levels of pain catastrophizing have been associated with a long-term worsening of OA pain [117].

Conversely, resilience characteristics may offset maladaptive psychosocial factors. For example, increased positive affect in people with knee OA predicts lower joint pain intensity and it is associated with attenuated temporal summation [118], a measure of amplified central nociceptive processing. Similarly, dispositional optimism is associated with lower depression symptoms and greater life satisfaction in people with OA [119], while higher levels of self-efficacy are associated with long-term stability or improvement in OA pain [117]. Finally, more social support has been associated with reduced pain intensity, less distress, and greater activity levels amongst those with chronic pain generally [120,121], and in people with OA specifically [122], while the OA pain and depression symptoms are less strongly correlated in the presence of social support [119].

1.3. Summary and Aims

OA pain involves a complex interplay of mechanisms, some of which relate to the underlying joint pathology and some of which are distinct—relating to the altered processing and interpretation of nociception in the central nervous system. To date, there are no established disease modifying interventions that can halt or reverse OA related cartilage loss or disease progression. Therefore, treatment is focused on alleviating pain and maintaining or improving physical and psychological function. Rehabilitation is widely recommended as first-line treatment for OA in evidence based clinical guidelines [123–125], as it is safer and, in many cases, more effective at reducing pain than the best established pharmacological interventions [126,127]. This paper provides a state-of-the-art overview of rehabilitation interventions for OA pain. In the sections below, we review the best evidence for rehabilitation—including self-management programs, exercise, weight loss, cognitive behavioral therapy, adjunct therapies, and the use of aids and devices. Next, we explore several promising directions for clinical practice, including novel education strategies to target unhelpful illness and treatment beliefs, methods to enhance the efficacy of exercise and innovative, brain-directed treatments. Finally, we discuss potential future research in areas, such as treatment adherence and personalized rehabilitation for OA pain.

2. State-of-the-Art Rehabilitation

In this section we focus on synthesizing evidence from international treatment guidelines, meta-analyses, systematic reviews, and, at times, recent randomized controlled trials. A non-systematic search of the literature was performed in PubMed, Scopus, and Google Scholar using the following search terms: rehabilitation, exercise, non-pharmacological, conservative, osteoarthritis, and pain, in order to achieve this. Where appropriate, we used 'systematic review', 'meta-analysis' and 'randomized controlled trial' filters. Additionally, several international treatment guidelines from the last decade were sourced and utilized.

Importantly, much of the evidence discussed in this section comes from studies in knee OA and, to a lesser extent, hip and hand OA. There may be key differences in the optimum rehabilitation strategies that were employed according to the joint(s) affected by OA. Where possible, we attempt to provide examples where the strength of evidence or recommendations differ according to the joint involved. However, until such time, as a sufficient number of high-quality studies are performed in people suffering from OA at other joints, some extrapolation from the available literature is necessary.

Furthermore, it is important to emphasize that the overall quality of the evidence considerably varies across interventions (Table 1). Where possible, we attempt to highlight the quality of the evidence in each section, as indicated in recent systematic reviews and international treatment guidelines. Finally, the nature of many of the treatments discussed means that the effective blinding of the intervention is difficult or, in some cases, impossible to achieve. Thus, as with any intervention, part of the therapeutic effect described is likely to be non-specific in nature.

2.1. Self-Management Programs

Given that OA is a chronic disease, its symptoms require long-term, habitual management. A passive coping style, through which people become behaviorally inhibited and avoid taking an active role in self-managing their pain, has been consistently related to poorer outcomes across various chronic pain disorders [128–130], including OA [131,132]. Several OA treatment guidelines recommend self-management interventions as a core component in the effective management of OA [123,133,134]. The notion that expectancy, belief, and motivation shape the pain experience and the accompanying behaviors that contribute to either chronic pain adaptation or disability is critical to the concept of self-management. Self-management interventions are programs that aim to teach people to take an active role in managing their condition through any combination of education, behavior change, and psychosocial coping skills [135]. For example, these interventions can include modules providing information regarding the health condition, healthcare resource utilization, stress management techniques, physical exercises, and interpersonal problem-solving skills. These programs can be heterogeneous in the implementation of specific strategies, but commonly try to counter unhelpful illness and treatment beliefs and impart transferable skills that empower individuals to effectively manage their symptoms long-term [136].

The existing evidence for self-management program efficacy in OA shows mixed outcomes. A meta-analysis pooling results from 13 trials found an overall small beneficial effect of self-management programs on pain reduction, but no significant impact on quality of life or physical function [137]. However, the authors found a specific pooled effect of pain reduction and quality of life improvement for self-management programs that contained exercise programs, which suggests the latter might be a key component for OA. Furthermore, Kroon and colleagues examined 29 studies comparing education-specific self-management interventions to other interventions for adults with OA. The authors found overall weak effect sizes for self-management programs that are focused on disease education over other treatments [138], which suggests that current education strategies may be suboptimal. Both reviews concluded that self-management programs vary widely in their content (e.g., focus on managing OA symptoms vs. holistic well-being), duration (e.g., single session vs. ongoing, weekly vs. monthly), and method of delivery (e.g., in-person vs. telehealth, individual vs. group, lay leader vs. healthcare professional), limiting conclusive evidence for their efficacy.

2.2. Exercise

Regular exercise is considered to be a core treatment for OA and it is universally recommended amongst treatment guidelines for all individuals with OA, regardless of their individual presentation [126,139,140]. Exercise has a number of potential benefits, including improving pain [126,141,142], physical function [143], and mood [144], as well as decreasing the risk of secondary health problems, including cardiovascular, metabolic, neurodegenerative, and bone disorders [145]. Exercise likely reduces OA pain by several different mechanisms, including increased central nervous system inhibition [146,147], local [148] and systemic [149] reductions in inflammation, psychosocial effects [150], and biomechanical effects at the affected joint [151].

Exercise for OA might include low impact aerobic exercise, such as walking or cycling, resistance training for muscle strengthening, stretching, and other forms of exercise, such as Tai Chi or Yoga. Importantly, exercise has very few adverse effects [152], does not appear to accelerate joint degeneration [152–154], and has similar or better effect sizes for OA pain as compared to commonly used analgesics, such as acetaminophen and non-steroidal anti-inflammatory drugs (NSAIDS) [126].

At this time, there is insufficient evidence to determine whether one type of exercise is superior, with systematic reviews suggesting that several different types of exercise are effective for OA [125–127,155]. Resistance training is the most studied type of exercise for individuals with OA. The strongest evidence for pain relief and improvements in function exists in people with knee and hip OA [141,142], with fewer high quality studies in hand OA [156]. Resistance training interventions can be home or clinic based, and should be undertaken for at least 2–4 months in order to maximize the clinical benefits [157]. Aerobic exercise is widely recommended in treatment guidelines [123,124,126,133,134,158,159], effectively relieves OA pain [127], and it may have additional benefits, such as promoting cardiovascular health and weight loss. However, the majority of RCTs that were conducted in OA populations include interventions that are not solely aerobic but have elements of strengthening and stretching to varying degrees [158]. Hence, their findings could be viewed as supporting the inclusion of aerobic exercise within a wider program of exercise. Other forms of exercise, such as tai chi, yoga, and whole body vibration, currently have less evidence to support them, with low to very low quality evidence that shows both positive and negative effects [125,160]. Some guidelines [124,126] have made conditional recommendations concerning land-based versus water-based interventions. Overall, there is greater support for land-based exercise that is based upon both the magnitude of effects in RCTs and the quality of evidence [125]. However, some individuals with hip or knee OA might be better suited or have a preference for water-based exercise for some parts of their rehabilitation program [124].

For exercise to be most successful, it must be of sufficient volume to elicit adaptations that relieve pain and improve physical function. Concerning resistance training, guidelines [157] highlight that pain relief can occur, irrespective of the equipment (dynamometers, weights, bands) utilized, the type of exercise (e.g., isokinetic, isotonic), and the muscle action (i.e., isometric, eccentric concentric) performed. Despite such a range of options, consideration should be given within the overall program to those exercises that more closely simulate the type of muscle activity utilized in the work tasks and/or activities that are required in the individual's daily life. Other parameters, such as the load, the number of repetitions within a set, the number of sets performed per session, the rest intervals between sets, and the frequency of sessions per week should all be carefully considered. For aerobic exercise, the intensity, type of exercise, how it is performed (e.g., continuous or in intervals), and frequency per week are all important. For aerobic and strengthening exercises, the suggested starting points for these training parameters are well described in the ACSM public health guidelines [161], with a recent clinical guideline [162] recommending these levels of exercise are embedded within standard care in people with OA. Specifically, a minimum of 150 min. moderate intensity or 75 min. vigorous intensity aerobic exercise per week is recommended (in bouts of at least 10 min). For resistance training, two sessions per week, with two sets of eight to 12 repetitions at a load of 60% to 70% of one repetition maximum can be recommended as a starting point [161]. A rest period of ≥48 h between resistance training sessions is suggested in order to optimize muscle hypertrophy [161].

The need for personalized, individually tailored exercise programs while taking into account a person's exercise preferences has been highlighted [124,163], as these are considered more likely to achieve long term exercise adherence [164]. Another key point concerning adherence is that education is often needed to emphasize that appropriate levels of exercise are safe, and while pain exacerbations may occur at times, these will reduce over the course of a training program [165] and people with OA will continue to benefit from ongoing exercise. It is recommended [162] that exercise regimes be provided by health care professionals with suitable backgrounds (e.g., physiotherapists) who regularly reassess progress and modify training parameters to limit and manage symptom exacerbations. The importance of progression has also been highlighted by Brosseau et al. [157] and Magni et al. [156], who noted that the majority of trials that did not find positive results for an exercise intervention had not implemented a program that continually reassessed and progressed the training volume over time.

Concerning the overall duration of the exercise program, one could argue that exercise should be considered as a lifestyle change and undertaken perennially. To date, most RCTs of exercise interventions involving people with OA have been undertaken over a two to four month period with few interventions extending past six months. While benefits can continue for several months, it is well known from the literature related to athletic training that when training is stopped completely, a detraining effect be observed within two to three weeks [166], and this decline steadily continues, depending upon factors, such as age and physical activity level. Importantly, there is evidence [166] that these declines in performance can be slowed with booster sessions that are undertaken less regularly (e.g., one training sessions every one to two weeks for resistance and aerobic exercise). Booster sessions may also be useful in promoting longer-term exercise adherence [167].

2.3. Weight Loss

Increased body weight is considered to be an important modifiable risk factor for the onset and progression of pain and radiographic findings [168–170] of OA, specifically at the knee and hip [124,171–173]. In symptomatic knee OA, this risk is doubled with every 3–4 kg/m^2 increase in Body Mass Index (BMI) [168]. Furthermore, obesity is associated with a systemic pro-inflammatory state that may accelerate joint degeneration [174] and increase the sensitization of the nociceptive system, thereby enhancing OA pain [175]. As a result, weight loss interventions are recommended by several international treatment guidelines for OA as part of the core treatment for people with knee and/or hip OA that are overweight or obese [123,124,126,133,134,140,159,169,176–180]. Furthermore, education regarding the importance of maintaining a healthy lifestyle and body weight is recommended for all people with OA [124].

Although a consensus regarding the BMI cut off for determining the target population for weight loss programs is lacking [180], weight loss is typically recommended in individuals presenting with symptomatic OA and a BMI ≥ 25 kg/m^2 [124,133,169,177] (pre-obesity BMI value, as defined by the World Health Organization [181]). Care should be taken when advising weight loss to older people (aged > 65 years) to ensure the maintenance of lean body mass and bone density [124,182].

The importance of weight loss programs is supported by moderate to high quality evidence reporting improvements in pain and disability after weight loss in people with knee OA [177,183–185]. More recently, a reduction in systemic inflammatory biomarkers has also been observed [186]. Ideally, weight loss interventions should comprise a combination of dietary advice and exercise [124,177,184,187–190], including explicit individual weight loss goals and problem solving regarding how to reach these goals [159,184,191,192]. The benefits of weight loss interventions are dose dependent—with higher amounts of weight loss resulting in larger benefits—starting at a minimum of 5–7.5% body weight loss [124,184,185,193].

Although the evidence for weight management programs is generally limited to knee OA, the systemic health benefits of weight loss and maintaining a healthy body weight are not negligible. Therefore, weight loss principles are most likely transferable to people with hip OA [134], in which being overweight is known to be a risk factor [124,171], and possibly also to individuals with OA in other joints [123,176].

2.4. Cognitive Behavioral Therapy

Cognitive behavioral therapy (CBT) is increasingly recognized as a valuable intervention for OA pain. A recent guideline [124] recommends CBT for selected people with knee and/or hip OA, particularly those with psychosocial comorbidities. Another recent treatment guideline specifically focused on arthritis pain management [125] concluded there is now moderate evidence supporting CBT for OA pain and recommended that appropriately selected individuals should receive both psychological and sleep interventions. CBT for pain generally involves the identification and facilitation of individually specific behavioral goals that promote activity and social engagement while minimizing withdrawal and guarding. Cognitive barriers to engagement in adaptive behaviors (e.g., pain catastrophizing) are also identified and systematically challenged in the course of CBT. While CBT for pain has been extensively investigated in a variety of chronic pain disorders, relatively fewer trials are available for OA [194]. A recent systematic review and meta-analysis identified 12 RCTs that examine psychological interventions in an OA population [195]. While heterogeneous in the focus of their treatment, overall, these studies demonstrated small reductions in pain and fatigue and moderate to large improvements in self efficacy and pain coping. Interestingly, despite focusing on non-pain symptoms, several RCTs that involve CBT interventions have also demonstrated modest efficacy for improving OA pain. For example, an online CBT intervention for depression in people with knee OA and comorbid depression significantly reduced depression symptoms, but also demonstrated a medium-sized effect on OA pain and function relative to treatment as usual [196]. Similarly, CBT for insomnia has been tested in several different cohorts of people with knee OA and comorbid insomnia. Smith et al. [197] demonstrated that CBT for insomnia improved wake after sleep onset—a key marker of sleep disruption—among people with OA. Statistically significant reductions in pain severity were observed through six-month follow-up, and improvements in wake after sleep onset predicted reduced pain at follow-up. Small to medium sized effects on pain were observed in another RCT of CBT for insomnia in people with knee OA and comorbid insomnia [198], as well as a larger population-based RCT of CBT for insomnia in people with knee OA recruited from primary care clinics [199]. Finally, Vitiello et al. [200] conducted a three-arm trial comparing CBT for pain with CBT for comorbid pain and insomnia symptoms and an education control in people with OA and comorbid insomnia. Interestingly, the mean pain levels were not significantly improved in any treatment condition by post intervention. However, in subgroup analyses, those individuals who had clinically meaningful improvements in insomnia symptoms (≥30% reduction) by post-intervention (two months) demonstrated significant long-term reductions in pain at both nine and 18-month follow-up. Thus, there is growing evidence that CBT interventions, whether directed at pain or at other problems, such as depression or sleep, can produce clinical benefits and should be considered in appropriate individuals.

2.5. Adjunct Treatments

Several OA treatment guidelines include recommendations regarding the use of adjunct treatments, such as manual therapy, thermal modalities, acupuncture, and electrotherapies [123,124,126,133]. The quality of evidence used in forming these recommendations is generally low quality, with a high risk of bias, and it is apparent that more studies involving these interventions are needed before strong conclusions can be drawn. Manual therapy (that may include joint mobilization/manipulation and massage) is generally not recommended as a stand-alone treatment [123,124,133,178], but a short course of manual therapy [124], provided as an adjunct treatment to facilitate engagement in active strategies, such as exercise, is recommended by several guidelines [123,124,178] and might enhance pain relief compared to exercise alone [201].

The use of thermal modalities, such as superficial heat or cold, may provide short-term relief of symptoms and are low cost, low risk interventions that can be incorporated into self-management, and are therefore widely recommended as adjunct treatments in several guidelines [123,124,178], despite low quality evidence supporting their use.

Some treatment guidelines recommend acupuncture, particularly for knee OA [178], but others recommend against it [123,124,133], as well conducted systematic reviews have typically shown that the benefits as compared to placebo are small and of questionable clinical importance [202,203]. There may be value over usual care for individuals with OA who have positive treatment expectations regarding acupuncture, although much of the clinical benefit may be due to non-specific effects [204].

The evidence for electrotherapies is mixed and it is limited by low quality studies with short follow up times. A recent systematic review [205] suggests that interferential and high frequency TENS may have some benefit, while evidence is generally lacking for other modalities. Several treatment guidelines recommend using TENS as an adjunct treatment [123,124,163,178]. The portability of TENS units, their relatively low cost, and their ability to be used at home as part of a self-management strategy or in combination with exercise makes this form of electrotherapy particularly attractive.

2.6. Aids and Devices

A large range of braces, insoles, and splints are available and marketed for individuals with OA. In general, these devices are designed to produce mechanical effects that decrease load on the OA affected joint or offer additional sensory input that may enhance proprioception and joint stability. There is generally low to very low evidence supporting their use and very little information that can be used clinically to determine which device may or may not be appropriate for a given individual [164].

Unloading braces have metal and soft materials, which are located or positioned to reduce joint forces during gait activities, particularly in knee OA. A recent treatment guideline [124] recommended that valgus unloading braces should not be offered for medial compartment OA. For lateral compartment OA, a decision to recommend either for or against the use of a varus unloading brace could not be made. These findings were similar to other treatment guidelines [123,125], where low quality evidence provided unclear to positive support of braces. Individuals with lower limb musculoskeletal conditions have long used canes (walking sticks). Based on low and very low evidence levels, these devices may be useful for some individuals with knee and/or hip OA, and they were conditionally recommended by some treatment guidelines [123,124].

For other types of support (e.g., elastic bandages/soft braces/tape) that are thought to primarily improve joint proprioception, a EULAR guidelines group [125] indicated that while there was low quality evidence, it was generally positive. With hand OA, splints are often utilized to manage pain, alignment, and instability issues, particularly at the thumb. Long term use (>3 months) of splints has been recommended for pain that is associated with thumb OA [163,206], with short term use and use in other joints considered to be ineffective [125,206]. Overall, the evidence supporting these recommendations is considered low quality.

Regarding footwear for lower limb OA, a recent treatment guideline [124] has recommended that unloading shoes, minimalist footwear, and rocker-sole shoes should not be offered to individuals with knee OA at this time, due to limited evidence supporting their efficacy. It was also thought that high heel shoes should be avoided but that shoes with additional shock absorbing properties might be suggested to some people. The support for shoe inserts is mixed, with recent treatment guidelines [124,125], finding low to very low evidence supporting lateral wedge shoe insoles for medial compartment OA and medial wedge insoles for lateral compartment OA with benefits ranging from unclear to positive.

Table 1. Best evidence table for the rehabilitation of people with osteoarthritis: Summary of the evidence and recommendations for practice.

Intervention	LoE	Summary of Evidence	Main Profession(s) Involved	Recommended by Recent Treatment Guidelines			Authors' Recommendations for Practice
				Yes [Ref]	No [Ref]	Uncertain/Not Included [Ref]	
Self-Management Programs							
	1A	Low to moderate quality evidence of no or small positive effect on pain, function and quality of life. Large degree of variability in delivery. Self-management programs that include exercise may be more effective.	General practitioner OR psychologist OR physiotherapist OR internet based	ACR [178] EULAR knee & hip [159] NICE [164] OARSI knee [126] PANLAR [16] EULAR hand [207] EULAR pain [125]	-	RACGP [124]	Provide education to enhance understanding of OA and its treatment in order to counter misconceptions that OA inevitably progresses, cannot be treated and that symptoms are closely related to imaging findings. Encourage active self-management and positive behavioral changes such as regular exercise, weight loss, good sleep hygiene and activity pacing. Avoid use of language such as "wear and tear" and "bone on bone" as this may perpetuate unhelpful illness and treatment beliefs.
Exercise							
	1A	Moderate to high quality evidence of a positive effect on pain and function in hip and knee OA that is sustained for several months. Low quality evidence for hand OA. Several different types of exercise may be effective (not clear which is best). Programs that progress exercise volume over time and deliver higher overall doses of exercise may be more effective.	Physiotherapist OR exercise physiologist	ACR [178] EULAR knee & hip [159] NICE [164] OARSI knee [126] PANLAR [163] EULAR hand [207] EULAR pain [125] RACGP [124]	-	-	A combination of resistance training and low impact aerobic exercise should be provided and tailored to the impairments, functional requirements and preferences of the individual. Consider water-based exercise in individuals who prefer it, or cannot tolerate land-based exercise. Provide education that exercise is safe and provide reassurance about potential symptom exacerbations. Exercise should continue for at least 8 weeks and training volume progressed regularly in order to maximize benefits. Provide booster sessions to minimize detraining effects and enhance long term exercise adherence.
Weight Loss							
	1A	Moderate to high quality evidence of dose dependent improvements in pain and function with weight loss in knee OA, with presumed benefits for hip OA and possibly other joints.	Dietician OR physiotherapist OR psychologist OR general practitioner	ACR [178] EULAR knee & hip [159] NICE [164] OARSI knee [126] PANLAR [163] EULAR pain [125] RACGP [124]	-	EULAR hand [207]	Target a minimum weight loss of 5–7.5% of body weight in all people with knee and/or hip OA who have a BMI of ≥ 25 kg/m^2. Greater weight loss will likely result in increased benefit. Provide education about the importance of maintaining a healthy body weight to people with a BMI of < 25 kg/m^2. Explicit weight loss goals and problem solving on how to achieve those goals should be planned in a patient centered, collaborative manner. Consider a combination of individualized strategies such as regular weight monitoring, increased physical activity, social support, meal plans, limiting portion size, reducing fat and sugar intake, time restricted feeding and addressing behavioral triggers to eating (e.g., stress, poor sleep). Combining weight loss with regular exercise will increase its benefits.

Table 1. Cont.

Intervention	LoE	Summary of Evidence	Main Profession(s) Involved	Recommended by Recent Treatment Guidelines			Authors' Recommendations for Practice
				Yes [Ref]	No [Ref]	Uncertain/Not Included [Ref]	
Cognitive Behavioral Therapy							
	1A	Low to moderate quality evidence that CBT has small positive effects on OA pain and fatigue and moderate to large positive effects on self efficacy and pain coping. Overall mixed (no to medium positive) effects on pain in trials of CBT for insomnia.	Psychologist OR internet based	ACR [178] EULAR pain [125] RACGP [124]	-	EULAR hand [207] PANLAR [165] OARSI knee [126] NICE [164] EULAR knee & hip [159]	Consider CBT if significant psychosocial comorbidities (e.g., depression) exist that may interfere with effective pain management and rehabilitation. Consider CBT based sleep interventions for people with OA who have co-morbid sleep problems. Consider CBT if psychological factors such as fear of movement and pain catastrophizing, are a barrier to physical function and engaging in exercise.
Adjunct Treatments							
Manual therapy	1A	Low quality evidence that manual therapy alone or in combination with exercise has short term positive effects on pain and function	Physiotherapist OR osteopath OR chiropractor	RACGP knee & hip [124] ACR [178] NICE [164] (all as an adjunct treatment only)		EULAR knee & hip [159] OARSI knee [126] PANLAR EULAR hand [207] EULAR pain [125]	Consider providing a time-limited course of manual therapy as an adjunct to exercise if the individual finds it beneficial.
Thermal modalities	1B	Low quality evidence that thermal modalities may provide short term positive effects on pain	Self-management OR physiotherapist OR general practitioner	PANLAR [165] (stand-alone) RACGP knee & hip [124] ACR [178] NICE [164] (all as an adjunct only)		EULAR knee & hip [159] EULAR hand [207] EULAR pain [125]	Consider the use of local hot or cold packs as a pain self-management strategy or as an adjunct to exercise if the individual finds this beneficial.
Acupuncture	1A	Low to moderate quality evidence of mixed (no to medium positive) effects on pain compared to sham acupuncture interventions.	Acupuncturist	ACR [178]	NICE [164] RACGP knee & hip [124]	EULAR knee & hip [159] OARSI knee [126] PANLAR [165] EULAR hand [207] EULAR pain [125]	Acupuncture is generally not recommended for the treatment of OA. Consider a time-limited course of acupuncture as an adjunct treatment only if the individual has positive treatment expectations.
Electro-therapy	1A	Low quality evidence that interferential and high-frequency TENS may have positive effects on pain and function. Limited evidence for other forms of electrotherapy.	Self-management OR physiotherapist OR general practitioner	ACR [178] NICE [164] PANLAR [165] RACGP knee & hip [124]		EULAR knee & hip [159] OARSI knee [126] EULAR hand [207] EULAR pain [125]	Consider the use of TENS as a pain self-management strategy or as an adjunct to exercise if the individual finds this beneficial.

Table 1. Cont.

Intervention	LoE	Summary of Evidence	Main Profession(s) Involved	Recommended by Recent Treatment Guidelines			Authors' Recommendations for Practice
				Yes [Ref]	No [Ref]	Uncertain/Not Included [Ref]	
Aids and Devices							
Unloading braces	1B	Limited, low quality evidence that unloading braces have no effect on pain or function in knee OA	Not discipline specific	NICE [164] OARSI knee [126]	RACGP knee & hip [124]	ACR [178] EULAR knee & hip [159] EULAR hand [207]	Unloading braces are not recommended in the treatment of OA.
Cane (walking stick)	2B	Limited, low quality evidence that the use of a cane has positive effects on pain and function in knee OA with possible benefits for other lower limb joints.	Not discipline specific	ACR [178] EULAR knee & hip [159] EULAR pain [125] RACGP knee & hip [124]		EULAR hand [207]	Consider the use of a cane (walking stick) in people with lower limb OA if the individual finds this beneficial or has notable problems with balance and mobility. The cane should be used on the contralateral side and adjusted to the height of the greater trochanter.
Soft braces	1A	Low quality evidence that soft braces have mixed (no to positive) effects on pain and function in knee OA	Not discipline specific	NICE [164] OARSI knee [126] PANLAR [163] EULAR pain [125]		ACR [178] EULAR knee & hip [159] EULAR hand [207]	Consider the use of a soft brace (e.g., neoprene brace, elastic sleeve) in people with knee OA if the individual finds this beneficial.
Splints	1A	Low quality evidence that long term use of splints have a positive effect on pain and function for thumb OA only. Limited evidence that one type of splint is better than any other.	Physiotherapist OR occupational therapist	ACR [178] NICE [164] EULAR hand [207] PANLAR [163] EULAR pain [125]		EULAR knee & hip [159] RACGP knee & hip [124] OARSI knee [126]	Consider the long term use (>3 months) of a splint for people with thumb OA only.
Footwear	1B	Limited, low quality evidence that specific footwear has no benefit on pain and function compared to standard footwear.	Not discipline specific	EULAR knee & hip [159] NICE [164] EULAR pain [125] OARSI knee [126]	RACGP knee & hip [124]	EULAR hand [207] ACR [178] PANLAR [163]	Specific footwear (e.g., minimalist footwear, rocker-sole shoes, unloading shoes) is not recommended in the treatment of OA. Consider the use of shoes with appropriate shock absorbing properties for people with lower limb OA.
Shoe Insoles	1B	Low quality evidence that medial wedge shoe insoles may provide positive effects on pain and function for lateral compartment knee OA. Low quality evidence that lateral wedge insoles for medial compartment knee OA have mixed (no to positive) effects on pain and function	Podiatrist OR physiotherapist	ACR [178] NICE [164] OARSI knee [126] PANLAR [163]	RACGP knee & hip [124]	EULAR knee & hip [159] EULAR hand [207]	Consider the use of medial wedge shoe insole for people with lateral compartment knee OA if the individual finds this beneficial. Lateral wedge shoe insoles are not recommended in the treatment of knee OA.

Level of Evidence (LoE): 1A: Systematic review of randomized controlled trials; 1B: Individual randomized controlled trials; 2A: Systematic review of cohort studies; 2B: Individual cohort study or low quality randomized controlled trials; 3A: Systematic review of case-control studies; 3B: individual case-control study; 4: Case-series; 5: Expert opinion. Quality of evidence is as reported in recent systematic reviews or international treatment guidelines. Abbreviations: LoE = Level of evidence; OA = osteoarthritis; Ref = Reference; CBT = Cognitive behavioral therapy.

3. Promising Directions for Clinical Practice

3.1. Improved Education Strategies to Address Maladaptive Pain-Related Beliefs

People with OA can display fear avoidance behaviors [16–18] that limit their engagement in effective rehabilitation strategies, such as regular exercise. A recent Cochrane review [207] has highlighted many of the unhelpful beliefs held by people with hip and knee OA that help to shape these behaviors. Many people describe being confused about the cause of their pain and bewildered by its variability and unpredictable nature [207]. Furthermore, as movement frequently increased their pain, they worried that this might be doing their joint further harm and described avoiding physical activity and exercise as a result [207]. These findings suggest a need for strategies tackling these maladaptive beliefs and behaviors.

Pain neuroscience education is a cognitive-based intervention that is aimed at reconceptualizing pain by de-emphasizing pathoanatomical content and focusing on other factors, such as the discordance between imaging findings and pain, peripheral and central sensitization, cognition, mood and lifestyle factors that may contribute to the development and persistence of pain, all within a biopsychosocial framework [208,209]. The use of this educational strategy in people with chronic pain in order to change pain related beliefs, improve health behaviors and—importantly—desensitize the central nervous system, is supported by high quality evidence [209–211]. Although pain neuroscience education has been studied in several chronic pain populations [211], the evidence in people with OA is still limited and mainly focused on people undergoing knee arthroplasty [212,213]. In these studies, positive effects of preoperative pain neuroscience education were found in terms of psychosocial measures (pain catastrophizing [212] and kinesiophobia [212,213]), pressure pain thresholds [213], and peoples' beliefs regarding their scheduled surgery [213].

As the evidence suggests that current education strategies for OA have limited success [138], a pain neuroscience approach might provide an alternative and more effective means of targeting unhelpful illness and treatment beliefs, particularly at the beginning of a rehabilitation program. This may help to reduce pain and psychological distress as well as facilitate engagement and adherence in exercise-based interventions. Such an approach might be particularly effective if the pain-relieving effects of exercise and its role in desensitizing the nociceptive system are specifically emphasized and incorporated into the education session(s), as this has been shown to enhance positive expectations and increase exercise induced pain relief [214].

3.2. Enhancing the Effectiveness of Resistance Training

The weakness of muscles adjacent to the painful joint(s) is a common feature of OA. Adequate muscle strength is required for many activities of daily living [215,216] and muscle weakness is a major factor contributing to OA related functional disability [217,218]. In the lower limb, muscles may also have a protective role, attenuating mechanical loading of the OA joint during gait and other activities [27,219]. There is some evidence that higher quadriceps muscle volume might protect against incident knee pain and ongoing cartilage loss [29,30] and recent findings suggest that the magnitude of quadriceps strength gains partially mediate the pain-relieving effect of resistance training in knee OA [220]. Unfortunately, muscle strength gains during resistance training are often compromised by arthrogenic muscle inhibition, an ongoing neural inhibition of muscle activation due to factors, such as joint effusion, nociception, and sensory loss [23,221–223]. This problem is widely recognized in knee OA [224], although arthrogenic muscle inhibition might also contribute to ongoing muscle weakness at other joints [225–228]. Importantly, it has been shown in people with OA that adjunct disinhibitory interventions, such as cryotherapy, TENS, and NSAIDS, can be used to reduce arthrogenic muscle inhibition [229,230] and, when used in conjunction with resistance training, might enhance muscle strength gains when compared to resistance training alone [230–232].

Another promising intervention that might enhance the efficacy of resistance training in OA is blood flow restriction training. Blood flow restriction training utilizes an inflatable cuff or band to partially occlude blood flow in the exercising muscles. Importantly, blood flow restriction allows exercise of very low load (e.g., 20–40% of 1RM) to produce significant gains in muscle strength and size [233], seemingly due to exaggerated metabolic stress when training the muscle(s) under partial occlusion. To date, blood flow restriction training has been largely applied in healthy populations [233], but it is an attractive intervention for OA, as it has the potential to accelerate muscle hypertrophy and strength gains while also notably reducing the mechanical load placed on the affected joint(s) during training—thus potentially minimizing exercise-induced flares in joint pain. Preliminary evidence in populations that are relevant to OA suggests that blood flow restriction training is associated with less pain during exercise [234–236] and may produce similar [234–237] or greater [238] gains in muscle strength than resistance training performed without blood flow restriction.

3.3. Brain Directed Treatments of Sensorimotor Networks

There is growing evidence of dysfunction in brain sensorimotor networks amongst people with OA, with observations of widespread tactile hypoaesthesia [239], reduced tactile acuity [240], body size distortions [41], neglect-like symptoms [42], altered primary somatosensory cortex volume [96], impaired implicit motor imagery performance [42,241], and both disinhibition [242] and reorganization [243] of the primary motor cortex. While the clinical implications of these changes are yet to be fully elucidated, there is evidence that some might be important treatment targets for OA pain. For example, recent RCTs provide preliminary evidence that non-invasive brain stimulation of the primary motor cortex may reduce OA pain, either when delivered alone or in combination with other interventions [244–247]. Furthermore, in other chronic pain conditions, sensory discrimination training has been used to reverse deficits in tactile acuity that are similar to those that were observed in OA [248,249]. These interventions have also been shown to reduce chronic pain intensity [248–251], with the magnitude of pain relief being strongly correlated to improvements in tactile acuity [249,250] and cortical sensory representation of the affected body part [250]. Finally, it has been shown that presenting a multisensory illusion of the painful OA joint(s) stretching or shrinking can produce immediate and, in some cases, substantial pain relief [40,252], and that this intervention can partially correct distorted size perceptions of the OA affected limb [41]. While still in its infancy, the use of brain directed treatments that target impaired sensorimotor networks is a promising clinical direction that might have important future implications in the rehabilitation of OA pain.

4. Promising Directions for Research

4.1. Personalized Treatment

In recent years, a number of studies have attempted to identify several distinct OA pain phenotypes or subgroups from a larger population [253–258]. The potential benefits of such an approach include the identification of key prognostic factors that predict treatment response and, ultimately, the development of more targeted treatments that are personalized to the individual and their dominant pain mechanism(s). For example, individuals with OA who have more pronounced central sensitization, as evidenced by increased temporal summation [259–264] and, in some cases, widespread pain sensitivity [265] and reduced conditioned pain modulation [261,266] may experience less pain relief and are at higher risk of persistent pain after peripherally targeted treatments, such as NSAIDs or total joint replacement surgery.

The identification of relevant OA pain phenotypes may also lead to improved rehabilitation strategies. For example, Fingleton et al. [267] have recently shown that the initial response to exercise in people with knee OA varies according to the baseline function of their endogenous descending pain inhibitory/facilitatory pathways—i.e., those with deficient conditioned pain modulation tended to experience increased pain after both aerobic and resistance exercise, while pain was reduced in those with intact conditioned pain modulation and in healthy controls. Studies such as this that explore within-group differences in OA may allow for better identification of likely non-responders to treatment and facilitate the development of alternative, more personalized strategies (e.g., the combination of centrally acting analgesics with exercise) to enhance clinical outcomes in these individuals.

Similarly, despite consistent evidence of the positive treatment effects of psychological therapies for OA, there is a gap between the strength of evidence for process-oriented measures and core outcomes. For example, whereas psychological therapies produce large effects on active coping, the effects on pain and function tend to be smaller [268]. One reason for this discrepancy might be the fact that a portion of people with OA have more pronounced central sensitization [89], which may be less responsive to traditional CBT and related psychosocial therapies [269]. Lumley & Schubiner [269] have recently proposed a novel treatment paradigm that is intended to target people with central sensitization by performing a detailed intake assessment and tailoring treatment with pain neuroscience education, cognitive therapy, mindfulness, behavioral desensitization, emotional expression, and interpersonal communication skills. An initial RCT in fibromyalgia patients [270] showed that this treatment approach outperformed traditional CBT in lowering the fibromyalgia symptoms and widespread pain. Future work is needed to similarly evaluate the differential efficacy between this novel pain treatment and traditional CBT for people with OA subtyped based on their degree of central sensitization.

4.2. New Ways of Understanding and Enhancing Treatment Adherence

Better adherence to rehabilitation interventions in OA is typically associated with greater symptom improvement [196,271–273]. However, previous work has documented poor to adequate adherence among this population [274–277]. Furthermore, current strategies that aimed at increasing adherence are not uniformly effective. A meta-analysis of adherence interventions found significant improvements in only 18 of the 42 included trials [278]. This low efficacy rate emphasizes the need for novel, more potent interventions to promote adherence to rehabilitation programs. The predictors and mechanisms of adherence to rehabilitation interventions in OA are not fully established. However, previous work suggests that motivation is a consistent predictor of treatment adherence in OA and across chronic pain conditions [279–284].

Although psychosocial factors predicting treatment motivation amongst those with chronic pain have been probed, physiological mechanisms potentially subserving these processes have not been examined. For example, a potentially important physiological mechanism of treatment motivation is mesocorticolimbic function [285]. This neural system—colloquially referred to as "the reward system"—has been extensively associated with motivational processes and reward learning in humans and animal models [286–289]. On behavioral tasks, individuals with chronic pain demonstrated altered reward learning [290–292] and reduced motivation [280,293] when compared to individuals without pain. Factors, such as depression and opioid use, are likely to further compound these effects. Neuroimaging data support these findings by demonstrating aberrant mesocorticolimbic system structure [96,294] and function during pain relief—potentially reflective of attenuated rewarding effects of analgesia [295–299]—and wakeful rest [300–302] among people with chronic pain.

It is possible that altered reward learning and attenuated rewarding effects of pain relief contribute to reductions in treatment motivation and the resultant adherence to rehabilitation. Future studies might examine the extent of the relationships among baseline treatment motivation, mesocorticolimbic function, and engagement in adaptive rehabilitation strategies, such as regular exercise. This question could be addressed while using a combination of neuroimaging, questionnaire, and ecological momentary assessment (e.g., daily diary) data. Such an approach might inform the development of adjunct interventions to bolster the rewarding effects of pain relief early in the course of rehabilitation (e.g., via non-invasive brain stimulation, endogenous reward system training) and promote better long-term adherence to rehabilitation interventions.

5. Conclusions

Treatment strategies for OA pain should be broadened beyond a simple focus on the affected joint(s). While joint directed treatments remain sensible, it is important to screen for, recognize, and appropriately manage other factors (e.g., central sensitization, psychosocial factors, sleep problems) that may be contributing to an individual's pain experience. Rehabilitation is considered first line treatment for OA pain. Core interventions that are widely recommended by evidence-based OA treatment guidelines include regular aerobic and resistance exercise, self-management programs, and, where appropriate, weight loss. A range of other options, such as manual therapy, thermal modalities, TENS, and joint braces/splints, may also be useful adjunct therapies, although there is currently less evidence supporting their use. CBT is increasingly recognized as a valuable treatment option for selected individuals and may have important clinical benefits for psychological and sleep related comorbidities. While further evidence is needed to support their clinical utility, novel treatment approaches, such as pain neuroscience education, the use of disinhibitory interventions to augment resistance training, blood flow restriction training, and brain directed treatments (e.g., illusory resizing and non-invasive brain stimulation) may play an important role in the future rehabilitation of OA pain. In addition, key avenues for future research include the development of personalized rehabilitation interventions and improved methods to both enhance treatment adherence and better understand its physiological underpinnings.

Author Contributions: Conceptualization: D.R. and E.H.; Literature search and data extraction: all authors; Writing, original draft preparation: all authors; Writing, review & editing: all authors; Supervision: D.R.

Funding: This research received no external funding.

Acknowledgments: Eva Huysmans is a PhD research fellow of the Research Foundation Flanders (FWO - 1108619N).

Conflicts of Interest: The authors declare no conflict of interest.

References

1. Lim, S.S.; Vos, T.; Flaxman, A.D.; Danaei, G.; Shibuya, K.; Adair-Rohani, H.; AlMazroa, M.A.; Amann, M.; Anderson, H.R.; Andrews, K.G. A comparative risk assessment of burden of disease and injury attributable to 67 risk factors and risk factor clusters in 21 regions, 1990–2010: A systematic analysis for the Global Burden of Disease Study 2010. *Lancet* **2012**, *380*, 2224–2260. [CrossRef]
2. Martel-Pelletier, J.; Barr, A.J.; Cicuttini, F.M.; Conaghan, P.G.; Cooper, C.; Goldring, M.B.; Goldring, S.R.; Jones, G.; Teichtahl, A.J.; Pelletier, J.-P. Osteoarthritis. *Nat. Rev. Dis. Primers* **2016**, *2*, 16072. [CrossRef] [PubMed]
3. Johnson, V.L.; Hunter, D.J. The epidemiology of osteoarthritis. *Best Pract. Res. Clin. Rheumatol.* **2014**, *28*, 5–15. [CrossRef] [PubMed]
4. Spector, T.D.; MacGregor, A.J. Risk factors for osteoarthritis: Genetics. *Osteoarthr. Cartil.* **2004**, *12* (Suppl. A), S39–S44. [CrossRef]
5. Felson, D.T.; Anderson, J.J.; Naimark, A.; Walker, A.M.; Meenan, R.F. Obesity and Knee Osteoarthritis: The Framingham Study. *Ann. Intern. Med.* **1988**, *109*, 18–24. [CrossRef] [PubMed]
6. Gelber, A.C.; Hochberg, M.C.; Mead, L.A.; Wang, N.-Y.; Wigley, F.M.; Klag, M.J. Body mass index in young men and the risk of subsequent knee and hip osteoarthritis1. *Am. J. Med.* **1999**, *6*, 542–548. [CrossRef]
7. Jensen, L.K. Hip osteoarthritis: Influence of work with heavy lifting, climbing stairs or ladders, or combining kneeling/squatting with heavy lifting. *Occup. Environ. Med.* **2008**, *65*, 6–19. [CrossRef]
8. Jensen, L.K. Knee osteoarthritis: Influence of work involving heavy lifting, kneeling, climbing stairs or ladders, or kneeling/squatting combined with heavy lifting. *Occup. Environ. Med.* **2008**, *65*, 72–89. [CrossRef]
9. Kaila-kangas, L.; Arokoski, J.; Impivaara, O.; Viikari-juntura, E.; Leino-arjas, P.; Luukkonen, R.; Heliövaara, M. Associations of hip osteoarthritis with history of recurrent exposure to manual handling of loads over 20 kg and work participation: A population-based study of men and women. *Occup. Environ. Med.* **2011**, *68*, 734–738. [CrossRef]
10. Madry, H.; Luyten, F.P.; Facchini, A. Biological aspects of early osteoarthritis. *Knee Surg. Sports Traumatol. Arthrosc.* **2012**, *20*, 407–422. [CrossRef]

11. Williams, D.A.; Farrell, M.J.; Cunningham, J.; Gracely, R.H.; Ambrose, K.; Cupps, T.; Mohan, N.; Clauw, D.J. Knee pain and radiographic osteoarthritis interact in the prediction of levels of self-reported disability. *Arthritis Care Res.* **2004**, *51*, 558–561. [CrossRef] [PubMed]
12. Rejeski, W.J.; Martin, K.; Ettinger, W.H.; Morgan, T. Treating disability in knee osteoarthritis with exercise therapy: A central role for self-efficacy and pain. *Arthritis Rheum.* **1998**, *11*, 94–101. [CrossRef]
13. Ayis, S.; Dieppe, P. The natural history of disability and its determinants in adults with lower limb musculoskeletal pain. *J. Rheumatol.* **2009**, *36*, 583–591. [CrossRef] [PubMed]
14. Moe, R.H.; Grotle, M.; Kjeken, I.; Hagen, K.B.; Kvien, T.K.; Uhlig, T. Disease impact of hand OA compared with hip, knee and generalized disease in specialist rheumatology health care. *Rheumatology* **2012**, *52*, 189–196. [CrossRef]
15. Grotle, M.; Hagen, K.; Natvig, B.; Dahl, F.; Kvien, T. Prevalence and burden of osteoarthritis: Results from a population survey in Norway. *J. Rheumatol.* **2008**, *35*, 677–684.
16. Scopaz, K.A.; Piva, S.R.; Wisniewski, S.; Fitzgerald, G.K. Relationships of Fear, Anxiety, and Depression With Physical Function in Patients With Knee Osteoarthritis. *Arch. Phys. Med. Rehabil.* **2009**, *90*, 1866–1873. [CrossRef]
17. Heuts, P.; Vlaeyen, J.; Roelofs, J.; de Bie, R.; Aretz, K.; van Weel, C.; van Schayck, O. Pain-related fear and daily functioning in patients with osteoarthritis. *Pain* **2004**, *110*, 228–235. [CrossRef]
18. Vincent, H.K.; Lamb, K.M.; Day, T.I.; Tillman, S.M.; Vincent, K.R.; George, S.Z. Morbid Obesity Is Associated with Fear of Movement and Lower Quality of Life in Patients with Knee Pain-Related Diagnoses. *PmR* **2010**, *2*, 713–722. [CrossRef]
19. Allen, K.; Renner, J.; Devellis, B.; Helmick, C.; Jordan, J. Osteoarthritis and sleep: The Johnston County Osteoarthritis Project. *J. Rheumatol.* **2008**, *35*, 1102–1107.
20. Hawker, G.; Gignac, M.; Badley, E.; Davis, A.; French, M.; Li, Y.; Perruccio, A.; Power, J.; Sale, J.; Lou, W. A longitudinal study to explain the pain-depression link in older adults with osteoarthritis. *Arthritis Care Res.* **2011**, *63*, 1382–1390. [CrossRef]
21. Dominick, K.L.; Ahern, F.M.; Gold, C.H.; Heller, D.A. Health-related quality of life and health service use among older adults with osteoarthritis. *Arthritis Care Res.* **2004**, *51*, 326–331. [CrossRef] [PubMed]
22. Abbott, J.H.; Usiskin, I.M.; Wilson, R.; Hansen, P.; Losina, E. The quality-of-life burden of knee osteoarthritis in New Zealand adults: A model-based evaluation. *PLoS ONE* **2017**, *12*, e0185676. [CrossRef] [PubMed]
23. Henriksen, M.; Rosager, S.; Aaboe, J.; Graven-Nielsen, T.; Bliddal, H. Experimental knee pain reduces muscle strength. *J. Pain* **2011**, *12*, 460–467. [CrossRef] [PubMed]
24. Rice, D.A.; McNair, P.J.; Lewis, G.N.; Mannion, J. Experimental knee pain impairs submaximal force steadiness in isometric, eccentric, and concentric muscle actions. *Arthritis Res. Ther.* **2015**, *1*, 1–6. [CrossRef]
25. Henriksen, M.; Graven-Nielsen, T.; Aaboe, J.; Andriacchi, T.P.; Bliddal, H. Gait changes in patients with knee osteoarthritis are replicated by experimental knee pain. *Arthritis Care Res.* **2010**, *62*, 501–509. [CrossRef]
26. Liikavainio, T.; Isolehto, J.; Helminen, H.J.; Perttunen, J.; Lepola, V.; Kiviranta, I.; Arokoski, J.P.; Komi, P.V. Loading and gait symmetry during level and stair walking in asymptomatic subjects with knee osteoarthritis: Importance of quadriceps femoris in reducing impact force during heel strike? *Knee* **2007**, *14*, 231–238. [CrossRef]
27. Mikesky, A.E.; Meyer, A.; Thompson, K.L. Relationship between quadriceps strength and rate of loading during gait in women. *J. Orthop. Res.* **2000**, *18*, 171–175. [CrossRef]
28. Amin, S.; Baker, K.; Niu, J.; Clancy, M.; Goggins, J.; Guermazi, A.; Grigoryan, M.; Hunter, D.J.; Felson, D.T. Quadriceps strength and the risk of cartilage loss and symptom progression in knee osteoarthritis. *Arthritis Rheum.* **2009**, *60*, 189–198. [CrossRef]
29. Segal, N.A.; Glass, N.A. Is quadriceps muscle weakness a risk factor for incident or progressive knee osteoarthritis? *Phys Sportsmed* **2011**, *39*, 44–50. [CrossRef]
30. Oiestad, B.E.; Juhl, C.B.; Eitzen, I.; Thorlund, J.B. Knee extensor muscle weakness is a risk factor for development of knee osteoarthritis. A systematic review and meta-analysis. *Osteoarthr. Cartil.* **2015**, *23*, 171–177. [CrossRef]
31. Hawker, G.A. Experiencing painful osteoarthritis: What have we learned from listening? *Curr. Opin. Rheumatol.* **2009**, *21*, 507–512. [CrossRef] [PubMed]

32. Cedraschi, C.; Delézay, S.; Marty, M.; Berenbaum, F.; Bouhassira, D.; Henrotin, Y.; Laroche, F.; Perrot, S. "Let's talk about OA pain": A qualitative analysis of the perceptions of people suffering from OA. Towards the development of a specific pain OA-related questionnaire, the Osteoarthritis Symptom Inventory Scale (OASIS). *PLoS ONE* **2013**, *8*, e79988. [CrossRef] [PubMed]
33. Moss, P.; Knight, E.; Wright, A. Subjects with knee osteoarthritis exhibit widespread hyperalgesia to pressure and cold. *PLoS ONE* **2016**, *11*, e0147526. [CrossRef] [PubMed]
34. Stamm, T.; van der Giesen, F.; Thorstensson, C.; Steen, E.; Birrell, F.; Bauernfeind, B.; Marshall, N.; Prodinger, B.; Machold, K.; Smolen, J. Patient perspective of hand osteoarthritis in relation to concepts covered by instruments measuring functioning: A qualitative European multicentre study. *Ann. Rheum. Dis.* **2009**, *68*, 1453–1460. [CrossRef]
35. Hawker, G.; Stewart, L.; French, M.; Cibere, J.; Jordan, J.; March, L.; Suarez-Almazor, M.; Gooberman-Hill, R. Understanding the pain experience in hip and knee osteoarthritis–an OARSI/OMERACT initiative. *Osteoarthr. Cartil.* **2008**, *16*, 415–422. [CrossRef] [PubMed]
36. Blikman, T.; Rienstra, W.; van Raay, J.J.; Dijkstra, B.; Bulstra, S.K.; Stevens, M.; van den Akker-Scheek, I. Neuropathic-like symptoms and the association with joint-specific function and quality of life in patients with hip and knee osteoarthritis. *PLoS ONE* **2018**, *13*, e0199165. [CrossRef]
37. Hochman, J.; Gagliese, L.; Davis, A.; Hawker, G. Neuropathic pain symptoms in a community knee OA cohort. *Osteoarthr. Cartil.* **2011**, *19*, 647–654. [CrossRef]
38. Hochman, J.; French, M.; Bermingham, S.; Hawker, G. The nerve of osteoarthritis pain. *Arthritis Care Res.* **2010**, *62*, 1019. [CrossRef]
39. Nishigami, T.; Mibu, A.; Tanaka, K.; Yamashita, Y.; Yamada, E.; Wand, B.M.; Catley, M.J.; Stanton, T.R.; Moseley, G.L. Development and psychometric properties of knee-specific body-perception questionnaire in people with knee osteoarthritis: The Fremantle Knee Awareness Questionnaire. *PLoS ONE* **2017**, *12*, e0179225. [CrossRef]
40. Stanton, T.R.; Gilpin, H.R.; Edwards, L.; Moseley, G.L.; Newport, R. Illusory resizing of the painful knee is analgesic in symptomatic knee osteoarthritis. *PeerJ* **2018**, *6*, e5206. [CrossRef]
41. Gilpin, H.R.; Moseley, G.L.; Stanton, T.R.; Newport, R. Evidence for distorted mental representation of the hand in osteoarthritis. *Rheumatology* **2014**, *54*, 678–682. [CrossRef] [PubMed]
42. Magni, N.E.; McNair, P.J.; Rice, D.A. Sensorimotor performance and function in people with osteoarthritis of the hand: A case–control comparison. *Semin. Arthritis Rheum.* **2018**, *47*, 676–682. [CrossRef] [PubMed]
43. Keefe, F.J.; Affleck, G.; France, C.R.; Emery, C.F.; Waters, S.; Caldwell, D.S.; Stainbrook, D.; Hackshaw, K.V.; Fox, L.C.; Wilson, K. Gender differences in pain, coping, and mood in individuals having osteoarthritic knee pain: A within-day analysis. *Pain* **2004**, *110*, 571–577. [CrossRef] [PubMed]
44. Bellamy, N.; Sothern, R.; Campbell, J.; Buchanan, W. Rhythmic variations in pain, stiffness, and manual dexterity in hand osteoarthritis. *Ann. Rheum. Dis.* **2002**, *61*, 1075. [CrossRef] [PubMed]
45. Parry, E.; Ogollah, R.; Peat, G. Significant pain variability in persons with, or at high risk of, knee osteoarthritis: Preliminary investigation based on secondary analysis of cohort data. *Bmc Musculoskelet. Disord.* **2017**, *18*, 80. [CrossRef] [PubMed]
46. Verkleij, S.P.; Hoekstra, T.; Rozendaal, R.M.; Waarsing, J.H.; Koes, B.W.; Luijsterburg, P.A.; Bierma-Zeinstra, S. Defining discriminative pain trajectories in hip osteoarthritis over a 2-year time period. *Ann. Rheum. Dis.* **2012**, *71*, 1517–1523. [CrossRef] [PubMed]
47. Nicholls, E.; Thomas, E.; van der Windt, D.; Croft, P.; Peat, G. Pain trajectory groups in persons with, or at high risk of, knee osteoarthritis: Findings from the Knee Clinical Assessment Study and the Osteoarthritis Initiative. *Osteoarthr. Cartil.* **2014**, *22*, 2041. [CrossRef]
48. Collins, J.; Katz, J.; Dervan, E.; Losina, E. Trajectories and risk profiles of pain in persons with radiographic, symptomatic knee osteoarthritis: Data from the osteoarthritis initiative. *Osteoarthr. Cartil.* **2014**, *22*, 622–630. [CrossRef]
49. Felson, D.T. Developments in the clinical understanding of osteoarthritis. *Arthritis Res. Ther.* **2009**, *11*, 203. [CrossRef]
50. Peters, T.J.; Sanders, C.; Dieppe, P.; Donovan, J. Factors associated with change in pain and disability over time. *Br. J. Gen. Pract.* **2005**, *55*, 205–211.

51. Leffondré, K.; Abrahamowicz, M.; Regeasse, A.; Hawker, G.A.; Badley, E.M.; McCusker, J.; Belzile, E. Statistical measures were proposed for identifying longitudinal patterns of change in quantitative health indicators. *J. Clin. Epidemiol.* **2004**, *57*, 1049–1062. [CrossRef] [PubMed]
52. Brandt, K.D. Pain, synovitis, and articular cartilage changes in osteoarthritis. *Semin Arthritis Rheum* **1989**, *18*, 77–80. [CrossRef]
53. Zimmermann, M. Pain mechanisms and mediators in osteoarthritis. *Semin Arthritis Rheum* **1989**, *18*, 22–29. [CrossRef]
54. Hunter, D.J.; McDougall, J.J.; Keefe, F.J. The symptoms of osteoarthritis and the genesis of pain. *Rheum. Dis. Clin. North Am.* **2008**, *34*, 623–643. [CrossRef] [PubMed]
55. Bartley, E.J.; Palit, S.; Staud, R. Predictors of Osteoarthritis Pain: The Importance of Resilience. *Curr. Rheumatol. Rep.* **2017**, *9*, 1–9. [CrossRef]
56. Hunter, D.; Guermazi, A.; Roemer, F.; Zhang, Y.; Neogi, T. Structural correlates of pain in joints with osteoarthritis. *Osteoarthr. Cartil.* **2013**, *9*, 1170–1178. [CrossRef]
57. Felson, D. The sources of pain in knee osteoarthritis. *Curr. Opin. Rheumatol.* **2005**, *17*, 624–628. [CrossRef]
58. Schaible, H.-G.; Richter, F.; Ebersberger, A.; Boettger, M.K.; Vanegas, H.; Natura, G.; Vazquez, E.; Segond von Banchet, G. Joint pain. *Exp. Brain Res.* **2009**, *196*, 153–162. [CrossRef]
59. Eitner, A.; Hofmann, G.; Schaible, H. Mechanisms of Osteoarthritic Pain. Studies in Humans and Experimental Models. *Front. Mol. Neurosci.* **2017**, *10*, 349. [CrossRef]
60. Hannan, M.; Felson, D.; Pincus, T. Analysis of the discordance between radiographic changes and knee pain in osteoarthritis of the knee. *J. Rheumatol.* **2000**, *27*, 1513.
61. Cubukcu, D.; Sarsan, A.; Alkan, H. Relationships between Pain, Function and Radiographic Findings in Osteoarthritis of the Knee: A Cross-Sectional Study. *Arthritis* **2012**, *2012*, 5. [CrossRef] [PubMed]
62. Duncan, R.; Peat, G.; Thomas, E.; Hay, E.; McCall, I.; Croft, P. Symptoms and radiographic osteoarthritis: Not as discordant as they are made out to be? *Ann. Rheum. Dis.* **2007**, *66*, 86. [CrossRef] [PubMed]
63. Neogi, T.; Felson, D.; Niu, J.; Nevitt, M.; Lewis, C.E.; Aliabadi, P.; Sack, B.; Torner, J.; Bradley, L.; Zhang, Y. Association between radiographic features of knee osteoarthritis and pain: Results from two cohort studies. *Bmj Br. Med J.* **2009**, 498–501. [CrossRef]
64. Kim, C.; Nevitt, M.C.; Niu, J.; Clancy, M.M.; Lane, N.E.; Link, T.M.; Vlad, S.; Tolstykh, I.; Jungmann, P.M.; Felson, D.T. Association of hip pain with radiographic evidence of hip osteoarthritis: Diagnostic test study. *Bmj* **2015**, 351. [CrossRef] [PubMed]
65. Bedson, J.; Croft, P.R. The discordance between clinical and radiographic knee osteoarthritis: A systematic search and summary of the literature. *Bmc Musculoskelet. Disord.* **2008**, *9*, 1–11. [CrossRef] [PubMed]
66. Dieppe, P.A.; Cushnaghan, J.; Shepstone, L. The Bristol 'OA500' study: Progression of osteoarthritis (OA) over 3 years and the relationship between clinical and radiographic changes at the knee joint. *Osteoarthr. Cartil.* **1997**, *5*, 87–97. [CrossRef]
67. Kumm, J.; Turkiewicz, A.; Zhang, F.; Englund, M. Structural abnormalities detected by knee magnetic resonance imaging are common in middle-aged subjects with and without risk factors for osteoarthritis. *Acta Orthop.* **2018**, *89*, 535–540. [CrossRef]
68. Barr, A.J.; Campbell, T.M.; Hopkinson, D.; Kingsbury, S.R.; Bowes, M.A.; Conaghan, P.G. A systematic review of the relationship between subchondral bone features, pain and structural pathology in peripheral joint osteoarthritis. *Arthritis Res. Ther.* **2015**, *1*, 1–36. [CrossRef]
69. Yusuf, E.; Kortekaas, M.; Watt, I.; Huizinga, T.; Kloppenburg, M. Do knee abnormalities visualised on MRI explain knee pain in knee osteoarthritis? A systematic review. *Ann. Rheum. Dis.* **2011**, *70*, 60. [CrossRef]
70. Roemer, F.; Frobell, R.; Hunter, D.; Crema, M.; Fischer, W.; Bohndorf, K.; Guermazi, A. MRI-detected subchondral bone marrow signal alterations of the knee joint: Terminology, imaging appearance, relevance and radiological differential diagnosis. *Osteoarthr. Cartil.* **2009**, *17*, 1115–1131. [CrossRef]
71. Alliston, T.; Hernandez, C.J.; Findlay, D.M.; Felson, D.T.; Kennedy, O.D. Bone marrow lesions in osteoarthritis: What lies beneath. *J. Orthop. Res.* **2018**, *36*, 1818–1825. [CrossRef] [PubMed]
72. Taljanovic, M.S.; Graham, A.R.; Benjamin, J.B.; Gmitro, A.F.; Krupinski, E.A.; Schwartz, S.A.; Hunter, T.B.; Resnick, D.L. Bone marrow edema pattern in advanced hip osteoarthritis: Quantitative assessment with magnetic resonance imaging and correlation with clinical examination, radiographic findings, and histopathology. *Skelet. Radiol.* **2008**, *37*, 423–431. [CrossRef] [PubMed]

73. Kuttapitiya, A.; Assi, L.; Laing, K.; Hing, C.; Mitchell, P.; Whitley, G.; Harrison, A.; Howe, F.A.; Ejindu, V.; Heron, C. Microarray analysis of bone marrow lesions in osteoarthritis demonstrates upregulation of genes implicated in osteochondral turnover, neurogenesis and inflammation. *Ann. Rheum. Dis.* **2017**, *76*, 1764–1773. [CrossRef] [PubMed]
74. Wang, X.; Hunter, D.; Jin, X.; Ding, C. The importance of synovial inflammation in osteoarthritis: Current evidence from imaging assessments and clinical trials. *Osteoarthr. Cartil.* **2018**, *26*, 165–174. [CrossRef]
75. Guermazi, A.; Niu, J.; Hayashi, D.; Roemer, F.W.; Englund, M.; Neogi, T.; Aliabadi, P.; McLennan, C.E.; Felson, D.T. Prevalence of abnormalities in knees detected by MRI in adults without knee osteoarthritis: Population based observational study (Framingham Osteoarthritis Study). *BMJ* **2012**, *345*, e5339. [CrossRef]
76. Kornaat, P.R.; Bloem, J.L.; Ceulemans, R.Y.; Riyazi, N.; Rosendaal, F.R.; Nelissen, R.G.; Carter, W.O.; Hellio Le Graverand, M.-P.; Kloppenburg, M. Osteoarthritis of the knee: Association between clinical features and MR imaging findings. *Radiology* **2006**, *239*, 811–817. [CrossRef]
77. Felson, D.T.; Chaisson, C.E.; Hill, C.L.; Totterman, S.M.; Gale, M.E.; Skinner, K.M.; Kazis, L.; Gale, D.R. The Association of Bone Marrow Lesions with Pain in Knee Osteoarthritis. *Ann. Intern. Med.* **2001**, *134*, 541–549. [CrossRef]
78. de Lange-Brokaar, B.; Ioan-Facsinay, A.; Yusuf, E.; Kroon, H.; Zuurmond, A.-M.; Stojanovic-Susulic, V.; Nelissen, R.; Bloem, J.; Kloppenburg, M. Evolution of synovitis in osteoarthritic knees and its association with clinical features. *Osteoarthr. Cartil.* **2016**, *24*, 1867–1874. [CrossRef]
79. Kornaat, P.R.; Kloppenburg, M.; Sharma, R.; Botha-scheepers, S.A.; Le Graverand, M.-p.H.; Coene, N.L.; Bloem, J.L.; Watt, I. Bone marrow edema-like lesions change in volume in the majority of patients with osteoarthritis; associations with clinical features. *Eur. Radiol.* **2007**, *17*, 3073–3078. [CrossRef]
80. Martindale, J.; Wilson, A.; Reeve, A.; Chessell, I.; Headley, P. Chronic secondary hypersensitivity of dorsal horn neurones following inflammation of the knee joint. *Pain* **2007**, *1*, 79–86. [CrossRef]
81. Drake, R.A.; Leith, J.; Almahasneh, F.; Martindale, J.; Wilson, A.; Lumb, B.; Donaldson, L.F. Periaqueductal grey EP3 receptors facilitate spinal nociception in arthritic secondary hypersensitivity. *J. Neurosci.* **2016**, *36*, 9026–9040. [CrossRef] [PubMed]
82. Havelin, J.; Imbert, I.; Cormier, J.; Allen, J.; Porreca, F.; King, T. Central sensitization and neuropathic features of ongoing pain in a rat model of advanced osteoarthritis. *J. Pain* **2016**, *17*, 374–382. [CrossRef] [PubMed]
83. Neugebauer, V.; Li, W. Differential sensitization of amygdala neurons to afferent inputs in a model of arthritic pain. *J. Neurophysiol.* **2003**, *89*, 716–727. [CrossRef] [PubMed]
84. Woolf, C.J. Central sensitization: Implications for the diagnosis and treatment of pain. *Pain* **2011**, *152*, S2–S15. [CrossRef] [PubMed]
85. Arendt-Nielsen, L.; Nie, H.; Laursen, M.B.; Laursen, B.S.; Madeleine, P.; Simonsen, O.H.; Graven-Nielsen, T. Sensitization in patients with painful knee osteoarthritis. *Pain* **2010**, *149*, 573–581. [CrossRef] [PubMed]
86. Imamura, M.; Imamura, S.T.; Kaziyama, H.H.; Targino, R.A.; Hsing, W.T.; De Souza, L.P.M.; Cutait, M.M.; Fregni, F.; Camanho, G.L. Impact of nervous system hyperalgesia on pain, disability, and quality of life in patients with knee osteoarthritis: A controlled analysis. *Arthritis Care Res.* **2008**, *59*, 1424–1431. [CrossRef]
87. Skou, S.T.; Graven-Nielsen, T.; Lengsoe, L.; Simonsen, O.; Laursen, M.B.; Arendt-Nielsen, L. Relating clinical measures of pain with experimentally assessed pain mechanisms in patients with knee osteoarthritis. *Scand. J. Pain* **2013**, *4*, 111–117. [CrossRef]
88. Lluch, E.; Torres, R.; Nijs, J.; Van Oosterwijck, J. Evidence for central sensitization in patients with osteoarthritis pain: A systematic literature review. *Eur. J. Pain* **2014**, *18*, 1367–1375. [CrossRef]
89. Finan, P.H.; Buenaver, L.F.; Bounds, S.C.; Hussain, S.; Park, R.J.; Haque, U.J.; Campbell, C.M.; Haythornthwaite, J.A.; Edwards, R.R.; Smith, M.T. Discordance between pain and radiographic severity in knee osteoarthritis: Findings from quantitative sensory testing of central sensitization. *Arthritis Rheum.* **2013**, *65*, 363–372. [CrossRef]
90. Baliki, M.N.; Geha, P.Y.; Jabakhanji, R.; Harden, N.; Schnitzer, T.J.; Apkarian, A.V. A preliminary fMRI study of analgesic treatment in chronic back pain and knee osteoarthritis. *Mol. Pain* **2008**, *4*, 47. [CrossRef]
91. Parks, E.L.; Geha, P.Y.; Baliki, M.N.; Katz, J.; Schnitzer, T.J.; Apkarian, A.V. Brain activity for chronic knee osteoarthritis: Dissociating evoked pain from spontaneous pain. *Eur. J. Pain* **2011**, *15*, 1–14. [CrossRef]
92. Gwilym, S.E.; Keltner, J.R.; Warnaby, C.E.; Carr, A.J.; Chizh, B.; Chessell, I.; Tracey, I. Psychophysical and functional imaging evidence supporting the presence of central sensitization in a cohort of osteoarthritis patients. *Arthritis Care Res.* **2009**, *61*, 1226–1234. [CrossRef] [PubMed]

93. Gwilym, S.E.; Filippini, N.; Douaud, G.; Carr, A.J.; Tracey, I. Thalamic atrophy associated with painful osteoarthritis of the hip is reversible after arthroplasty: A longitudinal voxel-based morphometric study. *Arthritis Rheum.* **2010**, *62*, 2930–2940. [CrossRef] [PubMed]
94. Kulkarni, B.; Bentley, D.E.; Elliott, R.; Julyan, P.J.; Boger, E.; Watson, A.; Boyle, Y.; El-Deredy, W.; Jones, A.K. Arthritic pain is processed in brain areas concerned with emotions and fear. *Arthritis Rheum.* **2007**, *56*, 1345–1354. [CrossRef] [PubMed]
95. Rodriguez-Raecke, R.; Niemeier, A.; Ihle, K.; Ruether, W.; May, A. Structural brain changes in chronic pain reflect probably neither damage nor atrophy. *PLoS ONE* **2013**, *8*, 1–8. [CrossRef] [PubMed]
96. Lewis, G.N.; Parker, R.S.; Sharma, S.; Rice, D.A.; McNair, P.J. Structural brain alterations before and after total knee arthroplasty: A longitudinal assessment. *Pain Med.* **2018**, *19*, 2166–2176. [CrossRef] [PubMed]
97. Bushnell, M.C.; Čeko, M.; Low, L.A. Cognitive and emotional control of pain and its disruption in chronic pain. *Nat. Rev. Neurosci.* **2013**, *14*, 502. [CrossRef]
98. Finan, P.H.; Goodin, B.R.; Smith, M.T. The association of sleep and pain: An update and a path forward. *J. Pain* **2013**, *14*, 1539–1552. [CrossRef]
99. Chen, Q.; Heinricher, M. Descending Control Mechanisms and Chronic Pain. *Curr. Rheumatol. Rep.* **2019**, *21*, 13. [CrossRef]
100. Vase, L.; Nikolajsen, L.; Christensen, B.; Egsgaard, L.; Arendt-Nielsen, L.; Svensson, P.; Staehelin, J.T. Cognitive-emotional sensitization contributes to wind-up-like pain in phantom limb pain patients. *Pain* **2011**, *152*, 157. [CrossRef]
101. Matre, D.; Casey, K.L.; Knardahl, S. Placebo-induced changes in spinal cord pain processing. *J. Neurosci.* **2006**, *26*, 559–563. [CrossRef] [PubMed]
102. Salomons, T.V.; Moayedi, M.; Erpelding, N.; Davis, K.D. a brief cognitive-behavioural intervention for pain reduces secondary hyperalgesia. *Pain* **2014**, *155*, 1446–1452. [CrossRef] [PubMed]
103. Dekker, J.; Lemmens, J.; Oostendorp, R.; Bijlsma, J. Pain and disability in patients with osteoarthritis of hip or knee: The relationship with articular, kinesiological, and psychological characteristics. *J. Rheumatol.* **1998**, *25*, 125–133.
104. Carragee, E.J.; Alamin, T.F.; Miller, J.L.; Carragee, J.M. Discographic, MRI and psychosocial determinants of low back pain disability and remission: A prospective study in subjects with benign persistent back pain. *Spine J.* **2005**, *1*, 24–35. [CrossRef]
105. Crombez, G.; Vlaeyen, J.W.; Heuts, P.H.; Lysens, R. Pain-related fear is more disabling than pain itself: Evidence on the role of pain-related fear in chronic back pain disability. *Pain* **1999**, *80*, 329–339. [CrossRef]
106. McCracken, L.M.; Iverson, G.L. Disrupted sleep patterns and daily functioning in patients with chronic pain. *Pain Res. Manag.* **2002**, *7*, 75–79. [CrossRef]
107. Smith, M.T.; Quartana, P.J.; Okonkwo, R.M.; Nasir, A. Mechanisms by which sleep disturbance contributes to osteoarthritis pain: A conceptual model. *Curr. Pain Headache Rep.* **2009**, *6*, 447–454. [CrossRef]
108. Campbell, C.M.; Buenaver, L.F.; Finan, P.; Bounds, S.C.; Redding, M.; McCauley, L.; Robinson, M.; Edwards, R.R.; Smith, M.T. Sleep, Pain Catastrophizing, and Central Sensitization in Knee Osteoarthritis Patients with and Without Insomnia. *Arthritis Care Res. (Hoboken)* **2015**, *67*, 1387–1396. [CrossRef]
109. Fu, K.; Makovey, J.; Metcalf, B.; Bennell, K.L.; Zhang, Y.; Asher, R.; Robbins, S.R.; Deveza, L.A.; Cistulli, P.A.; Hunter, D.J. Sleep Quality and Fatigue are Associated with Hip Osteoarthritis Pain Exacerbations: An Internet-Based Case-Crossover Study. *J. Rheumatol.* **2019**. [CrossRef]
110. Petrov, M.E.; Goodin, B.R.; Cruz-Almeida, Y.; King, C.; Glover, T.L.; Bulls, H.W.; Herbert, M.; Sibille, K.T.; Bartley, E.J.; Fessler, B.J.; et al. Disrupted sleep is associated with altered pain processing by sex and ethnicity in knee osteoarthritis. *J. Pain* **2015**, *16*, 478–490. [CrossRef]
111. Akin-Akinyosoye, K.; Frowd, N.; Marshall, L.; Stocks, J.; Fernandes, G.S.; Valdes, A.; McWilliams, D.F.; Zhang, W.; Doherty, M.; Ferguson, E.; et al. Traits associated with central pain augmentation in the Knee Pain In the Community (KPIC) cohort. *Pain* **2018**, *159*, 1035–1044. [CrossRef] [PubMed]
112. Parmelee, P.A.; Tighe, C.A.; Dautovich, N.D. Sleep disturbance in osteoarthritis: Linkages with pain, disability, and depressive symptoms. *Arthritis Care Res. (Hoboken)* **2015**, *67*, 358–365. [CrossRef] [PubMed]
113. Ho, K.K.N.; Ferreira, P.H.; Pinheiro, M.B.; Aquino Silva, D.; Miller, C.B.; Grunstein, R.; Simic, M. Sleep interventions for osteoarthritis and spinal pain: A systematic review and meta-analysis of randomized controlled trials. *Osteoarthr. Cartil.* **2019**, *27*, 196–218. [CrossRef] [PubMed]

114. Axford, J.; Butt, A.; Heron, C.; Hammond, J.; Morgan, J.; Alavi, A.; Bolton, J.; Bland, M. Prevalence of anxiety and depression in osteoarthritis: Use of the Hospital Anxiety and Depression Scale as a screening tool. *Clin. Rheumatol.* **2010**, *29*, 1277–1283. [CrossRef]
115. Burston, J.J.; Valdes, A.M.; Woodhams, S.G.; Mapp, P.I.; Stocks, J.; Watson, D.J.; Gowler, P.R.; Xu, L.; Sagar, D.R.; Fernandes, G. The impact of anxiety on chronic musculoskeletal pain and the role of astrocyte activation. *Pain* **2019**, *160*, 658. [CrossRef] [PubMed]
116. Cruz-Almeida, Y.; King, C.; Goodin, B.; Sibille, K.; Glover, T.; Riley, J.; Sotolongo, A.; Herbert, M.; Schmidt, J.; Fessler, B. Psychological profiles and pain characteristics of older adults with knee osteoarthritis. *Arthritis Care Res.* **2013**, *65*, 1786. [CrossRef] [PubMed]
117. Rayahin, J.E.; Chmiel, J.S.; Hayes, K.W.; Almagor, O.; Belisle, L.; Chang, A.H.; Moisio, K.; Zhang, Y.; Sharma, L. Factors Associated with Pain Experience Outcome in Knee Osteoarthritis. *Arthritis Care Res.* **2014**, *12*, 1828–1835. [CrossRef]
118. Finan, P.H.; Quartana, P.J.; Smith, M.T. Positive and negative affect dimensions in chronic knee osteoarthritis: Effects on clinical and laboratory pain. *Psychosom. Med.* **2013**, *75*, 463–470. [CrossRef]
119. Ferreira, V.; Sherman, A. The relationship of optimism, pain and social support to well-being in older adults with osteoarthritis. *Aging Ment. Health* **2007**, *11*, 89–98. [CrossRef]
120. Jamison, R.N.; Virts, K.L. The influence of family support on chronic pain. *Behav. Res. Ther.* **1990**, *28*, 283–287. [CrossRef]
121. Strating, M.; Suurmeijer, T.; van Schuur, W. Disability, social support, and distress in rheumatoid arthritis: Results from a thirteen-year prospective study. *Arthritis Rheum.* **2006**, *55*, 736. [CrossRef]
122. Sherman, A.M. Social relations and depressive symptoms in older adults with knee osteoarthritis. *Soc. Sci. Med.* **2003**, *56*, 247–257. [CrossRef]
123. The National Institute for Health and Care Excellence. *Osteoarthritis: Care and Management—Clinical Guideline*; National Institute for Health and Care Excellence: London, UK, 2014.
124. Royal Australian College of General Practitioners. *Guideline for the Management of Knee and Hip Osteoarthritis*, 2nd ed.; Royal Australian College of General Practitioners: Melbourne, Australia, 2018.
125. Geenen, R.; Overman, C.L.; Christensen, R.; Åsenlöf, P.; Capela, S.; Huisinga, K.L.; Husebø, M.E.P.; Köke, A.J.A.; Paskins, Z.; Pitsillidou, I.A.; et al. EULAR recommendations for the health professional's approach to pain management in inflammatory arthritis and osteoarthritis. *Ann. Rheum. Dis.* **2018**, *77*, 797–807. [CrossRef]
126. McAlindon, T.E.; Bannuru, R.R.; Sullivan, M.C.; Arden, N.K.; Berenbaum, F.; Bierma-Zeinstra, S.M.; Hawker, G.A.; Henrotin, Y.; Hunter, D.J.; Kawaguchi, H.; et al. OARSI guidelines for the non-surgical management of knee osteoarthritis. *Osteoarthr. Cartil.* **2014**, *22*, 363–388. [CrossRef]
127. Juhl, C.; Christensen, R.; Roos, E.M.; Zhang, W.; Lund, H. Impact of exercise type and dose on pain and disability in knee osteoarthritis: A systematic review and meta-regression analysis of randomized controlled trials. *Arthritis Rheumatol.* **2014**, *66*, 622–636. [CrossRef]
128. Evers, A.W.; Kraaimaat, F.W.; Geenen, R.; Jacobs, J.W.; Bijlsma, J.W. Pain coping and social support as predictors of long-term functional disability and pain in early rheumatoid arthritis. *Behav. Res. Ther.* **2003**, *41*, 1295–1310. [CrossRef]
129. McCracken, L.M.; Zayfert, C.; Gross, R.T. The Pain Anxiety Symptoms Scale: Development and validation of a scale to measure fear of pain. *Pain* **1992**, *50*, 67–73. [CrossRef]
130. Brown, G.; Nicassio, P. Development of a questionnaire for the assessment of active and passive coping strategies in chronic pain patients. *Pain* **1987**, *31*, 53. [CrossRef]
131. Steultjens, M.; Dekker, J.; Bijlsma, J. Coping, pain, and disability in osteoarthritis: A longitudinal study. *J. Rheumatol.* **2001**, *28*, 1068–1072.
132. Wesseling, J.J.; Bastick, A.A.; ten Wolde, S.; Kloppenburg, M.M.; Lafeber, F.F.; Bierma-Zeinstra, S.S.; Bijlsma, H.J. Identifying trajectories of pain severity in early symptomatic knee osteoarthritis: A 5-year followup of the cohort hip and cohort knee (CHECK) study. *J. Rheumatol.* **2015**, *42*, 1470–1477. [CrossRef]
133. American Academy of Orthopaedic Surgeons. *Treatment of Osteoarthritis of the knee: Evidence-Based Guideline*, 2nd ed.; American Academy of Orthopaedic Surgeons: Rosemont, IL, USA, 2013.

134. Zhang, W.; Nuki, G.; Moskowitz, R.W.; Abramson, S.; Altman, R.D.; Arden, N.K.; Bierma-Zeinstra, S.; Brandt, K.D.; Croft, P.; Doherty, M.; et al. OARSI recommendations for the management of hip and knee osteoarthritis: Part III: Changes in evidence following systematic cumulative update of research published through January 2009. *Osteoarthr. Cartil.* **2010**, *18*, 476–499. [CrossRef]

135. Lorig, K.R.; Holman, H.R. Self-management education: History, definition, outcomes, and mechanisms. *Ann. Behav. Med.* **2003**, *1*, 1–7. [CrossRef]

136. Mann, E.G.; LeFort, S.; VanDenKerkhof, E.G. Self-management interventions for chronic pain. *Pain Manag.* **2013**, *3*, 211. [CrossRef]

137. Smith, C.; Kumar, S.; Pelling, N. The effectiveness of self-management educational interventions for osteoarthritis of the knee. *Jbi Database Syst. Rev. Implement. Rep.* **2009**, *7*, 1091–1118. [CrossRef]

138. Kroon, F.P.; van der Burg, L.R.; Buchbinder, R.; Osborne, R.H.; Johnston, R.V.; Pitt, V. Self-management education programmes for osteoarthritis. *Cochrane Database Syst. Rev.* **2014**. [CrossRef]

139. Larmer, P.J.; Reay, N.D.; Aubert, E.R.; Kersten, P. Systematic Review of Guidelines for the Physical Management of Osteoarthritis. *Arch. Phys. Med. Rehabil.* **2014**, *95*, 375–389. [CrossRef]

140. Nelson, A.E.; Allen, K.D.; Golightly, Y.M.; Goode, A.P.; Jordan, J.M. A systematic review of recommendations and guidelines for the management of osteoarthritis: The chronic osteoarthritis management initiative of the U.S. bone and joint initiative. *Semin. Arthritis Rheum.* **2014**, *43*, 701–712. [CrossRef]

141. Fransen, M.; McConnell, S.; Harmer, A.R.; Van der Esch, M.; Simic, M.; Bennell, K.L. Exercise for osteoarthritis of the knee: A Cochrane systematic review. *Br. J. Sports Med.* **2015**, *49*, 1554–1557. [CrossRef]

142. Fransen, M.; McConnell, S.; Hernandez-Molina, G.; Reichenbach, S. Exercise for osteoarthritis of the hip. *Cochrane Database Syst. Rev.* **2014**. [CrossRef]

143. Li, Y.; Su, Y.; Chen, S.; Zhang, Y.; Zhang, Z.; Liu, C.; Lu, M.; Liu, F.; Li, S.; He, Z. The effects of resistance exercise in patients with knee osteoarthritis: A systematic review and meta-analysis. *Clin. Rehabil.* **2016**, *30*. [CrossRef]

144. Hoffman, M.D.; Hoffman, D.R. Does aerobic exercise improve pain perception and mood? A review of the evidence related to healthy and chronic pain subjects. *Curr. Pain Headache Rep.* **2007**, *11*, 93–97. [CrossRef]

145. Pedersen, B.K.; Saltin, B. Exercise as medicine: Evidence for prescribing exercise as therapy in 26 different chronic diseases. *Scand. J. Med. Sci. Sports* **2015**, *25*, 1–72. [CrossRef]

146. Sluka, K.A.; Frey-Law, L.; Bement, M.H. Exercise-induced pain and analgesia? Underlying mechanisms and clinical translation. *Pain* **2018**, *159*, S91–S97. [CrossRef]

147. Rice, D.; Nijs, J.; Kosek, E.; Wideman, T.; Hasenbring, M.I.; Koltyn, K.; Graven-Nielsen, T.; Polli, A. Exercise induced hypoalgesia in pain-free and chronic pain populations: State of the art and future directions. *J. Pain* **2019**. [CrossRef]

148. Helmark, I.C.; Mikkelsen, U.R.; Børglum, J.; Rothe, A.; Petersen, M.C.; Andersen, O.; Langberg, H.; Kjaer, M. Exercise increases interleukin-10 levels both intraarticularly and peri-synovially in patients with knee osteoarthritis: A randomized controlled trial. *Arthritis Res. Ther.* **2010**, *12*, R126. [CrossRef]

149. Runhaar, J.; Beavers, D.; Miller, G.; Nicklas, B.; Loeser, R.; Bierma-Zeinstra, S.; Messier, S. Inflammatory cytokines mediate the effects of diet and exercise on pain and function in knee osteoarthritis, independent of BMI. *Osteoarthr. Cartil.* **2019**, *27*, S453. [CrossRef]

150. Hurley, M.; Mitchell, H.; Walsh, N. In osteoarthritis, the psychosocial benefits of exercise are as important as physiological improvements. *Exerc. Sport Sci. Rev.* **2003**, *31*, 138–143. [CrossRef]

151. Saxby, D.; Lloyd, D. Osteoarthritis year in review 2016: Mechanics. *Osteoarthr. Cartil.* **2017**, *25*, 190–198. [CrossRef]

152. Foster, N.; Thomas, M.; Holden, M. Is long term physical activity safe for older adults with knee pain: A systematic review. *Osteoarthr. Cartil.* **2015**, *23*, 1445–1456.

153. Van Ginckel, A.; Hall, M.; Dobson, F.; Calders, P. Effects of long-term exercise therapy on knee joint structure in people with knee osteoarthritis: A systematic review and meta-analysis. *Semin Arthritis Rheum* **2019**, *48*, 941–949. [CrossRef]

154. Bricca, A.; Juhl, C.B.; Steultjens, M.; Wirth, W.; Roos, E.M. Impact of exercise on articular cartilage in people at risk of, or with established, knee osteoarthritis: A systematic review of randomised controlled trials. *Br. J. Sports Med.* **2018**. [CrossRef]

155. Roddy, E.; Zhang, W.; Doherty, M. Aerobic walking or strengthening exercise for osteoarthritis of the knee? A systematic review. *Ann. Rheum. Dis.* **2005**, *64*, 544. [CrossRef]

156. Magni, N.E.; McNair, P.J.; Rice, D.A. The effects of resistance training on muscle strength, joint pain, and hand function in individuals with hand osteoarthritis: A systematic review and meta-analysis. *Arthritis Res. Ther.* **2017**, *19*, 131. [CrossRef]
157. Brosseau, L.; Taki, J.; Desjardins, B.; Thevenot, O.; Fransen, M.; Wells, G.A.; Mizusaki Imoto, A.; Toupin-April, K.; Westby, M.; Alvarez Gallardo, I.C. The Ottawa panel clinical practice guidelines for the management of knee osteoarthritis. Part two: Strengthening exercise programs. *Clin. Rehabil.* **2017**, *31*, 596–611. [CrossRef]
158. Brosseau, L.; Taki, J.; Desjardins, B.; Thevenot, O.; Fransen, M.; Wells, G.A.; Mizusaki Imoto, A.; Toupin-April, K.; Westby, M.; Alvarez Gallardo, I.C.; et al. The Ottawa panel clinical practice guidelines for the management of knee osteoarthritis. Part three: Aerobic exercise programs. *Clin. Rehabil.* **2017**, *31*, 612–624. [CrossRef]
159. Fernandes, L.; Hagen, K.B.; Bijlsma, J.W.; Andreassen, O.; Christensen, P.; Conaghan, P.G.; Doherty, M.; Geenen, R.; Hammond, A.; Kjeken, I.; et al. EULAR recommendations for the non-pharmacological core management of hip and knee osteoarthritis. *Ann. Rheum Dis.* **2013**, *72*, 1125–1135. [CrossRef]
160. Brosseau, L.; Taki, J.; Desjardins, B.; Thevenot, O.; Fransen, M.; Wells, G.A.; Imoto, A.M.; Toupin-April, K.; Westby, M.; Gallardo, I.C.Á.; et al. The Ottawa panel clinical practice guidelines for the management of knee osteoarthritis. Part one: Introduction, and mind-body exercise programs. *Clin. Rehabil.* **2017**, *31*, 582–595. [CrossRef]
161. Garber, C.E.; Blissmer, B.; Deschenes, M.R.; Franklin, B.A.; Lamonte, M.J.; Lee, I.M.; Nieman, D.C.; Swain, D.P.; Medicine, A.C.o.S. American College of Sports Medicine position stand. Quantity and quality of exercise for developing and maintaining cardiorespiratory, musculoskeletal, and neuromotor fitness in apparently healthy adults: Guidance for prescribing exercise. *Med. Sci. Sports Exerc.* **2011**, *43*, 1334–1359. [CrossRef]
162. Rausch Osthoff, A.-K.; Niedermann, K.; Braun, J.; Adams, J.; Brodin, N.; Dagfinrud, H.; Duruoz, T.; Esbensen, B.A.; Günther, K.-P.; Hurkmans, E.; et al. 2018 EULAR recommendations for physical activity in people with inflammatory arthritis and osteoarthritis. *Ann. Rheum. Dis.* **2018**, *77*, 1251–1260. [CrossRef]
163. Rillo, O.; Riera, H.; Acosta, C.; Liendo, V.; Bolaños, J.; Monterola, L.; Nieto, E.; Arape, R.; Franco, L.M.; Vera, M.; et al. PANLAR Consensus Recommendations for the Management in Osteoarthritis of Hand, Hip, and Knee. *J. Clin. Rheumatol.* **2016**, *22*, 345–354. [CrossRef]
164. Conaghan, P.; Birrel, F.; Porcheret, M.; Doherty, M.; Dziedzic, K.; Bernstein, I.; Wise, E.; Whiting, T.; Cumming, J.; Frearson, R.; et al. *Osteoarthritis: Care and Management in Adults. Clinical Guideline 177*; National Clinical Guideline Centre: London, UK, 2014; pp. 1–498. Available online: Nice.org.uk/guidance/cg177 (accessed on 21 October 2019).
165. Sandal, L.; Roos, E.; Bøgesvang, S.; Thorlund, J. Pain trajectory and exercise-induced pain flares during 8 weeks of neuromuscular exercise in individuals with knee and hip pain. *Osteoarthr. Cartil.* **2016**, *4*, 589–592. [CrossRef] [PubMed]
166. McMaster, D.T.; Gill, N.; Cronin, J.; McGuigan, M. The development, retention and decay rates of strength and power in elite rugby union, rugby league and American football. *Sports Med.* **2013**, *43*, 367–384. [CrossRef]
167. Nicolson, P.J.A.; Bennell, K.L.; Dobson, F.L.; Van Ginckel, A.; Holden, M.A.; Hinman, R.S. Interventions to increase adherence to therapeutic exercise in older adults with low back pain and/or hip/knee osteoarthritis: A systematic review and meta-analysis. *Br. J. Sports Med.* **2017**, *51*, 791–799. [CrossRef]
168. Vrezas, I.; Elsner, G.; Bolm-Audorff, U.; Abolmaali, N.; Seidler, A. Case-control study of knee osteoarthritis and lifestyle factors considering their interaction with physical workload. *Int. Arch. Occup. Environ. Health* **2010**, *83*, 291–300. [CrossRef]
169. Tuncer, T.; Cay, F.H.; Altan, L.; Gurer, G.; Kacar, C.; Ozcakir, S.; Atik, S.; Ayhan, F.; Durmaz, B.; Eskiyurt, N.; et al. 2017 update of the Turkish League Against Rheumatism (TLAR) evidence-based recommendations for the management of knee osteoarthritis. *Rheumatol. Int.* **2018**, *38*, 1315–1331. [CrossRef]
170. Weiss, E. Knee osteoarthritis, body mass index and pain: Data from the Osteoarthritis Initiative. *Rheumatology (Oxf. Engl.)* **2014**, *53*, 2095–2099. [CrossRef]
171. Jiang, L.; Rong, J.; Wang, Y.; Hu, F.; Bao, C.; Li, X.; Zhao, Y. The relationship between body mass index and hip osteoarthritis: A systematic review and meta-analysis. *Jt. BoneSpine Rev. Du Rhum.* **2011**, *78*, 150–155. [CrossRef]
172. Blagojevic, M.; Jinks, C.; Jeffery, A.; Jordan, K.P. Risk factors for onset of osteoarthritis of the knee in older adults: A systematic review and meta-analysis. *Osteoarthr. Cartil.* **2010**, *18*, 24–33. [CrossRef]

173. Muthuri, S.G.; Hui, M.; Doherty, M.; Zhang, W. What if we prevent obesity? Risk reduction in knee osteoarthritis estimated through a meta-analysis of observational studies. *Arthritis Care Res. (Hoboken)* **2011**, *63*, 982–990. [CrossRef]
174. Wang, X.; Hunter, D.; Xu, J.; Ding, C. Metabolic triggered inflammation in osteoarthritis. *Osteoarthr. Cartil.* **2015**, *23*, 22–30. [CrossRef]
175. Lee, Y.C.; Lu, B.; Bathon, J.M.; Haythornthwaite, J.A.; Smith, M.T.; Page, G.G.; Edwards, R.R. Pain sensitivity and pain reactivity in osteoarthritis. *Arthritis Care Res. (Hoboken)* **2011**, *63*, 320–327. [CrossRef] [PubMed]
176. Collins, N.J.; Hart, H.F.; Mills, K.A.G. Osteoarthritis year in review 2018: Rehabilitation and outcomes. *Osteoarthr. Cartil.* **2019**, *27*, 378–391. [CrossRef] [PubMed]
177. *Department of Veterans Affairs/Department of Defense, Clinical Practice Guideline for the Non-Surgical Management of Hip & Knee Osteoarthritis*; Department of Veterans Affairs/Department of Defense: Washington, DC, USA, 2014.
178. Hochberg, M.C.; Altman, R.D.; April, K.T.; Benkhalti, M.; Guyatt, G.; McGowan, J.; Towheed, T.; Welch, V.; Wells, G.; Tugwell, P. American College of Rheumatology 2012 recommendations for the use of nonpharmacologic and pharmacologic therapies in osteoarthritis of the hand, hip, and knee. *Arthritis Care Res.* **2012**, *64*, 465–474. [CrossRef]
179. Combe, B.; Landewe, R.; Daien, C.I.; Hua, C.; Aletaha, D.; Alvaro-Gracia, J.M.; Bakkers, M.; Brodin, N.; Burmester, G.R.; Codreanu, C.; et al. 2016 update of the EULAR recommendations for the management of early arthritis. *Ann. Rheum Dis.* **2017**, *76*, 948–959. [CrossRef]
180. American Academy of Orthopaedic Surgeons. *Management of Osteoarthritis of the Hip: Evidence—Based Clinical Practice Guideline*; American Academy of Orthopaedic Surgeons: Rosemont, IL, USA, 2017.
181. World Health Organization. Global Strategy on Diet, Physical Activity and Health. Available online: https://www.who.int/dietphysicalactivity/childhood_what/en/ (accessed on 4 April 2019).
182. Hunter, G.R.; Plaisance, E.P.; Fisher, G. Weight loss and bone mineral density. *Curr. Opin. Endocrinol. DiabetesObes.* **2014**, *21*, 358–362. [CrossRef]
183. Christensen, R.; Astrup, A.; Bliddal, H. Weight loss: The treatment of choice for knee osteoarthritis? A randomized trial. *Osteoarthr. Cartil.* **2005**, *13*, 20–27. [CrossRef]
184. Messier, S.P.; Loeser, R.F.; Miller, G.D.; Morgan, T.M.; Rejeski, W.J.; Sevick, M.A.; Ettinger, W.H., Jr.; Pahor, M.; Williamson, J.D. Exercise and dietary weight loss in overweight and obese older adults with knee osteoarthritis: The Arthritis, Diet, and Activity Promotion Trial. *Arthritis Rheum.* **2004**, *50*, 1501–1510. [CrossRef]
185. Riddle, D.L.; Stratford, P.W. Body weight changes and corresponding changes in pain and function in persons with symptomatic knee osteoarthritis: A cohort study. *Arthritis Care Res. (Hoboken)* **2013**, *65*, 15–22. [CrossRef]
186. Messier, S.P.; Mihalko, S.L.; Legault, C.; Miller, G.D.; Nicklas, B.J.; DeVita, P.; Beavers, D.P.; Hunter, D.J.; Lyles, M.F.; Eckstein, F.; et al. Effects of intensive diet and exercise on knee joint loads, inflammation, and clinical outcomes among overweight and obese adults with knee osteoarthritis: The IDEA randomized clinical trial. *JAMA* **2013**, *310*, 1263–1273. [CrossRef]
187. Christensen, R.; Bartels, E.M.; Astrup, A.; Bliddal, H. Effect of weight reduction in obese patients diagnosed with knee osteoarthritis: A systematic review and meta-analysis. *Ann. Rheum Dis.* **2007**, *66*, 433–439. [CrossRef]
188. Tak, E.; Staats, P.; Van Hespen, A.; Hopman-Rock, M. The effects of an exercise program for older adults with osteoarthritis of the hip. *J. Rheumatol.* **2005**, *32*, 1106–1113. [PubMed]
189. Miller, G.D.; Nicklas, B.J.; Davis, C.; Loeser, R.F.; Lenchik, L.; Messier, S.P. Intensive weight loss program improves physical function in older obese adults with knee osteoarthritis. *Obesity (Silver Spring Md.)* **2006**, *14*, 1219–1230. [CrossRef] [PubMed]
190. Rejeski, W.J.; Focht, B.C.; Messier, S.P.; Morgan, T.; Pahor, M.; Penninx, B. Obese, older adults with knee osteoarthritis: Weight loss, exercise, and quality of life. *Health Psychol. Off. J. Div. Health Psychol. Am. Psychol. Assoc.* **2002**, *21*, 419–426. [CrossRef]
191. Foy, C.G.; Lewis, C.E.; Hairston, K.G.; Miller, G.D.; Lang, W.; Jakicic, J.M.; Rejeski, W.J.; Ribisl, P.M.; Walkup, M.P.; Wagenknecht, L.E. Intensive lifestyle intervention improves physical function among obese adults with knee pain: Findings from the Look AHEAD trial. *Obesity (Silver Spring Md.)* **2011**, *19*, 83–93. [CrossRef]

192. Witham, M.D.; Avenell, A. Interventions to achieve long-term weight loss in obese older people: A systematic review and meta-analysis. *Age Ageing* **2010**, *39*, 176–184. [CrossRef]
193. Atukorala, I.; Makovey, J.; Lawler, L.; Messier, S.P.; Bennell, K.; Hunter, D.J. Is There a Dose-Response Relationship Between Weight Loss and Symptom Improvement in Persons with Knee Osteoarthritis? *Arthritis Care Res. (Hoboken)* **2016**, *68*, 1106–1114. [CrossRef]
194. Babatunde, O.O.; Jordan, J.L.; Van der Windt, D.A.; Hill, J.C.; Foster, N.E.; Protheroe, J. Effective treatment options for musculoskeletal pain in primary care: A systematic overview of current evidence. *PLoS ONE* **2017**, *12*, e0178621. [CrossRef]
195. Zhang, L.; Fu, T.; Zhang, Q.; Yin, R.; Zhu, L.; He, Y.; Fu, W.; Shen, B. Effects of psychological interventions for patients with osteoarthritis: A systematic review and meta-analysis. *Psychol. Health Med.* **2018**, *23*, 1–17. [CrossRef]
196. O'moore, K.A.; Newby, J.M.; Andrews, G.; Hunter, D.J.; Bennell, K.; Smith, J.; Williams, A.D. Internet cognitive–behavioral therapy for depression in older adults with knee osteoarthritis: A randomized controlled trial. *Arthritis Care Res.* **2018**, *70*, 61–70. [CrossRef]
197. Smith, M.T.; Finan, P.H.; Buenaver, L.F.; Robinson, M.; Haque, U.; Quain, A.; McInrue, E.; Han, D.; Leoutsakis, J.; Haythornthwaite, J.A. Cognitive–behavioral therapy for insomnia in knee osteoarthritis: A randomized, double-blind, active placebo–controlled clinical trial. *Arthritis Rheumatol.* **2015**, *67*, 1221–1233. [CrossRef]
198. Vitiello, M.V.; Rybarczyk, B.; Von Korff, M.; Stepanski, E.J. Cognitive behavioral therapy for insomnia improves sleep and decreases pain in older adults with co-morbid insomnia and osteoarthritis. *J. Clin. Sleep Med.* **2009**, *5*, 355–362.
199. Vitiello, M.; McCurry, S.; Shortreed, S.; Baker, L.; Rybarczyk, B.; Keefe, F.; Von, M.K. Short-term improvement in insomnia symptoms predicts long-term improvements in sleep, pain, and fatigue in older adults with comorbid osteoarthritis and insomnia. *Pain* **2014**, *155*, 1547–1554. [CrossRef] [PubMed]
200. Vitiello, M.V.; McCurry, S.M.; Shortreed, S.M.; Balderson, B.H.; Baker, L.D.; Keefe, F.J.; Rybarczyk, B.D.; Von Korff, M. Cognitive-behavioral treatment for comorbid insomnia and osteoarthritis pain in primary care: The lifestyles randomized controlled trial. *J. Am. Geriatr. Soc.* **2013**, *61*, 947–956. [CrossRef]
201. Sampath, K.K.; Mani, R.; Miyamori, T.; Tumilty, S. The effects of manual therapy or exercise therapy or both in people with hip osteoarthritis: A systematic review and meta-analysis. *Clin. Rehabil.* **2016**, *30*, 1141–1155. [CrossRef] [PubMed]
202. Manheimer, E.; Cheng, K.; Wieland, L.S.; Shen, X.; Lao, L.; Guo, M.; Berman, B.M. Acupuncture for hip osteoarthritis. *Cochrane Database Syst. Rev.* **2018**, *5*, Cd013010. [CrossRef] [PubMed]
203. Manheimer, E.; Cheng, K.; Linde, K.; Lao, L.; Yoo, J.; Wieland, S.; van der Windt, D.A.; Berman, B.M.; Bouter, L.M. Acupuncture for peripheral joint osteoarthritis. *Cochrane Database Syst. Rev.* **2010**, Cd001977. [CrossRef] [PubMed]
204. Bennell, K.L.; Buchbinder, R.; Hinman, R.S. Physical therapies in the management of osteoarthritis: Current state of the evidence. *Curr. Opin. Rheumatol.* **2015**, *27*, 304–311. [CrossRef] [PubMed]
205. Zeng, C.; Li, H.; Yang, T.; Deng, Z.H.; Yang, Y.; Zhang, Y.; Lei, G.H. Electrical stimulation for pain relief in knee osteoarthritis: Systematic review and network meta-analysis. *Osteoarthr. Cartil.* **2015**, *23*, 189–202. [CrossRef]
206. Kloppenburg, M.; Kroon, F.P.; Blanco, F.J.; Doherty, M.; Dziedzic, K.S.; Greibrokk, E.; Haugen, I.K.; Herrero-Beaumont, G.; Jonsson, H.; Kjeken, I.; et al. 2018 update of the EULAR recommendations for the management of hand osteoarthritis. *Ann. Rheum Dis.* **2018**. [CrossRef]
207. Hurley, M.; Dickson, K.; Hallett, R.; Grant, R.; Hauari, H.; Walsh, N.; Stansfield, C.; Oliver, S. Exercise interventions and patient beliefs for people with hip, knee or hip and knee osteoarthritis: A mixed methods review. *Cochrane Database Syst. Rev.* **2018**, *4*, Cd010842. [CrossRef]
208. Goudman, L.; Huysmans, E.; Ickmans, K.; Nijs, J.; Moens, M.; Putman, K.; Buyl, R.; Louw, A.; Logghe, T.; Coppieters, I. A Modern Pain Neuroscience Approach in Patients Undergoing Surgery for Lumbar Radiculopathy: A Clinical Perspective. *Phys. Ther.* **2019**. [CrossRef] [PubMed]
209. Louw, A.; Diener, I.; Butler, D.S.; Puentedura, E.J. The effect of neuroscience education on pain, disability, anxiety, and stress in chronic musculoskeletal pain. *Arch. Phys. Med. Rehabil.* **2011**, *92*, 2041–2056. [CrossRef] [PubMed]

210. Van Oosterwijck, J.; Meeus, M.; Paul, L.; De Schryver, M.; Pascal, A.; Lambrecht, L.; Nijs, J. Pain physiology education improves health status and endogenous pain inhibition in fibromyalgia: A double-blind randomized controlled trial. *Clin. J. Pain* **2013**, *29*, 873–882. [CrossRef] [PubMed]
211. Watson, J.A.; Ryan, C.G.; Cooper, L.; Ellington, D.; Whittle, R.; Lavender, M.; Dixon, J.; Atkinson, G.; Cooper, K.; Martin, D.J. Pain Neuroscience Education for Adults with Chronic Musculoskeletal Pain: A Mixed-Methods Systematic Review and Meta-Analysis. *J. Pain* **2019**. [CrossRef] [PubMed]
212. Lluch, E.; Duenas, L.; Falla, D.; Baert, I.; Meeus, M.; Sanchez-Frutos, J.; Nijs, J. Preoperative Pain Neuroscience Education Combined with Knee Joint Mobilization for Knee Osteoarthritis: A Randomized Controlled Trial. *Clin. J. Pain* **2018**, *34*, 44–52. [CrossRef]
213. Louw, A.; Zimney, K.; Reed, J.; Landers, M.; Puentedura, E.J. Immediate preoperative outcomes of pain neuroscience education for patients undergoing total knee arthroplasty: A case series. *Physiother. Theory Pract.* **2018**, 1–11. [CrossRef]
214. Jones, M.D.; Valenzuela, T.; Booth, J.; Taylor, J.L.; Barry, B.K. Explicit Education About Exercise-Induced Hypoalgesia Influences Pain Responses to Acute Exercise in Healthy Adults: A Randomized Controlled Trial. *J. Pain* **2017**, *18*, 1409–1416. [CrossRef]
215. Ploutz-Snyder, L.L.; Manini, T.; Ploutz-Snyder, R.J.; Wolf, D.A. Functionally relevant thresholds of quadriceps femoris strength. *J. Gerontol. Ser. A Biol. Sci. Med Sci.* **2002**, *57*, B144–B152. [CrossRef]
216. Bacon, K.L.; Segal, N.A.; Oiestad, B.E.; Lewis, C.E.; Nevitt, M.C.; Brown, C.; LaValley, M.P.; McCulloch, C.E.; Felson, D.T. Thresholds in the relationship of quadriceps strength with functional limitations in women with knee osteoarthritis. *Arthritis Care Res. (Hoboken)* **2018**. [CrossRef]
217. Nur, H.; Sertkaya, B.S.; Tuncer, T. Determinants of physical functioning in women with knee osteoarthritis. *Aging Clin. Exp. Res.* **2018**, *30*, 299–306. [CrossRef]
218. Hall, M.; Wrigley, T.V.; Kasza, J.; Dobson, F.; Pua, Y.H.; Metcalf, B.R.; Bennell, K.L. Cross-sectional association between muscle strength and self-reported physical function in 195 hip osteoarthritis patients. *Semin. Arthritis Rheum* **2017**, *46*, 387–394. [CrossRef] [PubMed]
219. Ward, S.; Blackburn, J.; Padua, D.; Stanley, L.; Harkey, M.; Luc-Harkey, B.; Pietrosimone, B. Quadriceps Neuromuscular Function and Jump-Landing Sagittal-Plane Knee Biomechanics after Anterior Cruciate Ligament Reconstruction. *J. Athl. Train.* **2018**, *53*, 135. [CrossRef] [PubMed]
220. Hall, M.; Hinman, R.S.; Wrigley, T.V.; Kasza, J.; Lim, B.W.; Bennell, K.L. Knee extensor strength gains mediate symptom improvement in knee osteoarthritis: Secondary analysis of a randomised controlled trial. *Osteoarthr. Cartil.* **2018**, *26*, 495–500. [CrossRef] [PubMed]
221. Rice, D.; McNair, P.J.; Dalbeth, N. Effects of cryotherapy on arthrogenic muscle inhibition using an experimental model of knee swelling. *Arthritis Rheum.* **2009**, *61*, 78–83. [CrossRef] [PubMed]
222. Rice, D.A.; McNair, P.J. Quadriceps arthrogenic muscle inhibition: Neural mechanisms and treatment perspectives. *Semin Arthritis Rheum* **2010**, *40*, 250–266. [CrossRef] [PubMed]
223. Rice, D.A.; McNair, P.J.; Lewis, G.N. Mechanisms of quadriceps muscle weakness in knee joint osteoarthritis: The effects of prolonged vibration on torque and muscle activation in osteoarthritic and healthy control subjects. *Arthritis Res.* **2011**, *13*, R151. [CrossRef]
224. Pietrosimone, B.G.; Hertel, J.; Ingersoll, C.D.; Hart, J.M.; Saliba, S.A. Voluntary quadriceps activation deficits in patients with tibiofemoral osteoarthritis: A meta-analysis. *Pm R J. Inj. Funct. Rehabil.* **2011**, *3*, 153–162, quiz 162. [CrossRef]
225. Hurley, M.; O'Flanagan, S.; Newham, D. Isokinetic and isometric muscle strength and inhibition after elbow arthroplasty. *J. Orthop. Rhematology* **1991**, *4*, 83–95.
226. Freeman, S.; Mascia, A.; McGill, S. Arthrogenic neuromusculature inhibition: A foundational investigation of existence in the hip joint. *Clin. Biomech. (BristolAvon)* **2013**, *28*, 171–177. [CrossRef]
227. Hopkins, J.T.; Palmieri, R. Effects of ankle joint effusion on lower leg function. *Clin. J. Sport Med. Off. J. Can. Acad. Sport Med.* **2004**, *14*, 1–7. [CrossRef]
228. Muething, A.; Acocello, S.; Pritchard, K.A.; Brockmeier, S.F.; Saliba, S.A.; Hart, J.M. Shoulder-Muscle Activation in Individuals with Previous Shoulder Injuries. *J. Sport Rehabil.* **2015**, *24*. [CrossRef] [PubMed]
229. Pietrosimone, B.G.; Hart, J.M.; Saliba, S.A.; Hertel, J.; Ingersoll, C.D. Immediate effects of transcutaneous electrical nerve stimulation and focal knee joint cooling on quadriceps activation. *Med. Sci. Sports Exerc.* **2009**, *41*, 1175–1181. [CrossRef] [PubMed]

230. Petersen, S.G.; Beyer, N.; Hansen, M.; Holm, L.; Aagaard, P.; Mackey, A.L.; Kjaer, M. Nonsteroidal anti-inflammatory drug or glucosamine reduced pain and improved muscle strength with resistance training in a randomized controlled trial of knee osteoarthritis patients. *Arch. Phys. Med. Rehabil.* **2011**, *92*, 1185–1193. [CrossRef] [PubMed]
231. Pietrosimone, B.G.; Saliba, S.A.; Hart, J.M.; Hertel, J.; Kerrigan, D.C.; Ingersoll, C.D. Effects of transcutaneous electrical nerve stimulation and therapeutic exercise on quadriceps activation in people with tibiofemoral osteoarthritis. *J. Orthop. Sports Phys. Ther.* **2011**, *41*, 4–12. [CrossRef]
232. Hart, J.M.; Kuenze, C.M.; Diduch, D.R.; Ingersoll, C.D. Quadriceps muscle function after rehabilitation with cryotherapy in patients with anterior cruciate ligament reconstruction. *J Athl. Train* **2014**, *49*, 733–739. [CrossRef]
233. Loenneke, J.P.; Wilson, J.M.; Marín, P.J.; Zourdos, M.C.; Bemben, M.G. Low intensity blood flow restriction training: A meta-analysis. *Eur. J. Appl. Physiol.* **2012**, *5*, 1849–1859. [CrossRef]
234. Rodrigues, R.; Ferraz, R.B.; Kurimori, C.O.; Guedes, L.K.; Lima, F.R.; de Sa-Pinto, A.L.; Gualano, B.; Roschel, H. Low-load resistance training with blood flow restriction increases muscle function, mass and functionality in women with rheumatoid arthritis. *Arthritis Care Res. (Hoboken)* **2019**. [CrossRef]
235. Harper, S.A.; Roberts, L.M.; Layne, A.S.; Jaeger, B.C.; Gardner, A.K.; Sibille, K.T.; Wu, S.S.; Vincent, K.R.; Fillingim, R.B.; Manini, T.M.; et al. Blood-Flow Restriction Resistance Exercise for Older Adults with Knee Osteoarthritis: A Pilot Randomized Clinical Trial. *J. Clin. Med.* **2019**, *8*. [CrossRef]
236. Ferraz, R.B.; Gualano, B.; Rodrigues, R.; Kurimori, C.O.; Fuller, R.; Lima, F.R.; AL, D.E.S.-P.; Roschel, H. Benefits of Resistance Training with Blood Flow Restriction in Knee Osteoarthritis. *Med Sci Sports Exerc* **2018**, *50*, 897–905. [CrossRef]
237. Segal, N.; Davis, M.D.; Mikesky, A.E. Efficacy of Blood Flow-Restricted Low-Load Resistance Training For Quadriceps Strengthening in Men at Risk of Symptomatic Knee Osteoarthritis. *Geriatr. Orthop. Surg. Rehabil.* **2015**, *6*, 160–167. [CrossRef]
238. Segal, N.A.; Williams, G.N.; Davis, M.C.; Wallace, R.B.; Mikesky, A.E. Efficacy of blood flow-restricted, low-load resistance training in women with risk factors for symptomatic knee osteoarthritis. *Pm R J. Inj. Funct. Rehabil.* **2015**, *7*, 376–384. [CrossRef] [PubMed]
239. Wylde, V.; Palmer, S.; Learmonth, I.D.; Dieppe, P. Somatosensory abnormalities in knee OA. *Rheumatology (Oxf. Engl.)* **2012**, *51*, 535–543. [CrossRef] [PubMed]
240. Stanton, T.R.; Lin, C.W.; Bray, H.; Smeets, R.J.; Taylor, D.; Law, R.Y.; Moseley, G.L. Tactile acuity is disrupted in osteoarthritis but is unrelated to disruptions in motor imagery performance. *Rheumatol. (Oxf. Engl.)* **2013**, *52*, 1509–1519. [CrossRef] [PubMed]
241. Stanton, T.R.; Lin, C.W.; Smeets, R.J.; Taylor, D.; Law, R.; Lorimer Moseley, G. Spatially defined disruption of motor imagery performance in people with osteoarthritis. *Rheumatology (Oxf. Engl.)* **2012**, *51*, 1455–1464. [CrossRef] [PubMed]
242. Parker, R.S.; Lewis, G.N.; Rice, D.A.; McNair, P.J. The Association Between Corticomotor Excitability and Motor Skill Learning in People with Painful Hand Arthritis. *Clin. J. Pain* **2017**, *33*, 222–230. [CrossRef] [PubMed]
243. Shanahan, C.J.; Hodges, P.W.; Wrigley, T.V.; Bennell, K.L.; Farrell, M.J. Organisation of the motor cortex differs between people with and without knee osteoarthritis. *Arthritis Res.* **2015**, *17*, 164. [CrossRef]
244. Ahn, H.; Suchting, R.; Woods, A.J.; Miao, H.; Green, C.; Cho, R.Y.; Choi, E.; Fillingim, R.B. Bayesian analysis of the effect of transcranial direct current stimulation on experimental pain sensitivity in older adults with knee osteoarthritis: Randomized sham-controlled pilot clinical study. *J. Pain Res.* **2018**, *11*, 2071–2082. [CrossRef]
245. Chang, W.J.; Bennell, K.L.; Hodges, P.W.; Hinman, R.S.; Young, C.L.; Buscemi, V.; Liston, M.B.; Schabrun, S.M. Addition of transcranial direct current stimulation to quadriceps strengthening exercise in knee osteoarthritis: A pilot randomised controlled trial. *PLoS ONE* **2017**, *12*, e0180328. [CrossRef]
246. Ahn, H.; Woods, A.J.; Kunik, M.E.; Bhattacharjee, A.; Chen, Z.; Choi, E.; Fillingim, R.B. Efficacy of transcranial direct current stimulation over primary motor cortex (anode) and contralateral supraorbital area (cathode) on clinical pain severity and mobility performance in persons with knee osteoarthritis: An experimenter- and participant-blinded, randomized, sham-controlled pilot clinical study. *Brain Stimul.* **2017**, *10*, 902–909. [CrossRef]

247. da Graca-Tarrago, M.; Lech, M.; Angoleri, L.D.M.; Santos, D.S.; Deitos, A.; Brietzke, A.P.; Torres, I.L.; Fregni, F.; Caumo, W. Intramuscular electrical stimulus potentiates motor cortex modulation effects on pain and descending inhibitory systems in knee osteoarthritis: A randomized, factorial, sham-controlled study. *J. Pain Res.* **2019**, *12*, 209–221. [CrossRef]
248. Moseley, G.; Zalucki, N.; Wiech, K. Tactile discrimination, but not tactile stimulation alone, reduces chronic limb pain. *Pain* **2008**, *137*, 600–608. [CrossRef] [PubMed]
249. Moseley, G.L.; Wiech, K. The effect of tactile discrimination training is enhanced when patients watch the reflected image of their unaffected limb during training. *Pain* **2009**, *144*, 314–319. [CrossRef] [PubMed]
250. Flor, H.; Denke, C.; Schaefer, M.; Grusser, S. Effect of sensory discrimination training on cortical reorganisation and phantom limb pain. *Lancet* **2001**, *357*, 1763–1764. [CrossRef]
251. Wakolbinger, R.; Diers, M.; Hruby, L.A.; Sturma, A.; Aszmann, O.C. Home-Based Tactile Discrimination Training Reduces Phantom Limb Pain. *Pain Pract. Off. J. World Inst. Pain* **2018**, *18*, 709–715. [CrossRef] [PubMed]
252. Preston, C.; Newport, R. Analgesic effects of multisensory illusions in osteoarthritis. *Rheumatology (Oxf. Engl.)* **2011**, *50*, 2314–2315. [CrossRef]
253. Egsgaard, L.L.; Eskehave, T.N.; Bay-Jensen, A.C.; Hoeck, H.C.; Arendt-Nielsen, L. Identifying specific profiles in patients with different degrees of painful knee osteoarthritis based on serological biochemical and mechanistic pain biomarkers: A diagnostic approach based on cluster analysis. *Pain* **2015**, *156*, 96–107. [CrossRef]
254. Lluch, E.; Nijs, J.; Courtney, C.A.; Rebbeck, T.; Wylde, V.; Baert, I.; Wideman, T.H.; Howells, N.; Skou, S.T. Clinical descriptors for the recognition of central sensitization pain in patients with knee osteoarthritis. *Disabil. Rehabil.* **2018**, *40*, 2836–2845. [CrossRef]
255. Osgood, E.; Trudeau, J.J.; Eaton, T.A.; Jensen, M.P.; Gammaitoni, A.; Simon, L.S.; Katz, N. Development of a bedside pain assessment kit for the classification of patients with osteoarthritis. *Rheumatol. Int.* **2015**, *35*, 1005–1013. [CrossRef]
256. Kittelson, A.J.; Stevens-Lapsley, J.E.; Schmiege, S.J. Determination of Pain Phenotypes in Knee Osteoarthritis: A Latent Class Analysis Using Data From the Osteoarthritis Initiative. *Arthritis Care Res. (Hoboken)* **2016**, *68*, 612–620. [CrossRef]
257. Cardoso, J.S.; Riley, J.L., 3rd; Glover, T.; Sibille, K.T.; Bartley, E.J.; Goodin, B.R.; Bulls, H.W.; Herbert, M.; Addison, A.S.; Staud, R.; et al. Experimental pain phenotyping in community-dwelling individuals with knee osteoarthritis. *Pain* **2016**, *157*, 2104–2114. [CrossRef]
258. Frey-Law, L.A.; Bohr, N.L.; Sluka, K.A.; Herr, K.; Clark, C.R.; Noiseux, N.O.; Callaghan, J.J.; Zimmerman, M.B.; Rakel, B.A. Pain sensitivity profiles in patients with advanced knee osteoarthritis. *Pain* **2016**, *157*, 1988–1999. [CrossRef] [PubMed]
259. Rice, D.A.; Kluger, M.T.; McNair, P.J.; Lewis, G.N.; Somogyi, A.A.; Borotkanics, R.; Barratt, D.T.; Walker, M. Persistent postoperative pain after total knee arthroplasty: A prospective cohort study of potential risk factors. *Br. J. Anaesth.* **2018**, *121*, 804–812. [CrossRef] [PubMed]
260. Petersen, K.K.; Arendt-Nielsen, L.; Simonsen, O.; Wilder-Smith, O.; Laursen, M.B. Presurgical assessment of temporal summation of pain predicts the development of chronic postoperative pain 12 months after total knee replacement. *Pain* **2015**, *156*, 55–61. [CrossRef] [PubMed]
261. Petersen, K.K.; Graven-Nielsen, T.; Simonsen, O.; Laursen, M.B.; Arendt-Nielsen, L. Preoperative pain mechanisms assessed by cuff algometry are associated with chronic postoperative pain relief after total knee replacement. *Pain* **2016**, *157*, 1400–1406. [CrossRef]
262. Petersen, K.K.; Olesen, A.E.; Simonsen, O.; Arendt-Nielsen, L. Mechanistic pain profiling as a tool to predict the efficacy of 3-week nonsteroidal anti-inflammatory drugs plus paracetamol in patients with painful knee osteoarthritis. *Pain* **2019**, *160*, 486–492. [CrossRef]
263. Petersen, K.K.; Simonsen, O.; Laursen, M.B.; Arendt-Nielsen, L. The Role of Preoperative Radiologic Severity, Sensory Testing, and Temporal Summation on Chronic Postoperative Pain Following Total Knee Arthroplasty. *Clin. J. Pain* **2018**, *34*, 193–197. [CrossRef]
264. Izumi, M.; Petersen, K.K.; Laursen, M.B.; Arendt-Nielsen, L.; Graven-Nielsen, T. Facilitated temporal summation of pain correlates with clinical pain intensity after hip arthroplasty. *Pain* **2017**, *158*, 323–332. [CrossRef]

265. Wylde, V.; Sayers, A.; Odutola, A.; Gooberman-Hill, R.; Dieppe, P.; Blom, A.W. Central sensitization as a determinant of patients' benefit from total hip and knee replacement. *Eur. J. Pain (Lond. Engl.)* **2017**, *21*, 357–365. [CrossRef]
266. Edwards, R.R.; Dolman, A.J.; Martel, M.O.; Finan, P.H.; Lazaridou, A.; Cornelius, M.; Wasan, A.D. Variability in conditioned pain modulation predicts response to NSAID treatment in patients with knee osteoarthritis. *Bmc Musculoskelet Disord* **2016**, *17*, 284. [CrossRef]
267. Fingleton, C.; Smart, K.M.; Doody, C.M. Exercise-induced Hypoalgesia in People with Knee Osteoarthritis With Normal and Abnormal Conditioned Pain Modulation. *Clin. J. Pain* **2017**, *33*, 395–404. [CrossRef]
268. Dixon, K.E.; Keefe, F.J.; Scipio, C.D.; Perri, L.M.; Abernethy, A.P. Psychological interventions for arthritis pain management in adults: A meta-analysis. *Health Psychol. Off. J. Div. Health Psychol. Am. Psychol. Assoc.* **2007**, *26*, 241–250. [CrossRef] [PubMed]
269. Lumley, M.A.; Schubiner, H. Psychological Therapy for Centralized Pain: An Integrative Assessment and Treatment Model. *Psychosom Med.* **2019**, *81*, 114–124. [CrossRef] [PubMed]
270. Lumley, M.A.; Schubiner, H.; Lockhart, N.A.; Kidwell, K.M.; Harte, S.E.; Clauw, D.J.; Williams, D.A. Emotional awareness and expression therapy, cognitive behavioral therapy, and education for fibromyalgia: A cluster-randomized controlled trial. *Pain* **2017**, *158*, 2354–2363. [CrossRef] [PubMed]
271. Pisters, M.F.; Veenhof, C.; Schellevis, F.G.; Twisk, J.W.; Dekker, J.; De Bakker, D.H. Exercise adherence improving long-term patient outcome in patients with osteoarthritis of the hip and/or knee. *Arthritis Care Res. (Hoboken)* **2010**, *62*, 1087–1094. [CrossRef] [PubMed]
272. Roddy, E.; Doherty, M. Changing life-styles and osteoarthritis: What is the evidence? *Best Pr. Res. Clin. Rheumatol.* **2006**, *20*, 81–97. [CrossRef] [PubMed]
273. van Gool, C.H.; Penninx, B.W.; Kempen, G.I.; Rejeski, W.J.; Miller, G.D.; van Eijk, J.T.; Pahor, M.; Messier, S.P. Effects of exercise adherence on physical function among overweight older adults with knee osteoarthritis. *Arthritis Rheum.* **2005**, *53*, 24–32. [CrossRef] [PubMed]
274. Bennell, K.L.; Dobson, F.; Hinman, R.S. Exercise in osteoarthritis: Moving from prescription to adherence. *Best Pract. Res. Clin. Rheumatol.* **2014**, *28*, 93–117. [CrossRef]
275. Marks, R. Knee osteoarthritis and exercise adherence: A review. *Curr. Aging Sci.* **2012**, *5*, 72–83. [CrossRef]
276. Thorstensson, C.A.; Garellick, G.; Rystedt, H.; Dahlberg, L.E. Better Management of Patients with Osteoarthritis: Development and Nationwide Implementation of an Evidence-Based Supported Osteoarthritis Self-Management Programme. *Musculoskelet. Care* **2015**, *13*, 67–75. [CrossRef]
277. Brand, C.A. The role of self-management in designing care for people with osteoarthritis of the hip and knee. *Med J. Aust.* **2008**, *189*, S25–S28. [CrossRef]
278. Jordan, J.L.; Holden, M.A.; Mason, E.E.; Foster, N.E. Interventions to improve adherence to exercise for chronic musculoskeletal pain in adults. *Cochrane Database Syst. Rev.* **2010**, Cd005956. [CrossRef]
279. Jensen, M.P.; Nielson, W.R.; Kerns, R.D. Toward the development of a motivational model of pain self-management. *J. Pain* **2003**, *4*, 477–492. [CrossRef]
280. Damush, T.M.; Perkins, S.M.; Mikesky, A.E.; Roberts, M.; O'Dea, J. Motivational factors influencing older adults diagnosed with knee osteoarthritis to join and maintain an exercise program. *J. Aging Phys. Act.* **2005**, *13*, 45–60. [CrossRef] [PubMed]
281. Guite, J.W.; Kim, S.; Chen, C.P.; Sherker, J.L.; Sherry, D.D.; Rose, J.B.; Hwang, W.T. Pain beliefs and readiness to change among adolescents with chronic musculoskeletal pain and their parents before an initial pain clinic evaluation. *Clin. J. Pain* **2014**, *30*, 27–35. [CrossRef] [PubMed]
282. Dobson, F.; Bennell, K.L.; French, S.D.; Nicolson, P.J.; Klaasman, R.N.; Holden, M.A.; Atkins, L.; Hinman, R.S. Barriers and Facilitators to Exercise Participation in People with Hip and/or Knee Osteoarthritis: Synthesis of the Literature Using Behavior Change Theory. *Am. J. Phys. Med. Rehabil.* **2016**, *95*, 372–389. [CrossRef] [PubMed]
283. Biller, N.; Arnstein, P.; Caudill, M.A.; Federman, C.W.; Guberman, C. Predicting completion of a cognitive-behavioral pain management program by initial measures of a chronic pain patient's readiness for change. *Clin. J. Pain* **2000**, *16*, 352–359. [CrossRef] [PubMed]
284. Dorflinger, L.; Kerns, R.D.; Auerbach, S.M. Providers' roles in enhancing patients' adherence to pain self management. *Transl. Behav. Med.* **2013**, *3*, 39–46. [CrossRef]

285. Letzen, J.E.; Seminowicz, D.A.; Campbell, C.M.; Finan, P.H. Exploring the potential role of mesocorticolimbic circuitry in motivation for and adherence to chronic pain self-management interventions. *Neurosci. Biobehav. Rev.* **2019**, *98*, 10–17. [CrossRef]
286. Taylor, A.M.; Becker, S.; Schweinhardt, P.; Cahill, C. Mesolimbic dopamine signaling in acute and chronic pain: Implications for motivation, analgesia, and addiction. *Pain* **2016**, *157*, 1194. [CrossRef]
287. Salamone, J.D.; Pardo, M.; Yohn, S.E.; López-Cruz, L.; SanMiguel, N.; Correa, M. Mesolimbic dopamine and the regulation of motivated behavior. *Behav. Neurosci. Motiv.* **2015**, *27*, 231–257.
288. Heshmati, M.; Russo, S.J. Anhedonia and the Brain Reward Circuitry in Depression. *Curr. Behav. Neurosci. Rep.* **2015**, *3*, 146–153. [CrossRef] [PubMed]
289. Kato, T.; Ide, S.; Minami, M. Pain relief induces dopamine release in the rat nucleus accumbens during the early but not late phase of neuropathic pain. *Neurosci. Lett.* **2016**, *100*, 73–78. [CrossRef] [PubMed]
290. Martucci, K.T.; Borg, N.; MacNiven, K.H.; Knutson, B.; Mackey, S.C. Altered prefrontal correlates of monetary anticipation and outcome in chronic pain. *Pain* **2018**, *159*, 1494–1507. [CrossRef] [PubMed]
291. Kobinata, H.; Ikeda, E.; Zhang, S.; Li, T.; Makita, K.; Kurata, J. Disrupted offset analgesia distinguishes patients with chronic pain from healthy controls. *Pain* **2017**, *158*, 1951–1959. [CrossRef] [PubMed]
292. Flor, H.; Knost, B.; Birbaumer, N. The role of operant conditioning in chronic pain: An experimental investigation. *Pain* **2002**, *95*, 111–118. [CrossRef]
293. Anderson, R.J.; Hurley, R.W.; Staud, R.; Robinson, M.E. Cognitive-motivational influences on health behavior change in adults with chronic pain. *Pain Med.* **2016**, *17*, 1079–1093. [CrossRef] [PubMed]
294. Mansour, A.; Baliki, M.; Huang, L.; Torbey, S.; Herrmann, K.; Schnitzer, T.; Apkarian, A. Brain white matter structural properties predict transition to chronic pain. *Pain* **2013**, *154*, 2160–2168. [CrossRef] [PubMed]
295. Becerra, L.; Borsook, D. Signal valence in the nucleus accumbens to pain onset and offset. *Eur. J. Pain* **2008**, *12*, 866–869. [CrossRef]
296. Becerra, L.; Navratilova, E.; Porreca, F.; Borsook, D. Analogous responses in the nucleus accumbens and cingulate cortex to pain onset (aversion) and offset (relief) in rats and humans. *J. Neurophysiol.* **2013**, *110*, 1221. [CrossRef]
297. Baliki, M.N.; Geha, P.Y.; Fields, H.L.; Apkarian, A.V. Predicting value of pain and analgesia: Nucleus accumbens response to noxious stimuli changes in the presence of chronic pain. *Neuron* **2010**, *66*, 149–160. [CrossRef]
298. Leknes, S.; Lee, M.; Berna, C.; Andersson, J.; Tracey, I. Relief as a reward: Hedonic and neural responses to safety from pain. *PLoS ONE* **2011**, *6*, e17870. [CrossRef] [PubMed]
299. Zhang, S.; Li, T.; Kobinata, H.; Ikeda, E.; Ota, T.; Kurata, J. Attenuation of offset analgesia is associated with suppression of descending pain modulatory and reward systems in patients with chronic pain. *Mol Pain* **2018**, *14*. [CrossRef] [PubMed]
300. Letzen, J.E.; Boissoneault, J.; Sevel, L.S.; Robinson, M.E. Altered mesocorticolimbic functional connectivity in chronic low back pain patients at rest and following sad mood induction. *Brain Imaging Behav.* **2019**. [CrossRef] [PubMed]
301. Martikainen, I.K.; Nuechterlein, E.B.; Pecina, M.; Love, T.M.; Cummiford, C.M.; Green, C.R.; Stohler, C.S.; Zubieta, J.K. Chronic Back Pain Is Associated with Alterations in Dopamine Neurotransmission in the Ventral Striatum. *J. Neurosci. Off. J. Soc. Neurosci.* **2015**, *35*, 9957–9965. [CrossRef] [PubMed]
302. Ikeda, E.; Li, T.; Kobinata, H.; Zhang, S.; Kurata, J. Anterior insular volume decrease is associated with dysfunction of the reward system in patients with chronic pain. *Eur. J. Pain (Lond. Engl.)* **2018**, *22*, 1170–1179. [CrossRef] [PubMed]

 © 2019 by the authors. Licensee MDPI, Basel, Switzerland. This article is an open access article distributed under the terms and conditions of the Creative Commons Attribution (CC BY) license (http://creativecommons.org/licenses/by/4.0/).

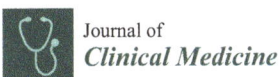

Article

Early Changes in Pain Acceptance Predict Pain Outcomes in Interdisciplinary Treatment for Chronic Pain

Thomas Probst [1,*], Robert Jank [1], Nele Dreyer [2], Stefanie Seel [2], Ruth Wagner [3], Klaus Hanshans [3], Renate Reyersbach [3], Andreas Mühlberger [2], Claas Lahmann [4] and Christoph Pieh [1]

1 Department for Psychotherapy and Biopsychosocial Health, Danube University Krems, 3500 Krems, Austria
2 Institute for Psychology, Regensburg University, 93053 Regensburg, Germany
3 Hospital Barmherzige Brüder, 93049 Regensburg, Germany
4 Department of Psychosomatic Medicine and Psychotherapy, University Medical Center Freiburg, Faculty of Medicine, University of Freiburg, 79106 Freiburg, Germany
* Correspondence: thomas.probst@donau-uni.ac.at

Received: 19 August 2019; Accepted: 26 August 2019; Published: 2 September 2019

Abstract: Studies have shown that pain acceptance is associated with a better pain outcome. The current study explored whether changes in pain acceptance in the very early treatment phase of an interdisciplinary cognitive-behavioral therapy (CBT)-based treatment program for chronic pain predict pain outcomes. A total of 69 patients with chronic, non-malignant pain (at least 6 months) were treated in a day-clinic for four-weeks. Pain acceptance was measured with the Chronic Pain Acceptance Questionnaire (CPAQ), pain outcomes included pain intensity (Numeric Rating Scale, NRS) as well as affective and sensory pain perception (Pain Perception Scale, SES-A and SES-S). Regression analyses controlling for the pre-treatment values of the pain outcomes, age, and gender were performed. Early changes in pain acceptance predicted pain intensity at post-treatment measured with the NRS (B = −0.04 (SE = 0.02); T = −2.28; $p = 0.026$), affective pain perception at post-treatment assessed with the SES-A (B = −0.26 (SE = 0.10); T = −2.79; $p = 0.007$), and sensory pain perception at post-treatment measured with the SES-S (B = −0.19 (SE = 0.08); T = −2.44; $p = 0.017$). Yet, a binary logistic regression analysis revealed that early changes in pain acceptance did not predict clinically relevant pre-post changes in pain intensity (at least 2 points on the NRS). Early changes in pain acceptance were associated with pain outcomes, however, the impact was beneath the threshold defined as clinically relevant.

Keywords: chronic pain; pain acceptance; early change; interdisciplinary pain treatment

1. Introduction

Chronic pain (CP) is a serious clinical problem [1]. In the United States, more than 100 million people suffer from CP and the annual costs for the society range between $560 and $635 billion [2]. As the presence of pain affects all aspects of an individual's functioning, an interdisciplinary approach incorporating the knowledge and skills of different healthcare providers is essential [3].

Interdisciplinary treatments for CP are based on the bio-psycho-social model of pain [4]. Such interdisciplinary treatments are conducted by a multi-professional team and address biological factors (e.g., medication, exercise), psychological factors (e.g., cognitions, emotions), as well as social factors (e.g., family, work) [4]. Several studies on CP showed that such interdisciplinary interventions are efficacious in randomized controlled trials [5,6] as well as effective under the conditions of routine care [7,8].

Psychotherapy is a central component in interdisciplinary pain treatments and cognitive-behavioral therapy (CBT) is the most often used [9]. Several meta-analyses and reviews have evaluated the efficacy of CBT for patients with CP [10]. A Cochrane review [11] revealed that CBT had statistically significant but small effects on pain and disability. The effects on mood and catastrophizing were moderate. These effects were compared with treatment-as-usual and wait-list control conditions. An integrative review of Knoerl et al. reported that CBT reduced pain intensity in 43% of the trials [12].

Another psychotherapeutic approach for the treatment of CP is Acceptance and Commitment Therapy (ACT; [13]). Acceptance and Commitment Therapy is a contextual form of CBT. Recent reviews reported that ACT is beneficial for patients with CP [14,15]. The ACT aims at increasing psychological flexibility (PF) and decreasing its counterpart psychological inflexibility [13,16]. While psychological inflexibility is associated with psychological problems or even psychiatric symptoms, PF is defined as the capacity to be in conscious and open contact with one's thoughts and feelings, and to behave according to one's values and goals [17]. Psychological flexibility consists of six core components (acceptance, cognitive defusion, self as a context, committed action, values, contact with the present moment) [18]. In the context of CP, pain acceptance is central to PF. Pain acceptance refers to the degree to which a patient is willing to live with pain or decides to get on with life despite pain. The Chronic Pain Acceptance Questionnaire (CPAQ; [19]) is a psychometrically sound instrument to operationalize pain acceptance and consists of a total scale and the following two subscales: Activity engagement and pain willingness. Activity engagement refers to the performance of personally valued activities, even in the presence of pain. Pain willingness refers to the willingness to give up attempts to control or avoid pain. Several studies on ACT for CP found that improvements in pain acceptance are associated with better pain outcomes [20–22]. Yet, two other studies suggest that pain acceptance is a change mechanism in other treatments as well and no ACT specific treatment process. These studies investigated whether improvements in pain acceptance are correlated with pain outcomes in interdisciplinary CBT-based treatments. Baranoff et al. [23] reported that pre-post improvements in pain acceptance were associated with improvements in almost all outcomes at the end of an interdisciplinary CBT-based treatment for CP. In another study on interdisciplinary CBT-based treatment for CP, Akerblom et al. [9] found that pain acceptance was not related to the outcome pain intensity but that it was the strongest mediator for the other outcome measures. These studies showed that improvements in pain acceptance play a crucial role for pain outcomes in different therapeutic approaches for CP. Baranoff et al. as well as Akerblom et al. assessed pain acceptance at pre-treatment, post-treatment, and at follow-up, but not during the interdisciplinary CBT-based treatment. To extend these previous findings, pain acceptance was monitored during interdisciplinary CBT-based treatment for CP in this project. The aim of the current study was to evaluate whether changes of pain acceptance in the very early treatment phase (first week) predict pain outcomes at post-treatment. We hypothesized that such early changes related to PF are predictors of pain outcomes at post-treatment, since early changes of variables related to psychological inflexibility (e.g., catastrophizing, depression, anxiety) have already been shown to be predictors of changes in pain and interference [24–27].

2. Materials and Method

2.1. Measurements

2.1.1. Pain Acceptance

Pain acceptance was measured with the Chronic Pain Acceptance Questionnaire (CPAQ [19,28]). The CPAQ consists of 20 items and has satisfactorily psychometric properties [19,28,29]. For the present study, only the total score of the CPAQ was analyzed. In the sample of the current study, the internal consistency at pre-treatment was Cronbachs Alpha $\alpha = 0.87$. Higher CPAQ scores indicate higher pain acceptance. Early changes in pain acceptance were operationalized as the difference between the CPAQ scores after the first treatment week and the CPAQ scores at the beginning of treatment. Differences were calculated so that more positive differences indicate more improvements in pain acceptance.

2.1.2. Pain Outcomes

Pain was measured with (1) an 11-point Numerical Rating Scale (NRS) and (2) the Pain Perception Scale. The NRS is a common self-rating instrument to measure pain intensity in patients with CP from 0 (no pain) to 10 (worst imaginable pain). The psychometric properties of the NRS have been investigated in several studies [30,31]. In the current study, self-ratings on average pain intensity were investigated. The Pain Perception Scale (SES) has 28 items and measures affective and sensory pain perception [32]. Both scales showed good internal consistencies in our sample at pre-treatment, with Cronbachs Alpha $\alpha = 0.93$ for the affective pain perception scale (SES-A) and Cronbachs $\alpha = 0.88$ for the sensory pain perception scale (SES-S). The pre-treatment and post-treatment scores of the NRS and SES were analyzed in the current study.

2.2. Study Sample

All patients taking part in the interdisciplinary CBT-based treatment for CP at the Hospital Barmherzige Brüder, Regensburg (Germany) between June 2014 and November 2015 were asked to participate in the study. During this time interval, N = 69 patients with CP were treated in a day-clinic setting for four weeks and all of them gave written informed consent to partake in this study. All patients suffered from chronic, non-malignant pain according to the ICD-10 diagnosis "chronic pain disorder with somatic and psychological factors (F45.41)". Of the patients, 36.2% had a comorbid depression diagnosis, 50.7% fulfilled the criteria for at least one comorbid psychiatric disorder.

2.3. Intervention

The interdisciplinary treatment was performed according to the pain treatment program "Marburger Schmerzbewältigungsprogramm" [33]. It is a CBT-based program for CP. The patients received treatment for four weeks. Each week treatment lasted from 8:00 a.m. to 4:00 p.m. between Monday and Thursday as well as from 08:00 a.m. to 01:15 p.m. at Friday. The treatment consisted of individual treatment as well as group therapy (closed groups; up to 8 patients per group). The interdisciplinary pain treatment was performed by a team of physicians, psychologists, physical therapists, occupational therapists, and social workers. The CBT component focused mainly on psychoeducation, the bio-psycho-social pain model, relaxation training, and directing the attention towards positive experiences in group sessions and individual sessions. The CBT-based group sessions took part four times per week, and the individual sessions once a week.

2.4. Statistical Analysis

All analyses were conducted with SPSS25. To evaluate pre-post changes of pain outcomes (NRS; SES-A; SES-S), we conducted paired t-tests and calculated effect sizes (d) according to the following formula: $(M_{prä} - M_{post})/SD_{prä}$. Effect sizes are interpreted as follows: $d \geq 0.20$ small effect, $d \geq 0.50$ medium effect, $d \geq 0.80$ large effect. Linear regression analyses (method selection "enter") were performed to address the research question whether early changes in pain acceptance predict pain outcomes at post-treatment. One linear regression model was performed for each pain outcome, i.e., either the NRS at post-treatment, or the SES-A at post-treatment, or the SES-S at post-treatment were the dependent variable. As predictors, we added early changes in pain acceptance, the pre-treatment scores of the respective pain outcome variable (to control for pre-treatment values), age, and gender. Moreover, a logistic regression analysis (method selection "enter") was performed to evaluate whether early changes in pain acceptance during the first treatment week predict clinically relevant changes in pain intensity from pre- to post-treatment (≥ 2 points improvement on the NRS from pre- to post-treatment) [34]. The dichotomized NRS (0 = pre-post NRS improvement < 2 points; 1 = pre-post NRS improvement ≥ 2 points) was the dependent variable, and predictors were early changes in pain acceptance, age, and gender. We included age and gender in the regression models, since they have been shown to influence pain outcomes in previous studies [35,36]. Moreover, Pearson correlation coefficients were calculated between the measures at pre-treatment to investigate potential overlap between the measures. The significance level was set at $p < 0.05$ and the statistical tests were performed two-tailed. Missing data were replaced by the average of the time series.

2.5. Ethical Consideration

The Ethics Committee of the University Clinic Regensburg approved the materials and methods for this study. All patients gave written informed consent.

3. Results

The sample comprised N = 69 patients with CP (49 females), who were on average M = 52.62 (standard deviation (SD) = 9.78) years old. The participants gave written informed consent to participate in the study, but during the study, some patients did not fill in the measures or dropped out from treatment. Table 1 shows how many patients filled in the applied measures.

Table 1. Number of patients filling in the questionnaires. N = 69.

Measure	Number of Patients Filling in the Measure N (%)
NRS pre-treatment	66 (96%)
NRS post-treatment	53 (77%)
SES-A pre-treatment	61 (88%)
SES-A post-treatment	52 (75%)
SES-S pre-treatment	62 (90%)
SES-S post-treatment	50 (72%)
CPAQ pre-treatment	52 (75%)
CPAQ after first treatment week	61 (88%)

Note: NRS = Numeric Rating Scale; SES-A = Affective Pain Perception Scale; SES-S = Sensory Pain Perception Scale; CPAQ = Chronic Pain Acceptance Questionnaire.

The correlations between the measures at pre-treatment are presented in Table 2. Pain intensity was positively correlated with affective pain perception ($r = 0.56$; $p < 0.001$) and with sensory pain perception ($r = 0.25$; $p = 0.040$). Affective and sensory pain perception were also positively correlated ($r = 0.57$; $p < 0.001$). Significantly negative correlations emerged between pain intensity and pain acceptance ($r = -0.27$; $p = 0.025$) as well as between affective pain perception and pain acceptance ($r = -0.48$; $p < 0.001$).

Table 2. Correlations between the measures at pre-treatment. N = 69.

		SES-A	SES-S	CPAQ
NRS	r	0.56	0.25	−0.27
	p-value	<0.001	0.040	0.025
SES-A	r		0.57	−0.48
	p-value		<0.001	<0.001
SES-S	r			−0.23
	p-value			0.061

Note: NRS = Numeric Rating Scale; SES-A = Affective Pain Perception Scale; SES-S = Sensory Pain Perception Scale.

Results of the analyses evaluating pre-post changes of the pain outcomes are presented in Table 3. Pain intensity improved ($t(68) = 5.82$; $p < 0.001$) with a large effect size of $d = 0.81$, affective pain perception improved ($t(68) = 4.43$; $p < 0.001$) with a medium effect size of $d = 0.60$, and sensory pain perception improved ($t(68) = 3.26$; $p = 0.002$) with a small effect size of $d = 0.41$.

Table 3. Pre–post changes in pain outcomes. N = 69.

	Pre-Treatment M (SD)	Post-Treatment M (SD)	Statistics	Effect Size
Pain intensity (NRS)	6.33 (1.62)	4.97 (1.65)	$t(68) = 5.82; p < 0.001$	$d = 0.84$
Affective Pain Perception (SES-A)	35.90 (9.60)	30.12 (10.21)	$t(68) = 4.43; p < 0.001$	$d = 0.60$
Sensory Pain Perception (SES-S)	31.94 (8.64)	28.38 (8.02)	$t(68) = 3.26; p = 0.002$	$d = 0.41$

Note: NRS = Numeric Rating Scale; SES-A = Affective Pain Perception Scale; SES-S = Sensory Pain Perception Scale; SD = standard deviation.

Three linear regression analysis were conducted to evaluate if early changes in pain acceptance predict the pain outcomes (NRS, SES-A, SES-S) at post-treatment. As can be seen in Table 4, early changes in pain acceptance were negatively correlated with the three pain outcomes. This means that early improvements in pain acceptance were associated with more favorable pain outcomes (i.e., less pain intensity, less affective pain perception, and less sensory pain perception at post-treatment), since higher values on the NRS, SES-A, and SES-S indicate more severe pain, whereas more positive CPAQ difference scores indicate larger early improvements in pain acceptance.

Table 4. Results of the multiple regression analyses testing early changes in pain acceptance as predictors of pain outcomes. N = 69.

	Unstandardized Coefficients B (SE)	Standardized Coefficients Beta	T	p-Value
Pain intensity (NRS)				
(Constant)	3.31 (1.21)		2.74	0.008
Early changes in pain acceptance (CPAQ)	−0.04 (0.02)	−0.27	−2.28	0.026
NRS pre-treatment	0.34 (0.12)	0.33	2.81	0.007
Age	−0.01 (0.02)	−0.06	−0.46	0.648
Gender	0.07 (0.43)	0.02	0.17	0.869
Affective Pain Perception (SES-A)				
(Constant)	22.45 (7.03)		3.20	0.002
Early changes in pain acceptance (CPAQ)	−0.26 (0.10)	−0.31	−2.79	0.007
SES-A pre-treatment	0.41 (0.11)	0.38	3.66	0.001
Age	−0.17 (0.11)	−0.16	−1.48	0.145
Gender	1.74 (2.43)	0.08	0.72	0.476
Sensory Pain Perception (SES-S)				
(Constant)	23.53 (6.21)		3.79	<0.001
Early changes in pain acceptance (CPAQ)	−0.19 (0.08)	−0.28	−2.44	0.017
SES-S pre-treatment	0.35 (0.10)	0.38	3.50	0.001
Age	−0.10 (0.09)	−0.12	−1.10	0.276
Gender	−0.53 (1.95)	−0.03	−0.27	0.787

Note: NRS = Numeric Rating Scale; SES-A = Affective Pain Perception Scale; SES-S = Sensory Pain Perception Scale; CPAQ = Chronic Pain Acceptance Questionnaire; SE = standard error.

Outcome pain intensity (NRS): R^2 was 0.17 (F(4, 64) = 3.34, $p = 0.015$). Early changes in pain acceptance predicted pain intensity at post-treatment (B = −0.04 (standard error (SE) = 0.02); T = −2.28; $p = 0.026$) when statistically controlling for pain intensity at pre-treatment (B = 0.34 (SE = 0.12); T = 2.81; $p = 0.007$), age (B = −0.01 (SE = 0.02); T = −0.46; $p = 0.648$), and gender (B = 0.07 (SE = 0.43); T = 0.17; $p = 0.869$).

Outcome affective pain perception (SES-A): R^2 reached 0.31 (F(4, 64) = 7.27, $p < 0.001$). Affective pain perception at post-treatment was predicted by early changes in pain acceptance (B = −0.26 (SE = 0.10); T = −2.79; $p = 0.007$) when statistically controlling for affective pain perception at pre-treatment (B = 0.41 (SE = 0.11); T = 3.66; $p = 0.001$), age (B = −0.17 (SE = 0.11); T = −1.48; $p = 0.145$), and gender (B = 1.74 (SE = 2.43); T = 0.72; $p = 0.476$).

Outcome sensory pain perception (SES-S): R^2 amounted to 0.27 (F(4, 64) = 5.91, $p < 0.001$). When statistically controlling for sensory pain perception at pre-treatment (B = 0.35 (SE = 0.10); T = 3.50; $p = 0.001$), age (B = −0.10 (SE = 0.09); T = −1.10; $p = 0.276$), and gender (B = −0.53 (SE = 1.95); T = −0.27; $p = 0.787$), sensory pain perception at post-treatment was predicted by early changes in pain acceptance (B = −0.19 (SE = 0.08); T = −2.44; $p = 0.017$).

For the outcome pain intensity, we calculated how many patients show a clinically relevant improvement from pre- to post-treatment of at least 2 points on the NRS [34]. N = 31 (45%) improved at least 2 points from pre- to post-treatment and N = 38 (55%) did not. A logistic regression analysis was performed to investigate whether early changes in pain acceptance predict clinically relevant pre-post changes in pain intensity. The results of this logistic regression (−2 Log-Likelihood = 90.77; Cox and Snell R-Quadrat = 0.06; Nagelkerkes R-Quadrat = 0.08) showed that early changes in pain acceptance do not predict clinically significant NRS changes (Exp(B) = 1.04; 95% confidence interval (CI): 0.99; 1.09; $p = 0.157$) when controlling for age (Exp(B) = 1.03; 95% CI: 0.98; 1.09; $p = 0.304$) and gender (Exp(B) = 1.07; 95% CI: 0.36; 3.25; $p = 0.900$).

4. Discussion

This study evaluated whether early changes in pain acceptance predict pain outcomes at the end of an interdisciplinary CBT-based treatment for CP. As pain outcomes, we evaluated pain intensity, affective pain perception, and sensory pain perception. The results showed that early changes in pain acceptance within the first treatment week were associated with less pain intensity, less affective pain perception, and less sensory pain perception at the end of an interdisciplinary pain program. However, clinically relevant changes in pain intensity from pre- to post-treatment were not predicted by early changes in pain acceptance.

Our results extend past research on pain acceptance in interdisciplinary CBT-based treatments for CP [9,23], which showed that changes in pain acceptance are associated with outcomes. Yet, the previous studies did not investigate pain acceptance in the early treatment phase. With regard to the pain outcome pain intensity, our results appear to be in contrast to another study [9] where the outcome pain intensity was not correlated with changes in pain acceptance. One explanation could be that Akerblom et al. [9] analyzed pre-post changes in pain acceptance, whereas we investigated early changes in pain acceptance during the first treatment week. It might be that the outcome pain intensity is predicted by early changes in pain acceptance but not by pre-post changes in pain acceptance. This speculation receives some support from pain studies showing that different predictors of the outcome can be found in the early and late treatment phase [24–27].

When interpreting our results, it should be kept in mind that pain acceptance is no explicit treatment target in CBT-based treatments. We can only speculate about the factors influencing early changes in pain acceptance. Possibly, non-specific common factors like the therapeutic alliance or hope might be associated with early changes in pain acceptance as these common factors have been discussed to play a role in the early phase of psychotherapy [37,38], but this needs to be further studied in the area of pain. It should also be kept in mind that some of the pain outcome measures (NRS, SES-A) were significantly correlated with the pain acceptance measure at pre-treatment. Therefore, the correlation between changes in pain acceptance and changes in pain intensity as well as changes in affective pain perception may be overstated. There are several further shortcomings to discuss. Although the external validity/generalizability of the results is positively influenced by the conditions of routine practice, the following points limit the generalizability. All patients had the ICD-10 diagnosis "chronic pain disorder with somatic and psychological factors (F45.41)" and it remains unclear how early changes in pain acceptance influence pain outcomes in patients with other forms of pain. The representativeness is further reduced by the rather small sample size (N = 69) as well as the relatively large amount of missing data. The sample is, for example, too small for a sound investigation of moderators between early changes in pain acceptance and pain outcomes. Future larger studies could include age and gender as moderators and investigate whether the effect of early changes in pain acceptance on pain outcomes interacts with age and gender. Besides CP, more than half of the patients had various, especially psychiatric diagnoses. Another limitation is that the diagnoses were made by the clinic team, but not with a structured or standardized clinical interview. Due to the naturalistic design we did not calculate a power analysis ahead of the study. We replaced missing data by the average of the time series. This approach leads to an overestimation of the effect compared to replacing missing post-treatment data with the pre-treatment values. Other strategies to handle missing data (e.g., Expectation-Maximization algorithm) might lead to different results. Furthermore, regression analysis does not allow drawing causal inferences and the internal validity of the results is rather low. A randomized controlled trial comparing a condition including a component to increase pain acceptance in the early treatment phase and a condition excluding this component would produce results of higher internal validity. Based on our results, one would expect that pain outcomes are better in the condition with the component to increase pain acceptance in the early treatment phase. A further limitation is that we only included pain acceptance as process variable. The inclusion of more process variables (e.g., pain catastrophizing) would have allowed to investigate whether early changes in one process variable are more or less important predictors of pain outcomes than early changes in other process variables. Another shortcoming is that pain intensity and pain perception were the solely outcomes in the current study and other outcomes such as functioning or patient satisfaction should also be integrated to evaluate treatments for CP [39]. Pain acceptance might also be an important outcome in treatments for CP and we analyzed pain acceptance as a process measure only. Furthermore, our results rely on self-report data and complementary assessments of more objective pain outcomes (e.g., quantitative sensory testing) would be welcome in future studies. Moreover, our definition of early change should be discussed in more detail. We investigated difference scores within the first week to investigate early changes in pain acceptance. The first treatment week might a suitable time frame to study early changes, but other studies defined the change from pre- to mid-treatment [25,26], or the change from pre-treatment to the third treatment week [24,40] as early change. It should also be mentioned that there are several other approaches to operationalize change rate [41] such as deviations from expected recovery curves [40], sudden gains [42] reliable change [43] or the method of percent of improvement [44]. Finally, we only investigated how early changes in pain acceptance influence the short-term outcome at the end of the interdisciplinary treatment for CP, but we do not know how the long-term outcome is predicted by early changes of pain acceptance due to the lack of follow-up assessments.

5. Conclusions

Early changes in pain acceptance are associated with continuous pain outcomes, but not with clinically relevant improvements in pain intensity.

Author Contributions: Conceptualization, T.P. and A.M.; methodology, T.P.; software, T.P., R.J., N.D. and S.S.; validation, A.M., C.L. and C.P.; formal analysis, T.P. and R.J.; investigation, N.D. and S.S.; resources, R.W., K.H., R.R., A.M. and C.P.; data curation, N.D. and S.S.; writing—original draft preparation, T.P. and R.J.; writing—review and editing, T.P. and C.P.; visualization, T.P.; supervision, T.P., A.M., C.L. and C.P.; project administration, T.P., N.D., S.S., R.W., K.H., R.R. and A.M.

Funding: The research was performed as a part of the employment of the authors. Open Access Funding by the University for Continuing Education Krems.

Acknowledgments: The data underlying the findings of the study are available from the corresponding author upon request.

Conflicts of Interest: The authors declare that there is no conflict of interest regarding the publication of this paper.

References

1. Gereau, R.W.; Sluka, K.A.; Maixner, W.; Savage, S.R.; Price, T.J.; Murinson, B.B.; Sullivan, M.D.; Fillingim, R.B. A pain research agenda for the 21st century. *J. Pain* **2014**, *15*, 1203–1214. [CrossRef] [PubMed]

2. Gaskin, D.J.; Richard, P. The economic costs of pain in the United States. *J. Pain* **2014**, *13*, 715–724. [CrossRef] [PubMed]
3. Interdisciplinary Pain Management. Available online: http://americanpainsociety.org/uploads/about/position-statements/interdisciplinary-white-paper.pdf (accessed on 31 May 2019).
4. Gatchel, R.J.; McGeary, D.D.; McGeary, C.A.; Lippe, B. Interdisciplinary chronic pain management: Past, present, and future. *Am. Psychol.* **2014**, *69*, 119–130. [CrossRef] [PubMed]
5. Kamper, S.J.; Apeldoorn, A.T.; Chiarotto, A.; Smeets, R.J.; Ostelo, R.W.; Guzman, J.; van Tulder, M.W. Multidisciplinary biopsychosocial rehabilitation for chronic low back pain. *Cochrane Database Syst. Rev.* **2014**, *9*, CD000963. [CrossRef] [PubMed]
6. Guzman, J.; Esmail, R.; Karjalainen, K.; Malmivaara, A.; Irvin, E.; Bombardier, C. Multidisciplinary rehabilitation for chronic low back pain: Systematic review. *BMJ* **2001**, *322*, 1511. [CrossRef] [PubMed]
7. Pieh, C.; Neumeier, S.; Loew, T.; Altmeppen, J.; Angerer, M.; Busch, V.; Lahmann, C. Effectiveness of a multimodal treatment program for somatoform pain disorder. *Pain Pract.* **2014**, *14*, E146–E151. [CrossRef] [PubMed]
8. Preis, M.A.; Vogtle, E.; Dreyer, N.; Seel, S.; Wagner, R.; Hanshans, K.; Reyersbach, R.; Pieh, C.; Muhlberger, A.; Probst, T. Long-term outcomes of a multimodal day-clinic treatment for chronic pain under the conditions of routine care. *Pain Res. Manag.* **2018**, *2018*, 9472104. [CrossRef]
9. Akerblom, S.; Perrin, S.; Rivano Fischer, M.; McCracken, L.M. The mediating role of acceptance in multidisciplinary cognitive-behavioral therapy for chronic pain. *J. Pain.* **2015**, *16*, 606–615. [CrossRef]
10. Ehde, D.M.; Dillworth, T.M.; Turner, J.A. Cognitive-behavioral therapy for individuals with chronic pain: Efficacy, innovations, and directions for research. *Am. Psychol.* **2014**, *69*, 153–166. [CrossRef]
11. Williams, A.C.; Eccleston, C.; Morley, S. Psychological therapies for the management of chronic pain (excluding headache) in adults. *Cochrane Database Syst. Rev.* **2012**, *11*, CD007407. [CrossRef]
12. Knoerl, R.; Lavoie Smith, E.M.; Weisberg, J. Chronic pain and cognitive behavioral therapy: An integrative review. *West. J. Nurs. Res.* **2016**, *38*, 596–628. [CrossRef] [PubMed]
13. Hayes, S.C. Acceptance and commitment therapy, relational frame theory, and the third wave of behavioral and cognitive therapies. *Behav. Ther.* **2016**, *47*, 869–885. [CrossRef] [PubMed]
14. Hughes, L.S.; Clark, J.; Colclough, J.A.; Dale, E.; McMillan, D. Acceptance and commitment therapy (ACT) for chronic pain: A systematic review and meta-analyses. *Clin. J. Pain.* **2017**, *33*, 552–568. [CrossRef] [PubMed]
15. Veehof, M.M.; Trompetter, H.R.; Bohlmeijer, E.T.; Schreurs, K.M. Acceptance- and mindfulness-based interventions for the treatment of chronic pain: A meta-analytic review. *Cogn. Behav. Ther.* **2016**, *45*, 5–31. [CrossRef] [PubMed]
16. Hayes, S.C.; Luoma, J.B.; Bond, F.W.; Masuda, A.; Lillis, J. Acceptance and commitment therapy: Model, processes and outcomes. *Behav. Res. Ther.* **2006**, *44*, 1–25. [CrossRef]
17. McCracken, L.M.; Morley, S. The psychological flexibility model: A basis for integration and progress in psychological approaches to chronic pain management. *J. Pain.* **2014**, *15*, 221–234. [CrossRef]
18. Hayes, S.C.; Strosahl, K.D.; Wilson, K.G. *Acceptance and commitment therapy: The Process and Practice of Mindful Change*, 2nd ed.; Guilford Publications: New York, NY, USA, 2011.
19. McCracken, L.M.; Vowles, K.E.; Eccleston, C. Acceptance of chronic pain: Component analysis and a revised assessment method. *Pain* **2004**, *107*, 159–166. [CrossRef]
20. Cederberg, J.T.; Cernvall, M.; Dahl, J.; von Essen, L.; Ljungman, G. Acceptance as a mediator for change in acceptance and commitment therapy for persons with chronic pain? *Int. J. Behav. Med.* **2016**, *23*, 21–29. [CrossRef]
21. Vowles, K.E.; McCracken, L.M. Acceptance and values-based action in chronic pain: A study of treatment effectiveness and process. *J. Consult. Clin. Psychol.* **2008**, *76*, 397–407. [CrossRef]
22. Lin, J.; Klatt, L.I.; McCracken, L.M.; Baumeister, H. Psychological flexibility mediates the effect of an online-based acceptance and commitment therapy for chronic pain: An investigation of change processes. *Pain* **2018**, *159*, 663–672. [CrossRef]
23. Baranoff, J.; Hanrahan, S.J.; Kapur, D.; Connor, J.P. Acceptance as a process variable in relation to catastrophizing in multidisciplinary pain treatment. *Eur. J. Pain.* **2013**, *17*, 101–110. [CrossRef]
24. Bergbom, S.; Boersma, K.; Linton, S.J. Both early and late changes in psychological variables relate to treatment outcome for musculoskeletal pain patients at risk for disability. *Behav. Res. Ther.* **2012**, *50*, 726–734. [CrossRef] [PubMed]

25. Wideman, T.H.; Adams, H.; Sullivan, M.J. A prospective sequential analysis of the fear-avoidance model of pain. *Pain* **2009**, *145*, 45–51. [CrossRef] [PubMed]
26. Burns, J.W.; Glenn, B.; Bruehl, S.; Harden, R.N.; Lofland, K. Cognitive factors influence outcome following multidisciplinary chronic pain treatment: A replication and extension of a cross-lagged panel analysis. *Behav. Res. Ther.* **2003**, *41*, 1163–1182. [CrossRef]
27. Burns, J.W.; Kubilus, A.; Bruehl, S.; Harden, R.N.; Lofland, K. Do changes in cognitive factors influence outcome following multidisciplinary treatment for chronic pain? A cross-lagged panel analysis. *J. Consult. Clin. Psychol.* **2003**, *71*, 81–91. [CrossRef] [PubMed]
28. Nilges, P.; Köster, B.; Schmidt, C.O. Schmerzakzeptanz – Konzept und Überprüfung einer deutschen Fassung des Chronic Pain Acceptance Questionnaire. *Der Schmerz* **2007**, *21*, 57–67. [CrossRef] [PubMed]
29. Reneman, M.F.; Dijkstra, A.; Geertzen, J.H.; Dijkstra, P.U. Psychometric properties of Chronic Pain Acceptance Questionnaires: A systematic review. *Eur. J. Pain* **2010**, *14*, 457–465. [CrossRef]
30. Jensen, M.P.; Turner, J.A.; Romano, J.M.; Fisher, L.D. Comparative reliability and validity of chronic pain intensity measures. *Pain* **1999**, *83*, 157–162. [CrossRef]
31. Ferreira-Valente, M.A.; Pais-Ribeiro, J.L.; Jensen, M.P. Validity of four pain intensity rating scales. *Pain* **2011**, *152*, 2399–2404. [CrossRef]
32. Geissner, E. Die Schmerzempfindungsskala SES–Ein differenziertes und veränderungssensitives Verfahren zur Erfassung chronischer und akuter Schmerzen. *Rehabilitation* **1995**, *34*, 35–43.
33. Basler, H.-D. *Psychologische Therapie bei Kopf- und Rückenschmerzen: Das Marburger Schmerzbewältigungsprogramm zur Gruppen- und Einzeltherapie*, 1st ed.; Quintessenz; MMV, Medizin-Verl.: München, Germany, 1998.
34. Farrar, J.T.; Young, J.P., Jr.; LaMoreaux, L.; Werth, J.L.; Poole, R.M. Clinical importance of changes in chronic pain intensity measured on an 11-point numerical pain rating scale. *Pain* **2001**, *94*, 149–158. [CrossRef]
35. Pieh, C.; Altmeppen, J.; Neumeier, S.; Loew, T.; Angerer, M.; Lahmann, C. Gender differences in outcomes of a multimodal pain management program. *Pain* **2012**, *153*, 197–202. [CrossRef] [PubMed]
36. Buchner, M.; Neubauer, E.; Zahlten-Hinguranage, A.; Schiltenwolf, M. Age as a predicting factor in the therapy outcome of multidisciplinary treatment of patients with chronic low back pain—a prospective longitudinal clinical study in 405 patients. *Clin. Rheumatol.* **2007**, *26*, 385–392. [CrossRef] [PubMed]
37. Lambert, M.J. Early response in psychotherapy: Further evidence for the importance of common factors rather than "placebo effects". *J. Clin. Psychol.* **2005**, *61*, 855–869. [CrossRef] [PubMed]
38. Ilardi, S.S.; Craighead, W.E. The role of nonspecific factors in cognitive-behavior therapy for depression. *Clin. Psychol-Sci. Pr.* **1994**, *1*, 138–155. [CrossRef]
39. Dworkin, R.H.; Turk, D.C.; Farrar, J.T.; Haythornthwaite, J.A.; Jensen, M.P.; Katz, N.P.; Kerns, R.D.; Stucki, G.; Allen, R.R.; Bellamy, N.; et al. Core outcome measures for chronic pain clinical trials: IMMPACT recommendations. *Pain* **2005**, *113*, 9–19. [CrossRef]
40. Haas, E.; Hill, R.D.; Lambert, M.J.; Morrell, B. Do early responders to psychotherapy maintain treatment gains? *J. Clin. Psychol.* **2002**, *58*, 1157–1172. [CrossRef]
41. Erekson, D.M.; Horner, J.; Lambert, M.J. Different lens or different picture? Comparing methods of defining dramatic change in psychotherapy. *Psychother. Res.* **2018**, *28*, 750–760. [CrossRef]
42. Stiles, W.B.; Leach, C.; Barkham, M.; Lucock, M.; Iveson, S.; Shapiro, D.A.; Iveson, M.; Hardy, G.E. Early sudden gains in psychotherapy under routine clinic conditions: Practice-based evidence. *J. Consult. Clin. Psychol.* **2003**, *71*, 14–21. [CrossRef]
43. Kleinstauber, M.; Lambert, M.J.; Hiller, W. Early response in cognitive-behavior therapy for syndromes of medically unexplained symptoms. *BMC Psychiatry* **2017**, *17*, 195. [CrossRef]
44. Hiller, W.; Schindler, A.C.; Lambert, M.J. Defining response and remission in psychotherapy research: A comparison of the RCI and the method of percent improvement. *Psychother. Res.* **2012**, *22*, 1–11. [CrossRef] [PubMed]

© 2019 by the authors. Licensee MDPI, Basel, Switzerland. This article is an open access article distributed under the terms and conditions of the Creative Commons Attribution (CC BY) license (http://creativecommons.org/licenses/by/4.0/).

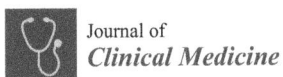

Article

Cost–Utility of Mindfulness-Based Stress Reduction for Fibromyalgia versus a Multicomponent Intervention and Usual Care: A 12-Month Randomized Controlled Trial (EUDAIMON Study)

Adrián Pérez-Aranda [1,2,3,4], Francesco D'Amico [5], Albert Feliu-Soler [1,2,3,*], Lance M. McCracken [6], María T. Peñarrubia-María [7,8,9], Laura Andrés-Rodríguez [1,2,3], Natalia Angarita-Osorio [1,2], Martin Knapp [5,8], Javier García-Campayo [3,10] and Juan V. Luciano [1,2,3,*]

1. Group of Psychological Research in Fibromyalgia & Chronic Pain (AGORA), Institut de Recerca Sant Joan de Déu, 08950 Esplugues de Llobregat, Spain
2. Teaching, Research & Innovation Unit, Parc Sanitari Sant Joan de Déu, 08830 Sant Boi de Llobregat, Spain
3. Primary Care Prevention and Health Promotion Research Network, RedIAPP, 28029 Madrid, Spain
4. Department of Clinical Psychology and Psychobiology (Section Personality, Assessment and Psychological Treatments), University of Barcelona, 08193 Barcelona, Spain
5. The London School of Economics and Political Science (LSE), London WC2A 2AE, UK
6. Department of Psychology, Uppsala University, SE-751 05 Uppsala, Sweden
7. Primary Health Centre Bartomeu Fabrés Anglada, SAP Delta Llobregat, Unitat Docent Costa de Ponent, Institut Català de la Salut, 08850 Gavà, Spain
8. Centre for Biomedical Research in Epidemiology and Public Health, CIBERESP, 28029 Madrid, Spain
9. Fundació IDIAP Jordi Gol I Gurina, 08007 Barcelona, Spain
10. Department of Psychiatry, Miguel Servet Hospital, Aragon Institute of Health Sciences (I+CS), 50009 Zaragoza, Spain
* Correspondence: a.feliu@pssjd.org (A.F.-S.); jvluciano@pssjd.org (J.V.L.); Tel.: +34-93-640-6350 (ext. 1-2540) (J.V.L.)

Received: 19 June 2019; Accepted: 17 July 2019; Published: 20 July 2019

Abstract: Fibromyalgia (FM) is a prevalent, chronic, disabling, pain syndrome that implies high healthcare costs. Economic evaluations of potentially effective treatments for FM are needed. The aim of this study was to analyze the cost–utility of Mindfulness-Based Stress Reduction (MBSR) as an add-on to treatment-as-usual (TAU) for patients with FM compared to an adjuvant multicomponent intervention ("FibroQoL") and to TAU. We performed an economic evaluation alongside a 12 month, randomized, controlled trial; data from 204 (68 per study arm) of the 225 patients (90.1%) were included in the cost–utility analyses, which were conducted both under the government and the public healthcare system perspectives. The main outcome measures were the EuroQol (EQ-5D-5L) for assessing Quality-Adjusted Life Years (QALYs) and improvements in health-related quality of life, and the Client Service Receipt Inventory (CSRI) for estimating direct and indirect costs. Incremental cost-effectiveness ratios (ICERs) were also calculated. Two sensitivity analyses (intention-to-treat, ITT, and per protocol, PPA) were conducted. The results indicated that MBSR achieved a significant reduction in costs compared to the other study arms ($p < 0.05$ in the completers sample), especially in terms of indirect costs and primary healthcare services. It also produced a significant incremental effect compared to TAU in the ITT sample (ΔQALYs = 0.053, $p < 0.05$, where QALYs represents quality-adjusted life years). Overall, our findings support the efficiency of MBSR over FibroQoL and TAU specifically within a Spanish public healthcare context.

Keywords: fibromyalgia; cost–utility; cost-effectiveness; quality-adjusted life years

1. Introduction

Fibromyalgia (FM) is a disabling syndrome of unknown etiology mainly characterized by chronic widespread musculoskeletal pain, fatigue, stiffness, sleep problems, perceived cognitive dysfunction, and mood disturbances [1]. It is usually diagnosed in women aged between 30 and 50 years old and has an estimated prevalence of around 2% in the general population [2,3]. Health-related quality of life is significantly lower for people with FM compared to the general population and similar or lower than those seen for other medical conditions such as osteoarthritis, rheumatoid arthritis, or osteoporosis [4].

FM is a costly syndrome for both healthcare funders and society in general. It is the chronic pain condition with the highest rates of unemployment, sick-leave, claims for incapacity benefits, work absenteeism, and per-patient costs [5]. FM patients' direct costs have been described as three times higher than those for patients with other pathologies but similar sociodemographic characteristics [6]. Regarding indirect costs, the range of women with FM who are able to preserve their jobs has been reported to be between 34% and 77% [7,8], and reducing work hours due to the impact of symptoms is a common practice among patients with FM [9]. Altogether, FM is second only to irritable bowel syndrome in its contribution to the approximately $300B in costs that inflammatory diseases and related chronic syndromes are expected to generate in the US in coming years [10]. There is a need, therefore, to optimize the development and the implementation of treatments for FM that, next to early accurate diagnoses and methods to support treatment-adherence, would help to address this burden [10].

To date, no cure has been found for FM, although different pharmacological (pregabalin and noradrenaline reuptake inhibitors) and non-pharmacological interventions (aerobic exercise, cognitive-behavioral therapy (CBT), multicomponent therapy, and "third-wave" CBT such as mindfulness-based interventions (MBIs) or Acceptance and Commitment Therapy (ACT)) have demonstrated some benefits for reducing the impact of the symptoms and increasing quality of life [11,12]. The pharmacological approach is most common for FM despite its limited effectiveness. In fact, non-pharmacological treatments appear to show effects in more separate symptom domains as compared with pharmacological treatments for FM [13].

A crucial aspect for including interventions such as those mentioned above in any health system is the balance between costs and benefits that each intervention produces. Policy-makers are faced with limited economic resources and therefore must prioritize among available alternatives. Cost-effectiveness analyses allow cost comparisons of different treatments in relation to the health improvement that each one produces [14]. The cost–utility analysis is a type of cost-effectiveness analysis that allows comparison of therapies across different pathologies, as it is based on quality-adjusted life years (QALYs), a measure that combines the length of survival and its quality, regardless of the illness. The value of a QALY ranges from 0 (death) to 1 (best imaginable health), although states deemed worse than death can have negative values. Thus, cost–utility is measured in costs per QALYs.

Unfortunately, to date, there have been few cost-effectiveness or cost–utility studies of effective interventions for FM, although interest in these has recently increased. To our knowledge, 12 studies have assessed the cost–utility of different treatments for FM [14–25]. Four of them focused on pharmacological treatments, concluding that both pregabalin [15,18,19] and duloxetine [20] would be cost-effective compared to other pharmacological options or placebo. Regarding non-pharmacological interventions, one study evaluated the cost–utility of a cognitive-educational treatment for FM and found that the group discussion component alone was more cost-effective as compared to adding a cognitive component [21]. However, further studies have found cognitive-behavioral interventions to be cost-effective. This includes Schröder et al. [25], who studied the long-term cost–utility of a CBT group compared to usual care in functional somatic syndromes such as FM and found that the intervention improved quality of life and reduced costs in the long term.

In another study, Luciano et al. [22] found that the multicomponent intervention FibroQoL, consisting of the combination of psychoeducation and training in relaxation, was cost-effective in the long-term compared to usual care. The same research group found that CBT was more cost-effective than recommended pharmacological treatment (RPT) and usual care due to significant reduction in direct costs, although it was not associated with significantly improved quality of life [23]. More recently, the same authors compared group ACT (GACT) to RPT and a waitlist control (WLC), and the cost–utility analysis favored GACT in comparison to RPT and WLC [14]. Even more recently, Hedman-Lagerlöf et al. [24] evaluated the cost-effectiveness of an internet-based exposure intervention for FM (to stimuli that elicit pain-related distress) compared to WLC and found that the intervention could be highly cost-effective, as each incremental responder generated an annual societal cost reduction of more than $15,000.

Certainly, some treatments show limited cost-effectiveness. For example, in studies of alternative treatments including aquatic training [17] and spa treatments [16], the first concluded that an eight month aquatic training was cost-effective compared to usual care, although some external variables (e.g., distance from the patients' homes or number of patients that participate in each session) could have a major impact on the cost of the intervention. The second found that the spa treatment improved the quality of life only temporarily but not in the long term and resulted in neither a significant decrease of health care consumption nor in productivity loss.

Regarding MBIs, economic evaluations are scarce and have been specially focused on depression and emotional unstable personality disorder [26] but not on FM. Economic evaluation of MBIs for FM seems particularly relevant because these interventions have demonstrated promising clinical results in previous studies [27–30], albeit with some methodological limitations, such as small sample sizes or lack of long-term follow-up assessments.

As a response to limitations of previous studies, the EUDAIMON study conducted in Spain recruited a large sample of patients with FM (N = 225) and employed a 12 month follow-up evaluation. Results showed superior efficacy of Mindfulness-Based Stress Reduction (MBSR) compared to the multicomponent intervention FibroQoL and to usual care [31]. MBSR led to improved functional impairment, FM-related symptoms, and other secondary outcomes (e.g., depressive and anxiety symptoms, perceived stress, pain catastrophizing, cognitive dysfunction) with moderate to large effect sizes at post-treatment assessment. Some of these improvements were partially lost in the long-term, probably due to reduced, intermittent, and non-structured practice of mindfulness once the eight week intervention finished.

The present study extends our earlier work on clinical efficacy of MBSR in patients with FM [31] and shows the results of an economic evaluation alongside the randomized controlled trial (RCT). Here, we compare for the first time the 12 month health care and societal costs as well as the 12 month cost–utility of MBSR compared to FibroQoL and usual care (passive control arm) in terms of QALY gains and increases in health-related quality of life in Spanish patients with FM.

2. Methods

2.1. Participants

Following a multi-stage recruitment process, a total of 225 adult patients diagnosed with FM according to the American College of Rheumatology (ACR) 1990 criteria [32] were recruited from the Rheumatology Service at Sant Joan de Déu Hospital (St. Boi de Llobregat, Spain) and participated in the EUDAIMON study between January 2016 and April 2018. As seen in Figure 1, the total sample was randomized into three study arms, as explained below. However, due to missing data in some of the baseline variables needed for the cost–utility analyses (i.e., EQ-5D VAS and/or FM-related medication costs), 21 patients were not included in the economic evaluation, and the final sample of this study consisted of 204 individuals with FM (68 per study arm).

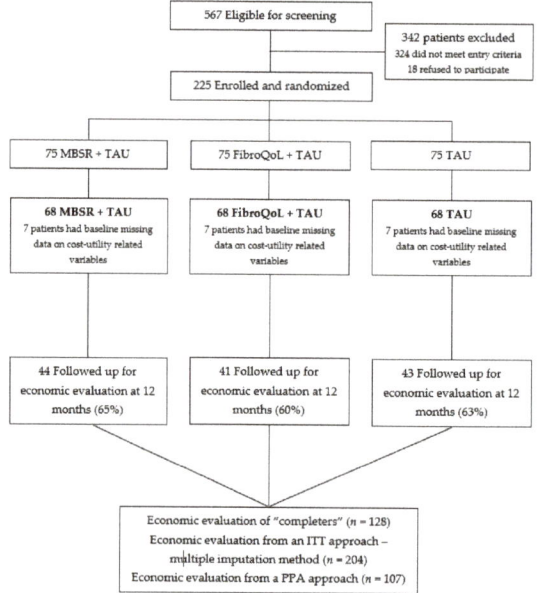

Figure 1. Trial flow chart describing the recruitment process of all three study arms. Note: MBSR = Mindfulness-Based Stress Reduction; TAU = Treatment-as-usual; ITT = intention-to-treat; PPA = Per protocol analysis.

2.2. Inclusion and Exclusion Criteria

All 567 potential participants underwent a phone screening to assess the following inclusion criteria: (1) aged between 18–65 years old; (2) able to understand Spanish language; and (3) provided informed consent to participate, and exclusion criteria: (1) participation in a concurrent treatment trial; (2) presence of cognitive impairment according to the Mini Mental State Examination (score < 27) [33]; (3) participation in psychological treatment during the last 12 months; (4) previous experience in meditation or other mind-body therapies; (5) presence of comorbid severe mental or medical disorders that could interfere with treatment; (6) pregnancy; and (7) involvement in ongoing litigation relating to FM.

Those participants meeting the eligibility criteria were scheduled for a first face-to-face interview in the hospital with a trained clinical psychologist blind to treatment allocation where inclusion criteria were checked again; if the criteria were fulfilled, the baseline evaluation started. The evaluations consisted of the administration of a battery of measures to assess different clinical outcomes (e.g., functional impairment, "fibromyalginess", anxiety and depression symptoms, pain catastrophizing, cognitive dysfunction, and perceived stress), process variables (e.g., mindfulness facets, self-compassion, and psychological inflexibility) and quality of life and cost-related outcomes (e.g., use of clinical services, medication, sick leaves, etc.). Moreover, during the baseline clinical interview, the Structured Clinical Interview for DSM-IV-Axis I Depressive disorders (SCID-I) was used to establish the diagnostic of a current episode of major depression, a previous episode of major depression, and/or dysthymia. See Pérez-Aranda et al. [31] for more detailed information.

2.3. Design

The study is registered at Clinicaltrials.gov under registration number NCT02561416. A 12 month RCT was performed with random allocation of the participants to 3 arms (using a computer-generated randomization list): MBSR added to treatment-as-usual (TAU); FibroQoL added to TAU; and TAU alone.

A detailed description of the study protocol can be found elsewhere [34]. In summary, all recruited patients signed an informed consent and participated voluntarily in the RCT. This included three assessments: at baseline, post-treatment (or 2 months after baseline, in the case of the participants allocated in the TAU condition), and at 12 months follow-up (48 weeks after randomization).

The study was approved by the Ethics Committee at the Sant Joan de Déu Foundation (PIC-102-15) and was performed in accordance with the ethical standards laid down in the 1964 Declaration of Helsinki and its following updates.

2.4. Interventions

2.4.1. MBSR

MBSR is a transdiagnostic program originally developed by Jon Kabat-Zinn [35] to help patients with chronic conditions. Mindfulness is defined as "the awareness that emerges through paying attention on purpose, in the present moment, and nonjudgmentally to the unfolding of experience" [36]. In MBSR, structured training in mindfulness is provided to help patients to relate to their physical and psychological conditions in more accepting and non-judgmental ways [37]. We used the MBSR protocol developed at the University of Massachusetts Medical School (USA) with minimal adaptations for our patients with FM attending to the characteristics of this population. The program consisted of eight weekly 2 h sessions and included the usual one half-day of silent retreat (6 h long session between weeks 6 and 7), although it was optional in our study. The book *Con rumbo propio* [38] and audiotapes were provided to facilitate practice at home, which is reinforced throughout the program and recorded in a practice log. The intervention was delivered in a group format (approximately 15 patients per group), and each group was conducted by a different properly trained MBSR instructor.

2.4.2. FibroQoL

The FibroQoL program is a multicomponent intervention developed by expert and multidisciplinary groups in Catalonia between 2006 and 2007. It was used as an active treatment comparator because it had previously demonstrated cost–utility compared to TAU for FM [22,39]. MBSR and FibroQoL were practically equivalent in terms of structure, which offers a comparison of MBSR to an active control that matches MBSR in non-specific factors but does not contain mindfulness techniques. FibroQoL consists of eight weekly 2 h sessions that are divided in two parts: four sessions of psychoeducation in which patients receive updated information about pathophysiology, diagnosis, and management of FM symptoms, and another four sessions of training in relaxation and self-hypnosis through different techniques with goals to generate a state of deep relaxation, achieve control over the body and pain, and imagine one's life in the future without pain [12]. Audiotapes were provided to facilitate practice at home. The recently published Beginner's Guide to Fibromyalgia [40] was also provided for giving updated information about FM syndrome. The intervention was delivered in a group format (15 patients per group), and one team formed by two psychologists, three family physicians, and a rheumatologist conducted the five groups.

2.4.3. TAU

Patients randomized to this arm received no additional active treatment over the study period but continued with their regular pattern of medication (if any). The usual treatment of FM typically includes analgesics, anxiolytics, opioids, antidepressants, and/or anti-inflammatories, and recommendations for practicing aerobic exercise regularly. For ethical reasons, participants allocated to TAU arm were offered participation in an MBI at the end of the study.

2.5. Outcome Measures

2.5.1. The EuroQol Questionnaire [41]

The five-level version of the EuroQol five-dimensional classification system (EQ-5D-5L) is a widely used health-related quality of life instrument with a non-disease-specific classification system that consists of two parts.

In the first part, the patient chooses one of five levels of severity (1 = no problems, 2 = mild problems, 3 = moderate problems, 4 = severe problems, 5 = extreme problems) in five domains: mobility, self-care, usual activities, pain, and anxiety/depression. The time frame is the day of reporting. The combination of the answers given to these domains results in 3125 (5^5) different health states. The utility scores are obtained from the EQ-5D classification system and are used to rate patients' health-related quality of life. This continuous variable includes negative values, which indicate a health state "worse than death", 0, which indicates a state "as bad as death", and 1, which represents "perfect health". This scale reflects the health status as described by the subject and is often the preferred method for economic evaluations from a general perspective. In order to derive the EQ-5D utility value from a set of EQ-5D-5L domains, there exist different sets of country-specific preference weights; in our case, these utility values were calculated using the Spanish tariffs of EQ-5D-5L [42], since they are more relevant to our decision-making context. EQ-5D utility values are then used to estimate QALYs, which represent a common measure to assess the outcomes associated with different treatments both in terms of patients' quality of life and survival [43]. In terms of QALYs, a year of perfect health is worth 1, and a year of less than perfect health is worth less than 1.

The second part of the questionnaire is a visual analogue scale (EQ VAS) on which participants record their current overall health status ranging from 0 (worst imaginable health) to 100 (best imaginable health).

2.5.2. The Client Service Receipt Inventory (CSRI) Spanish Version

The Client Service Receipt Inventory (CSRI) [44] was used to collect retrospective data on medication and service receipt. For medication intake, patients were asked to bring their daily medication prescriptions and the following information for FM-related drugs (i.e., analgesics, anti-inflammatories, opioids, antiepileptics, muscle relaxants, antidepressants, and anxiolytics) was recorded: the name of the drug, the dosage, the total number of prescription days, and the daily dosage consumed. Regarding service receipt, patients were asked about the total visits to emergency services, the total days of general inpatient hospital admissions, the number of diagnostic tests administered, and the total visits to general practitioner, nurse, social worker, psychologist, psychiatrist, group psychotherapy, and other community health care professionals, specifying in each case if these services were provided by the public or by the private sector. The CSRI was administered on two occasions: at baseline and at 12 month follow-up, both referring to the previous 12 months.

2.6. Statistical Analysis

The present economic evaluation is reported according to the Consolidated Health Economic Evaluation Reporting Standards statement [45] (see Table S1) and follows the Good Research Practices for Cost-Effectiveness Analysis Alongside Clinical Trials [46]. Statistical analyses were performed using STATA v13.0 (StataCorp, College Station, TX, USA) and SPSS v22 (SPSS Inc., Chicago, IL, USA).

We estimated costs from the healthcare and the government perspectives, taking the previous year as the time frame. Catalonia has full governance of health and social care and, as in every other Spanish region, healthcare is universal and publicly financed. The government perspective included direct healthcare costs assumed by the Catalan government (out-of-pocket costs and costs associated with private insurances were not included) and indirect costs related to productivity losses assumed by the Spanish government. The healthcare perspective included only direct healthcare costs. These costs were calculated by summing costs from medications, use of healthcare services, medical tests, and costs of the professionals delivering the MBSR and FibroQoL treatments. We calculated the cost of medications by consulting the price per milligram in the Vademecum International (Red Book; edition 2016) and included the value-added tax. Thus, we computed total costs of medications by multiplying the price per milligram by the total daily dose consumed (in milligrams) and the number of days that the pharmacological treatment was delivered. The SOIKOS database of health care costs [47] was the principal source of unit cost data for health services use and medical tests. The total cost of the MBSR and the FibroQoL treatments took into account the price per patient per group session for the health professional who provided the sessions. Attendance to MBSR and FibroQoL sessions was obtained by consulting professionals' records. The cost of treatment sessions and resources was considered equal across all sessions and groups, but the number of participants attending those sessions was not; therefore, MBSR and FibroQoL costs were dependent on the number of sessions attended by participants.

We calculated indirect costs (lost productivity) from the human capital approach. We multiplied the minimum daily wage in Spain for 2016 by the number of days on sick leave reported by each patient. Finally, we calculated total costs by summing the direct and the indirect costs. Unit costs are reported in Euros (€) based on 2016 prices. Table 1 displays the unit costs for the calculation of direct and indirect costs. Given that the time horizon was the previous year, it was not necessary to apply a discount to the costs.

Table 1. Unit costs used in the calculations of direct and indirect costs (Financial Year 2016; values in €).

Service (Unit)	Costs (€)
Health care	
General practitioner (per appointment)	36.97
Nurse/psychiatric nurse (per appointment)	34.13
Social worker (per appointment)	35.78
Clinical Psychologist (per appointment)	45.06
Psychiatrist (per appointment)	45.06
Other medical specialists (per appointment)	43.82
Accident & Emergency in hospital (per attendance)	99.34
Hospital stay (per night)	112
Diagnostic tests (range)	6.13–455.53
Pharmacological treatment (per daily dose) *	Various
MBSR & FibroQoL (per participant per group session)	45.06
Productivity loss	
Absenteeism from work (minimum daily wage)	21.8

Note: Unit costs were applied to each resource use to compute the total cost of resources used by each participant. All unit costs were for the year 2016. * The cost of prescribed medications was calculated by determining the price per milligram according to the Vademecum International (Red Book; edition 2016) and included the value-added tax.

The comparison between two intervention groups in the frame of an economic evaluation results in four potential scenarios: (1) the intervention costs less and is more effective than the alternative; (2) the intervention costs more and is less effective than the alternative; (3) the intervention costs less but is less effective than the alternative; and (4) the intervention costs more but is more effective than the alternative. The first two scenarios exhibit strong dominance; thus, the decision on which intervention to adopt is normally straightforward. For the other two scenarios, the decision depends on the incremental cost-effectiveness ratio (ICER), which is defined as the ratio between incremental costs and incremental effects measured on QALYs or EQ VAS points [48]. For considering the intervention cost-effective, each country establishes an investment ceiling, which in the case of Spain is €25,000 per QALY [14].

Our cost-effectiveness analyses were implemented using the Zellner's seemingly unrelated regression (SUR) model [49]. Estimates were performed using STATA's sureg command. Using the SUR method for cost-effectiveness purposes implies the use of a bivariate system of regressions that includes both costs and outcomes (with the latter being either QALYs or EQ VAS, depending on the model considered) as the dependent variables of the two separate equations, which are estimated jointly. The regressions of costs and outcomes are therefore part of two regressions on treatment allocation (i.e., whether they were assigned to MBSR, FibroQoL, or TAU) plus an additional set of control variables (measured at baseline): age, gender, marital status, education level, employment status, current episode of major depression, baseline costs, or baseline outcome, depending on the equation considered. Estimates of incremental cost and of incremental effect values using the SUR method described above were derived with 1000 bootstrap replications in order to address a possible skewness in the distribution of the dependent variables [50].

We assessed cost-effectiveness of the interventions using several different scenarios. In the first instance, we performed a complete case analysis (CCA), including only the 128 patients who were assessed both at baseline and at 12 month follow-up. Additional scenarios (sensitivity analysis) adopted instead intention-to-treat (ITT) and per protocol analysis (PPA) approaches. In order to be able to perform an ITT analysis, we needed to impute missing values for those variables that were missing at the 12 month follow-up. In order to do so, we used multiple imputation methods with the chained equations approach [51]. Variables that presented most missing values were, in particular, the EQ-5D-5L domains and the costs of the non-responders at 12 months follow-up. The imputation model, run on ten imputed datasets, included all the main sociodemographic and prognostic variables associated with the outcome variables and the other variables containing missing values. In the present study, patients who had baseline CSRI data ($n = 204$) comprised the ITT sample—missing baseline data were not imputed. Finally, the PPA scenario (2nd sensitivity analysis) was estimated on a sample that included only those who attended at least 6 treatment sessions out of 8, with a final sample size of 107 patients.

3. Results

In terms of descriptive statistics, no significant differences were observed between the three study arms in any outcome but the clinical diagnosis of "Current episode of major depression" and "Previous episode of major depression" based on the SCID-I (see Table 2), indicating that the MBSR group had fewer participants currently depressed compared to the other two groups. Considering that this variable could impact the economic evaluation, subsequent analyses were adjusted for "Current episode of major depression" among other covariates. Table 2 displays descriptive details for the sociodemographic variables of this sample.

Table 3 contains the descriptive statistics of costs and outcomes at baseline and at 12 month follow-up, split according to the three arms of the RCT, along with adjusted and unadjusted p values.

3.1. Baseline Costs

The analyses revealed that only the specialized health care services cost was significantly different among study arms (adjusted p value = 0.02), indicating that TAU was the most expensive group in this particular service with an average cost of approximately €660, higher than MBSR (approximately €540) and FibroQoL (approximately €400). However, the other costs did not show any significant difference, including direct and total costs.

3.2. Follow-Up Costs

For 12 month follow-up costs, we observed that primary health care services cost was significantly lower for the MBSR group (approximately €200) than for the FibroQoL (approximately €320) and for the TAU groups (approximately €360). Post hoc pairwise comparisons indicated that MBSR's primary health care costs were significantly lower than TAU's (adjusted p value = 0.002) and presented a marginal significance compared to the FibroQoL group (adjusted $p = 0.06$).

Table 2. Baseline characteristics of patients with Fibromyalgia (FM) by treatment group.

	MBSR (n = 68)	FibroQoL (n = 68)	TAU (n = 68)	p
Gender (women, %)	66 (97.1%)	67 (98.5%)	67 (98.5%)	0.78
Age, mean (SD)	52.63 (8.03)	54.44 (7.69)	53.16 (8.39)	0.4
Marital status, n (%)				
Single	2 (2.9%)	3 (4.4%)	1 (1.5%)	
Married/living with a partner	53 (77.9%)	50 (73.5%)	55 (80.9%)	0.59
Separated/divorced	11 (16.2%)	9 (13.2%)	10 (14.7%)	
Widowed	2 (2.9%)	6 (8.8%)	2 (2.9%)	
Education level, n (%)				
Illiterate	0 (0%)	1 (1.5%)	1 (1.5%)	
Did not graduate from primary school	4 (5.9%)	1 (1.5%)	4 (5.9%)	
Primary school	31 (45.6%)	37 (54.4%)	32 (47.1%)	0.21
Secondary school	31 (45.6%)	24 (35.3%)	28 (41.2%)	
University	0 (0%)	5 (7.4%)	3 (4.4%)	
Others	2 (2.9%)	0 (0%)	0 (0%)	
Employment status, n (%)				
Homemaker	10 (14.7%)	10 (14.7%)	4 (5.9%)	
Paid employment	19 (27.9%)	21 (30.9%)	19 (27.9%)	
Paid employment but in sick leave	6 (8.8%)	4 (5.9%)	4 (5.9%)	
Unemployed with subsidy	8 (11.8%)	9 (13.2%)	11 (16.2%)	0.47
Unemployed without subsidy	8 (11.8%)	15 (22.1%)	9 (13.2%)	
Retired/pensioner	9 (13.2%)	4 (5.9%)	10 (14.7%)	
Temporal disability	1 (1.5%)	2 (2.9%)	1 (1.5%)	
Others	7 (10.3%)	3 (4.4%)	10 (14.7%)	
Clinical variables				
Years of diagnosis, mean (SD)	14.46 (9.17)	11.28 (7.17)	13.68 (10.02)	0.14
Current episode of depression, n (%)	24 (35.3%)	39 (57.4%)	38 (55.9%)	0.02
Previous episode(s) of depression, n (%)	25 (36.8%)	20 (29.4%)	34 (50%)	0.04
Dysthymia, n (%)	14 (20.6%)	9 (13.2%)	8 (11.8%)	0.31
Daily FM-related medication				
Analgesics, n (%)	21 (30.9%)	21 (30.9%)	15 (22.1%)	0.42
Anti-inflammatory, n (%)	17 (25%)	17 (25%)	24 (35.3%)	0.31
Opioids, n (%)	25 (36.8%)	21 (30.9%)	17 (25%)	0.33
Antiepileptic, n (%)	13 (19.1%)	11 (16.2%)	14 (20.6%)	0.8
Muscle relaxant, n (%)	2 (2.9%)	5 (7.4%)	3 (4.4%)	0.48
Antidepressants, n (%)	35 (51.5%)	30 (44.1%)	26 (38.2%)	0.3
Anxiolytics, n (%)	30 (44.1%)	33 (48.5%)	31 (45.6%)	0.87

Table 3. Summary statistics of the costs (total and disaggregated in components) and outcomes according to treatment group.

	MBSR	FibroQoL	TAU	OMNIBUS Significance Test	
Baseline (N = 204)	n = 68	n = 68	n = 68	p	Adjusted p
Primary health care services	349.6 (325.8)	322.4 (282.8)	316.4 (269.6)	0.78	0.81
Specialized health care services	537.6 (438.1)	398.5 (411.9)	661.9 (674.8)	0.01	0.02
Medical tests	455.8 (462.8)	474.2 (634.7)	424.3 (480.4)	0.86	0.94
FM-related medications	307.6 (488.6)	204.3 (262.6)	171.6 (282.5)	0.15	0.19
Direct costs	1650.7 (1069.9)	1399.4 (1006.5)	1574.3 (1220.6)	0.35	0.39
Indirect costs	667.8 (1951.1)	669.7 (1569.6)	1144.8 (2953.1)	0.45	0.24
Total costs	2318.4 (2417.6)	2069.1 (2075.5)	2719.1 (3783.9)	0.45	0.18
Outcomes					
EQ-5D utility score (0 to 1)	0.50 (0.21)	0.48 (0.23)	0.53 (0.23)	0.44	0.28
EQ VAS (0 to 100) *	46.61 (21.82)	47.31 (19.91)	47.32 (18.51)	0.97	0.75
12-months Follow-up (N = 128)	n = 44	n = 41	n = 43		
Primary health care services	197.3 (233.4)	319.4 (312.3)	357.9 (301.8)	0.01	0.02
Specialized health care services	498 (485.3)	534.1 (552)	664.8 (754.3)	0.45	0.5
Medical tests	225.4 (360.3)	257.3 (280.4)	328.2 (417.6)	0.44	0.42
FM-related medications	235.9 (349.2)	189.8 (205.1)	255.4 (434.3)	0.56	0.58
Intervention (MBSR/FibroQoL)	702.5 (298.9)	578.1 (181.3)	0 (0)	0	0
Direct costs	1156.6 (938.3)	1300.6 (872.4)	1598.7 (1265.1)	0.17	0.13
Indirect costs	400.9 (1325.2)	714.6 (1905.8)	929.9 (2229.8)	0.36	0.1
Total costs	1557.5 (1626.9)	2015.2 (2122.1)	2528.7 (3017)	0.14	0.04
Outcomes					
EQ-5D utility score (0 to 1)	0.57 (0.25)	0.53 (0.27)	0.45 (0.26)	0.11	0.05
EQ VAS (0 to 100 points)	52.41 (23.06)	42.44 (21.16)	44.98 (19.85)	0.09	0.21
QALY (0 to 1, on the basis of EQ-5D utility score)	0.54 (0.18)	0.50 (0.20)	0.48 (0.22)	0.34	0.05

Note: Data are presented as mean € cost (SD), except where otherwise is stated. Covariates: age, gender, marital status, education level, employment status, duration of the illness since first diagnostic, current episode of major depression baseline costs, and baseline outcomes, depending on the analyses considered. The mean sessions attended per intervention were 5.3 for MBSR (no retreat included) and 5.8 for FibroQoL. Thirty-two participants (42.7%) attended to the optional mindfulness retreat. * One missing value was found in this variable. EQ-5D = EuroQol five-dimensional classification; EQ VAS = visual analogue scale; QALY = quality-adjusted life years.

Another marginal significance appeared in the post hoc pairwise comparisons for the variable "Medical tests costs", indicating that the MBSR group had a lower value than the TAU group (adjusted p value = 0.09). As could be expected, the intervention's cost was also significantly different between the groups, which could be attributed to one group (TAU) not receiving any intervention at all.

The comparisons regarding direct costs did not present statistical significance (adjusted p value = 0.13), although post hoc analyses revealed that the MBSR group, with cost at approximately €1160, was significantly lower than the TAU group, with cost at approximately €1600 (adjusted p value = 0.02).

Focusing on indirect costs, the analyses revealed no significant differences between the three groups (adjusted p value = 0.10), although the post hoc pairwise comparisons indicated that MBSR's associated indirect costs (approximately €400) were significantly lower than FibroQoL's (approximately €710, adjusted p value = 0.05) and TAU's (approximately €930, adjusted p value = 0.05).

Finally, the total costs were significantly different between the three study arms (adjusted p value = 0.04), as the MBSR group was less costly (approximately €1560) compared to the FibroQoL (approximately €2020) and the TAU groups (approximately €2530). Post hoc pairwise analyses showed that the MBSR group had significantly lower total costs compared to the FibroQoL (adjusted p value = 0.02) and the TAU groups (adjusted p value = 0.02).

3.3. Baseline Quality of Life Outcomes

Outcomes at baseline were very similar between the three groups, ranging from 0.48 to 0.53 for the EQ-5D utility scores and between 46 and 47 for the EQ VAS. The pairwise tests revealed no significant differences ($p > 0.05$ in every case).

3.4. Follow-Up Quality of Life Outcomes

At 12 month follow-up, the between group differences were significant overall for the EQ-5D utility score (adjusted p value = 0.05). The MBSR group had the highest value (0.57), and the TAU group had the lowest value (0.45). On the other hand, no significant differences were observed in the case of the EQ VAS (adjusted p value = 0.26). We calculated QALYs based on the EQ-5D utility score, and we found significant differences between the three groups (adjusted p value = 0.05).

3.5. Cost Utility Analysis from the Government Perspective

As shown in Table 4, MBSR was found to be dominant compared with TAU. The incremental costs (in €) were found to be significant in the base case analysis (completers) and the per-protocol analysis, ranging from approximately €−1030 to €−1110. On the other hand, the incremental effect was significant in the ITT analysis, in which 0.053 QALYs were gained with MBSR compared to TAU. The EQ VAS score, however, did not improve significantly in any case, despite ranging between 7 and 12.

When comparing the two active groups, MBSR showed a significantly lower incremental cost compared to FibroQoL using the completer sample (between €−70 and €−820), but no significant differences were observed in the incremental effects. Here, FibroQoL achieved a slightly better outcome in QALYs that translated into an ICER of €385,400/QALY, which cannot be considered a cost-effective result. Under the other two analyses, the incremental costs did not present any significant difference, ranging from €−540 to €−650. Regarding the incremental effects, they favored MBSR in all the cases, but neither the EQ-5D utility score nor the EQ VAS, which ranged from 7 to 12 depending on the sample used, showed any significant difference.

Finally, the comparison between FibroQoL and TAU indicated that the average incremental cost ranged between €−250 and €−460, with FibroQoL showing lower costs than TAU, although such difference was not found to be significant in any of the three samples considered. On the other hand, the incremental effect for QALYs was significant (0.056) using the completer sample, although the EQ VAS effect was slightly better for the TAU group, resulting in an ICER of €159/EQ VAS points gained, despite not being a significant difference. Under the two other analyses, the incremental effect was also non-statistically significant but favored the FibroQoL group.

Table 4. Incremental cost, effect, and cost-effectiveness ratios from the government perspective.

	Incremental Cost	Incremental Effect	ICER
	Mean	Mean	
	(95% Bootstrap CI)	(95% Bootstrap CI)	
MBSR vs TAU			
Completers (n = 128)			
QALY (EQ-5D)	**−1023.5** (−2024.7 to −270.5)	0.053 (−0.040 to 0.129)	MBSR dominant
EQ VAS (0-100) *	**−1072** (−2048.5 to −273.6)	7.89 (−1.72 to 18.69)	MBSR dominant
ITT (n = 204)			
QALY (EQ-5D)	−828.1 (−1699.4 to 43.2)	**0.053** (0.004 to 0.101)	MBSR dominant
EQ VAS (0-100) *	−855.2 (−1727.6 to 17.3)	7.13 (−0.52 to 14.79)	MBSR dominant
PPA (n = 107)			
QALY (EQ-5D)	**−1036.6** (−1894.3 to −178.9)	0.080 (-0.060 to 0.220)	MBSR dominant
EQ VAS (0–100) *	**−1108.6** (−1968.8 to −248.4)	12.23 (−2.33 to 26.78)	MBSR dominant
MBSR vs FibroQoL			
Completers (n = 128)			
QALY (EQ-5D)	**−770.8** (−1401.4 to −172.4)	-0.002 (-0.066 to 0.059)	€385,400/QALY
EQ VAS (0-100) *	**−822.5** (−1529.1 to −195)	9.46 (-0.84 to 20.35)	MBSR dominant
ITT (n = 204)			
QALY (EQ-5D)	−539.9 (−1214.6 to 134.8)	0.012 (−0.032 to 0.056)	MBSR dominant
EQ VAS (0-100) *	−575 (−1246.1 to 96.1)	6.68 (−1.01 to 14.37)	MBSR dominant
PPA (n = 107)			
QALY (EQ-5D)	−582.8 (−1269.1 to 103.4)	0.011 (−0.083 to 0.104)	MBSR dominant
EQ VAS (0-100) *	−651.6 (−1328 to 24.8)	12.08 (−3.62 to 27.78)	MBSR dominant
FibroQoL vs TAU			
Completers (n = 128)			
QALY (EQ-5D)	−252.7 (−1176.6 to 536)	**0.056** (0.006 to 0.172)	FibroQoL dominant
EQ VAS (0-100) *	−249.6 (−1164.5 to 654)	−1.57 (−6.71 to 10.44)	€159/EQ VAS
ITT (n = 204)			
QALY (EQ-5D)	−288.2 (−1307.9 to 731.6)	0.041 (−0.003 to 0.084)	FibroQoL dominant
EQ VAS (0-100) *	−280.1 (−1297 to 736.6)	0.45 (−7.31 to 8.22)	FibroQoL dominant
PPA (n = 107)			
QALY (EQ-5D)	−453.8 (−1290.3 to 382.8)	0.069 (-0.010 to 0.149)	FibroQoL dominant
EQ VAS (0-100) *	−456.9 (−1301 to 387.1)	0.15 (−9.47 to 9.76)	FibroQoL dominant

Note: Significant values ($p < 0.05$) are shown in **bold**. Covariates: gender, age, marital status, current episode of major depression, educational level, and employment status. * Analyses using the EQ VAS score as outcome were computed using one patient less in each case, due to missing data on this baseline variable. ICER = incremental cost-effectiveness ratios.

Figure 2 shows the degree of uncertainty around the differences in costs and QALYs between the groups from the government perspective in the completer sample.

3.6. Cost Utility Analysis from the Health Care Perspective

As shown in Table 5, results were in line with those found when considering the government perspective, whereas incremental costs varied given the different cost aggregated used for this part of the analysis.

When comparing MBSR and TAU, the first was again dominant as the incremental costs were significantly lower, ranging between approximately €−420 and €−490. The incremental effect observed for the QALYs was significant using the ITT sample (0.053, $p = 0.03$).

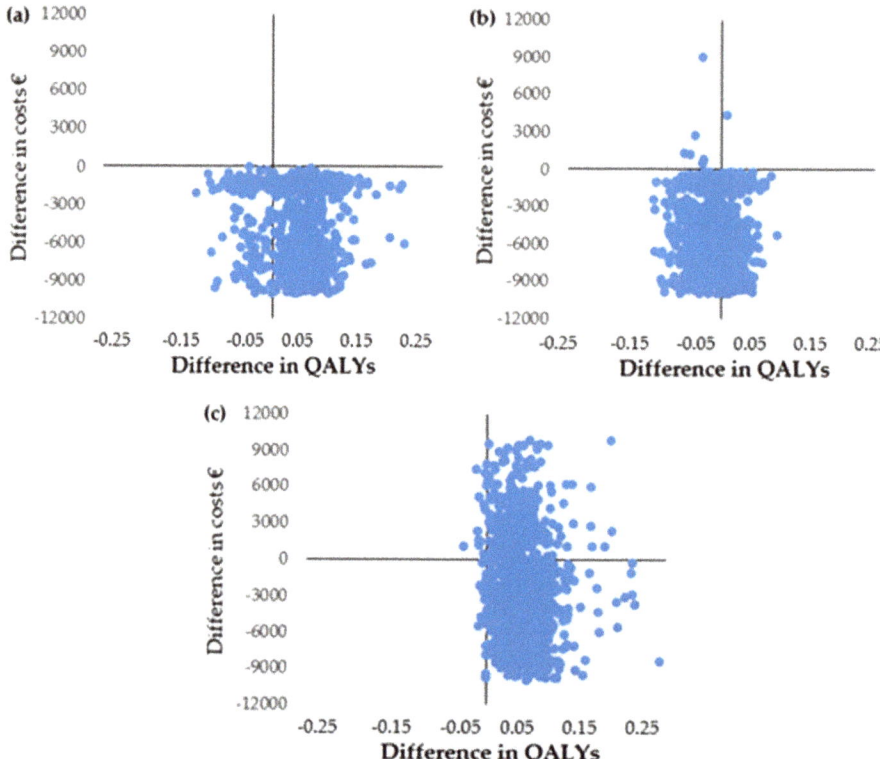

Figure 2. Cost–utility plane of 1000 bootstrap replicated incremental cost–utility from the government perspective (completer sample): (**a**) MBSR vs. TAU; (**b**) MBSR vs. FibroQoL; (**c**) FibroQoL vs. TAU.

Incremental costs of MBSR compared to FibroQoL ranged between €−120 and €−280 but were not found to be significantly different. Similarly, the incremental effects did not show any significant difference, although the EQ VAS score ranged from 7 to 12, depending on the sample. All the incremental effects favored MBSR but the incremental QALYs using the completer sample, which resulted in an ICER of €116,300/QALY gained and should not be considered a significant result.

Finally, the incremental costs of FibroQoL compared to TAU ranged between €−190 and €−320, but none of them were significant. The incremental effect in QALYs was found to be significant for the completer sample (0.056). All the incremental effects favored FibroQoL but the incremental EQ VAS using the completer sample, which resulted in an ICER of €121/EQ VAS points gained and should not be considered a significant result.

Although both scenarios presented similar results, it can be observed that, under the health care perspective, the MBSR group achieved a significant reduction in incremental costs compared to TAU in the three samples, including the ITT, which was not significant under the government perspective. On the other hand, the significant reduction in incremental costs of MBSR compared to FibroQoL taking the completer sample was lost when considering the health care perspective.

Figure S1 shows the degree of uncertainty around the differences in costs and QALYs between the groups from the health care perspective in the completer sample.

Table 5. Incremental cost, effect, and cost-effectiveness ratios from the health care perspective.

	Incremental Cost	Incremental Effect	ICER
	Mean	Mean	
	(95% Bootstrap CI)	(95% Bootstrap CI)	
MBSR vs. TAU			
Completers (n = 128)			
QALY (EQ-5D)	−420.7 (−883.8 to −34.9)	0.053 (−0.041 to 0.131)	MBSR dominant
EQ VAS (0–100) *	−464.8 (−884.2 to −63.3)	7.89 (−1.65 to 18.65)	MBSR dominant
ITT (n = 204)			
QALY (EQ-5D)	**−455.2 (−904.6 to −4.9)**	**0.053 (0.004 to 0.102)**	MBSR dominant
EQ VAS (0–100) *	**−483 (−929.5 to −36.5)**	7.14 (−0.49 to 14.77)	MBSR dominant
PPA (n = 107)			
QALY (EQ-5D)	−431.5 (−866.7 to 3.7)	0.080 (−0.060 to 0.220)	MBSR dominant
EQ VAS (0–100) *	**−493.6 (−914.9 to −72.2)**	12.22 (−2.57 to 27.02)	MBSR dominant
MBSR vs FibroQoL			
Completers (n = 128)			
QALY (EQ-5D)	−232.6 (−572 to 129.6)	−0.002 (−0.067 to 0.059)	116,300 €/QALY
EQ VAS (0–100) *	−275.2 (−629.2 to 96.7)	9.47 (−1.03 to 20.24)	MBSR dominant
ITT (n = 204)			
QALY (EQ-5D)	−236.2 (−551.8 to 79.5)	0.012 (−0.033 to 0.058)	MBSR dominant
EQ VAS (0–100) *	−265.2 (−573.9 to 43.6)	6.69 (−0.87 to 14.25)	MBSR dominant
PPA (n = 107)			
QALY (EQ-5D)	−117.6 (−505.4 to 270.1)	0.011 (−0.083 to 0.104)	MBSR dominant
EQ VAS (0–100) *	−174.2 (−551.3 to 202.8)	12.07 (−3.76 to 27.90)	MBSR dominant
FibroQoL vs TAU			
Completers (n = 128)			
QALY (EQ-5D)	−188 (−696.2 to 227.8)	**0.056 (0.007 to 0.173)**	FibroQoL dominant
EQ VAS (0–100) *	−189.6 (−625.8 to 259.4)	−1.57 (−10.49 to 6.68)	121 €/EQ VAS
ITT (n = 204)			
QALY (EQ-5D)	−219.1 (−656.3 to 218.1)	0.041 (−0.002 to 0.084)	FibroQoL dominant
EQ VAS (0–100) *	−217.8 (−655.9 to 220.3)	0.45 (−7.22 to 8.12)	FibroQoL dominant
PPA (n = 107)			
QALY (EQ-5D)	−313.9 (−747.9 to 120.2)	0.069 (−0.010 to 0.149)	FibroQoL dominant
EQ VAS (0–100) *	−319.4 (−748.8 to 110.1)	0.15 (−9.42 to 9.73)	FibroQoL dominant

Note: Significant values ($p < 0.05$) are shown in **bold**. Covariates: sex, age, marital status, current episode of major depression, educational level, and employment status. * Analyses using the EQ VAS score as outcome were computed using one patient less in each case due to missing data on this baseline variable.

4. Discussion

The primary aim of the present study was to analyze the cost–utility of MBSR in a sample of Spanish patients with FM, both from the government and the public health care system perspectives. The intervention was compared to an active control group (i.e., the multicomponent intervention FibroQoL) and to usual care, and the economic evaluation was performed in the context of a 12 month RCT.

The results of this study can be summarized as follows. MBSR (added to TAU) compared to TAU alone was associated with lower direct and total costs in people with FM at 12 month follow-up. This significant decrease of costs was mainly due to a reduction in the costs related to primary health care services and indirect costs during the follow-up period for the MBSR group. The incremental effect on quality of life, measured with QALYs, was significant when considering the ITT sample. Both from the health care and the government perspectives, all ICERs were dominant for MBSR independent of the approach (completers, ITT, or PPA) compared to TAU. These results are similar to those observed in previous studies, as other non-pharmacological interventions have been described as cost-effective when compared with usual care [14,22–25]. In line with Beard et al. [20], our findings point in the direction of considering that there is a large proportion of patients with FM who remain insufficiently treated with standard pharmacotherapy and could benefit from coadjuvant interventions such as MBSR.

When the two active groups (i.e., MBSR and FibroQoL, both added to TAU) were compared, the only significant difference was observed in the reduction of total costs under the government perspective in favor of MBSR (completers sample). This difference was based primarily on the reduction of indirect costs, as no significant reduction in direct costs was observed (i.e., health care perspective). Reducing indirect costs has been considered as one of the main target points for interventions addressed to chronic pain management [52]. As stated by Hedman-Lagerlöf et al. [24], it is possible that reduction of indirect costs was not only a consequence of reduced symptoms, but that engaging in work-related activities may in turn lead to improvements in FM symptoms. In addition, indirect costs derived from disability, unemployment, and/or early retirement have been associated with disease severity [53], and it would be interesting to update the rates of absenteeism and disability considering the recently proposed classification by Pérez-Aranda et al. [54], as this system already found significant differences in indirect costs among clusters that were not observed using the classical cut-off-based classification method. Considering that not all patients with FM respond equally to every treatment, including MBSR, as the current RCT proved, studying how effective the different, already validated interventions for FM are for each subtype of patient could be the next step toward the ideal of personalized medicine.

In terms of incremental effects on quality of life, no differences were found between MBSR and FibroQoL, indicating that both interventions achieved a similar effect in the long term. This tendency was already observed in the previous study based on this RCT [31], where MBSR was found as clearly more efficacious than FibroQoL at post-treatment, but only significant improvements in fibromyalginess (measured by the Fibromyalgia Survey Diagnostic Criteria [55]) and pain catastrophizing (measured by the Pain Catastrophising Scale [56]) were observed at 12 month follow-up.

It seems reasonable to believe that effects of MBSR on quality of life might show a similar long-term pattern as other outcomes, as it would be intimately related to some of the core FM symptoms (e.g., functional impairment, anxiety and depression, perceived stress, and perceived cognitive dysfunction). Based on what previous studies have demonstrated [57–60], this partial loss of effect in the long-term could be attributed to a reduction in the frequency of practice of mindfulness exercises once the intervention is over, which would imply that some FM symptoms and presumably quality of life are particularly practice-dependent. Therefore, finding ways to enhance the frequency and the quality of mindfulness home practice is an issue of great relevance to be studied in the future.

The comparison between FibroQoL and TAU indicated that the first produced a significant incremental effect on quality of life on the completers sample, although no significant reduction in costs was observed in any case beyond the perspective considered. Despite being dominant when compared to TAU, FibroQoL was not as superior as it had been in a previous RCT [22] in which the costs were reduced in a similar degree (approximately €−220), but the incremental quality of life was notably higher (0.12). A possible explanation would be that in the previous RCT, the recruited patients were already visited by the same professionals who conducted the FibroQoL program, which could have enhanced the therapeutic alliance, a relevant factor in any treatment context and particularly in a syndrome such as FM that is often associated with the experience of feeling stigmatized [61,62].

Considering previous findings on the cost–utility of different non-pharmacological interventions for FM, we can observe that some, such as the spa treatment or the aquatic training, achieved a significant incremental effect (0.04 and 0.131, respectively) but also higher incremental costs than usual care, resulting in ICERs which ranged between €8000 and more than €30,000 per QALY gained [16,17]. Other interventions, such as GACT [14], achieved a similar improvement in QALYs (0.05 compared to waiting list) as the one that MBSR achieved in the present study compared to TAU and reduced the costs considerably more (approximately €−1900). Also, GACT was dominant compared to recommended drugs under the health care perspective (approximately €−900). It is notable, however, that the GACT group did not consume any medication during the trial, which undoubtedly reduced associated costs. CBT, for its part, significantly reduced the costs compared to TAU (approximately €−2000) and recommended pharmacologic treatment (approximately €−2300), but no significant incremental effect was observed [23]. The STreSS program, however, also a cognitive-behavioral intervention, did achieve a significant incremental effect (0.035) compared to usual care as well as a significant cost reduction in the long term [25]. Finally, the internet-delivered exposure therapy assessed by Hedman-Largelöf et al. [24] not only achieved significant effects (0.07 QALYs gained) but also a great cost reduction (approximately €−5000) compared to usual care. When comparing the incremental effects achieved by the different interventions, one needs to bear in mind that the present study used the EQ-5D-5L, which has been associated with smaller changes in quality of life than the EQ-5D-3L [63], the version that most of the abovementioned studies used [14,17,22–24].

On the other hand, if we look at the cost–utility of MBIs for other medical conditions, the systematic review conducted by Duarte et al. [26] concluded that, despite positive results being found for depression and emotional unstable personality disorder, the small number of studies conducted (only five) and the heterogeneity in the interventions (four studies assessed Mindfulness-Based Cognitive Therapy and one MBSR) limited the generalizability of the findings. In this regard, our study extends the existing evidence of the cost–utility of MBIs in this case and for FM the first time.

Limitations

Some limitations of this study cannot be overlooked. First, given that the economic evaluation was not the primary objective when the original RCT was designed, an unexpectedly higher number of missing baseline data in economic- and quality of life-related variables emerged, invalidating 21 of the original 225 patients for the current study. Moreover, a considerably low follow-up rate (around 65%) added to more missing cost–utility-related data in the 12 month follow-up assessment and yielded a completer sample of only 128 patients. Even though regression models included bootstrapping with 1000 replications to address skewness within the data, the sample size in each study arm did not allow a robust estimation of costs, and confidence intervals were large in most cases; therefore, the results reported should be interpreted with caution.

Another limitation is that the randomization was not stratified by the presence of comorbid major depression, which resulted in the MBSR group having significantly fewer participants with a current episode of major depression compared to the other study arms. However, all reported analyses were performed after adjusting for this variable.

Although it could be thought that public registries would be a better way to collect data on health services use, self-reported data have been demonstrated to be of equal validity as registry-collected data in health-economic assessment [24]. In our study, the CSRI version included recall over a 12 month period, a commonly used time frame in which underreporting is usually more frequent than overreporting due to memory decay and memory biases such as reverse-telescoping (i.e., excluding some events from the recall period) [64]. Some authors, such as Bellón et al. [65], strongly recommend employing recall frames of at least 12 months to reduce memory biases present in patients' responses in short recall periods. We note that direct non-health care costs including out of pocket expenses, costs of paid and unpaid help, travel expenses, and over the counter medication and other treatment use (e.g., anti-constipation, vitamins, etc.) were not estimated.

Regarding the interventions, it needs to be considered that they were not fully equivalent. MBSR included an optional 6 h retreat, surely increasing the cost of the intervention, which accentuates the significant reduction in total costs that MBSR showed compared to FibroQoL. In terms of program completion, here defined as having attended to at least six of the eight sessions of each program (no retreat included in the case of MBSR), it was low (56% for MBSR and 65% for FibroQoL) but similar to what has been observed in FM intervention studies [28]. This continues to be a difficult problem to solve. Some authors have proposed strategies that could be implemented in further studies, such as written commitments from all participants or makeup classes for those who missed a session [66].

5. Conclusions

In summary, the results of the present work support that MBSR (added to TAU) is cost-effective compared with the multicomponent intervention FibroQoL (also added to TAU) and TAU alone. This is mainly because of a reduction in the 12 month follow-up incremental costs (€−1024 compared to TAU and €−771 compared to FibroQoL; government perspective, completers sample) produced essentially in primary health care services and indirect costs. Also, MBSR showed a significant incremental effect in quality of life compared to TAU using the ITT sample ($\Delta QALYs = 0.053$).

FM is a prevalent condition all around the world, however, our results are not necessarily generalizable to all FM patients (our sample has a very small representation of men) nor to other contexts—not only due to cultural differences but also importantly due to differences in how health care systems are organized in other countries. These results support the cost–utility of MBSR for FM, which is in line with previous findings regarding other non-pharmacological interventions such as forms of CBT and ACT. These interventions may have potential to be cost-effective not only for FM but also for treating other chronic pain conditions and/or central sensitivity syndromes (e.g., irritable bowel syndrome, chronic fatigue syndrome, and multiple chemical sensitivity), but this would need specific examination in future studies.

These findings add a substantial contribution to previous studies by presenting, for the first time, an economic evaluation of an MBI for FM. Nonetheless, they should be considered with caution as, among other limitations, the sample of each study arm did not allow robust estimations; if these results were supported by further studies, offering MBSR as a coadjuvant intervention to usual care should be considered as a therapeutic option in the public provision of healthcare.

Supplementary Materials: The following is available online at http://www.mdpi.com/2077-0383/8/7/1068/s1, Figure S1: Cost-utility plane of 1000 bootstrap replicated incremental cost–utility from the health care perspective (completer sample): (a) MBSR vs. TAU; (b) MBSR vs. FibroQoL; (c) FibroQoL vs. TAU. Table S1: CHEERS Checklist. Items to include when reporting economic evaluations of health interventions.

Author Contributions: Conceptualization, J.V.L. and A.P.-A.; methodology, F.D. and A.P.-A.; software, F.D.; validation, J.V.L., F.D. and A.P.-A.; formal analysis, F.D. and A.P.-A.; investigation, J.V.L.; resources, J.V.L.; data curation, L.A.-R., N.A.-O. and A.P.-A.; writing—original draft preparation, A.P.-A., F.D. and J.V.L.; writing—review and editing, A.F.-S., L.M.M., J.G.-C., M.T.P.-M. and M.K.; visualization, L.A.-R., N.A.-O. and M.T.P.-M.; supervision, M.K.; project administration, J.V.L. and A.F.-S.; funding acquisition, J.V.L.

Funding: The study has been funded in part by the Instituto de Salud Carlos III (ISCIII) of the Ministry of Economy and Competitiveness (Spain) through the Network for Prevention and Health Promotion in Primary Care (RD16/0007/0005 & RD16/0007/0012), by a grant for research projects on health from ISCIII (PI15/00383) cofinanced with European Union ERDF funds. The first listed author (A.P.-A.) has a FI predoctoral contract awarded by the Agency for Management of University and Research Grants (AGAUR; FI_B00754). The third listed author (A.F.-S.) has a "Sara Borrell" research contract from the ISCIII (CD16/00147). The sixth listed author (L.A.-R.) has a FI predoctoral contract awarded by the Agency for Management of University and Research Grants (AGAUR; FI_B00783). The last listed author (J.V.L.) has a "Miguel Servet" research contract from the ISCIII (CP14/00087).

Acknowledgments: The authors gratefully acknowledge the support of the staff and patients of the Department of Rheumatology at the Parc Sanitari Sant Joan de Déu Hospital.

Conflicts of Interest: The authors declare no conflict of interest. The funders had no role in the design of the study; in the collection, analyses, or interpretation of data; in the writing of the manuscript, or in the decision to publish the results.

References

1. Häuser, W.; Ablin, J.; Fitzcharles, M.-A.; Littlejohn, G.; Luciano, J.V.; Usui, C.; Walitt, B. Fibromyalgia. *Nat. Rev. Dis. Primers* **2015**, *1*, 15022. [CrossRef] [PubMed]
2. Heidari, F.; Afshari, M.; Moosazadeh, M. Prevalence of fibromyalgia in general population and patients, a systematic review and meta-analysis. *Rheumatol. Int.* **2017**, *37*, 1527–1539. [CrossRef] [PubMed]
3. Cabo-Meseguer, A.; Cerdá-Olmedo, G.; Trillo-Mata, J.L. Fibromyalgia: Prevalence, epidemiologic profiles and economic costs. *Med. Clin.* **2017**, *149*, 441–448. [CrossRef] [PubMed]
4. Hoffman, D.L.; Dukes, E.M. The health status burden of people with fibromyalgia: A review of studies that assessed health status with the SF-36 or the SF-12. *Int. J. Clin. Pract.* **2007**, *62*, 115–126. [CrossRef] [PubMed]

5. Leadley, R.M.; Armstrong, N.; Lee, Y.C.; Allen, A.; Kleijnen, J. Chronic Diseases in the European Union: The Prevalence and Health Cost Implications of Chronic Pain. *J. Pain Palliat. Care Pharmacother.* **2012**, *26*, 310–325. [CrossRef] [PubMed]
6. Berger, A.; Dukes, E.; Martin, S.; Edelsberg, J.; Oster, G. Characteristics and healthcare costs of patients with fibromyalgia syndrome. *Int. J. Clin. Pract.* **2007**, *61*, 1498–1508. [CrossRef]
7. Gerdle, B.; Björk, J.; Cöster, L.; Henriksson, K.; Henriksson, C.; Bengtsson, A. Prevalence of widespread pain and associations with work status: A population study. *BMC Musculoskelet. Disord.* **2008**, *9*, 102. [CrossRef]
8. Assefi, N.P.; Coy, T.V.; Uslan, D.; Smith, W.R.; Buchwald, D. Financial, occupational, and personal consequences of disability in patients with chronic fatigue syndrome and fibromyalgia compared to other fatiguing conditions. *J. Rheumatol.* **2003**, *30*, 804–808.
9. Henriksson, C.; Liedberg, G.; Gerdle, B. Women with fibromyalgia: Work and rehabilitation. *Disabil. Rehabil.* **2005**, *27*, 685–694. [CrossRef]
10. Wylezinski, L.S.; Gray, J.D.; Polk, J.B.; Harmata, A.J.; Spurlock, C.F. Illuminating an Invisible Epidemic: A Systemic Review of the Clinical and Economic Benefits of Early Diagnosis and Treatment in Inflammatory Disease and Related Syndromes. *J. Clin. Med.* **2019**, *8*, 493. [CrossRef]
11. Nüesch, E.; Häuser, W.; Bernardy, K.; Barth, J.; Jüni, P. Comparative efficacy of pharmacological and non-pharmacological interventions in fibromyalgia syndrome: Network meta-analysis. *Ann. Rheum. Dis.* **2013**, *72*, 955–962. [CrossRef] [PubMed]
12. Pérez-Aranda, A.; Barceló-Soler, A.; Andrés-Rodríguez, L.; Peñarrubia-María, M.T.; Tuccillo, R.; Borraz-Estruch, G.; García-Campayo, J.; Feliu-Soler, A.; Luciano, J.V. Description and narrative review of well-established and promising psychological treatments for fibromyalgia. *Mindfulness Compassion* **2017**, *2*, 112–129. [CrossRef]
13. Perrot, S.; Russell, I.J. More ubiquitous effects from non-pharmacologic than from pharmacologic treatments for fibromyalgia syndrome: A meta-analysis examining six core symptoms. *Eur. J. Pain* **2014**, *18*, 1067–1080. [CrossRef] [PubMed]
14. Luciano, J.V.; D'Amico, F.; Feliu-Soler, A.; McCracken, L.M.; Aguado, J.; Peñarrubia-María, M.T.; Knapp, M.; Serrano-Blanco, A.; García-Campayo, J. Cost-Utility of Group Acceptance and Commitment Therapy for Fibromyalgia Versus Recommended Drugs: An Economic Analysis Alongside a 6-Month Randomized Controlled Trial Conducted in Spain (EFFIGACT Study). *J. Pain* **2017**, *18*, 868–880. [CrossRef] [PubMed]
15. Lloyd, A.; Boomershine, C.S.; Choy, E.H.; Chandran, A.; Zlateva, G. The cost-effectiveness of pregabalin in the treatment of fibromyalgia: US perspective. *J. Med. Econ.* **2012**, *15*, 481–492. [CrossRef] [PubMed]
16. Zijlstra, T.R.; Braakman-Jansen, L.M.A.; Taal, E.; Rasker, J.J.; van de Laar, M.A.F.J. Cost-effectiveness of Spa treatment for fibromyalgia: General health improvement is not for free. *Rheumatology* **2007**, *46*, 1454–1459. [CrossRef] [PubMed]
17. Gusi, N.; Tomas-Carus, P. Cost-utility of an 8-month aquatic training for women with fibromyalgia: A randomized controlled trial. *Arthritis Res. Ther.* **2008**, *10*, R24. [CrossRef] [PubMed]
18. Choy, E.; Richards, S.; Bowrin, K.; Watson, P.; Lloyd, A.; Sadosky, A.; Zlateva, G. Cost effectiveness of pregabalin in the treatment of fibromyalgia from a UK perspective. *Curr. Med. Res. Opin.* **2010**, *26*, 965–975. [CrossRef]
19. Arreola Ornelas, H.; Rosado Buzzo, A.; García, L.; Dorantes Aguilar, J.; Contreras Hernández, I.; Mould Quevedo, J.F. Cost-effectiveness Analysis of Pharmacologic Treatment of Fibromyalgia in Mexico. *Reumatol. Clín.* **2012**, *8*, 120–127. [CrossRef]
20. Beard, S.M.; Roskell, N.; Le, T.K.; Zhao, Y.; Coleman, A.; Ang, D.; Lawson, K. Cost effectiveness of duloxetine in the treatment of fibromyalgia in the United States. *J. Med. Econ.* **2016**, *14*, 463–476. [CrossRef]
21. Goossens, M.E.; Rutten-van Mölken, M.P.; Leidl, R.M.; Bos, S.G.; Vlaeyen, J.W.; Teeken-Gruben, N.J. Cognitive-educational treatment of fibromyalgia: A randomized clinical trial. II. Economic evaluation. *J. Rheumatol.* **1996**, *23*, 1246–1254. [PubMed]
22. Luciano, J.V.; Sabes-Figuera, R.; Cardeñosa, E.; Peñarrubia-María, M.T.; Fernández-Vergel, R.; García-Campayo, J.; Knapp, M.; Serrano-Blanco, A. Cost-utility of a psychoeducational intervention in fibromyalgia patients compared with usual care: An economic evaluation alongside a 12-month randomized controlled trial. *Clin. J. Pain* **2013**, *29*, 702–711. [CrossRef] [PubMed]
23. Luciano, J.V.; D'Amico, F.; Cerdà-Lafont, M.; Peñarrubia-María, M.T.; Knapp, M.; Cuesta-Vargas, A.I.; Serrano-Blanco, A.; García-Campayo, J. Cost-utility of cognitive behavioral therapy versus U.S. Food and

Drug Administration recommended drugs and usual care in the treatment of patients with fibromyalgia: An economic evaluation alongside a 6-month randomized controlled trial. *Arthritis Res. Ther.* **2014**, *16*, 451. [CrossRef] [PubMed]
24. Hedman-Lagerlöf, M.; Hedman-Lagerlöf, E.; Ljótsson, B.; Wicksell, R.K.; Flink, I.; Andersson, E. Cost-Effectiveness and Cost-Utility of Internet-Delivered Exposure Therapy for Fibromyalgia: Results from a Randomized, Controlled Trial. *J. Pain* **2019**, *20*, 47–59. [CrossRef] [PubMed]
25. Schröder, A.; Ørnbøl, E.; Jensen, J.S.; Sharpe, M.; Fink, P. Long-term economic evaluation of cognitive-behavioural group treatment versus enhanced usual care for functional somatic syndromes. *J. Psychosom. Res.* **2017**, *94*, 73–81. [CrossRef] [PubMed]
26. Duarte, R.; Lloyd, A.; Kotas, E.; Andronis, L.; White, R. Are acceptance and mindfulness-based interventions 'value for money'? Evidence from a systematic literature review. *Br. J. Clin. Psychol.* **2018**, *58*, 187–210. [CrossRef] [PubMed]
27. Schmidt, S.; Grossman, P.; Schwarzer, B.; Jena, S.; Naumann, J.; Walach, H. Treating fibromyalgia with mindfulness-based stress reduction: Results from a 3-armed randomized controlled trial. *Pain* **2011**, *152*, 361–369. [CrossRef]
28. Sephton, S.E.; Salmon, P.; Weissbecker, I.; Ulmer, C.; Floyd, A.; Hoover, K.; Studts, J.L. Mindfulness meditation alleviates depressive symptoms in women with fibromyalgia: Results of a randomized clinical trial. *Arthritis Rheum.* **2007**, *57*, 77–85. [CrossRef]
29. Van Gordon, W.; Shonin, E.; Dunn, T.J.; Garcia-Campayo, J.; Griffiths, M.D. Meditation awareness training for the treatment of fibromyalgia syndrome: A randomized controlled trial. *Br. J. Health Psychol.* **2017**, *22*, 186–206. [CrossRef]
30. Cash, E.; Salmon, P.; Weissbecker, I.; Rebholz, W.N.; Bayley-Veloso, R.; Zimmaro, L.A.; Floyd, A.; Dedert, E.; Sephton, S.E. Mindfulness Meditation Alleviates Fibromyalgia Symptoms in Women: Results of a Randomized Clinical Trial. *Ann. Behav. Med.* **2015**, *49*, 319–330. [CrossRef]
31. Pérez-Aranda, A.; Feliu-Soler, A.; Montero-Marín, J.; García-Campayo, J.; Andrés-Rodríguez, L.; Borràs, X.; Rozadilla-Sacanell, A.; Peñarrubia-María, M.T.; Angarita-Osorio, N.; McCracken, L.M.; et al. A randomized controlled efficacy trial of Mindfulness-Based Stress Reduction compared to an active control group and usual care for fibromyalgia: The eudaimon study. *Pain* **2019**, in press.
32. Wolfe, F.; Smythe, H.A.; Yunus, M.B.; Bennett, R.M.; Bombardier, C.; Goldenberg, D.L.; Tugwell, P.; Campbell, S.M.; Abeles, M.; Clark, P.; et al. The american college of rheumatology 1990 criteria for the classification of fibromyalgia. *Arthritis Rheum.* **1990**, *33*, 160–172. [CrossRef] [PubMed]
33. Lobo, A.; Saz, P.; Marcos, G.; Día, J.L.; de la Cámara, C.; Ventura, T.; Morales Asín, F.; Fernando Pascual, L.; Montañés, J.A.; Aznar, S. Revalidation and standardization of the cognition mini-exam (first Spanish version of the Mini-Mental Status Examination) in the general geriatric population. *Med. Clin.* **1999**, *112*, 767–774.
34. Feliu-Soler, A.; Borràs, X.; Peñarrubia-María, M.T.; Rozadilla-Sacanell, A.; D'Amico, F.; Moss-Morris, R.; Howard, M.A.; Fayed, N.; Soriano-Mas, C.; Puebla-Guedea, M.; et al. Cost-utility and biological underpinnings of Mindfulness-Based Stress Reduction (MBSR) versus a psychoeducational programme (FibroQoL) for fibromyalgia: A 12-month randomised controlled trial (EUDAIMON study). *BMC Complement. Altern. Med.* **2016**, *16*, 81. [CrossRef] [PubMed]
35. Kabat-Zinn, J. An outpatient program in behavioral medicine for chronic pain patients based on the practice of mindfulness meditation: Theoretical considerations and preliminary results. *Gen. Hosp. Psychiatry* **1982**, *4*, 33–47. [CrossRef]
36. Kabat-Zinn, J. Mindfulness-based interventions in context: Past, present, and future. *Clin. Psychol. Sci. Pract.* **2003**, *10*, 144–156. [CrossRef]
37. Keng, S.L.; Smoski, M.J.; Robins, C.J. Effects of mindfulness on psychological health: A review of empirical studies. *Clin. Psychol. Rev.* **2011**, *31*, 1041–1056. [CrossRef]
38. Martín Asuero, A. *Con Rumbo Propio Disfruta de la Vida Sin Estrés*; Plataforma: Curia, Portugal, 2010; ISBN 841-5-11-5008.
39. Luciano, J.V.; Martínez, N.; Peñarrubia-María, M.T.; Fernández-Vergel, R.; García-Campayo, J.; Verduras, C.; Blanco, M.E.; Jiménez, M.; Ruiz, J.M.; Del Hoyo, Y.L.; et al. Effectiveness of a psychoeducational treatment program implemented in general practice for fibromyalgia patients: A randomized controlled trial. *Clin. J. Pain* **2011**, *27*, 383–391. [CrossRef]

40. Belenguer-Prieto, R.; Carbonell-Baeza, A.; García-Campayo, J.; Luciano, J.V.; Martín-Nogueras, A.M.; Martínez-Lavín, M.; Muñoz-Espinalt, E.; Pastor-Mira, M.A.; Peñacoba, C.; Calandre, E.; et al. Beginner's Guide to Fibromyalgia. Available online: http://www.fibro.info/guideen.pdf (accessed on 1 January 2019).
41. Herdman, M.; Gudex, C.; Lloyd, A.; Janssen, M.; Kind, P.; Parkin, D.; Bonsel, G.; Badia, X. Development and preliminary testing of the new five-level version of EQ-5D (EQ-5D-5L). *Qual. Life Res.* **2011**, *20*, 1727–1736. [CrossRef]
42. Badia, X.; Roset, M.; Montserrat, S.; Herdman, M.; Segura, A. The Spanish version of EuroQol: A description and its applications. European Quality of Life scale. *Med. Clin.* **1999**, *112*, 79–85.
43. Stone, G.; Hutchinson, A.; Corso, P.; Teutsch, S.; Fielding, J.; Carande-Kulis, V.; Briss, P. Understanding and using the economic evidence. In *The Guide to Community Preventive Services: What Works to Promote Health?* Oxford University Press: Oxford, UK, 2005; pp. 449–463.
44. Vázquez-Barquero, J.; Gaite, L.; Cuesta, M.; Garcia-Usieto, E.; Knapp, M.; Beecham, J. Spanish version of the CSRI: A mental health cost evaluation interview. *Arch. Neuobiol.* **1997**, *60*, 171–184.
45. Husereau, D.; Drummond, M.; Petrou, S.; Carswell, C.; Moher, D.; Greenberg, D.; Augustovski, F.; Briggs, A.H.; Mauskopf, J.; Loder, E. Consolidated Health Economic Evaluation Reporting Standards (CHEERS) statement. *Eur. J. Health Econ.* **2013**, *14*, 367–372. [CrossRef]
46. Ramsey, S.D.; Willke, R.J.; Glick, H.; Reed, S.D.; Augustovski, F.; Jonsson, B.; Briggs, A.; Sullivan, S.D. Cost-effectiveness analysis alongside clinical trials II—An ISPOR good research practices task force report. *Value Health* **2015**, *18*, 161–172. [CrossRef]
47. Base de Datos de Costes Sanitarios SOIKOS Barcelona: Oblikue Consulting. Base de Datos de Costes Sanitarios eSALUD Barcelona. 2016. Available online: http://www.oblikue.com/en/esalud.html (accessed on 1 April 2019).
48. Richardson, G.; Manca, A. Calculation of quality adjusted life years in the published literature: A review of methodology and transparency. *Health Econ.* **2004**, *13*, 1203–1210. [CrossRef]
49. Greene, W. *Econometric Analysis*; Prentice Hall: Englewood Cliffs, NJ, USA, 2003.
50. Briggs, A.H.; Wonderling, D.E.; Mooney, C.Z. Pulling cost-effectiveness analysis up by its bootstraps: A non-parametric approach to confidence interval estimation. *Health Econ.* **1997**, *6*, 327–340. [CrossRef]
51. Royston, P.; White, I. Multiple Imputation by Chained Equations (MICE): Implementation in Stata. *J. Stat. Softw.* **2015**, *45*, 1–20. [CrossRef]
52. Becker, A. Health economics of interdisciplinary rehabilitation for chronic pain: Does it support or invalidate the outcomes research of these programs? *Curr. Pain Headache Rep.* **2012**, *16*, 127–132. [CrossRef]
53. Schaefer, C.; Chandran, A.; Hufstader, M.; Baik, R.; McNett, M.; Goldenberg, D.; Gerwin, R.; Zlateva, G. The comparative burden of mild, moderate and severe Fibromyalgia: Results from a cross-sectional survey in the United States. *Health Qual. Life Outcomes* **2011**, *9*, 71. [CrossRef]
54. Pérez-Aranda, A.; Andrés-Rodríguez, L.; Feliu-Soler, A.; Núñez, C.; Stephan-Otto, C.; Pastor-Mira, M.A.; López-Roig, S.; Peñacoba, C.; Calandre, E.P.; Slim, M.; et al. Clustering a large Spanish sample of patients with fibromyalgia using the FIQR. *Pain* **2019**, *160*, 908–921. [CrossRef]
55. Häuser, W.; Jung, E.; Erbslöh-Möller, B.; Gesmann, M.; Kühn-Becker, H.; Petermann, F.; Langhorst, J.; Weiss, T.; Winkelmann, A.; Wolfe, F. Validation of the Fibromyalgia Survey Questionnaire within a Cross-Sectional Survey. *PLoS ONE* **2012**, *7*, e37504. [CrossRef]
56. Sullivan, M.J.L.; Bishop, S.R.; Pivik, J. The Pain Catastrophizing Scale: Development and validation. *Psychol. Assess.* **1995**, *7*, 524–532. [CrossRef]
57. Pradhan, E.K.; Baumgarten, M.; Langenberg, P.; Handwerger, B.; Gilpin, A.K.; Magyari, T.; Hochberg, M.C.; Berman, B.M. Effect of Mindfulness-Based stress reduction in rheumatoid arthritis patients. *Arthritis Rheum.* **2007**, *57*, 1134–1142. [CrossRef]
58. Parsons, C.E.; Crane, C.; Parsons, L.J.; Fjorback, L.O.; Kuyken, W. Home practice in Mindfulness-Based Cognitive Therapy and Mindfulness-Based Stress Reduction: A systematic review and meta-analysis of participants' mindfulness practice and its association with outcomes. *Behav. Res. Ther.* **2017**, *95*, 29–41. [CrossRef]
59. Mathew, K.L.; Whitford, H.S.; Kenny, M.A.; Denson, L.A. The Long-Term Effects of Mindfulness-Based Cognitive Therapy as a Relapse Prevention Treatment for Major Depressive Disorder. *Behav. Cogn. Psychother.* **2010**, *38*, 561–576. [CrossRef]

60. Carmody, J.; Baer, R.A. Relationships between mindfulness practice and levels of mindfulness, medical and psychological symptoms and well-being in a mindfulness-based stress reduction program. *J. Behav. Med.* **2008**, *31*, 23–33. [CrossRef]
61. Hayes, S.M.; Myhal, G.C.; Thornton, J.F.; Camerlain, M.; Jamison, C.; Cytryn, K.N.; Murray, S. Fibromyalgia and the Therapeutic Relationship: Where Uncertainty Meets Attitude. *Pain Res. Manag.* **2010**, *15*, 385–391. [CrossRef]
62. Album, D.; Westin, S. Do diseases have a prestige hierarchy? A survey among physicians and medical students. *Soc. Sci. Med.* **2008**, *66*, 182–188. [CrossRef]
63. Hernandez Alava, M.; Wailoo, A.; Grimm, S.; Pudney, S.; Gomes, M.; Sadique, Z.; Meads, D.; O'Dwyer, J.; Barton, G.; Irvine, L. EQ-5D-5L versus EQ-5D-3L: The Impact on Cost Effectiveness in the United Kingdom. *Value Health* **2018**, *21*, 49–56. [CrossRef]
64. Bhandari, A.; Wagner, T. Self-Reported Utilization of Health Care Services: Improving Measurement and Accuracy. *Med. Care Res. Rev.* **2006**, *63*, 217–235. [CrossRef]
65. Bellón, J.Á.; Lardelli, P.; de Dios Luna, J.; Delgado, A. Validity of self reported utilisation of primary health care services in an urban population in Spain. *J. Epidemiol. Community Health* **2000**, *54*, 544–551. [CrossRef]
66. Wang, C.; Schmid, C.H.; Rones, R.; Kalish, R.; Yinh, J.; Goldenberg, D.L.; Lee, Y.; McAlindon, T. A Randomized Trial of Tai Chi for Fibromyalgia. *N. Engl. J. Med.* **2010**, *363*, 743–754. [CrossRef]

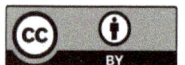

© 2019 by the authors. Licensee MDPI, Basel, Switzerland. This article is an open access article distributed under the terms and conditions of the Creative Commons Attribution (CC BY) license (http://creativecommons.org/licenses/by/4.0/).

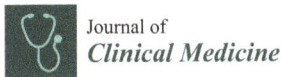

Article

Motor Imagery and Action Observation of Specific Neck Therapeutic Exercises Induced Hypoalgesia in Patients with Chronic Neck Pain: A Randomized Single-Blind Placebo Trial

Luis Suso-Martí [1,2], Jose Vicente León-Hernández [1,3], Roy La Touche [1,3,4,5,*], Alba Paris-Alemany [1,3,4,5] and Ferran Cuenca-Martínez [1,3]

[1] Motion in Brains Research Group, Institute of Neuroscience and Sciences of the Movement (INCIMOV), Centro Superior de Estudios Universitarios La Salle, Universidad Autónoma de Madrid, 28023 Madrid, Spain
[2] Department of Physiotherapy, Universidad CEU Cardenal Herrera, CEU Universities, 46115 Valencia, Spain
[3] Departamento de Fisioterapia, Centro Superior de Estudios Universitarios La Salle, Universidad Autónoma de Madrid, 28023 Madrid, Spain
[4] Instituto de Neurociencia y Dolor Craneofacial (INDCRAN), 28008 Madrid, Spain
[5] Instituto de Investigación Sanitaria del Hospital Universitario La Paz (IdiPAZ), 28046 Madrid, Spain
* Correspondence: roylatouche@yahoo.es; Tel.: +34-91-740-19-80; Fax: +34-91-357-17-30

Received: 15 June 2019; Accepted: 9 July 2019; Published: 12 July 2019

Abstract: The aim of the present study was to explore the pain modulation effects of motor imagery (MI) and action observation (AO) of specific neck therapeutic exercises both locally, in the cervical region, and remotely. A single-blind, placebo clinical trial was designed. A total of 30 patients with chronic neck pain (CNP) were randomly assigned to an AO group, MI group, or placebo observation (PO) group. Pain pressure thresholds (PPTs) of C2/C3, trapezius muscles, and epicondyle were the main outcome variables. Secondary outcomes included heart rate measurement. Statistically significant differences were observed in PPTs of the cervical region in the AO and MI groups between the preintervention and first postintervention assessment. Significant differences were found in the AO group in the epicondyle between the preintervention, first and second post-intervention assessments. Regarding heart rate response, differences were found in the AO and MI groups between the preintervention and average intervention measurements. AO and MI induce immediate pain modulation in the cervical region and AO also induces remote hypoalgesia. OA appears to lead to greater pain modulation as well as a greater heart rate response, however, both should be clinically considered in patients with CNP.

Keywords: motor imagery; action observation; chronic neck pain; pain modulation; pain neuroscience; musculoskeletal pain

1. Introduction

Chronic neck pain (CNP) is a common musculoskeletal disorder with a high prevalence, and is the fourth leading condition that generates significant disability [1,2]. Patients with CNP usually present disturbances in postural control or neuromuscular control of the deep neck muscles associated with the onset of the condition [3,4]. Therefore, specific neck therapeutic exercise (SNTE) training of the deep neck musculature is widely used and might reduce pain and disability in patients with CNP compared with other types of conservative treatment [5].

SNTE has also been shown to induce immediate pain modulation, similar to the hypoalgesia induced by aerobic or isometric exercise [6,7]. Therefore, a central mechanism might be responsible for pain modulation after exercise [8]. On the other hand, the mental practice paradigms of motor simulation, such as action observation (AO) and motor imagery (MI), have recently been developed as a neurocognitive treatment tool for chronic pain [9,10]. MI is defined as a dynamic mental process of an action, without its actual motor execution [11]. AO evokes an internal, real-time motor simulation of the movements that the observer perceives visually [12]. Both mental practice paradigms trigger the activation of the neurocognitive mechanisms that underlie the planning and execution of voluntary movements in a manner that resembles how the action is performed in real life [13–15]. AO and MI might involve an autonomic nervous system (ANS) response. It has been shown that both MI and AO lead to changes in the ANS that cause sympathetic responses, and the neurophysiological base appears to be centrally controlled [16–18].

In recent years, both of these mental processes have been used in the acquisition of new motor gestures, range-of-motion enhancements, or for chronic pain management [19–21]. Despite the similarities of mental practice and exercise, it is uncertain whether MI or OA can induce immediate pain modulation in a similar manner as real exercise in patients with CNP, which would open new treatment approaches for these patients.

The aim of the present study was to explore the pain modulatory effects of MI and AO of SNTE in the cervical region. Our objective was to evaluate the hypoalgesic effects induced by MI and AO, both locally, in the cervical region, and remotely [6]. We hypothesized that MI and AO strategies would induce hypoalgesia and would be associated with an increase in heart rate, whereas a placebo observation (PO) did not.

2. Methods

2.1. Study Design

This study was a randomized, placebo clinical trial, with patient and evaluator blind, planned and conducted in accordance with Consolidated Standards of Reporting Trials (CONSORT) requirements, and was approved by a university ethics committee, with number CSEULS-PI-026/2019, Madrid, Spain.

This study was registered in the United States Randomized Trials Registry on clinicaltrial.gov (trial registry number: NCT03905577). All patients completed the informed consent document prior to the study.

2.2. Recruitment of Participants

The participants had been referred to the primary care physiotherapy service, had been diagnosed with CNP by their family doctor, and met the study's inclusion criteria at one physiotherapy center. Participants were recruited between April 2019 and May 2019.

The inclusion criteria were as follows: (a) men and women aged between 18 and 65 years; and (b) a medical diagnosis of CNP with at least six months of neck pain symptoms. Exclusion criteria included the following: (a) patients with rheumatic diseases, cervical hernia or radicular pain, cervical whiplash syndrome, neck surgeries, or a history of arthrodesis; (b) systemic diseases; (c) vision, hearing, or vestibular problems; or (d) severe trauma or a traffic accident that had an impact on the cervical area.

All data were collected at the La Salle University Center for Advanced Studies. All the participants were given an explanation of the study procedures, which were planned according to the ethical standards of the Helsinki Declaration.

2.3. Randomization

Randomization was performed using a computer-generated random sequence table with a non-balanced three-block design (GraphPad Software, Inc., San Diego, CA, USA). An independent researcher generated the randomization list, and a member of the research team who was not involved in the assessment of the participants or the intervention was in charge of the randomization and

2.4. Blinding

The assessments and treatments were performed by various therapists. The evaluator was blinded to the participants' group assignment. All the intervention procedures were performed by the same physiotherapist who had experience in the field and was blinded to the purpose of the study. Patients were blinded to their group allocation. In addition, a different researcher, blinded to the objectives of the study, performed the data analysis.

2.5. Interventions

2.5.1. Action Observation Group

Patients in this group observed two SNTE typically used in the treatment of patients with CNP. Both exercises were based on the motor gesture of craniocervical flexion (Figure 1). Patients in the AO group performed the observation through a video of the continuous performance of both exercises repeatedly during two series of 1 min for each exercise, with a total duration of 4 min. The participants were seated with a laptop in front of them.

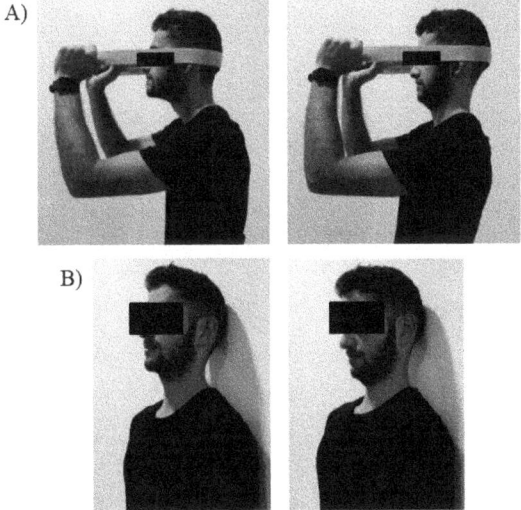

Figure 1. Specific therapeutic neck exercises included in the intervention. (**A**) Flexion-extension resistance exercise. (**B**) Cranio–cervical flexion exercise.

The first exercise involved a resistance deep muscle contraction by performing continuous the cranio-cervical flexo-extension gesture with the resistance of an elastic band (Figure 1A). The second exercise consisted of maintaining the cervical spine in a neutral position in a sitting position and performing a deep muscle contraction to flatten the curve of the neck by nodding with the head. This task involves flexion of the cranium on the cervical spine with the deep cervical muscle contraction (Figure 1B). Patients were instructed to just observe both movements on the monitor without executing or imagining any movement.

2.5.2. Motor Imagery Group

The patients in this group performed a motor imagery protocol of the same cervical exercises observed by the AO group (Figure 1). Patients were instructed on the movements they had to imagine by showing both exercises and the auditive precise instructions for each movement during the intervention. Next, they were instructed to perform a guided third-person mental task of visual motor imagery. For this intervention, the participants were guided by the therapist to imagine the SNTE, trying to form a visual mental image or picture of both movements and attempting to visualize the movement as clear and vivid as possible. The MI intervention of both exercises was performed during two series of 1 min for each exercise, with a total duration of 4 min.

2.5.3. Placebo Observation Group

Patients in this group underwent a PO protocol. A video composed of only nature landscape clips was visualized for 4 min, without visualizing any motor gesture. This kind of PO protocol has been used in previous research [22,23].

2.6. Outcomes

2.6.1. Primary Outcomes

Pressure Pain Thresholds

A pressure pain threshold (PPT) is defined as the minimal amount of pressure at which a sense of pressure first changes to pain. The mechanical pressure algometer (Wagner Instruments, Greenwich, CT, USA) used in this study consisted of a round rubber disk (area 1 cm^2) attached to a pressure (force) gauge. The gauge displayed values in kilograms, but because the surface of the rubber tip was 1 cm^2, the readings were expressed in kg/cm^2. The range of the pressure algometer values was from 0 to 10 kg, in 0.1 kg intervals. The pressure was applied at a rate of 0.31 kg/s [24]. Previous studies have reported an intraexaminer reliability of this procedure ranging from 0.6–0.97, whereas the interexaminer reliability ranged from 0.4–0.98 [25].

PPTs were tested in four different locations. These sites included the angle of both the upper fibers of the left and right trapezius muscles (5–8 cm superior medial from the superior angle of the scapula), the zygapophyseal joint of C2/C3, and the nondominant lateral epicondyle. All the assessments were performed in a quiet room. In order to familiarize the participants with the test procedure, pressure was first applied to an area that would not be tested during the study. Three consecutive measurements of the PPT at the four locations at intervals of 30 s and the mean of these three trials was used for the data analysis [25].

2.6.2. Secondary Outcomes

Heart Rate

Heart rate (HR) was measured to determine how the patients were engaging in the interventions, because HR is under autonomic nervous system control. The heart rate was recorded to quantify the changes produced during the performance of the mental motor practice. The Garmin Forerunner VR 225 is a commercially available wrist-worn heart rate monitor that uses an optical green light sensor to detect pulse rate, which represents HR. The Garmin Forerunner VR 225 was programmed with the participants' sex, age, weight, and height, and was fitted on the left forearm, according to the user manual. Previous studies have shown moderate to strong validity of the Garmin Forerunner VR 225 versus traditional electrocardiography measures (Pearson r = 0.650–0.868).

Motor Imagery Ability

The movement imagery questionnaire-revised (MIQ-R) is an eight-item self-report inventory used to assess visual and kinesthetic motor imagery ability. Four different movements are included in the MIQ-R, which is comprised of four visual and four kinesthetic items. For each item, participants read a description of the movement. They then physically performed the movement and were instructed to resume the starting position after finishing the movement and before performing the mental task, which was to imagine the movement visually or kinesthetically. Next, each participant rated the ease or difficulty of generating the mental image on a seven-point scale, in which 7 indicated "very easy to see/feel" and 1 "very difficult to see/feel." The internal consistencies of the MIQ-R have been adequate, with Cronbach's α coefficients ranging above 0.84 for the total scale, 0.80 for the visual subscale, and 0.84 for the kinesthetic subscale [26].

Mental Chronometry

Mental chronometry (MC) is a reliable measure that has been widely used to record objective measurements of the ability to create mental motor images [27–29]. To assess MC, the time dedicated to imagining each task of MIQ-R questionnaire was first recorded using a stopwatch. The time interval between the command to start the task (given by the evaluator) and the verbal response at the conclusion of the task (given by the participant) was recorded. After the motor imagery task, the participants were asked to execute the real movement of the task, and the time dedicated to performing each task was recorded using a stopwatch. Both time measurements were taken to obtain the temporal congruence between both tasks. During motor imagery, spatial and temporal information were similar to those of the physical execution, suggesting that the time taken to imagine the movement would be similar to that needed for its real execution. MC was used to measure the temporal congruence between real and imagined movements [28,30].

Pain-Related Fear of Movement

Pain-related fear of movement was assessed using the 11-item Spanish version of the Tampa Scale for Kinesiophobia, whose reliability and validity have been demonstrated [31]. The Tampa Scale for Kinesiophobia consists of two subscales, one related to fear of activity and the other related to fear of harm. The final score can range between 11 and 44 points, with higher scores indicating greater perceived kinesiophobia [31].

Pain Catastrophizing

The Spanish version of the Pain Catastrophizing Scale assesses the degree of pain catastrophizing and is a reliable and valid form of measurement. It is composed of 13 items, with a three-factor structure of rumination, magnification, and helplessness that must be answered with a numeric value between 0 (not at all) and 4 (all the time), with a maximum score of 52 points, with higher scores indicating greater pain catastrophizing [32].

Neck Disability

Disability was measured using the Spanish-validated Neck Disability Index (NDI), which consists of 10 items related to daily functional activities. Each question is measured on a scale from 0 (no disability) to 5, and an overall score out of 100 is calculated by adding each item score together and multiplying it by two. A higher NDI score indicates a patient's greater perceived disability due to neck pain. It has been shown to have high "test–retest" reliability and to have appropriate psychometric properties [33].

Physical Activity Level

The level of physical activity was objectified through the International Physical Activity Questionnaire, which allows the participants to be divided into three groups according to their level of activity: high, moderate, and low or inactive [34]. This questionnaire has shown acceptable validity and psychometric properties for measuring total physical activity.

Visual Analogue Scale

A visual analogue scale (VAS) was used to measure pain intensity. The VAS is a 100-mm line with two endpoints representing the extreme states "no pain" and "the maximum pain imaginable". It has been shown to have good retest reliability (r = 0.94, $p < 0.001$) [35,36].

2.7. Procedures

Each participant completed an informed consent document to participate in the study, in addition to a set of questionnaires to complete before starting the intervention. These questionnaires included psychometrics forms and a questionnaire about age, sex, medication, anthropometric measures, pain duration, and the predominant pain location. The psychological variables were evaluated with self-assessments and the pain intensity by VAS. Then, MIQ-R and mental chronometry were assessed. The preintervention PPT measurements were made at the four sites by an external assessor, in random order. Subsequently, an initial HR measurement was performed. The Garmin Forerunner VR 225 monitor was placed, the patients lay down for five minutes, and then sat upright for two more minutes. In both positions, the patients were instructed to maintain a comfortable position and relaxed breathing, with the aim of obtaining a baseline HR measurement. The first measurement was taken at the end of seven minutes, just before the start of the intervention (preintervention measure). At this time and in a sitting position, patients performed the AO protocol, MI or PO, according to the randomized group. HR measurements were taken during the intervention. A measurement was recorded every 15 s for four minutes; subsequently, the average of all the measurements was recorded (intervention average measure). The postintervention HR was recorded at the end of the four minutes of the intervention (postintervention measurement). Immediately after the intervention, a blinded evaluator measured the PPTs in all four locations (post-1). Following this, patients were asked to sit relaxed and comfortably, without movement, for 10 min, and the PPTs were again measured (post-2).

2.8. Statistical Analysis

The statistical data analysis was performed using statistical SPSS software version 22.0 (SPSS Inc., Chicago, IL, USA). The normality of the variables was evaluated by the Shapiro–Wilk test. Descriptive statistics were used to summarize the data for continuous variables and are presented as mean ± standard deviation, 95% confidence interval. Additionally, we compared age, weight, and height between groups with a one-way ANOVA to explore whether the groups were homogeneous at baseline. The chi-squared test was used for the categorical variables that were presented as frequency and percentage. A mixed model analysis of variance (ANOVA) was conducted to study the effect of the between-participant "treatment group" factor in each of the three categories (AO, MI, and placebo) and the within-participant "time" factor, also in each of the three categories (i.e., pre-, post-1, and post-2), of all the dependent variables except for the HR. For the HR, the difference between the preintervention measurement, average intervention measurement, and the immediate postintervention measurement was evaluated (pre-, average intervention, post-1). A post hoc analysis with Bonferroni correction was performed in the case of significant ANOVA findings for multiple comparisons between variables. Effect sizes (d) were calculated according to Cohen's method, in which the magnitude of the effect was classified as small (0.20–0.49), moderate (0.50–0.79), or large (>0.8) [37]. The α level was set at 0.05 for all tests.

3. Results

A total of 30 patients with CNP were included and were randomly allocated into three groups of 10 participants per group (Figure 2). There were no adverse events reported in either group. All the variables presented a normal distribution. No statistically significant differences were found between groups for any of the primary variables, demographic data, or self-report variables at baseline between the groups, except for educational level ($p < 0.05$) (Tables 1 and 2).

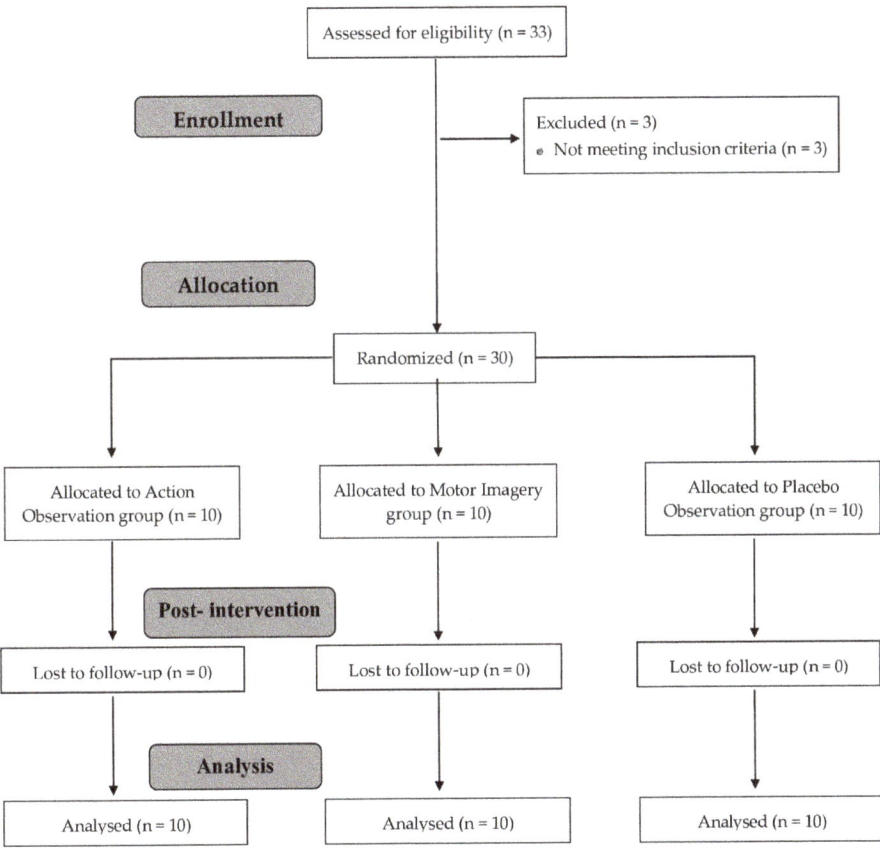

Figure 2. Study flow chart.

Table 1. Descriptive statistics of sociodemographic data.

Measures	AO Group (n = 10)	MI Group (n = 10)	PO Group (n = 10)	p Value
Age	33.5 ± 14.25	30.6 ± 11.53	27.70 ± 6.39	0.520
Height (cm)	171.9 ± 0.80	173.10 ± 0.70	174 ± 0.40	0.798
Weight (kg)	66.7 ± 7.97	68.70 ± 4.8	69.5 ± 8.26	0.672
Pain intensity (VAS)	68.9 ± 13.95	75 ± 7.73	70.8 ± 9.36	0.437
Pain duration (month)	27.9 ± 17.99	26.2 ± 12.45	17.4 ± 10.05	0.212
Sex				0.875
Male	5 (50)	5 (50)	4 (40)	
Female	5 (50)	5 (50)	6 (60)	
Educational Level				0.03
Secondary education	3 (30)	5 (50)	0 (00)	
College education	7 (70)	5 (50)	10 (100)	
Marital Status				0.136
Single	7 (70)	3 (30)	5 (50)	
Married	3 (30)	4 (40)	4 (40)	
Divorced	0 (0)	3 (30)	1 (0)	
Pain Location				0.530
Right	5 (50)	2 (20)	2 (20)	
Left	3 (30)	5 (50)	4 (40)	
Both	2 (20)	3 (30)	4 (40)	

Values are presented as mean ± standard deviation or number (%); MI: motor imagery; AO: action observation; PO: placebo observation; VAS: visual analogue scale.

Table 2. Descriptive statistics of self-reported and psychosocial data.

Measures	AO Group (n = 10)	MI Group (n = 10)	PO Group (n = 10)	p Value
PCS	31 ± 5.9	32.2 ± 6.71	33.1 ± 5.65	0.745
TSK-11	32.3 ± 6	33 ± 4.85	31.3 ± 3.93	0.633
NDI	30.5 ± 3.62	29.8 ± 3.82	32.1 ± 4.48	0.430
IPAQ	1760.6 ± 483.51	1713.85 ± 500.3	1785.7 ± 659.17	0.958
MIQ-R	47.4 ± 4.77	47.3 ± 7.86	48 ± 4.52	0.960
MC	3.65 ± 3.96	4.39 ± 5.7	4.71 ± 4.52	0.879

Values are presented as mean ± standard deviation or number (%); MI: motor imagery; AO: action observation; PO: placebo observation; PCS: Pain Catastrophizing Scale; TSK: Tampa Scale of Kinesiophobia; NDI: Neck Disability Index; IPAQ: International Physical Activity Questionnaires; MIQ-R: Movement Imagery Questionnaire-Revised; MC: Mental Chronometry.

3.1. Primary Outcomes

3.1.1. Pressure Pain Threshold

C2/C3

The ANOVA revealed significant changes in the C2/C3 PPT measurement during group*time ($F = 3.04$, $p = 0.025$, $\eta^2 = 0.185$) and time ($F = 10.74$, $p < 0.01$, $\eta^2 = 0.285$). The post hoc analysis revealed significant intragroup differences (Table 3). Statistically significant differences were observed between the preintervention assessment and the post-1 intervention in the AO and MI groups, with a moderate effect size ($p < 0.001$, $d = 0.74$, and $p = 0.004$, $d = 0.68$, respectively) (Figure 3).

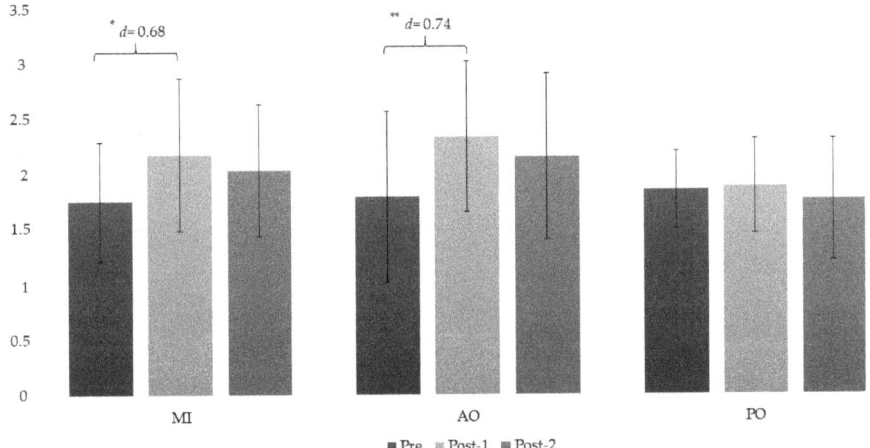

Figure 3. Changes in the pressure pain threshold (PPT) C2/C3 measurement. *: $p < 0.05$; **: $p < 0.001$; AO: action observation; MI: motor imagery group; PO: placebo observation group; Pre: pre-intervention measurement; Post-1: first post intervention measurement (immediately after intervention); Post-2: second post intervention measurement (10 min after intervention).

Table 3. Results of the PPT outcomes.

Measure	Group	Mean ± SD			Mean Difference (95% CI); Effect Size (d) (a) Pre–Post 1 (b) Pre–Post 2 (c) Post 1–Post 2
		Pre	Post-1	Post-2	
PPT (C2/C3)	MI	1.75 ± 0.54	2.17 ± 0.69	2.03 ± 0.60	(a) −0.41 * (−0.71 to 0.12); d = 0.68 (b) −0.27 (−0.66 to 0.11); d = 0.49 (c) 0.14 (−0.83 to 0.37); d = 0.21
	AO	1.79 ± 0.77	2.33 ± 0.68	2.15 ± 0.75	(a) −0.54 ** (−0.84 to −0.25); d = 0.74 (b) −0.36 (−0.75 to 0.02); d = 0.47 (c) 0.18 (−0.05 to 0.40); d = 0.25
	PO	1.85 ± 0.35	1.88 ± 0.43	1.76 ± 0.55	(a) −0.02 (−0.02 to 0.75); d = 0.07 (b) 0.09 (0.29 to 0.48); d = 0.19 (c) 0.11 (−0.11 to 0.33); d = 0.24
Mean difference (95% CI) Effect size (d)					
	MI-AO	−0.03 (−0.69 to 0.63); d = 0.06	−0.16 (−0.86 to 0.54); d = 0.23	−0.13 (−0.85 to 0.60); d = 0.17	
	MI-PO	−0.10 (−0.76 to 0.56); d = 0.22	0.29 (−0.41 to 0.99); d = 0.5	0.27 (−0.46 to 0.99); d = 0.47	
	AO-PO	−0.07 (−0.73 to 0.59); d = 0.1	0.46 (−0.24 to 1.11); d = 0.79	−0.39 (−0.34 to 1.12); d = 0.59	
PPT (RT)	MI	1.83 ± 0.89	2.32 ± 0.99	1.97 ± 0.73	(a) −0.49 * (−0.93 to −0.04); d = 0.52 (b) −0.14 (−0.60 to 0.32); d = 0.17 (c) 0.35 (−0.22 to 0.72); d = 0.40
	AO	1.86 ± 0.81	2.41 ± 1.16	2.26 ± 0.1.14	(a) −0.55 * (−0.99 to −0.11); d = 0.54 (b) −0.40 (−0.86 to 0.07); d = 0.40 (c) 0.16 (−0.21 to 0.52); d = 0.13
	PO	2.03 ± 0.59	1.86 ± 0.55	1.76 ± 0.34	(a) 0.17 (−0.28 to 0.61); d = 0.29 (b) 0.27 (−0.19 to 0.74); d = 0.56 (c) 0.11 (−0.26 to 0.47); d = 0.21
Mean difference (95% CI) Effect size (d)					
	MI-AO	−0.02 (−0.91 to 0.86); d = 0.03	−0.09 (−1.15 to 0.98); d = 0.08	0.28 (−1.2 to 0.63); d = −0.40	
	MI-PO	−0.20 (−1.08 to 0.68); d = 0.26	0.46 (−0.61 to 1.52); d = 0.57	0.21 (−0.70 to 1.13); d = 0.36	
	AO-PO	−0.18 (−1.06 to 0.71); d = 0.23	0.54 (−0.52 to 1.61); d = 0.6	0.49 (−0.42 to 1.41); d = 0.59	

Table 3. Cont.

Measure	Group	Mean ± SD			Mean Difference (95% CI); Effect Size (d) (a) Pre–Post 1 (b) Pre–Post 2 (c) Post 1–Post 2
		Pre	Post-1	Post-2	
PPT (LT)	MI	1.85 ± 0.77	2.30 ± 0.89	2.09 ± 0.69	(a) −0.46 * (−0.85 to −0.07); d = 0.54 (b) −0.24 (−0.66 to 0.17); d = 0.32 (c) 0.21 (−0.17 to 0.60); d = 0.26
	AO	2.01 ± 0.70	2.78 ± 0.85	2.38 ± 0.99	(a) −0.78 ** (−1.16 to −0.39); d = 0.99 (b) −0.37 (−0.79 to 0.04); d = 0.43 (c) −0.40 * (0.02 to 0.79); d = 0.43
	PO	1.78 ± 0.39	1.67 ± 0.41	1.68 ± 0.33	(a) 0.10 (−0.28 to 0.49); d = 0.27 (b) 0.09 (−0.32 to 0.51); d = 0.27 (c) 0.01 (−0.39 to 0.38); d = 0.02
Mean difference (95% CI) Effect size (d)					
MI-AO		−0.16 (−0.90 to 0.57); d = 0.21	−0.48 (−1.34 to 0.38); d = 0.55	−0.29 (−1.12 to 0.53) d =0.33	
MI-PO		−0.06 (−0.67 to 0.80) d = 0.11	0.63 (−0.23 to 1.49), d = 0.90	0.40 (−0.42 to 1.22); d = 0.75	
AO-PO		0.23 (0.51 to 0.96); d = 0.40	1.11 ** (0.25 to 1.96); d = 1.66	0.69 (−0.13 to 1.51); d = 0.94	
PPT (Epicondyle)	MI	2.88 ± 0.74	3.16 ± 0.81	2.95 ± 0.78	(a) −0.29 (−0.60 to −0.01); d = 0.36 (b) −0.08 (−0.21 to 0.62); d = 0.09 (c) 0.21 (−0.21 to 0.62); d = 0.26
	AO	2.47 ± 0.70	3.1 ± 0.62	3.02 ± 0.84	(a) −0.64 ** (−0.95 to −0.33); d = 0.95 (b) −0.56 * (−0.96 to −0.15); d = 0.71 (c) 0.07 (−0.49 to 0.34); d = 0.11
	PO	3.05 ± 0.54	2.87 ± 0.79	2.61 ± 0.85	(a) 0.18 (−0.13 to 0.49); d = 0.26 (b) 0.44 * (0.03 to 0.84); d = 0.62 (c) 0.25 (−0.67 to 0.16); d = 0.31
Mean difference (95% CI) Effect size (d)					
MI-AO		0.41 (−0.35 to 1.16); d = 0.56	−0.06 (−0.79 to 0.91); d = 0.08	−0.07 (−1.01 to 0.87) d = 0.08	
MI-PO		−0.18 (−0.94 to 0.58) d = 0.26	0.30 (−0.55 to 1.15), d= 0.36	0.34 (−0.59 to 1.28); d = 0.41	
AO-PO		−0.58 (−1.34 to 0.18); d = 0.92	0.24 (−0.61 to 1.09); d = 0.32	0.41 (−0.53 to 1.35); d = 0.48	

* p < 0.05; ** p < 0.001. AO: action observation group; MI: motor imagery group; PO: placebo observation group; PPT: pressure pain threshold; RT: right trapezius measurement; LT: left trapezius measurement; pre: preintervention measurement; Post-1: first post intervention measurement (immediately after intervention); Post-2: second post intervention measurement (10 min after intervention).

Right Trapezius Muscle

The ANOVA revealed significant changes in the right trapezius muscle PPT measurement during group*time (F = 3.42, p = 0.014, η^2 = 0.202) and time (F = 4.75, p = 0.013, η^2 = 0.15) The post hoc analysis revealed significant intragroup differences (Table 3). Statistically significant differences were observed between the preintervention assessment and the post-1 intervention in the AO and MI groups, with a moderate effect size (p = 0.012, d = 0.54, and p = 0.028, d = 0.52, respectively) (Figure 4).

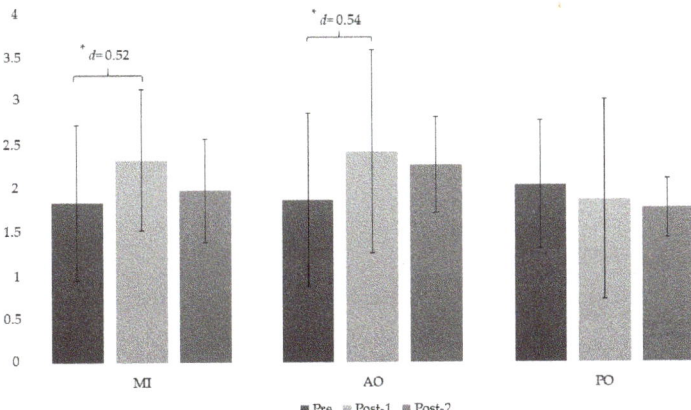

Figure 4. Changes in the PPT right trapezius measurement. *: $p < 0.05$; AO: action observation; MI: motor imagery group; PO: placebo observation group; Pre: pre-intervention measurement; Post-1: first post intervention measurement (immediately after intervention); Post-2: second post intervention measurement (10 min after intervention).

Left Trapezius Muscle

The ANOVA revealed significant changes in the left trapezius muscle PPT measurement during group*time ($F = 4.16$, $p = 0.005$, $\eta^2 = 0.235$) and time ($F = 8.92$, $p < 0.001$, $\eta^2 = 0.248$). The post hoc analysis revealed significant intragroup differences between the preintervention assessment and the post-1 measurement, with a large effect size ($p < 0.001$, $d = 0.99$), and between the post-1 and the post-2 assessments in the AO group, with a moderate effect size ($p = 0.037$, $d = 0.43$) (Table 3). In addition, statistically significant differences were observed in the MI group between the preintervention assessment and the post-1 measurement, with a moderate effect size ($p = 0.015$, $d = 0.54$). Finally, statistically significant differences were found between the AO and PO groups, with a large effect size ($p < 0.001$, $d = 1.66$) (Figure 5).

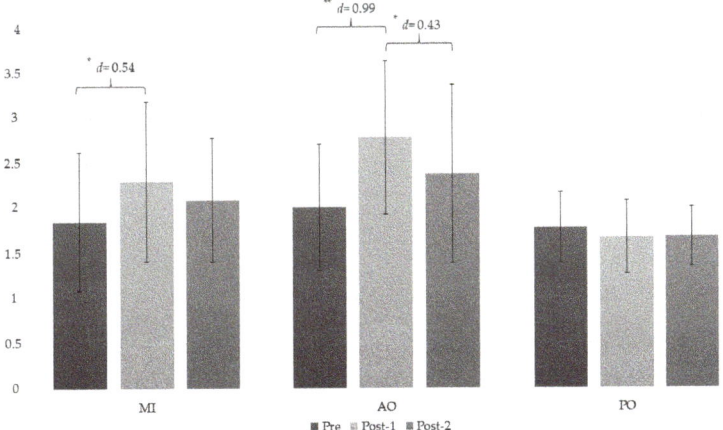

Figure 5. Changes in the PPT left trapezius measurement. *: $p < 0.05$; **: $p < 0.001$; AO: action observation; MI: motor imagery group; PO: placebo observation group; Pre: pre-intervention measurement; Post-1: first post intervention measurement (immediately after intervention); Post-2: second post intervention measurement (10 min after intervention).

Lateral Epicondyle

The ANOVA revealed significant changes in the lateral epicondyle PPT measurement during group*time ($F = 6.4, p < 0.001, \eta^2 = 0.321$) and time ($F = 4.44, p = 0.016, \eta^2 = 0.141$). The post hoc analysis revealed significant intragroup differences only in the AO group (Table 3). Statistically significant differences were observed between the preintervention assessment and the post-1 measurement, with a large effect size ($p < 0.001, d = 0.95$), and between the pre-intervention assessment and the post-2 measurement, with a moderate effect size ($p = 0.005, d = 0.71$). In addition, intra-group differences were found in the PO group between the preintervention and post-2 intervention measurements, with a moderate effect size ($p = 0.032, d = 0.62$) (Figure 6).

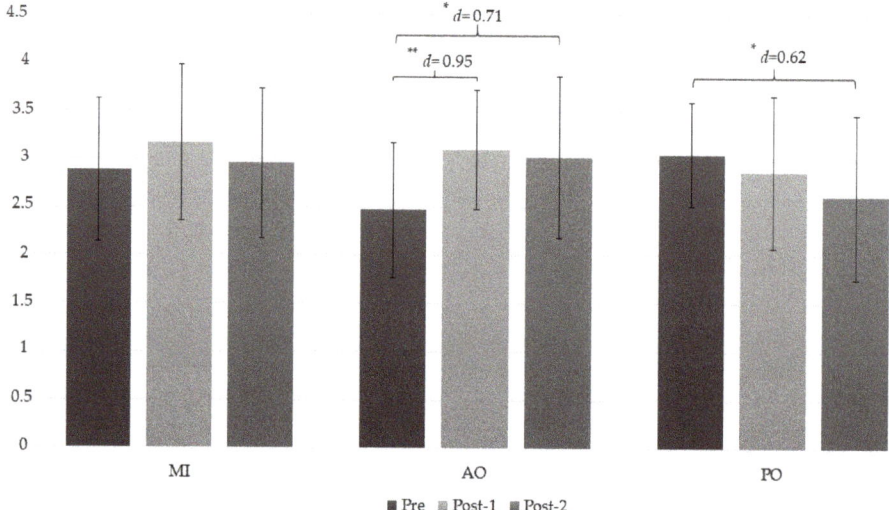

Figure 6. Changes in the PPT epicondyle measurement. *: $p < 0.05$; **: $p < 0.001$; AO: action observation; MI: motor imagery group; PO: placebo observation group; Pre: pre-intervention measurement; Post-1: first post intervention measurement (immediately after intervention); Post-2: second post intervention measurement (10 min after intervention).

3.2. Secondary Outcomes

Heart Rate

The ANOVA revealed significant changes in heart rate during group*time ($F = 18.52, p < 0.001, \eta^2 = 0.578$) and time ($F = 85.74, p < 0.001, \eta^2 = 0.761$). The post hoc analysis revealed significant intragroup differences in the MI and AO groups between the preintervention assessment and the intervention average assessment ($p < 0.001$ in both groups, $d = 0.48$ and $d = 0.67$, respectively). Statistically significant differences were observed between the preintervention assessment and the postintervention measurement, with a large effect size in the AO and MI groups ($p < 0.001$ in both groups, $d = 1.3$ and $d = 0.84$, respectively). In addition, in both groups, statistically significant differences were found between the intervention average measurement and postintervention measurement ($p < 0.001$ in both groups, $d = 0.42$ and $d = 0.7$, respectively).

Statistically significant intergroup differences were found between the AO and PO groups in the intervention average measurement ($p < 0.001; d = 1.4$). In addition, significant intergroup differences were found in the postintervention measurement between the MI and AO groups, with a large effect size ($p = 0.042, d = 1.10$), and between the AO and PO groups ($p = 0.001, d = 1.92$) (Table 4).

Table 4. Results of heart rate measurement.

Measure	Group	Mean ± SD			Mean Difference (95% CI); Effect Size (d). (a) Pre-Intervention (b) Pre–Post (c) Intervention–Post
		Pre	Intervention	Post	
HR	MI	72.3 ± 5.38	74.84 ± 4.99	77.3 ± 6.4	(a) −2.54 ** (−4.09 to −0.97) d = 0.48 (b) −5 ** (−7.15 to −2.85); d = 0.84 (c) −2.47 ** (−3.74 to −1.2) d = 0.42
	AO	75.7 ± 6.77	80.08 ± 6.24	84.8 ± 7.19	(a) −4.38 ** (−5.94 to −2.82) d = 0.67 (b) −9.1 ** (−11.24 to −6.95); d = 1.3 (c) −4.72 ** (−5.99 to −3.45) d = −0.7
	PO	71.6 ± 5.42	72.12 ± 5.05	72.6 ± 5.4	(a) −0.52 (−2.08 to 1.04) d = −0.09 (b) −1 (−0.73 to 2.73); d = −0.18 (c) −0.48 (−1.75 to 0.79); d = −0.09
Mean difference (95% CI) Effect size (d)					
	MI-AO	−3.4 (−10.13 to 3.33); d = −0.55	−5.24 (−11.48 to 0.99); d = −0.92	−7.5 * (−14.77 to −0.23); d = 1.10	
	MI-PO	−0.7 (−6.02 to 7.43); d = −0.12	2.72 (−3.52 to 8.95); d = −0.54	4.7 (−2.57 to 11.97); d = −0.79	
	AO-PO	−4.1 (−2.63 to 10.82); d = −0.66	7.96 * (1.73 to 14.19); d = 1.4	12.2 ** (−19.47 to −4.93); d = 1.92	

* $p < 0.05$; ** $p < 0.001$. AO: action observation group; MI: motor imagery group; PO: placebo observation group; HR: heart rate; pre: preintervention measure; intervention: average intervention measure; post: postintervention measure.

4. Discussion

The aim of the present study was to explore the immediate modulatory pain effects of MI and AO of SNTE in the cervical and remote regions. Our results show that both MI and AO induced an immediate pain modulation response in the cervical region (post-1), however, it was not sustained in the second measurement after the intervention. In the epicondyle, only AO induced pain reduction between the preintervention measurement and both postintervention measurements. AO and MI interventions provoked an increase in HR, however, AO showed significant differences in comparison with the PO and MI groups.

Exercise-induced hypoalgesia is a well-documented phenomenon. Although most research has demonstrated modulating effects on pain by aerobic exercise, O'Leary et al. have shown that performing SNTEs, similar to those employed in the present study, produced local hypoalgesic responses in the cervical region [6]. According to the literature, AO and MI might provoke cortical activations similar to the real movement execution; thus, it is possible that the overlapping of cortical areas between real execution and mental practice could explain our findings [38,39]. In this regard, Beinert et al. found no differences in PPTs between performing and imagining motor control exercises of the flexor neck musculature in patients with neck pain. These data suggest that there is probably a top-down central mechanism responsible for hypoalgesia, according to our results [40]. However, Beinert et al. found no differences in the PPTs of the cervical region after an MI or AO intervention of the articular position error task [41]. These controversial data appear to be related to the imagined or observed task. It is possible that if the selected movement is able to trigger pain or fear responses in patients during real execution, the pain modulation response might be lower if it is performed mentally. This result has also been found in studies using functional magnetic resonance, that show the activation of cortical areas related to pain processing after the mental practice of painful movements [42]. In this regard, Forkmann et al. examined the relationship between painful stimuli and cortical encoding of visual stimuli [43]. Their results showed that when a visual stimulus was accompanied with a painful input, there was a decrease in the activity of the hippocampus associated with a lower encoding of the visual stimulus. It is possible that if an imagined or observed painful movement activates brain areas similar to a real painful stimulus, the coding of visual information might also be influenced, affecting pain modulation.

In addition to the pain-trigger responses, another relevant factor could be pain-related fear. Previous research has shown that high levels of fear of movement directly affect the periaqueductal gray through the amygdala, which might have a direct negative effect on endogenous pain modulation [44].

The study by de-la-Puente-Ranea et al. showed hypoalgesic responses after complete cervical rotation movements in patients with CNP, although this movement could be considered painful or fear-associated in these patients [45]. However, the levels of patients' fear of movement were low, and it is possible that low fear of movement levels could influence these results in a manner opposite to the aforementioned findings of Beinert et al. We therefore suggest that MI and AO might produce relevant hypoalgesic responses, but it is necessary to consider factors such as pain-related fear or the possible pain-trigger responses related to the imagined or observed movement.

A relevant finding of the present study is that MI and AO produced pain modulation responses compared to PO. This finding is important because previous studies have suggested that distraction might be a mechanism involved in pain modulation produced by mental practice [46,47]. Although in the present study no immersive strategies were used that could provoke greater distraction, other mechanisms are required to explain the hypoalgesia induced by mental practice. In addition to the aforementioned top-down mechanism, additional hypotheses have been proposed concerning interactions between pain modulation and heart rate, which were also found in this study, suggesting a systemic pain modulatory effect. Previous research has investigated manual therapy hypoalgesia models, showing that hypoalgesia is related to increased ANS activity [48,49]. In addition, patients with chronic pain experience maladaptive neuroplastic changes that could lead to impaired cortical-motor representation and diminished cortical excitability [50,51]. In this regard, previous studies have shown that both AO and MI can cause an increase in cortical representation and excitability, influencing areas such as the primary motor cortex or the dorsal premotor cortex [52,53]. Larsen et al. showed that MI and AO could induce an increase in cortical excitability, which was associated with a decrease in pain perception [54]. These findings are consistent with those obtained by Volz et al., in which pain modulation was observed after AO training, which was associated with increased cortical excitability of the motor cortex. This outcome is also directly related to the neural networks related to pain modulation through corticothalamic networks, as well as changes in neural plasticity [55,56].

On the other hand, our results showed that the AO provoked greater local and remote hypoalgesic responses and triggered a higher HR increase compared with MI. Possible differences between AO and MI remain unclear and more research is needed. HR is under autonomic control, which could give an estimate of the physiological responses produced by both interventions, although other measurements, such as skin conductance or temperature, are necessary to establish whether AO or MI caused increased activity of the autonomic nervous system. However, one of the main difficulties in interventions with mental motor practice is to know if the patient was engaging to the intervention in the correct form. Our HR date showed that in both groups, patients were engaged in the intervention, although in the AO group the HR increase was higher compared to the MI group. One potential factor that could influence this outcome is the exercises selected for the intervention. The selection of these exercises was based on their extensive clinical application, the pain modulation effects found with their real execution, and the intent to prevent fear in their execution. Fear responses to movements perceived as dangerous have been associated with increases in ANS activity and pain intensity [57,58]. However, a significant point to note is that MI requires a good ability to imagine and is less effective in people with poorer imaginative ability [59]. Some aspects, such as imagining the body segment movement, the complexity or familiarity of the movement, as well as levels of physical activity, have all been related to MI performance ability. SNTE exercises are highly difficult to imagine, due to the fact that they require motor learning of unknown, complex, and high precision movements. This could result in less mental effort performed by patients in the MI group, due to their inability to imagine the exercises, and less effort is associated with decreased ANS responses and might therefore be associated with decreased hypoalgesic responses [60,61]. Another hypothesis in this aspect is that the difficulty in imagining the exercises could provoke a mental stress in the patients of the MI group that could be related to the hypoalgesia. The stress-inducing hypoalgesia phenomenon has been previously reported in the scientific literature and may be an alternative explanation to the results obtained [62]. In addition, patients with chronic pain have a decreased ability to create mental motor images, which could also be related to our results [63].

4.1. Clinical Implications

The results of the present study showed that AO and MI could provoke pain modulatory effects in the cervical region. The implementation of mental practice in patients with persistent pain, is highly relevant, as they could be performed in clinical environments where in the early stages, it is not possible to perform motor gestures in a real way due to the presence of pain or psychosocial variables, like fear of movement. These tools offer opportunities to improve the different stages of rehabilitation for patients with dysfunctional and maladaptive pain. In addition, this approach could increase the effectiveness of the current treatments, thus, they should be considered due to their simple implementation and cost-effectiveness in everyday daily routines or clinical practice. In addition, mental practice may have additional positive effects on motor learning or increase patient adherence to exercising the rehabilitation process. Future studies should continue to investigate the benefits of AO and MI in patients with chronic pain, as well as their implementation in clinical practice.

4.2. Limitations

This study presents some limitations. First, the sample size was small, and thus, the results should be considered with caution. In addition, the results have only been considered in the short term, and the duration and type of intervention might have been insufficient for greater increases in pain modulation in patients with CNP, especially in the MI group. Second, changes in clinical pain were not evaluated. Longer mental practice interventions may determine changes in clinical pain, which is certainly a very relevant aspect. More research is needed to determine the role of mental practice in pain modulation in patients with chronic pain.

5. Conclusions

Both the AO and MI of specific neck exercises are able to induce immediate pain modulation of the cervical region. Although both strategies led to increases in PPTs, AO appears to have led to greater local and remote pain modulation, as well as a greater response from the ANS. More research is needed in this area on the role and additional benefits of mental practice in terms of pain modulation and its implementation in clinical practice.

Author Contributions: Conceptualization, L.S.-M., F.C.-M. and R.L.T.; Methodology, L.S.-M. and F.C.-M.; Software, N/A; Validation, L.S.-M., J.V.L.-H. and R.L.T.; Formal Analysis, L.S.-M., F.C.-M. and R.L.T.; Investigation, L.S.-M. and J.V.L.-H.; Resources L.S.-M. and F.C.-M.; Data Curation, F.C.-M and J.V.L.-H.; Writing–Original Draft Preparation, L.S.-M., F.C.-M, J.V.L.-H. and R.L.T.; Writing–Review & Editing, L.S.-M, A.P.-A., J.V.L.-H. and R.L.T.; Visualization, L.S.-M., F.C.-M and J.V.L.-H.; Supervision, L.S.-M., J.V.L.-H., A.P.-A. and R.L.T.; Project Administration, R.L.T and A.P.-A.; Funding Acquisition, N/A.

Acknowledgments: We thank La Salle University Center for Advanced Studies for making this study possible, as well as all the participants in the study.

Conflicts of Interest: The authors declare that they have no conflicts of interest. This study did not receive any specific grant from funding agencies in the public, commercial, or not-for-profit sectors.

References

1. Vos, T.; Flaxman, A.D.; Naghavi, M.; Lozano, R.; Michaud, C.; Ezzati, M.; Shibuya, K.; Salomon, J.A.; Abdalla, S.; Aboyans, V.; et al. Years lived with disability (YLDs) for 1160 sequelae of 289 diseases and injuries 1990–2010: A systematic analysis for the Global Burden of Disease Study 2010. *Lancet* **2012**, *380*, 2163–2196. [CrossRef]
2. Manchikanti, L.; Singh, V.; Datta, S.; Cohen, S.P.; Hirsch, J.A. Comprehensive review of epidemiology, scope, and impact of spinal pain. *Pain Phys.* **2009**, *12*, E35–E70.

3. Falla, D.; Farina, D. Neuromuscular adaptation in experimental and clinical neck pain. *J. Electromyogr. Kinesiol.* **2008**, *18*, 255–261. [CrossRef] [PubMed]
4. Falla, D.; Jull, G.; Hodges, P.W. Feedforward activity of the cervical flexor muscles during voluntary arm movements is delayed in chronic neck pain. *Exp. Brain Res.* **2004**, *157*, 43–48. [CrossRef] [PubMed]
5. Martin-Gomez, C.; Sestelo-Diaz, R.; Carrillo-Sanjuan, V.; Navarro-Santana, M.J.; Bardon-Romero, J.; Plaza-Manzano, G. Motor control using cranio-cervical flexion exercises versus other treatments for non-specific chronic neck pain: A systematic review and meta-analysis. *Musculoskelet. Sci. Pract.* **2019**, *42*, 52–59. [CrossRef] [PubMed]
6. O'Leary, S.; Falla, D.; Hodges, P.W.; Jull, G.; Vicenzino, B. Specific Therapeutic Exercise of the Neck Induces Immediate Local Hypoalgesia. *J. Pain* **2007**, *8*, 832–839. [CrossRef] [PubMed]
7. Koltyn, K.F. Analgesia following exercise: A review. *Sports Med.* **2000**, *29*, 85–98. [CrossRef] [PubMed]
8. Koltyn, K.F.; Brellenthin, A.G.; Cook, D.B.; Sehgal, N.; Hillard, C. Mechanisms of Exercise-Induced Hypoalgesia. *J. Pain* **2014**, *15*, 1294–1304. [CrossRef]
9. Jeannerod, M. Neural Simulation of Action: A Unifying Mechanism for Motor Cognition. *NeuroImage* **2001**, *14*, S103–S109. [CrossRef]
10. Mulder, T. Motor imagery and action observation: Cognitive tools for rehabilitation. *J. Neural Transm.* **2007**, *114*, 1265–1278. [CrossRef]
11. Decety, J. The neurophysiological basis of motor imagery. *Behav. Brain Res.* **1996**, *77*, 45–52. [CrossRef]
12. Buccino, G. Action observation treatment: A novel tool in neurorehabilitation. *Philos. Trans. R. Soc. B Boil. Sci.* **2014**, *369*, 20130185. [CrossRef] [PubMed]
13. Wright, D.J.; Williams, J.; Holmes, P.S. Combined action observation and imagery facilitates corticospinal excitability. *Front. Hum. Neurosci.* **2014**, *8*, 951. [CrossRef] [PubMed]
14. Lotze, M.; Montoya, P.; Erb, M.; Hülsmann, E.; Flor, H.; Klose, U.; Birbaumer, N.; Grodd, W. Activation of Cortical and Cerebellar Motor Areas during Executed and Imagined Hand Movements: An fMRI Study. *J. Cogn. Neurosci.* **1999**, *11*, 491–501. [CrossRef] [PubMed]
15. Decety, J. Do imagined and executed actions share the same neural substrate? *Cogn. Brain Res.* **1996**, *3*, 87–93. [CrossRef]
16. Collet, C.; Di Rienzo, F.; El Hoyek, N.; Guillot, A.; Hoyek, N. Autonomic nervous system correlates in movement observation and motor imagery. *Front. Hum. Neurosci.* **2013**, *7*, 415. [CrossRef] [PubMed]
17. Decety, J.; Jeannerod, M.; Durozard, D.; Baverel, G. Central activation of autonomic effectors during mental simulation of motor actions in man. *J. Physiol.* **1993**, *461*, 549–563. [CrossRef]
18. Bolliet, O.; Collet, C.; Dittmar, A. Observation of action and autonomic nervous system responses 1. *Percept. Mot. Skill* **2005**, *101*, 195–202. [CrossRef]
19. Maciver, K.; Lloyd, D.M.; Kelly, S.; Roberts, N.; Nurmikko, T. Phantom limb pain, cortical reorganization and the therapeutic effect of mental imagery. *Brain* **2008**, *131*, 2181–2191. [CrossRef]
20. Hoyek, N.; Di Rienzo, F.; Collet, C.; Hoyek, F.; Guillot, A. The therapeutic role of motor imagery on the functional rehabilitation of a stage II shoulder impingement syndrome. *Disabil. Rehabil.* **2014**, *36*, 1113–1119. [CrossRef]
21. Moseley, G.L.; Moseley, L. Graded motor imagery for pathologic pain: A randomized controlled trial. *Neurology* **2006**, *67*, 2129–2134. [CrossRef] [PubMed]
22. Bang, D.-H.; Shin, W.-S.; Kim, S.-Y.; Choi, J.-D. The effects of action observational training on walking ability in chronic stroke patients: A double-blind randomized controlled trial. *Clin. Rehabil.* **2013**, *27*, 1118–1125. [CrossRef] [PubMed]
23. Buccino, G.; Arisi, D.; Gough, P.; Aprile, D.; Ferri, C.; Serotti, L.; Tiberti, A.; Fazzi, E. Improving upper limb motor functions through action observation treatment: A pilot study in children with cerebral palsy. *Dev. Med. Child Neurol.* **2012**, *54*, 822–828. [CrossRef] [PubMed]
24. Chesterton, L.S.; Sim, J.; Wright, C.C.; Foster, N.E. Interrater Reliability of Algometry in Measuring Pressure Pain Thresholds in Healthy Humans, Using Multiple Raters. *Clin. J. Pain* **2007**, *23*, 760–766. [CrossRef] [PubMed]
25. Takala, E.P. Pressure pain threshold on upper trapezius and levator scapulae muscles. Repeatability and relation to subjective symptoms in a working population. *Scand. J. Rehabil. Med.* **1990**, *22*, 63–68. [PubMed]
26. Campos, A.; González, M.Á. Spanish version of the revised movement image questionnaire (MIQ-R): Psychometric properties and validation. *Rev. Psicol. Deporte* **2010**, *19*, 265–275.

27. Guillot, A.; Collet, C. Duration of Mentally Simulated Movement: A Review. *J. Mot. Behav.* **2005**, *37*, 10–20. [CrossRef]
28. Malouin, F.; Richards, C.L.; Durand, A.; Doyon, J. Reliability of Mental Chronometry for Assessing Motor Imagery Ability After Stroke. *Arch. Phys. Med. Rehabil.* **2008**, *89*, 311–319. [CrossRef]
29. Williams, S.E.; Guillot, A.; Di Rienzo, F.; Cumming, J. Comparing self-report and mental chronometry measures of motor imagery ability. *Eur. J. Sport Sci.* **2015**, *15*, 703–711. [CrossRef]
30. Guillot, A.; Hoyek, N.; Louis, M.; Collet, C. Understanding the timing of motor imagery: Recent findings and future directions. *Int. Rev. Sport Exerc. Psychol.* **2012**, *5*, 3–22. [CrossRef]
31. Gómez-Pérez, L.; López-Martínez, A.E.; Ruiz-Párraga, G.T. Psychometric Properties of the Spanish Version of the Tampa Scale for Kinesiophobia (TSK). *J. Pain* **2011**, *12*, 425–435. [CrossRef] [PubMed]
32. Campayo, J.G.; Rodero, B.; Alda, M.; Sobradiel, N.; Montero, J.; Moreno, S. [Validation of the Spanish version of the Pain Catastrophizing Scale in fibromyalgia]. *Med. Clín.* **2008**, *131*, 487–492.
33. Ortega, J.A.A.; Martínez, A.D.D.; Ruiz, R.A. Validación de una versión española del Índice de Discapacidad Cervical. *Med. Clín.* **2008**, *130*, 85–89. [CrossRef]
34. Roman-Viñas, B.; Serra-Majem, L.; Hagströmer, M.; Ribas-Barba, L.; Sjöström, M.; Segura-Cardona, R. International Physical Activity Questionnaire: Reliability and validity in a Spanish population. *Eur. J. Sport Sci.* **2010**, *10*, 297–304. [CrossRef]
35. Bijur, P.E.; Silver, W.; Gallagher, E.J. Reliability of the Visual Analog Scale for Measurement of Acute Pain. *Acad. Emerg. Med.* **2001**, *8*, 1153–1157. [CrossRef] [PubMed]
36. Ostelo, R.W.; Deyo, R.A.; Stratford, P.; Waddell, G.; Croft, P.; Von Korff, M.; Bouter, L.M.; Henrica, C. Interpreting Change Scores for Pain and Functional Status in Low Back Pain. *Spine* **2008**, *33*, 90–94. [CrossRef] [PubMed]
37. Cohen, J. *Statistical Power Analysis for the Behavioral Sciences*; Lawrence Erlbaum Associates: Hillsdale, NJ, USA, 1988.
38. Hardwick, R.M.; Caspers, S.; Eickhoff, S.B.; Swinnen, S.P. Neural correlates of action: Comparing meta-analyses of imagery, observation, and execution. *Neurosci. Biobehav. Rev.* **2018**, *94*, 31–44. [CrossRef]
39. Hétu, S.; Grégoire, M.; Saimpont, A.; Coll, M.-P.; Eugène, F.; Michon, P.-E.; Jackson, P.L. The neural network of motor imagery: An ALE meta-analysis. *Neurosci. Biobehav. Rev.* **2013**, *37*, 930–949. [CrossRef]
40. Beinert, K.; Sofsky, M.; Trojan, J. Train the brain! Immediate sensorimotor effects of mentally-performed flexor exercises in patients with neck pain. A pilot study. *Eur. J. Phys. Rehabil. Med.* **2019**, *55*, 63–70. [CrossRef]
41. Beinert, K.; Preiss, S.; Huber, M.; Taube, W. Cervical joint position sense in neck pain. Immediate effects of muscle vibration versus mental training interventions: A RCT. *Eur. J. Phys. Rehabil. Med.* **2015**, *51*, 825–832.
42. Beinert, K.; Mouthon, A.; Keller, M.; Mouthon, M.; Annoni, J.M.; Taube, W. Neural Correlates of Maladaptive Pain Behavior in Chronic Neck Pain—A Single Case Control fMRI Study. *Pain Physician* **2017**, *20*, E115–E125. [PubMed]
43. Forkmann, K.; Wiech, K.; Ritter, C.; Sommer, T.; Rose, M.; Bingel, U. Pain-Specific Modulation of Hippocampal Activity and Functional Connectivity during Visual Encoding. *J. Neurosci.* **2013**, *33*, 2571–2581. [CrossRef] [PubMed]
44. Meier, M.L.; Stämpfli, P.; Humphreys, B.K.; Vrana, A.; Seifritz, E.; Schweinhardt, P. The impact of pain-related fear on neural pathways of pain modulation in chronic low back pain. *PAIN Rep.* **2017**, *2*, 1. [CrossRef] [PubMed]
45. De-La-Puente-Ranea, L.; García-Calvo, B.; La Touche, R.; Fernández-Carnero, J.; Gil-Martínez, A. Influence of the actions observed on cervical motion in patients with chronic neck pain: A pilot study. *J. Exerc. Rehabil.* **2016**, *12*, 346–354. [CrossRef]
46. Hayashi, K.; Aono, S.; Shiro, Y.; Ushida, T. Effects of Virtual Reality-Based Exercise Imagery on Pain in Healthy Individuals. *BioMed Res. Int.* **2019**, *2019*, 5021914. [CrossRef] [PubMed]
47. Peerdeman, K.; Van Laarhoven, A.; Bartels, D.; Peters, M.; Evers, A.; Laarhoven, A. Placebo-like analgesia via response imagery. *Eur. J. Pain* **2017**, *21*, 1366–1377. [CrossRef] [PubMed]
48. Paungmali, A.; O'Leary, S.; Souvlis, T.; Vicenzino, B. Hypoalgesic and Sympathoexcitatory Effects of Mobilization with Movement for Lateral Epicondylalgia. *Phys. Ther.* **2003**, *83*, 374–383. [CrossRef] [PubMed]
49. Vicenzino, B.; Collins, D.; Benson, H.; Wright, A. An investigation of the interrelationship between manipulative therapy-induced hypoalgesia and sympathoexcitation. *J. Manip. Physiol. Ther.* **1998**, *21*, 448–453.

50. Schabrun, S.M.; Elgueta-Cancino, E.L.; Hodges, P.W. Smudging of the Motor Cortex is Related to the Severity of Low Back Pain. *Spine* **2017**, *42*, 1172–1178. [CrossRef] [PubMed]
51. Le Pera, D.; Graven-Nielsen, T.; Valeriani, M.; Oliviero, A.; Di Lazzaro, V.; Tonali, P.A.; Arendt-Nielsen, L. Inhibition of motor system excitability at cortical and spinal level by tonic muscle pain. *Clin. Neurophysiol.* **2001**, *112*, 1633–1641. [CrossRef]
52. Caspers, S.; Zilles, K.; Laird, A.R.; Eickhoff, S.B. ALE meta-analysis of action observation and imitation in the human brain. *Neuroimage* **2010**, *50*, 1148–1167. [CrossRef] [PubMed]
53. Buccino, G.; Binkofski, F.; Fink, G.R.; Fadiga, L.; Fogassi, L.; Gallese, V.; Seitz, R.J.; Zilles, K.; Rizzolatti, G.; Freund, H.J. Action observation activates premotor and parietal areas in a somatotopic manner: An fMRI study. *Eur. J. Neurosci.* **2001**, *13*, 400–404. [CrossRef] [PubMed]
54. Larsen, D.B.; Graven-Nielsen, T.; Boudreau, S.A. Pain-induced reduction in corticomotor excitability is counteracted by combined action-observation and motor imagery. *J. Pain* **2019**. [CrossRef] [PubMed]
55. Castillo Saavedra, L.; Mendonca, M.; Fregni, F. Role of the primary motor cortex in the maintenance and treatment of pain in fibromyalgia. *Med. Hypotheses* **2014**, *83*, 332–336. [CrossRef] [PubMed]
56. Volz, M.S.; Suarez-Contreras, V.; Portilla, A.L.S.; Illigens, B.; Bermpohl, F.; Fregni, F. Movement observation-induced modulation of pain perception and motor cortex excitability. *Clin. Neurophysiol.* **2015**, *126*, 1204–1211. [CrossRef] [PubMed]
57. Shimo, K.; Ueno, T.; Younger, J.; Nishihara, M.; Inoue, S.; Ikemoto, T.; Taniguchi, S.; Ushida, T. Visualization of Painful Experiences Believed to Trigger the Activation of Affective and Emotional Brain Regions in Subjects with Low Back Pain. *PLoS ONE* **2011**, *6*, e26681. [CrossRef] [PubMed]
58. La Touche, R.; Pérez-González, A.; Suso-Martí, L.; Paris-Alemany, A.; Cuenca-Martínez, F. Observing neck movements evokes an excitatory response in the sympathetic nervous system associated with fear of movement in patients with chronic neck pain. *Somatosens. Mot. Res.* **2018**, *35*, 162–169. [CrossRef] [PubMed]
59. Patterson, D.R.; Hoffman, H.G.; Palacios, A.G.; Jensen, M.J. Analgesic effects of posthypnotic suggestions and virtual reality distraction on thermal pain. *J. Abnorm. Psychol.* **2006**, *115*, 834–841. [CrossRef] [PubMed]
60. Decety, J.; Jeannerod, M.; Germain, M.; Pastene, J. Vegetative response during imagined movement is proportional to mental effort. *Behav. Brain Res.* **1991**, *42*, 1–5. [CrossRef]
61. Cuenca-Martínez, F.; Suso-Martí, L.; Grande-Alonso, M.; Paris-Alemany, A.; La Touche, R. Combining motor imagery with action observation training does not lead to a greater autonomic nervous system response than motor imagery alone during simple and functional movements: A randomized controlled trial. *PeerJ* **2018**, *6*, e5142. [CrossRef]
62. Butler, R.K.; Finn, D.P. Stress-induced analgesia. *Prog. Neurobiol.* **2009**, *88*, 184–202. [CrossRef] [PubMed]
63. Breckenridge, J.D.; Ginn, K.A.; Wallwork, S.B.; McAuley, J.H. Do People With Chronic Musculoskeletal Pain Have Impaired Motor Imagery? A Meta-analytical Systematic Review of the Left/Right Judgment Task. *J. Pain* **2019**, *20*, 119–132. [CrossRef] [PubMed]

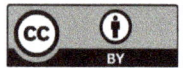

© 2019 by the authors. Licensee MDPI, Basel, Switzerland. This article is an open access article distributed under the terms and conditions of the Creative Commons Attribution (CC BY) license (http://creativecommons.org/licenses/by/4.0/).

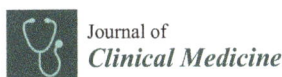

Article

Moderate and Stable Pain Reductions as a Result of Interdisciplinary Pain Rehabilitation—A Cohort Study from the Swedish Quality Registry for Pain Rehabilitation (SQRP)

Åsa Ringqvist [1], Elena Dragioti [2], Mathilda Björk [3], Britt Larsson [2] and Björn Gerdle [2,*]

1. Department of Neurosurgery and Pain Rehabilitation, Skåne University Hospital, SE-221 85 Lund, Sweden; asa.ringqvist@skane.se
2. Pain and Rehabilitation Centre, and Department of Medical and Health Sciences, Linköping University, SE-581 85 Linköping, Sweden; elena.dragioti@liu.se (E.D.); britt.larsson@liu.se (B.L.)
3. Department of Social and Welfare Studies, Linköping University, SE-602 21 Norrköping, Sweden; mathilda.bjork@liu.se
* Correspondence: bjorn.gerdle@liu.se; Tel: +46-763-927-191

Received: 10 June 2019; Accepted: 20 June 2019; Published: 24 June 2019

Abstract: Few studies have investigated the real-life outcomes of interdisciplinary multimodal pain rehabilitation programs (IMMRP) for chronic pain. This study has four aims: investigate effect sizes (ES); analyse correlation patterns of outcome changes; define a multivariate outcome measure; and investigate whether the clinical self-reported presentation pre-IMMRP predicts the multivariate outcome. To this end, this study analysed chronic pain patients in specialist care included in the Swedish Quality Registry for Pain Rehabilitation for 22 outcomes (pain, psychological distress, participation, and health) on three occasions: pre-IMMRP, post-IMMRP, and 12-month follow-up. Moderate stable ES were demonstrated for pain intensity, interference in daily life, vitality, and health; most other outcomes showed small ES. Using a Multivariate Improvement Score (MIS), we identified three clusters. Cluster 1 had marked positive MIS and was associated with the overall worst situation pre-IMMRP. However, the pre-IMMRP situation could only predict 8% of the variation in MIS. Specialist care IMPRPs showed moderate ES for pain, interference, vitality, and health. Outcomes were best for patients with the worst clinical presentation pre-IMMRP. It was not possible to predict who would clinically benefit most from IMMRP.

Keywords: chronic pain; musculoskeletal pain; patient care team; rehabilitation; treatment outcome

1. Introduction

Pain is an unpleasant experience with complex interactions between sensorimotoric, affective, and cognitive brain networks. As such, pain, especially chronic pain, is influenced by and interacts with physical, psychological, social, and contextual factors [1–3]. One-fifth of the European population has moderate to severe chronic pain conditions [4]. These conditions are associated with psychological distress, low health, sick leave, and high socioeconomic costs [5]. Therefore, a biopsychosocial (BPS) framework should be considered in clinical practice [6–8].

Unlike single/unimodal interventions, interdisciplinary multimodal pain rehabilitation programs (IMMRPs) for chronic pain—an interdisciplinary treatment according to the International Association for the Study of Pain (IASP)—distinguish themselves as well-coordinated complex interventions. Typically, IMMRPs are based on cognitive behavioural therapy (CBT) models (including Acceptance Commitment Therapy, ACT) and are administered over several weeks to months [9–12]. The Swedish programs generally include group activities such as pain education, supervised physical activity, training in simulated environments, and CBT coordinated by an interdisciplinary team (e.g., physician, occupational therapist, physiotherapist, psychologist, and social worker) based on a BPS framework [9–12]. The components of IMMRP are most often chosen based on the available evidence for unimodal interventions for chronic pain, for example, with respect to education, exercise, psychological interventions, and interventions for return to work. The core goals of rehabilitation programs in general [13] and especially for patients with chronic pain [14] are broad and multifactorial in combination with the individualised goals of the patient. These include increased ability to participate in valued activities such as work. Hence, IMMRP is a complex intervention [13,15] and, unlike pharmacological intervention, focusses on the whole person rather than just biochemical processes, implying complex patient conditions matched with complex IMMRPs [16,17]. The components of IMMRP can be active independently or interdependently [15], resulting in a combination of effects explained by known and unknown mechanisms. The effects are assumed to be greater than the sum of its components [18].

Systematic reviews (SRs) have generally reported higher efficacy both on a general level and for specific outcomes of IMMRP compared with single-treatment or treatment-as-usual programs [10,12,19–23]. SRs and Randomised Controlled Trials (RCTs) may be associated with risk for bias resulting from, for example, an unrepresentative selection of patients and researcher allegiance [24–26]. Thus, it is necessary to investigate whether the evidence obtained from SRs and RCTs can be replicated within a consecutive non-selected flow of patients in practice settings using prospective observational cohort study designs such as practice-based evidence (PBE). PBE has also been applied in the field of rehabilitation research [27]. The importance of such an approach is also emphasised in the real-effectiveness medicine framework [28]. IMMRPs are time consuming and expensive, even when most of the activities are group-based. From an ethical, individual, and socioeconomic perspective, it is indeed remarkable to note the lack of studies investigating effect sizes (ES) in patient populations in real-life practice settings. A recent study from two Swedish university clinics reported effect sizes of 0.51–0.61 (i.e., moderate ES) for two pain intensity variables at 12-month follow-up [29]. These effect sizes should be confirmed in larger studies based not only on patients at university hospitals, but also on specialist units in general. It would be motivating for patients to endure increases in pain, which is often observed in clinical practise during the start-up period of rehabilitation characterised by an increase in activity levels, if it were known that the long-term effects include the reduction of pain levels.

Complex interventions such as IMMRP should have several outcomes measured at multiple levels and strategies for handling multiple outcomes [17,30]. IMMRPs are evaluated using many outcomes. For example, one SR including 46 RCTs reported nine outcomes per RCT (median) [10]. However, outcomes are not usually divided into primary and secondary outcomes [10]. In addition, although it is most likely that changes in several of the selected outcomes are correlated, most SRs of IMMRPs evaluate the outcomes as independent from each other. Patterns of potential correlations (i.e., multivariate correlation patterns) are mainly unknown/uninvestigated, even though they could give valuable information regarding how to optimise IMMRPs. Hence, there is a need to develop clinically applicable ways to evaluate the multiple outcomes of MMPRs both for individual patients and within research studies.

The above knowledge gaps motivated this PBE study of chronic pain patients based on patient reported outcome measures (PROMs) from the Swedish Quality Registry for Pain Rehabilitation (SQRP) [31]. This registry offers an opportunity to investigate clinical outcomes and patterns of change, since all the relevant specialist care units throughout Sweden deliver data to SQRP. Hence, this PBE study has the general aim of investigating the effects of IMMRP in specialist care in Sweden considering the multivariate complexity of outcomes. We hypothesised that IMMRP in special care is associated with small-to-medium ES, that changes in outcomes generally are intercorrelated, and that the baseline situation (pre-IMMRP) can predict the multivariate outcomes. More specifically, we defined the following four aims:

- To investigate the outcome effect sizes of IMMRP immediately post-IMMRP and at 12-month follow-up.
- To analyse the multivariate correlation patterns of changes in outcomes of IMMRP: pre-IMMRP versus post IMMRP and pre-IMMRP versus 12-month follow-up.
- To define a multivariate outcome measure of IMMRP.
- To investigate if the clinical self-reported presentation pre-IMMRP can predict the multivariate outcome measure.

2. Materials and Methods

2.1. The Swedish Quality Registry for Pain Rehabilitation (SQRP)

The SQRP, recognised by the Swedish Association of Local Authorities and Regions, receives data from all specialist care units in Sweden [31]. The SQRP is based on PROM questionnaires that capture biopsychosocial data such as the patient's background, pain distribution and intensity, pain-related cognitions, and psychological distress symptoms (e.g., depression and anxiety), as well as activity/participation aspects and health-related quality of life variables. Patients complete the PROM questionnaires on up to three occasions: (1) during assessment at the first visit to the unit (pre-IMMRP); (2) immediately after the IMMRP (post-IMMRP); and (3) at the 12-month follow-up (FU) after IMMRP discharge (12-month FU).

2.2. Subjects

This study included SQRP data from women and men ≥18 years old with complex chronic (≥3 months) non-malignant pain who were referred to specialist pain and rehabilitation units (i.e., specialist care centres) between 2008–2016. These patients can be characterised as complex, as their health profiles included psychiatric comorbidities such as depression and anxiety, low levels of acceptance, high levels of kinesiophobia, decreased working life and participation in social activities, and/or did not respond to routine pharmacological/physiotherapeutic treatments delivered in a monodisciplinary fashion. Strict inclusion and exclusion criteria for inclusion in the registry is not available, since this is a registry study of patients with complex chronic pain conditions referred from mainly the primary care to specialist care in Sweden. A minority of patients were referred from other specialist clinics e.g., orthopedic and rheumatology clinics. The following general inclusion criteria for IMMRP were used: (i) disabling chronic pain (on sick leave or experiencing major interference in daily life due to chronic pain); (ii) age 18 years and above; (iii) no further medical investigations needed; and (iv) written consent to participate and attend IMMRP. General exclusion criteria for IMMRP included severe psychiatric morbidity, abuse of alcohol and/or drugs, diseases that did not allow physical exercise, and specific pain conditions with other treatment options available (i.e., red flags).

The proportions of patients within primary health care with chronic pain conditions are not exactly known, but 10–20% are estimates [32,33]. Furthermore, the proportion of chronic pain patients within primary health care that are referred to specialist clinics is not known.

The study was conducted in accordance with the Helsinki Declaration and Good Clinical Practice and approved by the Ethical Review Board in Linköping (Dnr: 2015/108-31). All the participants received written information about the study and gave their written consent.

2.3. Variables

Background variables that were collected pre-IMMRP and symptom-related self-reported variables that were collected at all three times (pre, post, and 12-month FU) were used in the analyses. The variables and instruments used are mandatory for the units registering their data with the SQRP.

Background Variables

The following background variables were collected: age (years), gender (man or woman), education level, and country of birth. Education level was dichotomised into university and the other alternatives (i.e., upper secondary school, elementary school, or other); this variable was labelled as University. Country of birth was dichotomised as from Europe and outside Europe and labelled as Outside-Europe. In addition, self-reported pain duration (days), persistent pain duration (days), and number of days off work (Days no work) were obtained.

Pain distribution was registered using 36 predefined anatomical areas (18 on the front and 18 on the back of the body) and the patients registered the areas with pain: (1) head/face, (2) neck, (3) shoulder, (4) upper arm, (5) elbow, (6) forearm, (7) hand, (8) anterior aspect of chest, (9) lateral aspect of chest, (10) belly, (11) sexual organs, (12) upper back, (13) low back, (14) hip/gluteal area, (15) thigh, (16) knee, (17) shank, and (18) foot. The number of areas with pain (range: 1–36) were summed, and the obtained variable was denoted as the Pain Region Index (PRI).

2.4. Repeated Self-Reported Measures

For reports of the psychometric aspects of the self-reported measures, the reader is referred to other studies summarising these [7,34–36].

2.4.1. Pain Aspects

Pain intensity average during the previous seven days was registered using a 0–10 (0 = no pain and 10 = worst possible pain) numeric rating scale (NRS)—NRS-7days.

2.4.2. The Multidimensional Pain Inventory (MPI)

MPI is a 61-item self-report questionnaire that measures the psychosocial, cognitive, and behavioural effects of chronic pain [37,38]. Part 1 consists of five scales: Pain severity—measuring several aspects of the pain experience (MPI-Pain-severity); Interference—pain-related interference in everyday life (MPI-Pain-interfer); Perceived Life Control (MPI-LifeCon); the level of affective distress (MPI-Distress); and Social Support—perceived support from a spouse or significant others (MPI-SocSupp). Part 2 assesses the perception of responses to displays of pain and suffering from significant others and consists of three scales: Punishing Responses (MPI-Punish); Solicitous Responses (MPI-Solict); and Distracting Responses (MPI-Distract). Part 3 measures to what extent the patients participate in various activities using four scales. These scales can be combined into a composite scale—the General Activity Index (MPI-GAI)—which was used in the present study [39].

2.4.3. Psychological Distress Variables

Symptoms of anxiety and depression were registered using the Hospital Anxiety and Depression Scale (HADS) [40,41]. This instrument comprises seven items in each of two subscales: depression (HADS-D) and anxiety (HADS-A) symptoms. Both subscale scores have a range of 0 to 21. A score of 7 or less in each subscale indicates a non-case, a score of 8–10 indicates a possible case, and a score of 11 or more indicates an almost definite case [40].

2.4.4. The Short Form Health Survey (SF36)

The Short Form Health Survey (SF36) attempts to represent multidimensional health concepts and measurements of the full range of health states, including levels of well-being and personal evaluations of health [42]. Scores are standardised into eight dimensions with a scale from 0 to 100 where higher scores indicate a better perception of health [42]: (1) physical functioning (sf36-pf), physical activity level including activities of daily living; (2) role limitations due to physical functioning (sf36-rp), to what extent physical health limits the performance of work and other regular activities; (3) bodily pain (sf36-bp), pain and related disability; (4) general health (sf36-gh), evaluation of health situation;

(5) vitality (sf36-vt), how rested and energetic; (6) social functioning (sf36-sf), disturbances of social life due to physical or mental illness; (7) role limitations due to emotional problems (sf36-re), difficulties in performing work or other regular activities due to emotional problems; and (8) mental health (sf36-mh), anxiety and depressive symptoms. Based on the eight scales, a physical summary component and a mental (psychological) summary component can be calculated, but these two summary component variables were not used in the present study.

2.4.5. The European Quality of Life Instrument (EQ-5D)

The European Quality of Life Instrument (EQ-5D) captures a patient's perceived state of health [43–45]. The first part of the instrument defines five dimensions: mobility, self-care, usual activities, pain/discomfort, and anxiety/depression. Each of these were measured at three levels. An EQ-5D-index is derived by applying a formula that essentially attaches values (weights) to each of the levels in each dimension. The collection of index values (weights) for all the possible EQ-5D states is called a value set. Most EQ-5D value sets have been obtained from a standardised valuation exercise where a representative sample of the general population in a country/region is asked to place a value on EQ-5D health states. The EQ5D also measures the self-estimation of today's health according to a 100-point scale, which is a thermometer-like scale (EQ-VAS) with defined end points (high values indicate good health and low values indicate bad health).

2.4.6. Estimations of Changes in Pain and in Life Situation

The patients post-IMMRP and at the 12-month FU estimated the degree of positive change in pain (Change-pain) and in their ability to handle life situations in general (Change-life situation). The Change-pain item was rated on a five-point Likert scale from markedly increased pain (0) to markedly decreased pain (4). The Change-life situation item was rated on a five-point Likert scale from markedly worsened (0) to markedly improved (4).

2.5. Statistics

All the statistics were performed using the statistical package IBM SPSS Statistics (version 24.0) and SIMCA-P+ (version 15.0; Umetrics Inc., Umeå, Sweden). A probability of <0.001 (two-tailed) was accepted as the criteria for significance due to the large number of subjects.

The text and tables generally report the mean value ± one standard deviation (±1 SD) together with a median and range of continuous variables. Percentages (%) are reported for categorical variables. The detailed analyses also report 95% confidence intervals (95% CI). SQRP uses predetermined rules when handling single missing items of a scale or a subscale; details about this have been reported elsewhere [29]. To compare groups, we used Student's t-test for unpaired observations, analysis of variance (ANOVA with post hoc test if significant difference), and Chi square test. Effect sizes (ES; Cohen's d) for within-group analysis were computed using a calculator when appropriate (https://webpower.psychstat.org/models/means01/effectsize.php). Hedges' g, which provides a measure of effect size weighted according to the relative size of each sample, was used for between ES using a calculator (https://www.socscistatistics.com/effectsize/default3.aspx). The absolute effect size was considered very large for values ≥ 1.3, large for values between 0.80–1.29, moderate for values between 0.50–0.79, small for values between 0.20–0.49, and insignificant for values < 0.20 [46].

Common methods such as logistic regression (LR) and multiple linear regression (MLR) can quantify the level of relations of individual factors but disregard interrelationships among different factors and thereby ignore system-wide aspects [47]. Moreover, such methods assume variable independence when interpreting results [48], and there are several risks when considering one variable at a time [49]. To account for our aims, the problems related to handling missing data (see below), and the risks associated with multicollinearity problems (see above), we used advanced multivariate analyses (MVDA).

Hence, using SIMCA-P+, we applied advanced Principal Component Analysis (PCA) for the multivariate correlation analyses of all investigated variables and Orthogonal Partial Least Square Regressions (OPLS) for the multivariate regressions. These techniques do not require normal distributions of the included variables [50]. Note that the PCA of SIMCA-P+ differs considerably from the simpler version implemented (e.g., the version used in SPSS).

PCA extracts and displays systematic variation in the data matrix. All the variables were log transformed before the statistical analyses if data were skewed. Using PCA, we analysed the multivariate correlation pattern for the changes in the 22 outcome variables for all the subjects. Note that changes in outcomes are calculated so that a positive value indicates an improvement. A cross-validation technique was used to identify nontrivial components (p). Variables loading on the same component p were correlated, and variables with high loadings but with opposing signs were negatively correlated. Variables with high absolute loadings were considered significant. The obtained components are per definition not correlated and are arranged in decreasing order with respect to explained variation. The loading plot reports the multivariate relationships between variables. A corresponding plot reporting the relationships between subjects (i.e., t-scores) can also be used (score plot), and each subject receives a score (t) for each of the significant components. The t-score was used to calculate a Multivariate Improvement Score (MIS). R^2 describes the goodness of fit—the fraction of sum of squares of all the variables explained by a principal component [51]. Q^2 describes the goodness of prediction—the fraction of the total variation of the variables that can be predicted using principal component cross-validation methods [51]. Outliers were identified using two methods: score plots in combination with Hotelling's T^2 and distance to model in the X-space. No extreme outliers were detected.

OPLS was used for the longitudinal multivariate regression analyses of the t-scores of the PCA mentioned above using pre-IMMRP data (i.e., baseline data) [51]. The variable influence on projection (VIP) indicates the relevance of each X-variable pooled over all dimensions and Y-variables—the group of variables that best explain Y. VIP ≥ 1.0 was considered significant if VIP had a 95% jack-knife uncertainty confidence interval non-equal to zero. p(corr) was used to note the direction of the relationship (positive or negative). This is the loading of each variable scaled as a correlation coefficient, and thus standardising the range from −1 to +1. [50] p(corr) is stable during iterative variable selection and comparable between models [50]. Thus, a variable/regressor was considered significant when VIP > 1.0. For each regression, we report R^2, Q^2, and the p-value of a cross-validated analysis of variance (CV-ANOVA). SIMCA-P+ uses the Non-linear Iterative Partial Least Squares (NIPALS) algorithm to handle missing data: maximum 50% missing data for variables/scales and maximum 50% missing data for subjects.

To identify clusters based on the t-scores of the PCA mentioned above, we performed hierarchical clustering analysis (HCA). Based on the identified clusters (subgroups) defined by HCA, we performed partial least squares discriminant analysis (PLS-DA). In addition, we applied a bottom–up HCA to the principal component score vectors using the default Ward linkage criterion to identify relevant subgroups of patients. HCA can find subtle clusters in the multivariate space. In the resulting dendrogram, clusters were identified and, based on these groups, we performed PLS-DA using group belonging as the Y-variable and the psychometric data as predictors (X-variables). The PLS-DA model was computed to identify associations between the X-variables and the subgroups. Based on the HCA defined clusters, traditional inferential statistics (ANOVA including post hoc tests when appropriate) were computed using SPSS.

3. Results

3.1. Background Data

There were 14,666 chronic pain patients registered in the SQRP that fulfilled the inclusion criteria: chronic pain; >18 years of age; and completed the SQRP questionnaire before and on at least one of the two time points after the IMMRP. More than half (60%) of the patients answering the questionnaires pre-IMMRP and post-IMMRP also answered the questionnaires at 12-m FU. Most of the patients (76.3%) were women, 25.2% had studied at university, and 10.4% were born outside of Europe. More men were born outside Europe (men: 13.4% versus women: 9.5%; Chi^2 = 43.437, $p < 0.001$), and fewer men had university education (men: 18.0% versus women: 27.4%; Chi^2 = 123.672; $p < 0.001$). Continuous background variables are shown in Table 1. Women were slightly younger than men (42.9 ± 10.7 versus 44.5 ± 10.7; $p < 0.001$) and reported more spreading of pain according to PRI (15.4 ± 8.8 versus 10.8 ± 7.0; $p < 0.001$). The other variables in Table 2 were not affected by gender.

Table 1. Continuous background variables; mean ± SD and 95% confidence intervals (95% CI).

Variables	Mean ± SD	95% CI Lower Bound	95% CI Upper Bound
Age (years)	43.2 ± 10.7	43.3	43.9
Days no work	1055 ± 2461	968	1095
Pain duration	3057 ± 3341	2970	3170
Persistent pain duration	2368 ± 2980	2239	2414
PRI	15.4 ± 8.6	15.1	15.6

Notes: SD = standard deviation; CI = confidence intervals; PRI = Pain Region Index.

Table 2. Outcome variables at baseline (pre-IMMRP) and immediately after IMMRP (post-IMMRP). Statistical comparisons are presented furthest to the right together with effects sizes (i.e., Cohen's d). Effect sizes in bold were moderate, i.e., Cohen's d ≥ 0.50. IMMRP: interdisciplinary multimodal pain rehabilitation programs.

Baseline vs. After IMMRP		Pre-IMMRP		Post-IMMRP			
	N	Mean	SD	Mean	SD	p-Value	Cohen's d
NRS-7days	14,146	6.86	1.72	5.95	2.09	<0.001	0.45
HADS-A	14,774	9.00	4.76	7.78	4.55	<0.001	0.32
HADS-D	14,772	8.49	4.44	6.70	4.31	<0.001	0.47
MPI-Pain-severity	14,692	4.39	0.93	3.87	1.16	<0.001	**0.52**
MPI-Pain-interfer	14,552	4.38	1.02	3.94	1.19	<0.001	0.49
MPI-LifeCon	14,687	2.72	1.10	3.30	1.18	<0.001	0.47
MPI-Distress	14,697	3.46	1.26	2.89	1.38	<0.001	0.42
MPI-Socsupp	14,618	4.16	1.34	3.95	1.35	<0.001	0.21
MPI-punish	13,054	1.74	1.36	1.72	1.33	0.037	0.02
MPI-protect	12,999	2.98	1.40	2.85	1.38	<0.001	0.12
MPI-distract	13,048	2.54	1.19	2.56	1.17	0.043	0.02
MPI-GAI	14,676	2.44	0.84	2.63	0.82	<0.001	0.26
EQ-5D-index	13,989	0.26	0.31	0.39	0.33	<0.001	0.40
EQ-VAS	13,777	41.22	19.09	50.99	21.38	<0.001	0.44
sf36-pf	14,253	52.76	20.58	57.67	21.17	<0.001	0.30
sf36-rp	13,945	12.53	24.40	22.46	33.12	<0.001	0.30
sf36-bp	14,268	24.36	14.49	32.96	17.41	<0.001	**0.52**
sf36-gh	13,988	41.70	20.22	46.69	21.88	<0.001	0.29
sf36-vt	14,206	23.95	18.48	35.67	22.76	<0.001	**0.54**
sf36-sf	14,229	47.29	25.19	54.93	25.91	<0.001	0.30
sf36-re	13,701	42.77	42.92	51.15	43.48	<0.001	0.18
sf36-mh	14,194	55.03	21.35	62.55	21.55	<0.001	0.38

NRS-7days = Pain intensity as measured by a numeric rating scale for the previous seven days; HADS = Hospital Anxiety and Depression Scale; MPI = Multidimensional Pain Inventory; EQ-5D-index = The index of the European quality of life instrument; EQ-VAS = The European quality of life instrument thermometer-like scale; sf36 = The Short Form (36) Health Survey. For explanations of the subscale abbreviations, see Methods.

3.2. Pairwise Comparisons of Repeated Measures

The results for pre-IMMRP and post-IMMRP are shown in Table 2. Significant improvements were generally found except for two of the three scales of the second part of the MPI. In addition, the comparisons between pre-IMMRP and the 12-month FU generally revealed significant improvements except for one of the scales on the second part of the MPI (Table 3). Some outcomes were associated with moderate effect sizes. For the pre-IMMRP versus post-IMMRP comparisons, three variables had moderate effects sizes: MPI-pain-severity, sf36-bp, and sf36-vt (Table 2). At the 12-month FU, MPI-pain-severity and sf36-bp were associated with moderate effect sizes; this was also the case for MPI-pain-interference and EQ5d-index (Table 3). However, generally small effect sizes were found for the significant improvements (Tables 2 and 3). The variables of the second part of the MPI had insignificant effect sizes both post-IMMRP and 12-month FU.

Table 3. Outcome variables at baseline (pre-IMMRP) and at the 12-month follow-up (FU). Statistical comparisons are presented furthest to the right together with effects sizes (i.e., Cohen's d). Effect sizes in bold were moderate (i.e., Cohen's d ≥ 0.50).

Baseline vs. 12-Month Follow-Up		Pre IMMRP		12-Month FU			
	N	Mean	SD	Mean	SD	p-Value	Cohen's d
NRS-7days	8568	6.84	1.72	5.78	2.32	<0.001	0.47
HADS-A	8865	8.73	4.69	7.38	4.70	<0.001	0.33
HADS-D	8865	8.18	4.37	6.74	4.66	<0.001	0.35
MPI-Pain-severity	8904	4.36	0.91	3.71	1.33	<0.001	**0.56**
MPI-Pain-interfer	8829	4.34	1.02	3.73	1.37	<0.001	**0.54**
MPI-LifeCon	8871	2.77	1.10	3.28	1.27	<0.001	0.40
MPI-Distress	8889	3.42	1.27	2.92	1.45	<0.001	0.35
MPI-Socsupp	8830	4.17	1.33	3.77	1.42	<0.001	0.35
MPI-punish	7824	1.69	1.34	1.69	1.35	0.676	0.01
MPI-protect	7784	2.96	1.39	2.78	1.40	<0.001	0.16
MPI-distract	7811	2.52	1.17	2.45	1.17	<0.001	0.06
MPI-GAI	8859	2.47	0.83	2.64	0.86	<0.001	0.20
EQ-5D-index	8844	0.27	0.31	0.44	0.34	<0.001	**0.50**
EQ-VAS	8607	41.90	19.29	52.96	22.87	<0.001	0.46
sf36-pf	8459	53.07	20.30	59.73	22.57	<0.001	0.36
sf36-rp	8301	13.07	24.91	27.74	36.32	<0.001	0.39
sf36-bp	8458	24.60	14.11	35.41	20.05	<0.001	**0.56**
sf36-gh	8342	42.59	20.49	47.35	23.52	<0.001	0.25
sf36-vt	8441	24.96	18.79	34.41	23.85	<0.001	0.41
sf36-sf	8459	48.95	25.50	57.66	27.05	<0.001	0.32
sf36-re	8159	44.69	43.17	55.60	43.53	<0.001	0.22
sf36-mh	8435	56.34	21.15	62.70	22.53	<0.001	0.30

NRS-7days = Pain intensity as measured by a numeric rating scale for the previous seven days; HADS = Hospital Anxiety and Depression Scale; MPI = Multidimensional Pain Inventory; EQ-5D-index = The index of the European quality of life instrument; EQ-VAS = The European quality of life instrument thermometer-like scale; sf36 = The Short Form (36); Health Survey; FU = Follow-up. For explanations of the subscale abbreviations see Methods.

3.3. Patients Not Participating in the 12-Month FU

There were only small differences between those reporting PROM data at the 12-month FU and those not reporting their situation pre-IMMRP (Supplementary Table S1). Although those not reporting had a somewhat worse situation for most of the PROM variables, the differences were of no clinical importance.

3.4. Estimations of Changes in Pain and in Life Situation

At both post-IMMRP and 12-month FU, most patients reported that their pain situation had improved as well as their ability to handle their life situation (Table 4).

Table 4. Estimations of pain situation (Change-pain) and in the ability to handle life situation in general (Change-life situation) made immediately after IMMRP (post-IMMRP) and at the 12-month FU.

Change-Pain	Post-IMMRP		12-Month FU	
	n	%	n	%
0. Markedly increased pain	447	3.2	225	2.6
1. Partially increased pain	1517	11	590	6.9
2. No change	4008	29.1	2905	34
3. Partially diminished pain	6178	44.9	3662	42.8
4. Markedly diminished pain	1607	11.7	1174	13.7
Total	13 757	100	8 556	100
Change-Life situation	**Post-IMMRP**		**12-Month FU**	
	n	%	n	%
0. Markedly deteriorated	74	0.5	108	1.3
1. Partially deteriorated	248	1.8	282	3.3
2. No change	1923	13.9	1615	18.8
3. Partially improved	8412	60.9	4628	54
4. Markedly improved	3161	22.9	1937	22.6
Total	13 818	100	8 570	100

FU = Follow-up.

3.5. Multivariate Correlation Pattern of Changes in Outcomes

PCAs of the changes (i.e., the difference) were performed for pre-IMMRP versus post-IMMRP and pre-IMMRP versus 12-month FU. Significant models were achieved for both analyses (Table 5). Similar patterns were obtained for the first significant component of the two PCAs (Table 5). The first component of both analyses, reflecting the most important variations, showed that changes in HAD-D, MPI-pain-severity, MPI-pain interference, MPI-control, MPI-distress, sf-36-bp, sf-36-vt, sf-36-sf, and sf36-mh were most important and intercorrelated significantly. Hence, it was obvious that the changes in outcome variables are intercorrelated. That is, rather than representing 22 independent variables, the multivariate analyses show that most changes in these variables are highly intercorrelated.

At 12-month FU, the PCA also identified two additional components (Table 5). The second component mainly reflected the intercorrelation pattern between the social support scale of the MPI and the scales of part 2 of the MPI. A third significant component only explaining 6% of the variation in the dataset was also obtained in the analysis of changes at the 12-month follow-up versus baseline (Table 5).

The loading plot (i.e., the intercorrelations between variables of the two most important components for the changes pre IMMRP versus 12-month FU) is shown in Figure 1 (Figure 1a is a graphic presentation of the first two components reported in Table 5). Figure 1b shows the corresponding score plot (i.e., the relationships between subjects/patients). Each patient can be described with a score (*t*-score) for each significant component. Patients with high positive *t*-scores on the first component show prominent changes in the important variables constituting the first component, whereas patients near zero do not benefit, and patients with negative *t*-scores (located to the left in the score plot) deteriorate in the multivariate context. Hence, the *t*-score of the first component of both analyses can be considered as a Multivariate Improvement Score, in the following denoted MIS-post-IMMRP and MIS-12-month FU.

Table 5. Principal component analysis (PCA) of changes pre-IMMRP vs. post-IMMRP (left part) and pre-IMMRP vs. 12-month FU (right part). The significant components (p) are shown. Absolute loadings ≥ 0.25 are shown in bold to facilitate interpretation. Changes in outcomes are calculated so that a positive value indicates an improvement.

	Changes Pre-IMMRP vs. Post-IMMRP	Changes Pre-IMMRP vs. 12-Month FU		
	p[1]	p[1]	p[2]	p[3]
diff-NRS-7days	0.23	0.23	−0.15	**0.29**
diff-HADS-A	0.23	0.22	0.19	**−0.33**
diff-HADS-D	**0.26**	**0.25**	0.17	−0.24
diff-MPI-Pain-sever	**0.27**	**0.27**	−0.16	**0.26**
diff-MPI-Pain-interfer	**0.26**	**0.28**	−0.11	0.10
diff-MPI-LifeCon	**0.26**	**0.25**	0.09	−0.05
diff-MPI-distress	**0.27**	**0.26**	0.13	−0.21
diff-MPI-SOCsupp	−0.03	−0.07	**0.41**	0.21
diff-MPI-punish	0.07	0.08	**0.32**	0.11
diff-MPI-protect	−0.02	−0.02	**0.51**	**0.33**
diff-MPI-distract	0.01	0.00	**0.45**	**0.36**
diff-MPI-GAI	0.12	0.15	0.00	0.07
diff-EQ-5D-index	0.22	0.22	−0.07	0.12
diff-EQ-VAS	0.22	0.23	−0.03	0.09
diff-sf36-pf	0.20	0.21	−0.14	0.20
diff-sf36-rp	0.19	0.21	−0.10	0.17
diff-sf36-bp	**0.26**	**0.27**	−0.15	**0.25**
diff-sf36-gh	0.21	0.21	0.02	0.02
diff-sf36-vt	**0.27**	**0.26**	0.03	−0.03
diff-sf36-sf	**0.25**	0.24	0.05	−0.09
diff-sf36-re	0.18	0.17	0.13	**−0.26**
diff-sf36-mh	**0.27**	**0.25**	0.21	**−0.30**
R^2	0.31	0.36	0.10	0.06
Q^2	0.25	0.31	0.04	0.02
N	14,666	8851		

diff = change in a certain variable; *p* = principal component; NRS-7days = Pain intensity as measured by a numeric rating scale for the previous seven days; HADS = Hospital Anxiety and Depression Scale; MPI = Multidimensional Pain Inventory; EQ-5D-index = The index of the European quality of life instrument; EQ-VAS = The European quality of life instrument thermometer-like scale; sf36 = The Short Form (36) Health Survey; FU = Follow-up. For explanations of the subscale abbreviations see Methods.

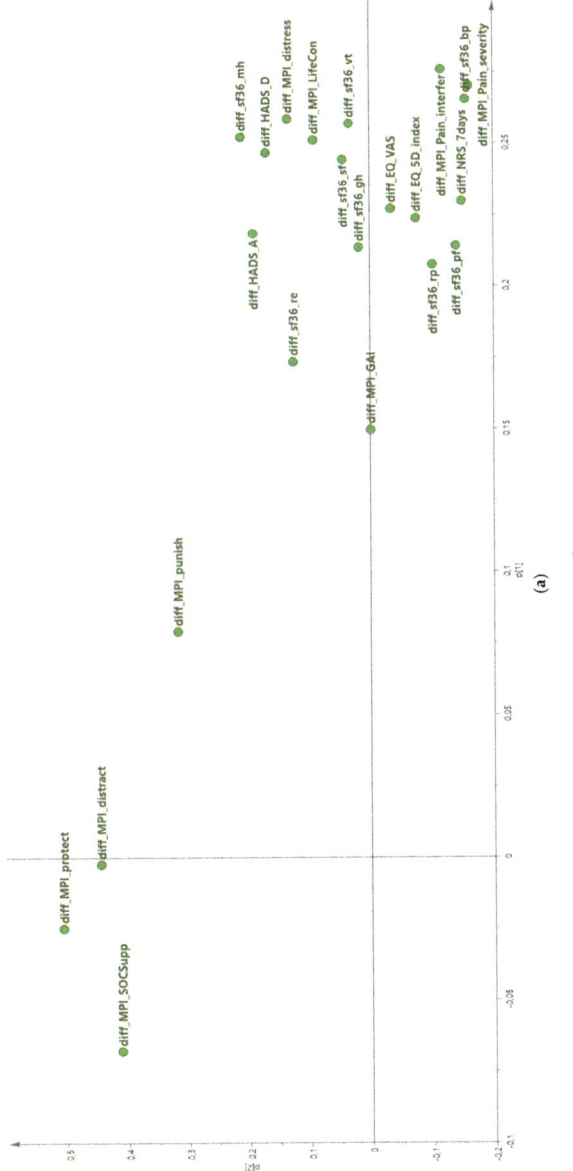

Figure 1. *Cont.*

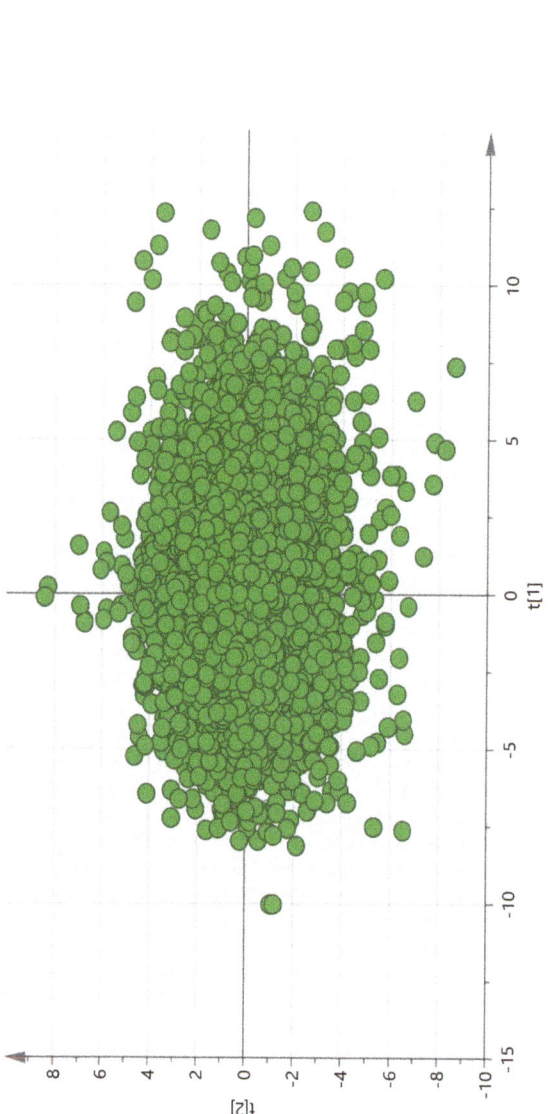

Figure 1. Loading plot of changes (pre-IMMRP vs. 12-month follow-up) in the 22 outcome variables—i.e., the relationships between the changes (**a**) and score plot ((**b**); the relationships between the patients). diff = change in a certain variable; NRS-7days = Pain intensity as measured by a numeric rating scale for the previous seven days; HADS = Hospital Anxiety and Depression Scale; MPI = Multidimensional Pain Inventory; EQ-5D-index = The index of the European quality of life instrument; EQ-VAS = The European quality of life instrument thermometer-like scale; sf36 = The Short Form (36) Health Survey; For explanations of the subscale abbreviations, see Methods.

3.6. Identification of Subgroups Based on the Multivariate Improvement Scores (MIS)

An HCA based on MIS-post-IMMRP was performed. Three subgroups/clusters were identified. Based on the HCA, a PLS-DA model with two predictive components was obtained with group belonging as the Y-variable (R^2 = 0.35; Q^2 = 0.35; CV-ANOVA $p < 0.001$; $n = 14,666$). Using a similar approach, we performed an HCA based on MIS-12-month FU. This analysis identified three subgroups/clusters. Based on the HCA, a PLS-DA model with two predictive components was obtained with group belonging as the Y-variable (R^2 = 0.37; Q^2 = 0.37; CV-ANOVA $p < 0.001$; $n = 8851$).

The MIS (i.e., t-score) showed clear positive values (i.e., improvements) for cluster 1 and negative scores (i.e., deterioration) for cluster 3 (Tables 6 and 7). Cluster 2 was an intermediary cluster with overall slightly positive improvements. Prominent effect sizes in the pairwise comparisons were observed post-IMMRP: cluster 1 versus cluster 2 = 3.33; cluster 1 versus cluster 3 = 5.36; and cluster 2 versus cluster 3 = 2.77; 12-month FU: cluster 1 versus cluster 2 = 2.92; cluster 1 versus cluster 3 = 4.99; and cluster 2 versus cluster 3 = 2.34. Thus, distinct differences in improvement levels were detected between the three clusters.

To facilitate the understanding of the identified clusters, the clusters were compared for the variables in each PCA (Tables 6 and 7). The three clusters differed significantly for all changes according to the ANOVAs performed. The post hoc tests showed that 20 of the 22 changes post-IMMRP differed significantly between all three clusters. The corresponding figure at 12-month FU was 21 of 22 changes.

The estimations of changes in pain (Change-pain) and in management of life (Change-life situation) were not included in the PCAs and thus not included in the calculations of MIS. However, these estimations showed a similar pattern: the most prominent positive changes were in cluster 1, and the least positive changes were in cluster 3 (Tables 6 and 7).

In the next step, the identified three clusters of both analyses were compared for their pre-IMMRP values (Tables 8 and 9). For the clusters obtained post-IMMRP (Table 8), small irrelevant cluster differences existed for age. The proportion with university education was significantly highest in cluster 1 and lowest in cluster 3, although the differences were small. Generally, cluster 1 was associated with the worst situation for the most variables followed longitudinally except for social support, two of the scales of Section 2 of the MPI, and sf36-pf. In contrast, cluster 3 had the best situation, and cluster 2 was intermediate (Table 8). A very similar pattern was found when using the clusters obtained from the 12-month FU (Table 9).

Table 6. Clusters from hierarchical clustering analysis (HCA) based on Multivariate Improvement Score (MIS) (*t*-scores) of the first component of the PCA for the changes in outcomes from pre-IMMRP to post-IMMRP (denoted *MIS post-IMMRP*). To facilitate understanding, the changes for all the outcomes are shown (mean, SD, and 95% confidence interval). The two bottom rows show the estimations of changes (not included in PCA and the calculation of MIS).

Variables	Cluster 1 (15.0%)					Cluster 2 (54.1%)					Cluster 3 (30.8%)					ANOVA	Post Hoc
	N	Mean	SD	95% CI LB	95% CI UB	N	Mean	SD	95% CI LB	95% CI UB	N	Mean	SD	95% CI LB	95% CI UB	*p*-Value	
MIS post-IMMRP	2205	*4.37*	*1.61*	*4.31*	*4.44*	7938	*0.33*	*1.08*	*0.30*	*0.35*	4523	*−2.74*	*1.16*	*−2.78*	*−2.71*	*<0.001*	*all different*
diff-NRS-7days	2086	3.04	2.05	2.95	3.13	7511	1.01	1.69	0.97	1.04	4267	−0.28	1.58	−0.32	−0.23	<0.001	all different
diff-HADS-A	2191	5.12	3.72	4.96	5.28	7873	1.59	3.08	1.52	1.66	4458	−1.30	3.24	−1.39	−1.20	<0.001	all different
diff-HADS-D	2188	5.93	3.55	5.78	6.08	7869	2.24	2.95	2.17	2.30	4462	−0.96	3.04	−1.05	−0.87	<0.001	all different
diff-MPI-Pain-severity	2185	1.77	1.02	1.73	1.82	7874	0.56	0.74	0.54	0.58	4500	−0.17	0.69	−0.19	−0.15	<0.001	all different
diff-MPI-Pain-interfer	2173	1.53	0.99	1.49	1.57	7811	0.50	0.70	0.48	0.51	4453	−0.17	0.66	−0.18	−0.15	<0.001	all different
diff-MPI-LifeCon	2189	1.94	1.05	1.89	1.98	7861	0.71	0.96	0.69	0.73	4491	−0.33	0.99	−0.36	−0.30	<0.001	all different
diff-MPI-distress	2187	2.18	1.17	2.13	2.23	7869	0.71	1.02	0.69	0.73	4487	−0.46	1.05	−0.49	−0.43	<0.001	all different
diff-MPI-SOCsupp	2180	−0.34	1.12	−0.39	−0.30	7828	−0.24	0.98	−0.26	−0.21	4462	−0.11	0.98	−0.14	−0.08	<0.001	all different
diff-MPI-punish	1991	0.39	1.20	0.34	0.45	7016	0.04	1.12	0.02	0.07	4008	−0.20	1.15	−0.24	−0.17	<0.001	all different
diff-MPI-protect	1988	−0.18	1.17	−0.23	−0.13	6984	−0.14	1.00	−0.17	−0.12	3989	−0.05	1.05	−0.09	−0.02	<0.001	cl1 NE cl2, cl2 NE cl3
diff-MPI-distract	1992	0.11	1.10	0.06	0.16	7012	0.00	0.96	−0.03	0.02	4006	0.01	1.03	−0.02	0.04	<0.001	cl1 NE cl2, cl3
diff-MPI-GAI	2187	0.57	0.82	0.53	0.60	7866	0.23	0.68	0.21	0.24	4489	−0.06	0.69	−0.08	−0.03	<0.001	all different
diff-EQ-5D-index	2105	0.44	0.30	0.43	0.45	7494	0.16	0.28	0.15	0.17	4205	−0.07	0.28	−0.08	−0.06	<0.001	all different
diff-EQ-VAS	2068	30.51	19.66	29.66	31.36	7409	11.61	18.58	11.19	12.03	4126	−3.84	19.15	−4.42	−3.25	<0.001	all different
diff-sf36-pf	2147	18.74	16.97	18.02	19.46	7644	6.02	13.63	5.72	6.33	4324	−3.83	14.22	−4.25	−3.40	<0.001	all different
diff-sf36-rp	2110	39.93	39.28	38.25	41.60	7513	10.46	29.70	9.79	11.13	4215	−5.96	25.56	−6.74	−5.19	<0.001	all different
diff-sf36-bp	2146	28.04	16.27	27.35	28.73	7663	9.72	12.96	9.43	10.01	4323	−2.93	12.38	−3.30	−2.56	<0.001	all different
diff-sf36-gh	2126	21.06	17.59	20.31	21.81	7529	6.05	14.51	5.72	6.37	4235	−4.89	14.57	−5.33	−4.45	<0.001	all different
diff-sf36-vt	2139	37.45	18.74	36.65	38.24	7626	13.58	17.26	13.19	13.96	4311	−4.20	16.16	−4.69	−3.72	<0.001	all different
diff-sf36-sf	2146	34.26	22.17	33.32	35.20	7652	10.12	20.39	9.66	10.58	4324	−9.86	21.10	−10.49	−9.23	<0.001	all different
diff-sf36-re	2087	43.52	44.58	41.60	45.43	7390	11.98	43.21	11.00	12.97	4121	−15.81	42.02	−17.09	−14.52	<0.001	all different
diff-sf36-mh	2139	29.61	17.48	28.86	30.35	7620	10.12	14.90	9.78	10.45	4307	−8.01	15.89	−8.49	−7.54	<0.001	all different
Change-Pain	2059	3.28	0.69	3.25	3.31	7280	2.53	0.87	2.51	2.55	4015	2.08	0.93	2.05	2.11	<0.001	all different
Change-Life situation	2067	3.51	0.58	3.48	3.53	7315	3.07	0.63	3.05	3.08	4032	2.76	0.72	2.74	2.79	<0.001	all different

LB = Lower Bound; UB = Upper Bound; diff = change in a certain variable; NRS-7days = Pain intensity as measured by a numeric rating scale for the previous seven days; HADS = Hospital Anxiety and Depression Scale; MPI = Multidimensional Pain Inventory; EQ-5D-index = The index of the European quality of life instrument; EQ-VAS = The European quality of life instrument thermometer-like scale; sf36 = The Short Form (36) Health Survey. For explanations of the subscale abbreviations, see Methods.

Table 7. Clusters from HCA based on MIS (*t*-scores) of the first component of the PCA for the changes in outcomes from pre-IMMRP to 12-month FU (denoted as *MIS 12-m FU*). To facilitate understanding, the changes for all the outcomes are shown (mean, SD, and 95% confidence interval). The two bottom rows show the estimations of changes (not included in PCA and the calculation of MIS).

Variables	Cluster 1 (12.4%)					Cluster 2 (46.6%)					Cluster 3 (41.0%)					ANOVA	Post Hoc
	N	Mean	SD	95% CI LB	UB	N	Mean	SD	95% CI LB	UB	N	Mean	SD	95% CI LB	UB	*p*-Value	
MIS -12-*m* FU	**1099**	**5.01**	**1.78**	**4.90**	**5.11**	**4123**	**0.78**	**1.35**	**0.74**	**0.82**	**3629**	**−2.43**	**1.39**	**−2.47**	**−2.38**	**<0.001**	**all different**
diff-NRS-7days	1031	3.67	2.15	3.54	3.80	3876	1.46	1.89	1.40	1.52	3435	−0.16	1.66	−0.21	−0.10	<0.001	all different
diff-HADS-A	1095	5.72	3.84	5.49	5.95	4087	2.06	3.34	1.96	2.16	3588	−0.80	3.53	−0.91	−0.68	<0.001	all different
diff-HADS-D	1096	6.13	3.75	5.90	6.35	4086	2.39	3.13	2.29	2.48	3588	−1.05	3.39	−1.16	−0.94	<0.001	all different
diff-MPI-Pain-severity	1092	2.30	1.14	2.24	2.37	4108	0.88	0.90	0.85	0.91	3619	−0.09	0.76	−0.12	−0.07	<0.001	all different
diff-MPI-Pain-interfer	1092	2.30	1.14	2.24	2.37	4108	0.88	0.90	0.85	0.91	3589	−0.14	0.74	−0.17	−0.12	<0.001	all different
diff-MPI-LifeCon	1086	2.27	1.10	2.21	2.34	4076	0.83	0.85	0.81	0.86	3604	−0.25	1.05	−0.28	−0.21	<0.001	all different
diff-MPI-distress	1091	2.10	1.10	2.03	2.16	4095	0.75	1.00	0.71	0.78	3618	−0.38	1.13	−0.41	−0.34	<0.001	all different
diff-MPI-SOCsupp	1086	−0.69	1.25	−0.77	−0.62	4081	−0.60	1.16	−0.64	−0.57	3583	−0.10	1.04	−0.13	−0.07	<0.001	all different
diff-MPI-punish	979	0.57	1.19	0.50	0.65	3633	−0.02	1.22	−0.06	0.02	3194	−0.13	1.22	−0.18	−0.09	<0.001	all different
diff-MPI-protect	980	−0.23	1.24	−0.31	−0.15	3616	−0.35	1.20	−0.39	−0.31	3173	0.03	1.09	−0.01	0.06	<0.001	all different
diff-MPI-distract	981	0.02	1.15	−0.05	0.10	3627	−0.22	1.09	−0.25	−0.18	3188	0.08	1.02	0.04	0.11	<0.001	Cl.NE cl3, cl2 NE cl3
diff-MPI-GAI	1090	0.76	0.95	0.70	0.82	4094	0.26	0.73	0.23	0.28	3613	−0.11	0.73	−0.14	−0.09	<0.001	all different
diff-EQ-5D-index	1048	0.53	0.30	0.51	0.55	3886	0.25	0.30	0.24	0.26	3351	−0.04	0.30	−0.05	−0.03	<0.001	all different
diff-EQ-VAS	1022	36.06	20.47	34.80	37.32	3833	16.27	19.82	15.64	16.89	3316	−3.31	19.66	−3.98	−2.64	<0.001	all different
diff-sf36-pf	1054	26.77	19.09	25.61	27.92	3953	10.00	15.13	9.53	10.47	3445	−3.31	15.24	−3.81	−2.80	<0.001	all different
diff-sf36-rp	1043	57.34	39.51	54.94	59.74	3889	19.15	14.30	18.07	20.22	3365	−3.69	27.14	−4.60	−2.77	<0.001	all different
diff-sf36-bp	1054	37.44	19.56	36.26	38.63	3954	14.29	14.79	13.83	14.75	3444	−1.33	13.03	−1.76	−0.89	<0.001	all different
diff-sf36-gh	1044	25.26	19.09	24.10	26.42	3908	7.78	16.33	7.26	8.29	3388	−5.04	15.87	−5.57	−4.50	<0.001	all different
diff-sf36-vt	1054	40.71	19.72	39.52	41.91	3951	13.32	17.83	12.77	13.88	3433	−4.60	16.67	−5.16	−4.05	<0.001	all different
diff-sf36-sf	1053	40.73	23.26	39.32	42.14	3958	14.43	21.21	13.77	15.09	3445	−7.66	22.38	−8.40	−6.91	<0.001	all different
diff-sf36-re	1031	53.10	44.27	50.40	55.81	3849	17.22	45.08	15.79	18.64	3277	−9.79	45.59	11.35	−8.22	<0.001	all different
diff-sf36-mh	1054	32.77	18.81	31.64	33.91	3948	10.62	16.33	10.11	11.13	3430	−6.66	17.25	−7.24	−6.09	<0.001	all different
Change-Pain	1049	3.32	0.74	3.28	3.37	3887	2.72	0.81	2.69	2.75	3373	2.20	0.85	2.17	2.22	<0.001	all different
Change-Life situation	1049	3.52	0.64	3.48	3.56	3901	3.05	0.70	3.03	3.08	3375	2.62	0.83	2.59	2.65	<0.001	all different

LB = Lower Bound; UB = Upper Bound; diff = change in a certain variable; NRS-7days = Pain intensity as measured by a numeric rating scale for the previous seven days; HADS = Hospital Anxiety and Depression Scale; MPI = Multidimensional Pain Inventory; EQ-5D-index = The index of the European quality of life instrument; EQ-VAS = The European quality of life instrument thermometer-like scale; sf36 = The Short Form (36) Health Survey. For explanations of the subscale abbreviations, see Methods.

Table 8. Pre-IMMRP values for the three clusters based on MIS obtained post-IMMRP.

Baseline Variables	Cluster 1					Cluster 2					Cluster 3					ANOVA	Post Hoc
	N	Mean	SD	95% CI LB	95% CI UB	N	Mean	SD	95% CI LB	95% CI UB	N	Mean	SD	95% CI LB	95% CI UB	p-Value	
Gender	2205	0.22	0.41	0.20	0.23	7938	0.24	0.43	0.23	0.25	4523	0.25	0.43	0.24	0.26	0.014	NA
Age	2205	42.7	11.2	42.2	43.2	7938	43.5	10.7	43.3	43.8	4523	43.0	10.6	42.7	43.3	0.001	cl1 NE cl3, cl2 NE cl3
Outside-Europe	2185	0.11	0.31	0.09	0.12	7877	0.10	0.30	0.09	0.10	4484	0.11	0.32	0.10	0.12	0.011	NA
University	2168	0.28	0.45	0.26	0.29	7826	0.26	0.44	0.25	0.27	4445	0.23	0.42	0.22	0.24	0.000	cl1 NE cl2, cl2 NE cl3
Days no work	716	889	2912	675	1102	2976	1037	2311	954	1120	1774	1152	2502	1036	1269	0.045	NA
PRI	2205	13.8	8.3	13.4	14.1	7938	14.4	8.3	14.2	14.6	4523	14.5	8.3	14.3	14.7	0.002	NA
NRS-7days	2158	7.1	1.7	7.0	7.2	7801	6.9	1.7	6.8	6.9	4440	6.7	1.7	6.7	6.8	0.000	all different
HADS-A	2199	10.4	4.7	10.2	10.6	7891	9.0	4.7	8.9	9.1	4494	8.2	4.6	8.1	8.4	0.000	all different
HADS-D	2197	9.6	4.4	9.4	9.8	7892	8.6	4.4	8.5	8.7	4494	7.7	4.3	7.6	7.9	0.000	all different
MPI-Pain-severity	2193	4.5	0.9	4.5	4.6	7895	4.4	0.9	4.4	4.4	4510	4.3	0.9	4.3	4.3	0.000	all different
MPI-Pain-interfer	2187	4.6	1.0	4.6	4.6	7853	4.4	1.0	4.4	4.4	4485	4.3	1.0	4.2	4.3	0.000	all different
MPI-LifeCon	2195	2.4	1.1	2.4	2.5	7880	2.7	1.1	2.7	2.7	4502	2.9	1.1	2.9	3.0	0.000	all different
MPI-Distress	2191	3.9	1.2	3.9	4.0	7891	3.5	1.3	3.5	3.5	4502	3.2	1.3	3.1	3.2	0.000	all different
MPI-Socsupp	2190	4.2	1.4	4.2	4.3	7861	4.2	1.3	4.1	4.2	4488	4.1	1.4	4.1	4.2	0.005	NA
MPI-punish	2069	1.9	1.5	1.8	1.9	7319	1.8	1.4	1.7	1.8	4169	1.7	1.3	1.6	1.7	0.000	all different
MPI-protect	2065	3.0	1.5	2.9	3.1	7295	2.9	1.4	2.9	3.0	4158	3.0	1.4	2.9	3.0	0.136	NA
MPI-distract	2069	2.6	1.2	2.5	2.6	7312	2.5	1.2	2.5	2.5	4168	2.5	1.2	2.5	2.6	0.075	NA
MPI-GAI	2193	2.4	0.8	2.4	2.4	7885	2.4	0.8	2.4	2.5	4500	2.5	0.8	2.5	2.5	0.000	cl1 NE cl2, cl2 NE cl3
EQ-5D-index	2126	0.2	0.3	0.2	0.2	7587	0.3	0.3	0.2	0.3	4277	0.3	0.3	0.3	0.3	0.000	all different
EQ-VAS	2097	38.0	18.2	37.2	38.8	7529	40.7	19.0	40.3	41.1	4224	43.9	19.4	43.3	44.5	0.000	all different
sf36-pf	2151	52.1	21.0	51.2	52.9	7683	52.8	20.6	52.3	53.2	4349	53.2	20.2	52.6	53.8	0.119	NA
sf36-rp	2139	9.0	19.8	8.2	9.9	7629	11.8	23.8	11.3	12.4	4283	15.3	26.8	14.5	16.1	0.000	all different
sf36-bp	2151	21.1	13.8	20.5	21.7	7694	24.1	14.3	23.8	24.4	4347	26.4	14.6	26.0	26.8	0.000	all different
sf36-gh	2139	39.8	20.0	38.9	40.6	7610	41.4	20.1	41.0	41.9	4299	43.3	20.4	42.7	43.9	0.000	all different
sf36-vt	2151	19.7	16.6	19.0	20.4	7679	23.3	18.4	22.9	23.7	4347	27.3	19.0	26.7	27.8	0.000	all different
sf36-sf	2151	40.0	23.7	39.0	41.0	7690	46.6	24.9	46.1	47.2	4348	52.1	25.3	51.4	52.9	0.000	all different
sf36-re	2126	30.6	39.6	28.9	32.2	7549	41.6	42.6	40.7	42.6	4220	50.6	43.6	49.3	51.9	0.000	all different
sf36-mh	2151	47.3	20.7	46.5	48.2	7672	54.5	21.2	54.0	54.9	4343	60.1	20.5	59.4	60.7	0.000	all different

LB = Lower Bound; UB = Upper Bound; NA = not applicable; NRS-7days = Pain intensity as measured by a numeric rating scale for the previous seven days; HADS = Hospital Anxiety and Depression Scale; MPI = Multidimensional Pain Inventory; EQ-5D-index = The index of the European quality of life instrument; EQ-VAS = The European quality of life instrument thermometer-like scale; sf36 = The Short Form (36) Health Survey; PRI = Pain Region Index. For explanations of the subscale abbreviations, see Methods.

Table 9. Pre-IMMRP values for the three clusters based on MIS obtained at 12-month FU.

		Cluster 1						Cluster 2						Cluster 3				ANOVA	Post Hoc
				95% CI						95% CI						95% CI			
Baseline Variables	N	Mean	SD	LB	UB	N	Mean	SD	LB	UB	N	Mean	SD	LB	UB			p-Value	
Gender	1099	0.24	0.43	0.21	0.26	4123	0.21	0.41	0.20	0.22	3629	0.25	0.43	0.24	0.27	<0.001	all different
Age	1099	41.9	11.1	41.2	42.5	4123	43.7	11.1	43.4	44.0	3629	44.2	10.4	43.8	44.5	<0.001	all different
Outside-Europe	1088	0.09	0.29	0.07	0.11	4091	0.08	0.28	0.08	0.09	3606	0.10	0.30	0.09	0.11	0.012	NA
University	1079	0.29	0.45	0.26	0.31	4060	0.27	0.45	0.26	0.29	3567	0.23	0.42	0.21	0.24	<0.001	all different except cl2 vs. cl3
Days no work	358	661	2587	392	930	1409	1046	2339	923	1168	1323	1270	2604	1130	1411	<0.001	all different
PRI	1099	12.8	8.0	12.3	13.2	4123	14.2	8.3	14.0	14.5	3629	14.8	8.3	14.5	15.1	<0.001	all different
NRS-7days	1071	7.0	1.7	6.9	7.1	4049	6.8	1.7	6.8	6.9	3574	6.8	1.7	6.8	6.9	0.049	NA
HADS-A	1096	9.7	4.7	9.4	10.0	4101	8.7	4.7	8.6	8.9	3606	8.4	4.6	8.3	8.6	<0.001	all different
HADS-D	1096	8.8	4.4	8.6	9.1	4102	8.2	4.3	8.1	8.3	3606	8.0	4.4	7.9	8.1	<0.001	all different
MPI-Pain-severity	1094	4.5	0.9	4.4	4.5	4114	4.4	0.9	4.3	4.4	3625	4.3	0.9	4.3	4.4	<0.001	cl1NE cl2, cl2 NE cl1, cl3
MPI-Pain-interfer	1093	4.5	0.9	4.5	4.6	4101	4.4	1.0	4.3	4.4	3609	4.3	1.0	4.2	4.3	<0.001	all different
MPI-LifeCon	1096	2.5	1.1	2.5	2.6	4113	2.8	1.1	2.7	2.8	3614	2.9	1.1	2.8	2.9	<0.001	all different
MPI-Distress	1095	3.8	1.2	3.8	3.9	4114	3.4	1.3	3.4	3.5	3621	3.3	1.3	3.2	3.3	<0.001	all different
MPI-Socsupp	1090	4.3	1.3	4.2	4.4	4097	4.2	1.3	4.2	4.3	3604	4.1	1.4	4.1	4.1	<0.001	all different
MPI-punish	1036	1.8	1.4	1.7	1.9	3833	1.7	1.3	1.6	1.7	3355	1.7	1.3	1.7	1.8	0.047	NA
IMP-protect	1038	3.0	1.4	2.9	3.1	3824	2.9	1.4	2.9	3.0	3341	2.9	1.4	2.9	3.0	0.583	NA
MPI-distract	1039	2.6	1.2	2.5	2.6	3831	2.6	1.2	2.5	2.6	3352	2.5	1.2	2.4	2.5	0.003	NA
MPI-GAI	1094	2.4	0.9	2.4	2.5	4108	2.5	0.8	2.5	2.5	3623	2.5	0.8	2.5	2.5	0.071	NA
EQ-5D-index	1058	0.2	0.3	0.2	0.2	3935	0.3	0.3	0.3	0.3	3407	0.3	0.3	0.3	0.3	<0.001	all different
EQ-VAS	1037	39.2	18.2	38.1	40.3	3905	41.3	19.2	40.7	42.0	3389	43.1	19.6	42.4	43.7	<0.001	all different
sf36-pf	1056	51.9	20.4	50.7	53.1	3969	53.0	20.4	52.4	53.7	3459	53.4	20.1	52.7	54.1	0.120	NA
sf36-rp	1053	8.5	20.6	7.2	9.7	3938	12.4	24.1	11.6	13.1	3417	15.3	26.9	14.4	16.2	<0.001	all different
sf36-bp	1058	21.5	13.3	20.7	22.3	3974	24.4	14.2	23.9	24.8	3461	25.9	14.0	25.4	26.3	<0.001	all different
sf36-gh	1052	43.1	21.0	41.8	44.4	3944	42.6	20.5	42.0	43.2	3424	42.3	20.3	41.7	43.0	0.556	NA
sf36-vt	1058	21.4	17.8	20.3	22.5	3972	24.7	19.1	24.1	25.3	3452	26.3	18.6	25.7	26.9	<0.001	all different
sf36-sf	1056	42.4	24.2	40.9	43.9	3976	48.2	25.6	47.4	49.0	3458	51.9	25.2	51.0	52.7	<0.001	all different
sf36-re	1046	32.1	40.3	29.7	34.5	3906	44.0	43.2	42.7	45.4	3363	49.1	43.2	47.6	50.5	<0.001	all different
sf36-mh	1058	49.6	20.9	48.3	50.9	3970	56.0	21.0	55.3	56.7	3451	58.7	20.9	58.0	59.4	<0.001	all different

LB = Lower Bound; UB = Upper Bound; NA = not applicable; NRS-7days = Pain intensity as measured by a numeric rating scale for the previous seven days; HADS = Hospital Anxiety and Depression Scale; MPI = Multidimensional Pain Inventory; EQ-5D-index = The index of the European quality of life instrument; EQ-VAS = The European quality of life instrument thermometer-like scale; sf36 = The Short Form (36) Health Survey; PRI = Pain Region Index. For explanations of the subscale abbreviations, see Methods.

3.7. Longitudinal Regression of MIS Using Baseline Data

The outcome data at baseline (pre-IMMRP) together with the background variables were used to regress MIS-post-IMMRP and MIS-12-month FU (Table 10). For both MIS, psychological distress variables were the most important regressors, but life impact variables, pain aspects, and health and vitality aspects contributed significantly. The directions of the correlations revealed that a more severe clinical situation (e.g., psychological distress, lack of control, low vitality and health, pain interference, and high pain intensity) were associated with high MIS (i.e., multivariate improvements). Although the obtained regressions were highly significant according to the CV-ANOVA, the explained variations in MIS were less than 10% ($R^2 = 0.08$ in both analyses). Hence, most of the variations in the two MIS were not possible to predict.

Similar analyses for each of the clusters (Supplementary Tables S2 and S3) revealed that regressions were highly significant, but only explained a minority of the variations in MIS. Although the relative importance of the variables pre-IMMRP differed somewhat between the three clusters, no marked differences existed; that is, psychological distress aspects were the most important post-IMMRP (Supplementary Table S2). For the 12-month FU, somewhat more pronounced differences existed between the clusters: in cluster 2, the pain intensity aspects were the most important for MIS, and in cluster 1 and cluster 3, psychological distress variables together with pain interference were the most important for MIS.

Table 10. Orthogonal Partial Least Square Regressions (OPLS) regressions of MIS post-IMMRP (left part) and at 12-month FU (right part) using the variables pre-IMMRP as regressors. Variables in bold type are significant regressors.

Post-IMMRP Variables Pre-IMMRP	VIP	p(corr)	12-Month FU Variables Pre-IMMRP	VIP	p(corr)
sf36-mh	1.80	−0.80	**sf36-mh**	1.63	−0.62
MPI-Distress	1.72	0.76	**MPI-Distress**	1.59	0.61
HADS-D	1.56	0.68	**sf36-sf**	1.44	−0.53
MPI-LifeCon	1.48	−0.65	**sf36-re**	1.39	−0.54
HADS-A	1.48	0.65	**MPI-LifeCon**	1.35	−0.49
sf36-sf	1.47	−0.63	**HADS-D**	1.34	0.46
sf36-re	1.43	−0.64	**HADS-A**	1.28	0.46
sf36-vt	1.27	−0.54	**MPI-Pain-interfer**	1.26	0.39
MPI-Pain-interfer	1.26	0.45	**Persistent-Pain-duration**	1.16	−0.46
EQ-5D-index	1.12	−0.41	**Pain duration**	1.15	−0.45
sf36-bp	1.07	−0.35	**EQ-5D-index**	1.14	−0.37
MPI-Pain-severity	1.05	0.28	**sf36-bp**	1.11	−0.35
EQ-VAS	1.04	−0.39	**sf36-vt**	1.11	−0.36
sf36-gh	0.95	−0.30	MPI-Pain-severity	0.99	0.21
NRS-7days	0.88	0.20	EQ-VAS	0.97	−0.28
sf36-pf	0.87	−0.07	sf36-rp	0.96	−0.37
sf36-rp	0.80	−0.33	PRI	0.95	−0.26
PRI	0.72	−0.09	sf36-gh	0.87	−0.10
MPI-GAI	0.68	−0.20	NRS-7days	0.81	0.11
MPI-punish	0.59	0.25	Days no work	0.80	−0.31
Outside-Europe	0.45	−0.01	sf36-pf	0.76	−0.05
Days no work	0.44	−0.16	Age	0.75	−0.30
University	0.43	0.12	MPI-GAI	0.72	−0.22
Persistent Pain duration	0.42	−0.16	University	0.54	0.18
MPI-protect	0.41	−0.04	MPI-punish	0.43	0.12
Pain duration	0.38	−0.15	Outside-Europe	0.39	−0.03
MPI-Socsupp	0.32	−0.05	MPI-protect	0.31	0.03
MPI-distract	0.29	−0.01	MPI-distract	0.26	0.06
Age	0.23	−0.10	MPI-Socsupp	0.22	0.07
Gender	0.04	−0.01	Gender	0.10	−0.04

Table 10. Cont.

Post-IMMRP Variables Pre-IMMRP	VIP	p(corr)	12-Month FU Variables Pre-IMMRP	VIP	p(corr)
R^2	0.08		R^2	0.08	
Q^2	0.08		Q^2	0.07	
n	14 657		n	7 976	
CV-ANOVA p-value	<0.001		CV-ANOVA p-value	<0.001	

VIP (VIP > 1.0 is significant) and p (corr) are reported for each regressor. The sign of p (corr) indicates the direction of the correlation with the dependent variable (+ = positive correlation; − = negative correlation). The four bottom rows of each regression report R^2, Q^2, and p-value of the CV-ANOVA and number of patients included in the regression (n). NRS-7days = Pain intensity as measured by a numeric rating scale for the previous seven days; HADS = Hospital Anxiety and Depression Scale; MPI = Multidimensional Pain Inventory EQ-5D-index = The index of the European quality of life instrument; EQ-VAS = The European quality of life instrument thermometer-like scale; sf36 = The Short Form (36) Health Survey; PRI = Pain Region Index. For explanations of the subscale abbreviations see Methods.

4. Discussions

The major findings of the present large PROM study from SQRP are listed below:

- Moderate long-term ES were found for pain intensity (MPI Pain severity and SF-36 bodily pain), interference in daily life (MPI Interference), and state of health (EQ-5D-index); most other variables showed small ES. Vitality also displayed moderate effect sizes immediately after IMMRP but fell slightly under cut-off for moderate change at 12-month follow-up. The majority of the 22 investigated outcomes were significantly improved.
- Significant intercorrelations between changes in pain intensity, interference, control, psychological distress, and mental health were confirmed. The changes in 22 outcomes reflected one (pre-IMMRP versus post-IMMRP) or three (pre-IMMRP versus 12-month follow-up) latent components (groups of variables).
- The outcomes were best for patients with the worst self-reported clinical presentation pre-IMMRP. Based on a defined multivariate improvement score (MIS), three clusters were identified. Cluster 1—overall, the worst situation pre-IMMRP—showed positive multivariate improvements in outcomes. Cluster 3—deteriorated—showed negative scores. Cluster 2, the intermediate cluster, was associated with overall slightly positive multivariate improvements.
- Certain variables (especially psychological distress and life impact variables, pain, and health and vitality aspects) pre-IMMRP were associated with improvements according to MIS both post-IMMRP and at 12-month FU. However statistically significant, the pre-IMMRP situation could only explain a small part of the variation in MIS (8%); therefore, for clinical use, it was not possible to predict those who would benefit most from IMMRP.

The outcome variables mandatory in SQRP and presented in the present study are in good agreement with the BSP model of chronic pain and the outcome domains presented by the Initiative on Methods, Measurement, and Pain Assessment in Clinical Trials (IMMPACT) [7,52] and the Validation and Application of a patient-relevant core set of outcome domains to assess multimodal PAIN therapy (VAPAIN) [14] initiatives.

The present study was not primarily designed to evaluate the efficacy of IMMRP, which requires RCTs and SRs/meta-analyses. However, our results for the repeated measurements (Tables 2 and 3) of chronic pain patients in real-life practice settings are in agreement with the positive evidence for IMMRPs reported in SRs [10–12] and in other studies [22,23,53]. As such, the small to moderate ES are noteworthy as these patients, who receive pain rehabilitation in specialist care centres, often have tried other treatments for their chronic pain with no or little effect. That is, these patients have severe problems and relative treatment resistance. Interestingly, the changes in outcomes with moderate ES are broad and not limited to a single outcome domain, and the most stable moderate ES were demonstrated for pain intensity aspects with moderate improvement both immediately after

IMMRPs and at 12-month follow-up. Pain interference demonstrated moderate ES improvement at 12-month follow-up, and vitality was moderately improved immediately after IMMRPs. Both objective registrations (e.g., sick-leave registrations and actigraphic recordings [54]) and subjective PROM data may be important for understanding the efficacy of IMMRPs. Very recently, a SQRP study using a subgroup of the same cohort of patients reported that sick leave benefits according to the Swedish Social Insurance Agency decreased as a consequence of IMMRP [55]. Hence, both PROM data and objective sick leave data indicate clinically important positive changes in response to IMMRPs for patients in real-life practice settings. As a comparison, SRs conclude that common pharmacological treatments—e.g., paracetamol, non-steroidal anti-inflammatory drugs, and opioids—for patients with chronic pain have no effects, small effects, and/or lack of long-term follow-up effects [56–58].

The present study reported medium ES for two of three pain intensity variables both post-IMMRP and at 12-month FU (i.e., for MPI-pain-severity and sf36-bp); the third pain intensity variable had effect sizes near medium ES. These results contrasted some SRs reporting of no evidence for efficacy with respect to pain intensity [10,11]. However, not all RCTs of IMMRP included pain intensity outcomes, since the interventions are not focused on the pain itself but rather on its consequences [10,11]. Obviously, many pain patients consider pain intensity improvement to be the most important aspect of treatments [59]. However, changing this perspective is considered important in IMMPRs, since focusing on pain reduction in many cases leads to short-sighted attempts to control pain, and this may, when not successful, lead to increased physical and psychological disability and reduced life quality [60,61]. Thus, specialist care IMMRPs in Sweden have largely adopted the idea of introducing acceptance as a cornerstone of the psychological component of IMMRP (i.e., the willingness to have the experiences of pain as it is and to encourage patients to set up activity-related rehabilitation goals and risk initial pain flare-ups). This also means that patients are advised against establishing pain reduction goals. Thus, it could be considered problematic to communicate the present results showing medium effect sizes in real-world practice settings on pain. On the other hand, it may also be ethically problematic if both clinical practice and research ignore the reports and wishes of the patients regarding pain intensity. However, health care providers should not underestimate their patients' ability to grasp, once explained, the complex pain experience. Therefore, health care providers should emphasise pain education, including descriptions of the affective and cognitive elements of pain as rational for the different components of IMMRPs, and stress the need to experiment with new behaviours and risk short-term pain flare-ups. Since the results are obtained in this context, no change in clinical practise as far as pain communication is called for.

SRs of IMMRP report that it is an effective intervention with small to moderate effects for patients with chronic pain conditions [11,12,62,63]. The present results concerning ES agree with most SRs of IMMRP, but it may also be appropriate to compare with ES results reported in other clinical studies. The moderate ES for two of the pain intensity variables agree with studies in clinical routine care (n = 65–395), and therefore, for long-term follow-up (6–12 months), such studies report small (Cohen's d: 0.20–0.33 [64,65]) to moderate (Cohen's d: 0.59–0.70 [26,66,67]) ES for pain intensity. For psychological distress variables, these studies agree with the present results: they generally found small ES for long-term follow-up (i.e., Cohen's d = 0–0.38 for depressive symptoms [26,64,65] and Cohen's d = 0.22–0.34 for anxiety) [26,65]. In a recent RCT comparing transdiagnostic emotion-focused exposure treatment (Hybrid) and Internet-delivered pain management treatment (ICBT) for chronic pain patients with comorbid anxiety and depression, we found that within group ES pre versus follow-up for pain interference were reported both for hybrid (ES = 1.17) and for ICBT (ES = 0.65) compared the present effect size of 0.49 [68]. However, the patients were not exclusively recruited from specialist care (i.e., clinical departments of pain rehabilitation); they were also recruited via advertisements in local newspapers and social media [68], and the numbers investigated were considerably smaller. An important observation from the present study is that moderate ES found at 12-month follow-up covered broad aspects (e.g., pain intensity, interference in daily life, and perceived health).

The number of outcomes in IMMRPs in RCTs are generally high, which reasonably reflects the broad goals of the complex intervention. The present study used 22 outcomes that are mandatory in SQRP measured on up to three occasions (i.e., pre-IMMRP, post-IMMRP, and 12-month follow-up). PCA was applied to handle the pattern of changes in potentially intercorrelated outcomes as suggested by the Medical Research Council of the United Kingdom [69]. From these analyses, it can be concluded that changes in pain intensity, pain interference, psychological distress, vitality, etc. were positively intercorrelated (Table 5). In fact, our study showed that the changes in the majority of the 22 outcomes are significantly intercorrelated. Hence, the changes in these variables cannot be considered independent of each other. As a consequence of this observation, the appropriateness to evaluate changes in outcomes separately, as done in a recent SR [70], must be questioned, since the treatment was not designed to target only a single outcome. Moreover, the ES must be seen in this complex context. Thus, small changes in many outcomes may be more important than one prominent change in a single or few outcomes. Furthermore, the Grading of Recommendations Assessment, Development and Evaluation (GRADE) used for evidence ratings in SRs may not adequately describe the evidence base of complex interventions [71]. Different definitions of positive outcomes of IMMRP interventions exist (e.g., the majority of outcomes had to be significantly better than for the control intervention) [10,11]. Another approach was that the authors of the SR predetermined primary and secondary outcomes and what was necessary to classify an intervention as positive before reviewing the RCTs [12].

The presented PCAs also highlight that it may be possible to reduce the number of outcome variables, since several of these appear to measure similar aspects of the chronic pain condition. The fact that 22 outcomes were analysed (Tables 2 and 3) may raise an issue of multiple comparisons. In such situations, Bonferroni corrections are frequently used [72,73]. This is a conservative approach when the number of tests increases [72,74,75], the chances to detect real treatment effects decrease, and corrections were designed for corrections of *independent* comparisons [74]. The latter is obviously not present for most changes in outcome variables according to the PCAs performed (Table 5). Hierarchal or 'gatekeeping' procedures do not require adjustment for multiplicity [73], but require a natural hierarchy of the outcomes, as such a hierarchy is not obvious for IMMRP, as discussed above. Another approach is that outcomes are combined into a single composite outcome (i.e., a composite outcome consists of two or more component outcomes) [76], but this may be problematic with respect to missing cases and when the components of the composite endpoint are measured on different scales (i.e., non-commensurate outcomes) [76]. However, some multivariate methods such as PCA and OPLS can handle non-commensurate outcomes [76]. We used advanced PCA, including the NIPALS algorithm, to handling missing data and non-commensurate outcomes. We calculated the t-scores for the most relevant latent factor (component). Hence, we defined an objective Multivariate Improvement Score (MIS; the t-score of the first PCA component), which on an individual patient level defines the multivariate improvement; a positive MIS indicates multivariate improvements because of IMMRP.

Three clearly separated clusters based on MIS were identified. On a group level, clusters 1 and 2 were associated with various degrees of improvements, whereas cluster 3 showed negative MIS, indicating deterioration. Although the greater improvement in cluster 1 can be interpreted as a sign of regression to the mean and that these patients did not benefit from IMMRP more than cluster 2, this cluster still improves from IMMRP at least as well as those with e.g., less severe psychological distress symptoms (clusters 2 and 3). This may seem unexpected, but it is important to recognise that addressing psychological symptoms with CBT is an important component of IMMRPs. The patients at post-IMMRP and 12-month follow-up estimated the degree of positive change in pain (i.e., Change-pain) and the ability to handle life situation in general (i.e., Change-life situation). Most patients reported improvements according to both the Change-pain and Change-life situations (Table 4). Relatively small proportions of the patients reported worse situations post-IMMRP and at the 12-month follow-up, which are results that agree with other studies [29,77,78]. These two variables have retrospective elements even though they are not explicitly expressed. There are several problems with such items in general—e.g., desirability and memory aspects, recall time [79–81], and in treatment context (e.g., overly optimistic assessments) [82]. However, on a general level, these estimations and the two MIS variables (Tables 6 and 7) agreed.

We found that cluster 1, which had high MIS values (i.e., prominent improvements), had a more severe clinical picture at baseline/pre-IMMRP than those with lower MIS (i.e., less improvements). These results agree with another SQRP study ($N > 35,000$) that identified clusters based on the clinical presentation at assessment (decision not taken about participation in IMMRP); the study found that patients with the most severe clinical situation who later participated in IMMRP had the most prominent improvements in six investigated outcomes [34]. Although IMMRP has been commended for its effectiveness ('of all approaches to the treatment of chronic pain, none has a stronger evidence basis for efficacy, cost-effectiveness, and lack of iatrogenic complications') [83], both this and our recent study [34] indicate that not all patients show important improvements in several domains of outcome after IMMRP. Both this and our previous study identified a large subgroup of patients that do not seem to significantly benefit from IMMRP. Presumably, these patients—in the present study, those with negative MIS (i.e., cluster 3)—need other interventions. In a relative context, they have a somewhat less complicated self-reported clinical picture pre-IMMRP than those in clusters 1 and 2, even though they are referred to specialist care and hence represent patients with complex needs.

The longitudinal regressions of MIS using background variables and pre-IMMRP data as regressors were significant (Table 10). A blend of variables was important; psychological distress variables were most important, but life impact variables, pain aspects, and health and vitality aspects contributed. Our results appear to be in line with a recent meta-analysis on prognostic factors for IMMRP outcome, demonstrating that both pre-treatment general emotional distress and pain-specific cognitive behavioural factors are related to worse long-term (>6 months) physical functioning [84]. Unfortunately, these regressions cannot be used clinically, since they only explained 8% of variations in MIS. Although the prediction does not work clinically, this and a previous study from our group give clear indications that patients with a severe clinical situation benefit from IMMRP [34].

4.1. Important Clinical Implications

Outcomes of IMMRP in real-life practice settings agree with the conclusions from SRs. Partly in contrast to SRs, this registry study of patients managed within specialist care found that pain intensity was positively affected because of IMMRP. It was also obvious that not all patients benefit from IMMRP. Hence, there is a need to develop better matching between clinical presentation and participation in MMRP in real-life practice settings. Moreover, the intercorrelations of most changes in outcomes also opens up the possibility of reducing the number of outcome variables and hereby reduce the burden upon patients included in the SQRP.

4.2. Strengths and Limitations

This study's strengths include a large number of patients with complex chronic pain conditions with a nation-wide representation. However, these patients were referred to specialist clinics and thus represent a selection of the most difficult cases, so our results cannot be generalised to other settings. Another strength was the use of MVDA methods such as PCA and OPLS to handle correlation patterns, repeated measures, and regressions when there were obvious risks for multicollinearity. Changes in the social context may have changed and influenced the longitudinal analyses; however, we used validated and well-known instruments. Repeated evaluations using PROM questionnaires in treatment studies may be problematic [85]. Thus, the changes that the patient undergo because of the intervention (i.e., IMMRP) may affect the interpretations of the questions when presented at follow-up. The fact that no control group or treatment-as-usual group was available, which ethically is complicated to arrange for a registry of real-life practice patients, might have influenced our interpretation of changes after IMMRP. Data for the time period 2008–2016 from the SQRP was used in the present study, and changes in the content of IMMRP may have occurred. Unfortunately, no data concerning such changes are available.

5. Conclusions

This large-scale study of IMMRPs in real life practise settings demonstrates significant outcome changes in almost all measures. Most short-term and long-term effect sizes were small, but interestingly, moderate long-term effect sizes were demonstrated for pain, pain interference in daily life, and perceived health. In addition, patients reporting higher levels of perceived disability and suffering displayed greater improvement.

Supplementary Materials: The following are available online at http://www.mdpi.com/2077-0383/8/6/905/s1, Table S1: Pre-IMMRP situation for patients reporting their outcomes at 12-m FU and those not reporting their outcomes at 12-m FU, Table S2: OPLS regressions of MIS at post IMMRP in the three clusters, Table S3: OPLS regressions of MIS at 12-month FU in the three clusters.

Author Contributions: Conceptualization, Å.R., E.D., M.B., B.L. and B.G.; Data curation, Å.R. and B.G.; Formal analysis, B.L. and B.G.; Methodology, Å.R., M.B. and B.G.; Validation, E.D.; Writing—original draft, B.G.; Writing—review & editing, Å.R., E.D., M.B. and B.L. All authors commented on different versions of the manuscript and all authors have approved the final version of the manuscript.

Funding: This study was supported by external funding from the Swedish Research Council (2018-02470), County Council of Östergötland (forsknings-ALF; LIO-608021), and AFA insurance (140340). AFA Insurance, a commercial founder, is owned by Sweden's labour market parties: The Confederation of Swedish Enterprise, the Swedish Trade Union Confederation (LO), and The Council for Negotiation and Co-operation (PTK). They insure employees in the private sector, municipalities, and county councils. AFA Insurance does not seek to generate a profit, which implies that no dividends are paid to shareholders. The sponsors of the study had no role in study design, data collection, data analysis, data interpretation, writing of the report, or the decision to submit for publication. The authors had full access to all the data in the study and had final responsibility for the decision to submit for publication.

Acknowledgments: The authors are very grateful for valuable comments from Marcelo Rivano Fischer, PhD.

Conflicts of Interest: The authors declare no conflict of interest.

List of Abbreviations

ACT	Acceptance Commitment Therapy
ANOVA	Analysis of Variance
BPS	biopsychosocial
CBT	Cognitive Behavioral Therapy
Change-pain	positive change in pain
Change-life situation	change in ability to handle life situations in general
CI	confidence interval
CV-ANOVA	ANOVA of the cross-validated residuals
ES	effect size
EQ-5D	European Quality of Life instrument
EQ-5D-index	index of EQ-5D based on five items
EQ-VAS	health scale of EQ-5D
FU	follow-up
GRADE	Grading of Recommendations Assessment, Development and Evaluation
HADS	Hospital Anxiety and Depression Scale
HADS-A	Hospital Anxiety and Depression Scale—anxiety subscale
HADS-D	Hospital Anxiety and Depression Scale—depression subscale
HCA	Hierarchical Clustering Analysis
HR-QoL	health-related quality of life
IASP	the International Association for the Study of Pain
IMMPACT	the Initiative on Methods, Measurement, and Pain Assessment in Clinical Trials
IMMRP	Interdisciplinary Multimodal Pain Rehabilitation Program

LR	logistic regression
MIS	Multivariate Improvement Score
MLR	multiple linear regression
MPI	Multidimensional Pain Inventory
MPI-Pain-severity	MPI subscale concerning pain severity
MPI-Pain-interfer	MPI subscale concerning pain-related interference
MPI-Distress	MPI-SocSupp affective distress
MPI-LifeCon	MPI subscale concerning life control
MPI-SocSupp	MPI subscale concerning social support
MPI-Punish	MPI subscale concerning punishing responses
MPI-Solict	MPI subscale concerning solicitous responses
MPI-Distract	MPI subscale concerning distracting responses
MPI-GAI	MPI subscale General Activity Index
MVDA	advanced multivariate analysis
NIPALS	Non-linear Iterative Partial Least Squares
NRS	Numeric Rating Scale
NRS-7days	average pain intensity the last week
OPLS	Orthogonal Partial Least Square Regression
Outside-Europe	born outside Europe
PBE	practice-based evidence
P(corr)	loading scaled as a correlation coefficient between −1.0 and +1.0
PCA	Principal Component Analysis
PLS-DA	partial least square discriminant analysis
PRI	Pain Region Index
PROM	patient reported outcome measures
RCT	Randomised Controlled Trial
SQRP	Swedish Quality Registry for Pain Rehabilitation
sf36	Short Form Health Survey
sf36-pf	sf36 subscale concerning physical functioning
sf36-rp	sf36 subscale concerning role limitations due to physical functioning
sf36-bp	sf36 subscale concerning bodily pain
sf36-gh	sf36 subscale concerning general health
sf36-vt	sf36 subscale concerning vitality
sf36-sf	sf36 subscale concerning social functioning
sf36-re	sf36 subscale concerning role limitations due to emotional problems
sf36-mh	sf36 subscale concerning mental health
SR	systematic review
University	University education
VAPAIN	Validation and Application of a patient-relevant core set of outcome domains to assess multimodal PAIN therapy
VIP	variable influence on projection

References

1. Linton, S.J.; Bergbom, S. Understanding the link between depression and pain. *Scand. J. Pain* **2011**, *2*, 47–54. [CrossRef] [PubMed]
2. Ossipov, M.H.; Dussor, G.O.; Porreca, F. Central modulation of pain. *J. Clin. Investig.* **2010**, *120*, 3779–3787. [CrossRef] [PubMed]
3. Gatchel, R.J.; Peng, Y.B.; Peters, M.L.; Fuchs, P.N.; Turk, D.C. The biopsychosocial approach to chronic pain: Scientific advances and future directions. *Psychol. Bull.* **2007**, *133*, 581–624. [CrossRef]
4. Breivik, H.; Collett, B.; Ventafridda, V.; Cohen, R.; Gallacher, D. Survey of chronic pain in Europe: Prevalence, impact on daily life, and treatment. *Eur. J. Pain* **2006**, *10*, 287. [CrossRef] [PubMed]
5. Bergman, S. *Chronic Musculoskeletal Pain: A Multifactorial Process*; Lund University: Lund, Sweden, 2001.
6. World Health Organization (WHO). *International Classification of Functioning, Disability and Health (ICF)*; World Health Organization: Geneva, Switzerland, 2001.

7. Dworkin, R.H.; Turk, D.C.; Farrar, J.T.; Haythornthwaite, J.A.; Jensen, M.P.; Katz, N.P.; Kerns, R.D.; Stucki, G.; Allen, R.R.; Bellamy, N.; et al. Core outcome measures for chronic pain clinical trials: IMMPACT recommendations. *Pain* **2005**, *113*, 9–19. [CrossRef] [PubMed]
8. Fillingim, R.B. Individual Differences in Pain: Understanding the Mosaic that Makes Pain Personal. *Pain* **2017**, *158*, S11–S18. [CrossRef] [PubMed]
9. Bennett, M.; Closs, S. Methodological issues in nonpharamacological trials for chronic pain. *Pain Clin. Updates* **2010**, *18*, 1–6.
10. Swedish Council on Health Technology Assessment (SBU). *Methods for Treatment of Chronic Pain a Systematic Review of the Literature*; SBU-Rapport; Swedish Council on Health Technology Assessment: Stockholm, Sweden, 2006; Volume 177, (In Swedish: Metoder för behandling av långvarig smärta: En systematisk litteraturöversikt).
11. Swedish Council on Health Technology Assessment (SBU). *Rehabilitation of Chronic Pain*; SBU-Rapport; Swedish Council on Health Technology Assessment: Stockholm, Sweden, 2010; Volume 198, (In Swedish: Rehabilitering vid långvarig smärta. En systematisk litteraturöversikt).
12. Scascighini, L.; Toma, V.; Dober-Spielmann, S.; Sprott, H. Multidisciplinary treatment for chronic pain: A systematic review of interventions and outcomes. *Rheumatology* **2008**, *47*, 670–678. [CrossRef] [PubMed]
13. Wade, D.T. Describing rehabilitation interventions. *Clin. Rehabil.* **2005**, *19*, 811–818. [CrossRef]
14. Kaiser, U.; Kopkow, C.; Deckert, S.; Neustadt, K.; Jacobi, L.; Cameron, P.; De Angelis, V.; Apfelbacher, C.; Arnold, B.; Birch, J.; et al. Developing a core outcome-domain set to assessing effectiveness of interdisciplinary multimodal pain therapy: The VAPAIN consensus statement on core outcome-domains. *Pain* **2017**, *159*, 673–683. [CrossRef] [PubMed]
15. Campbell, M.; Fitzpatrick, R.; Haines, A.; Kinmonth, A.L.; Sandercock, P.; Spiegelhalter, D.; Tyrer, P. Framework for design and evaluation of complex interventions to improve health. *BMJ* **2000**, *321*, 694–696. [CrossRef] [PubMed]
16. Paterson, C.; Baarts, C.; Launsø, L.; Verhoef, M.J. Evaluating complex health interventions: A critical analysis of the 'outcomes' concept. *BMC Complement. Altern. Med.* **2009**, *9*, 18. [CrossRef] [PubMed]
17. Shiell, A.; Hawe, P.; Gold, L. Complex interventions or complex systems? Implications for health economic evaluation. *BMJ* **2008**, *336*, 1281–1283. [CrossRef] [PubMed]
18. Hawe, P.; Shiell, A.; Riley, T. Complex interventions: How "out of control" can a randomised controlled trial be? *BMJ* **2004**, *328*, 1561–1563. [CrossRef] [PubMed]
19. Weiner, S.S.; Nordin, M. Prevention and management of chronic back pain. *Best Pract. Res. Clin. Rheumatol.* **2010**, *24*, 267–279. [CrossRef] [PubMed]
20. Kamper, S.J.; Apeldoorn, A.T.; Chiarotto, A.; Smeets, R.J.E.M.; Ostelo, R.W.J.G.; Guzman, J.; Van Tulder, M.W.; Van Tulder, M. Multidisciplinary biopsychosocial rehabilitation for chronic low back pain: Cochrane systematic review and meta-analysis. *BMJ* **2015**, *350*, h444. [CrossRef] [PubMed]
21. Norlund, A.; Ropponen, A.; Alexanderson, K. Multidisciplinary interventions: Review of studies of return to work after rehabilitation for low back pain. *J. Rehabil. Med.* **2009**, *41*, 115–121. [CrossRef] [PubMed]
22. Busch, H.; Bodin, L.; Bergström, G.; Jensen, I.B. Patterns of sickness absence a decade after pain-related multidisciplinary rehabilitation. *Pain* **2011**, *152*, 1727–1733. [CrossRef] [PubMed]
23. Jensen, I.B.; Busch, H.; Bodin, L.; Hagberg, J.; Nygren, A.; Bergström, G. Cost effectiveness of two rehabilitation programmes for neck and back pain patients: A seven year follow-up. *Pain* **2009**, *142*, 202–208. [CrossRef] [PubMed]
24. Munder, T.; Brütsch, O.; Leonhart, R.; Gerger, H.; Barth, J. Researcher allegiance in psychotherapy outcome research: An overview of reviews. *Clin. Psychol. Rev.* **2013**, *33*, 501–511. [CrossRef]
25. Margison, F.R.; Barkham, M.; Evans, C.; McGrath, G.; Clark, J.M.; Audin, K.; Connell, J. Measurement and psychotherapy. Evidence-based practice and practice-based evidence. *Br. J. Psychiatry* **2000**, *177*, 123–130. [CrossRef] [PubMed]
26. Preis, M.A.; Vögtle, E.; Dreyer, N.; Seel, S.; Wagner, R.; Hanshans, K.; Reyersbach, R.; Pieh, C.; Mühlberger, A.; Probst, T. Long-Term Outcomes of a Multimodal Day-Clinic Treatment for Chronic Pain under the Conditions of Routine Care. *Pain Res. Manag.* **2018**. [CrossRef] [PubMed]
27. Whiteneck, G.G.; Gassaway, J. SCIRehab Uses Practice-Based Evidence Methodology to Associate Patient and Treatment Characteristics with Outcomes. *Arch. Phys. Med. Rehabil.* **2013**, *94*, S67–S74. [CrossRef] [PubMed]

28. Malmivaara, A. Assessing the effectiveness of rehabilitation and optimizing effectiveness in routine clinical work. *J. Rehabil. Med.* **2018**, *50*, 849–851. [CrossRef] [PubMed]
29. Gerdle, B.; Molander, P.; Stenberg, G.; Stålnacke, B.-M.; Enthoven, P. Weak outcome predictors of multimodal rehabilitation at one-year follow-up in patients with chronic pain—A practice based evidence study from two SQRP centres. *BMC Musculoskelet. Disord.* **2016**, *17*, 287. [CrossRef]
30. Craig, P.; Dieppe, P.; MacIntyre, S.; Michie, S.; Nazareth, I.; Petticrew, M. Medical Research Council Guidance. Developing and evaluating complex interventions: The new Medical Research Council guidance. *BMJ* **2008**, *337*, a1655. [CrossRef]
31. Bromley Milton, M.; Borsbo, B.; Rovner, G.; Lundgren-Nilsson, A.; Stibrant-Sunnerhagen, K.; Gerdle, B. Is Pain Intensity Really That Important to Assess in Chronic Pain Patients? A Study Based on the Swedish Quality Registry for Pain Rehabilitation (SQRP). *PLoS ONE* **2013**, *8*, e65483. [CrossRef]
32. Hasselström, J.; Liu-Palmgren, J.; Rasjö-Wrååk, G.; Liu-Palmgren, J.; Rasjö-Wrååk, G. Prevalence of pain in general practice. *Eur. J. Pain* **2002**, *6*, 375–385. [CrossRef]
33. Mäntyselkä, P.; Kumpusalo, E.; Ahonen, R.; Kumpusalo, A.; Kauhanen, J.; Viinamäki, H.; Halonen, P.; Takala, J. Pain as a reason to visit the doctor: A study in Finnish primary health care. *Pain* **2001**, *89*, 175–180. [CrossRef]
34. Gerdle, B.; Åkerblom, S.; Brodda Jansen, G.; Enthoven, P.; Ernberg, M.; Dong, H.-J.; Stålnacke, B.; Äng, B.; Boersma, K. Who benefit from multimodal rehabilitation—An exploration of pain, psychological distress and life impacts in over 35,000 chronic pain patients identified in the Swedish Quality Registry for Pain Rehabilitation (SQRP). *J. Pain Res.* **2019**, *12*, 891–908. [CrossRef]
35. Rovner, G.S.; Sunnerhagen, K.S.; Björkdahl, A.; Gerdle, B.; Börsbo, B.; Johansson, F.; Gillanders, D. Chronic pain and sex-differences; women accept and move, while men feel blue. *PLoS ONE* **2017**, *12*, 0175737. [CrossRef] [PubMed]
36. Bernfort, L.; Gerdle, B.; Husberg, M.; Levin, L.-A. People in states worse than dead according to the EQ-5D UK value set: Would they rather be dead? *Qual. Life Res.* **2018**, *27*, 1827–1833. [CrossRef] [PubMed]
37. Turk, D.C.; Rudy, T.E. Toward an empirically derived taxonomy of chronic pain patients: Integration of psychological assessment data. *J. Consult. Clin. Psychol.* **1988**, *56*, 233–238. [CrossRef] [PubMed]
38. Turk, D.C.; Rudy, T.E. Towards a comprehensive assessment of chronic pain patients. *Behav. Res. Ther.* **1987**, *25*, 237–249. [CrossRef]
39. Bergström, G.; Jensen, I.B.; Bodin, L.; Linton, S.J.; Nygren, A.L.; Carlsson, S.G. Reliability and factor structure of the Multidimensional Pain Inventory—Swedish Language Version (MPI-S). *Pain* **1998**, *75*, 101–110. [CrossRef]
40. Zigmond, A.S.; Snaith, R.P. The Hospital Anxiety and Depression Scale. *Acta Psychiatr. Scand.* **1983**, *67*, 361–370. [CrossRef]
41. Bjelland, I.; Dahl, A.A.; Haug, T.T.; Neckelmann, D. The validity of the Hospital Anxiety and Depression Scale. *J. Psychosom. Res.* **2002**, *52*, 69–77. [CrossRef]
42. Sullivan, M.; Karlsson, J.; Ware, J. The Swedish 36 Health survey. Evaluation of data quality, scaling assumption, reliability and construct validity across general populations in Sweden. *Soc. Sci. Med.* **1995**, *41*, 1349–1358. [CrossRef]
43. EuroQol Group. EuroQol—A new facility for the measurement of health-related quality of life. *Health Policy* **1990**, *16*, 199–208. [CrossRef]
44. Brooks, R. EuroQol: The current state of play. *Health Policy* **1996**, *37*, 53–72. [CrossRef]
45. Dolan, P.; Sutton, M.; Sutton, M. Mapping visual analogue scale health state valuations onto standard gamble and time trade-off values. *Soc. Sci. Med.* **1997**, *44*, 1519–1530. [CrossRef]
46. Bäckryd, E.; Persson, E.B.; Larsson, A.I.; Fischer, M.R.; Gerdle, B. Chronic pain patients can be classified into four groups: Clustering-based discriminant analysis of psychometric data from 4665 patients referred to a multidisciplinary pain centre (a SQRP study). *PLoS ONE* **2018**, *13*, e0192623. [CrossRef] [PubMed]
47. Jansen, J.J.; Szymanska, E.; Hoefsloot, H.C.; Jacobs, D.M.; Strassburg, K.; Smilde, A.K. Between Metabolite Relationships: An essential aspect of metabolic change. *Metabolomics* **2012**, *8*, 422–432. [CrossRef] [PubMed]
48. Pohjanen, E.; Thysell, E.; Jonsson, P.; Eklund, C.; Silfver, A.; Carlsson, I.-B.; Lundgren, K.; Moritz, T.; Svensson, M.B.; Antti, H. A Multivariate Screening Strategy for Investigating Metabolic Effects of Strenuous Physical Exercise in Human Serum. *J. Proteome Res.* **2007**, *6*, 2113–2120. [CrossRef] [PubMed]

49. Eriksson, L.; Byrne, T.; Johansson, E.; Trygg, J.; Vikström, C. *Multi—And Megavariate Data Analysis—Basic Principles and Applications*, 3rd ed.; Umetrics Academy: Umeå, Sweden, 2013.
50. Wheelock Åsa, M.; Wheelock, C.E. Trials and tribulations of 'omics data analysis: Assessing quality of SIMCA-based multivariate models using examples from pulmonary medicine. *Mol. BioSyst.* **2013**, *9*, 2589. [CrossRef] [PubMed]
51. Eriksson, L.; Johansson, E.; Kettaneh-Wold, N.; Trygg, J.; Wikström, C.; Wold, S. *Multi—And Megavariate Data Analysis: Part I and II*, 2nd ed.; Umetrics AB: Umeå, Sweden, 2006.
52. Turk, D.C.; Dworkin, R.H.; Allen, R.R.; Bellamy, N.; Brandenburg, N.; Carr, D.B.; Cleeland, C.; Dionne, R.; Farrar, J.T.; Galer, B.S.; et al. Core outcome domains for chronic pain clinical trials: IMMPACT recommendations. *Pain* **2003**, *106*, 337–345. [CrossRef] [PubMed]
53. Norrefalk, J.; Ekholm, K.; Linder, J.; Borg, K.; Ekholm, J. Evaluation of a multiprofessional rehabilitation programme for persistent musculoskeletal-related pain: Economic benefits of return to work. *Acta Derm. Venereol.* **2008**, *40*, 15–22. [CrossRef] [PubMed]
54. Matthias, M.S.; Miech, E.J.; Myers, L.J.; Sargent, C.; Bair, M.J. There's more to this pain than just pain: How patients' understanding of pain evolved during a randomized controlled trial for chronic pain. *J. Pain* **2012**, *13*, 571–578. [CrossRef] [PubMed]
55. Rivano-Fischer, M.; Persson, E.; Stålnacke, B.; Schult, M.; Löfgren, M. Return to work after interdisciplinary pain rehabilitation: One- and two-years follow-up based on the Swedish Quality Registry for pain rehabilitation. *J. Rehabil. Med.* **2019**, *51*, 281–289. [CrossRef] [PubMed]
56. Busse, J.W.; Wang, L.; Kamaleldin, M.; Craigie, S.; Riva, J.J.; Montoya, L.; Mulla, S.M.; Lopes, L.C.; Vogel, N.; Chen, E.; et al. Opioids for Chronic Noncancer Pain: A Systematic Review and Meta-analysis. *JAMA* **2018**, *320*, 2448–2460. [CrossRef] [PubMed]
57. Enthoven, W.T.; Roelofs, P.D.; Deyo, R.A.; Van Tulder, M.W.; Koes, B.W. Non-steroidal anti-inflammatory drugs for chronic low back pain. *Cochrane Database Syst. Rev.* **2016**, *2*, 012087. [CrossRef] [PubMed]
58. Saragiotto, B.T.; Machado, G.C.; Ferreira, M.L.; Pinheiro, M.B.; Abdel Shaheed, C.; Maher, C.G. Paracetamol for low back pain. *Cochrane Database Syst. Rev.* **2016**. [CrossRef] [PubMed]
59. Henry, S.G.; Bell, R.A.; Fenton, J.J.; Kravitz, R.L. Goals of Chronic Pain Management: Do Patients and Primary Care Physicians Agree and Does It Matter? *Clin. J. Pain* **2017**, *33*, 955–961. [CrossRef] [PubMed]
60. Thompson, M.; McCracken, L.M. Acceptance and Related Processes in Adjustment to Chronic Pain. *Curr. Pain Headache Rep.* **2011**, *15*, 144–151. [CrossRef] [PubMed]
61. McCracken, L.M.; Zhao-O'Brien, J.; Zhao-O'Brien, J. General psychological acceptance and chronic pain: There is more to accept than the pain itself. *Eur. J. Pain* **2010**, *14*, 170–175. [CrossRef] [PubMed]
62. Skelly, A.; Chou, R.; Dettori, J.; Turner, J.; Friedly, J.; Rundell, S.; Fu, R.; Brodt, E.; Wasson, N.; Winter, C.; et al. *Noninvasive Nonpharmacological Treatment for Chronic Pain: A Systematic Review [Internet]*; Agency for Healthcare Research and Quality (US): Rockville, MD, USA, 2018.
63. Salathé, C.R.; Melloh, M.; Crawford, R.; Scherrer, S.; Boos, N.; Elfering, A. Treatment Efficacy, Clinical Utility, and Cost-Effectiveness of Multidisciplinary Biopsychosocial Rehabilitation Treatments for Persistent Low Back Pain: A Systematic Review. *Glob. Spine J.* **2018**, *8*, 872–886. [CrossRef] [PubMed]
64. Ruscheweyh, R.; Dany, K.; Marziniak, M.; Gralow, I. Basal Pain Sensitivity does not Predict the Outcome of Multidisciplinary Chronic Pain Treatment. *Pain Med.* **2015**, *16*, 1635–1642. [CrossRef] [PubMed]
65. Borys, C.; Lutz, J.; Strauss, B.; Altmann, U. Effectiveness of a Multimodal Therapy for Patients with Chronic Low Back Pain Regarding Pre-Admission Healthcare Utilization. *PLoS ONE* **2015**, *10*, 0143139. [CrossRef] [PubMed]
66. Letzel, J.; Angst, F.; Weigl, M.B. Multidisciplinary biopsychosocial rehabilitation in chronic neck pain: A naturalistic prospective cohort study with intraindividual control of effects and 12-month follow-up. *Eur. J. Phys. Rehabil. Med.* **2018**, in press. [CrossRef]
67. Moradi, B.; Hagmann, S.; Zahlten-Hinguranage, A.; Caldeira, F.; Putz, C.; Rosshirt, N.; Schonit, E.; Mesrian, A.; Schiltenwolf, M.; Neubauer, E. Efficacy of multidisciplinary treatment for patients with chronic low back pain: A prospective clinical study in 395 patients. *J. Clin. Rheumatol.* **2012**, *18*, 76–82. [CrossRef]
68. Boersma, K.; Södermark, M.; Hesser, H.; Flink, I.; Gerdle, B.; Linton, S. The efficacy of a transdiagnostic emotion-focused exposure treatment for chronic pain patients with comorbid anxiety and depression: A randomized controlled trial. *Pain* **2019**, in press. [CrossRef] [PubMed]

69. Craig, P.; Dieppe, P.; Macintyre, S.; Michie, S.; Nazareth, I.; Petticrew, M. Developing and Evaluating Complex Interventions: New Guidance. 2008. Available online: https://www.researchgate.net/publication/32899190_Developing_and_Evaluating_Complex_Interventions_New_Guidance_Online (accessed on 4 June 2019).
70. Kamper, S.J.; Apeldoorn, A.T.; Chiarotto, A.; Smeets, R.J.; Ostelo, R.W.J.G.; Guzman, J.; Van Tulder, M.W. Multidisciplinary biopsychosocial rehabilitation for chronic low back pain. *Cochrane Database Syst. Rev.* **2014**, *350*. [CrossRef] [PubMed]
71. Movsisyan, A.; Melendez-Torres, G.; Montgomery, P. Outcomes in systematic reviews of complex interventions never reached "high" GRADE ratings when compared with those of simple interventions. *J. Clin. Epidemiol.* **2016**, *78*, 22–33. [CrossRef] [PubMed]
72. Feise, R.J. Do multiple outcome measures require p-value adjustment? *BMC Med. Res. Methodol.* **2002**, *2*, 8. [CrossRef]
73. Turk, D.C.; Dworkin, R.H.; McDermott, M.P.; Bellamy, N.; Burke, L.B.; Chandler, J.M.; Cleeland, C.S.; Cowan, P.; Dimitrova, R.; Farrar, J.T.; et al. Analyzing multiple endpoints in clinical trials of pain treatments: IMMPACT recommendations. *Pain* **2008**, *139*, 485–493. [CrossRef] [PubMed]
74. Bagiella, E. Clinical Trials in Rehabilitation: Single or Multiple Outcomes? *Arch. Phys. Med. Rehabil.* **2009**, *90*, S17–S21. [CrossRef] [PubMed]
75. Tyler, K.M.; Normand, S.L.; Horton, N.J. The use and abuse of multiple outcomes in randomized controlled depression trials. *Contemp. Clin. Trials* **2011**, *32*, 299–304. [CrossRef] [PubMed]
76. Teixeira-Pinto, A.; Mauri, L. Msc Statistical Analysis of Noncommensurate Multiple Outcomes. *Circ. Cardiovasc. Qual. Outcomes* **2011**, *4*, 650–656. [CrossRef]
77. Boonstra, A.M.; Reneman, M.F.; Waaksma, B.R.; Schiphorst Preuper, H.R.; Stewart, R.E. Predictors of multidisciplinary treatment outcome in patients with chronic musculoskeletal pain. *Disabil. Rehabil.* **2015**, *37*, 1242–1250. [CrossRef]
78. Morley, S.; Williams, A.; Hussain, S. Estimating the clinical effectiveness of cognitive behavioural therapy in the clinic: Evaluation of a CBT informed pain management programme. *Pain* **2008**, *137*, 670–680. [CrossRef]
79. Pina-Sánchez, J.; Koskinen, J.; Plewis, I. *Measurement Error in Retrospective Reports of Unemployment*; CCSR Working Paper; The Cathie Marsh Centre for Census and Survey Research, University of Manchester: Manchester, UK, 2012; pp. 1–56.
80. Bernard, H.R.; Killworth, P.; Kronenfeld, D.; Sailer, L. The Problem of Informant Accuracy: The Validity of Retrospective Data. *Annu. Rev. Anthropol.* **1984**, *13*, 495–517. [CrossRef]
81. Van Der Vaart, W.; Van Der Zouwen, J.; Dijkstra, W. Retrospective questions: Data quality, task difficulty, and the use of a checklist. *Qual. Quant.* **1995**, *29*, 299–315. [CrossRef]
82. Schwartz, N. Retrospective and concurrent self-reports: The rationale for real-time data capture. In *The Science of Real-Time Data CAPTURE: Self-Reports in Health Research*; Oxford University Press: New York, NY, USA, 2007; pp. 11–26.
83. Schatman, M. Interdisciplinary Chronic Pain Management: International Perspectives. *Pain Clin. Updates* **2012**, *20*, 1–6.
84. Tseli, E.; Stalnacke, B.M.; Boersma, K.; Enthoven, P.; Gerdle, B.; Ang, B.O.; Grooten, W.J.A. Prognostic Factors for Physical Functioning After Multidisciplinary Rehabilitation in Patients with Chronic Musculoskeletal Pain: A Systematic Review and Meta-analysis. *Clin. J. Pain* **2018**, *35*, 148. [CrossRef] [PubMed]
85. Westlander, G. Refined use of standardized self-reporting in intervention studies (In Swedish: Förfinad användning av standardiserad självrapportering i interventionstudier). *Soc. Tidskr.* **2004**, *2*, 168–181.

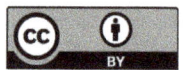

© 2019 by the authors. Licensee MDPI, Basel, Switzerland. This article is an open access article distributed under the terms and conditions of the Creative Commons Attribution (CC BY) license (http://creativecommons.org/licenses/by/4.0/).

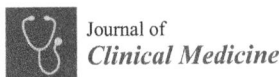

Article

Dissociation and Pain-Catastrophizing: Absorptive Detachment as a Higher-Order Factor in Control of Pain-Related Fearful Anticipations Prior to Total Knee Arthroplasty (TKA)

Matthias Vogel [1,*,†], Martin Krippl [2,†], Lydia Frenzel [1], Christian Riediger [3], Jörg Frommer [1], Christoph Lohmann [3] and Sebastian Illiger [3]

1. Universitätsklinik für Psychosomatische Medizin und Psychotherapie der Otto-von-Guericke-Universität Magdeburg, Leipziger Straße 44, 39120 Magdeburg, Germany; Lydia.frenzel@med.ovgu.de (L.F.); joerg.frommer@med.ovgu.de (J.F.)
2. Institut für Psychologie der Otto-von-Guericke-Universität Magdeburg, Universitätsplatz 2, Geb. 24, 39106 Magdeburg, Germany; martin.krippl@ovgu.de
3. Universitätsklinik für Orthopädie der Otto-von-Guericke-Universität Magdeburg, Leipziger Straße 44, 39120 Magdeburg, Germany; christian.riediger@med.ovgu.de (C.R.); christoph.lohmann@med.ovgu.de (C.L.); sebastian.illiger@med.ovgu.de (S.I.)
* Correspondence: matthias.vogel@med.ovgu.de; Tel.: +49-391-6714200
† These authors contributed equally.

Received: 9 March 2019; Accepted: 10 May 2019; Published: 16 May 2019

Abstract: Total Knee Arthroplasty (TKA) is the ultima-ratio therapy for knee-osteoarthritis (OA), which is a paradigmatic condition of chronic pain. A hierarchical organization may explain the reported covariation of pain-catastrophizing (PC) and dissociation, which is a trauma-related psychopathology. This study tests the hypotheses of an overlap and hierarchical organization of the two constructs, PC and dissociation, respectively, using the Western Ontario and McMaster Universities Osteoarthritis Index (WOMAC), the Childhood Trauma Screener (CTS), a shortened version of the Dissociative Experiences Scale (FDS-20), the Brief Symptom Inventory (BSI-18), the Pain-Catastrophizing Scale (PCS), and the Tampa Scale of Kinesiophobia (TSK) in 93 participants with knee-OA and TKA. Non-parametric correlation, linear regression, and an exploratory factor analysis comprising the PCS and the FDS-20 in aggregate were run. The three factors: (1) PC factor, (2) absorptive detachment, and (3) conversion altogether explained 60% of the variance of the two scales. Dissociative factors were related to childhood trauma, and the PC-factor to knee-pain. The latter was predicted by absorptive detachment, i.e., disrupted perception interfering with the integration of trauma-related experiences possibly including invasive surgery. Absorptive detachment represents negative affectivity and is in control of pain-related anxieties (including PC). The clinical associations of trauma, psychopathology, and maladaptation after TKA may be reflections of this latent hierarchical organization of trauma-related dissociation and PC.

Keywords: total knee arthroplasty (TKA); pain-catastrophizing; dissociation; hierarchical structure

1. Introduction

1.1. Hierarchy of Pain-Related Anxieties

The cognitive behavioral construct of pain-catastrophizing (PC) refers to "an exaggerated negative mental set brought to bear during actual or anticipated painful experience" [1]. It is known to exert a direct influence on a patient's response to the experience of pain [2]. Moreover, being a content-specific (i.e., pain-related) construct, PC overlaps with other constructs of negative affectivity (e.g., generic constructs of anxiety, aggression, and alienation) [3]. Therefore, Vancleef et al. [3] have reinforced the notion of a hierarchical structure of pain-related negative emotional constructs [4], in which content-specific constructs directly related to pain reside in close vicinity to the actual experience of pain. On the contrary, generic constructs of (negative) affectivity function as higher-order factors in the control of content-specific anxiety. For example, a common factorization of PC and higher order negative affect, as well as coping strategies, revealed a functional hierarchy involving PC and illness focused coping [5]. Likewise, Kleiman et al. [6] corroborated the hierarchical model by means of a factor analytic study examining the factor structure of measures of negative affect and content-related anxieties, including PC in aggregate. Those authors extracted one common factor termed sensitivity to pain traumatization, which represents a pain-related stress reaction of a posttraumatic character (e.g., intrusive thoughts, avoidance, and arousal). Dissociative phenomena are entangled with negative affect as well, partly as a result of their emotionally destabilizing potential [7], partly by virtue of their negative affective nature, which led Watson and Clark [8] and Lilienfeld et al. [4] to subsume alienation (i.e., derealisation/depersonalization) under negative affect. Likewise, Tellegen [9] and Patrick and Kramer [10] conceptualized alienation (or estrangement) and absorption as components of negative affectivity. Therefore, not surprisingly, high negative affectivity is linked to dissociative phenomena in the frame of posttraumatic stress disorder (PTSD) [11]. Not least, Kleiman et al. [6] postulate symptoms of emotional numbing (i.e., pain-related emotional detachment) to be reflective of such posttraumatic symptomatology, which occurs in response to pain. Similar to the factor analytic studies in personality disorder research, those studies indicate the possibility of explaining the covariation among the observed pain-related variables through the use of latent constructs, brought to light by factor analysis [12], also with regards to research on chronic pain and its nested psychological correlates. The knowledge of such systematic interactions between PC, which is an important predictor of postoperative pain [13], and posttraumatic symptomatology likely offers hints on adequate psychotherapeutic strategies, as well. For example, dissociative symptoms, if proven to contribute to chronic pain, would call for a trauma-specific therapy also in this context.

1.2. Dissociation and Pain-Catastrophizing

The DSM-5 defines dissociative symptomatology as the disruption of and /or discontinuity in the normal integration of consciousness, memory, identity, emotion, perception, body representation, motor control, and behavior [14]. Dissociation has been hypothesized as a survival mechanism for surviving a trauma (e.g., sexual) [15]. Holmes et al. [16] have suggested distinct classes of dissociative symptoms, namely detachment–dissociation and compartmentalization–dissociation, at which the former is characterized by a sense of separation from the body, self, and environment, whereas the latter reflects the temporary loss of deliberate control over distinct systems, e.g., memory [17]. Regarding chronic pain, dissociation is believed to serve to minimize memories of traumatic events, including the minimization or magnification of the pain perception (the pain focus) [18]. Dissociative symptoms are frequent in trauma-related psychiatric disorders [19], and, in addition, also occur in pain-prone medical conditions, such as Osteoarthritis (OA) and rheumatoid arthritis [20]. Likewise, PC is linked to chronic pain and to worse outcomes of OA-related arthroplasty [21]. Notably, preoperative PC increases pain perception by means of magnifying pain focus [22], and preoperative pain, in turn, is a strong predictor of the postoperative algofunction (AF) [23], i.e., the combined status regarding knee-pain and knee function.

1.3. Psychosomatic Aspects of Osteoarthritis and Total Knee Arthroplasty

OA is a degenerative joint disease causing pain and stiffness, is among the leading causes of chronic pain and disability [24], and serves well as an example of the progressive, complex, and multifaceted nature of chronic pain [25]. TKA represents the ultimate therapeutic option for OA of the knee. However, about a quarter of the patients undergoing TKA experience neither pain-relief nor functional restoration after TKA without there being any detectable medical cause [26]. Moreover, OA is known to coincide with depression, anxiety, and PC, with exactly these psychological circumstances signifying greater pain even after TKA [27]. Those reports correspond well to the prediction of postoperative outcomes by personality characteristics, such as neuroticism or borderline personality [13,28]. Moreover, chronic pain is connected to specific anxieties related to pain, which include kinesiophobia in addition to PC. The fear avoidance model of chronic pain posits a circular interaction between the pain focus (that is PC), the perception of pain as well as the fear of movement and re-injury. As a result, the individual is prompted to withdraw from activity and social surroundings to the effect of reduced participation, a less healthy lifestyle, and worsened pain [28].

1.4. Linking Pain-Catastrophizing and Dissociation

Experimental research [29] suggests an overlap between PC and dissociation, and theoretical considerations [30] do so regarding catastrophic cognitions and dissociative experiences. This assumption is based on the notion that symptoms, be it dissociation or chronic pain, are perceived and processed in accordance to the meaning which the individual ascribes to them. Specifically, according to Ehlers and Steil [30], the co-occurrence of helplessness and detachment dissociation serves to maintain mental control by preventing exposure to feared material. This theorizing is consistent with the results of Gómez-Pérez et al. [29], who demonstrated the simultaneous elicitation of PC and dissociative experiences through a cold pressor task, thus suggesting each of the idiosyncratic meanings of those symptoms to be mutually influenced. Given the relationship of PC and dissociation with chronic pain, both likely contribute to the adaptation to chronic pain, possibly based on an underlying hierarchical structure [3]. Interestingly, researchers have found PC and chronic pain to be linked to childhood abuse [31], paralleling the respective associations between dissociation and prior trauma [32].

Considering the relationship between PC and childhood trauma, on the one hand, and between dissociation and chronic pain on the other, let alone with the hierarchical model in mind, the question arises as to how those symptoms are connected. Lynn et al. [33] and Giesbrecht et al. [34] have proposed the action of cognitive processes in dissociation, which may find its reflection in a clinical population treated for chronic pain in the form of an interaction and functional hierarchy between the two constructs [3]. The present study tests the hypothesis of an overlap between dissociation and PC in patients with end-stage knee-OA and chronic pain scheduled for TKA, who are known to be put under an enormous stress by the imminence of knee-surgery, hypothesizing an overlap which, in addition, is structured by distinguishable categories of dissociation interacting with the respective categories of pain-catastrophizing as predicted by the hierarchical model of pain-related negative affective constructs [4]. We therefore investigate the hierarchically structured organization possibly underlying PC and dissociation in people with chronic pain scheduled for TKA by means of an exploratory factor analysis. This is based on the assumption that dissociation would function equivalently to higher-order constructs of negative affect. Moreover, we assume pain-related anxieties, including PC and kinesiophobia, to be hierarchically nested, thus possibly lending an explanation to the covariation of the two constructs by the identification of a latent construct [12]. The rationale behind this procedure is to improve our theoretical understanding of psychological dispositions, including childhood trauma and its (adult) correlate, dissociation, for the chronicity of TKA-related pain.

2. Materials and Methods

All procedures performed in this study were in accordance with the ethical standards of the institutional and/or national research committee and with the 1964 Helsinki declaration and its later amendments or comparable ethical standards. Informed consent was obtained from all individual participants included in the study.

2.1. Sample

A previous study [35] reported a moderate correlation (r = 0.32) between the Dissociative Experiences Scale [36] and the Cognitive Failure Questionnaire [37]. Given that the PC is also reflecting a cognitive construct, we used this finding as the basis of our power calculation, which we conducted by means of G*power (Version 3.1.9.2) [38], arriving at the minimum sample size of $n = 74$ (two-tailed, power = 80).

However, 98 patients (53% female) with an average age of 64.64 (±10.55) years (males: 64.27 ± 9.87, females: 64.98 ± 11.22) scheduled for elective primary TKA for OA were consecutively included in the present study. The study was approved by the local Institutional Review Board. Inclusion was based on the aspect of primary TKA for OA and age > 18, while exclusion pertained to the presence of records of major psychiatric illness. The assessment took place only one to two days before the operation for the sake of which participants were admitted to the orthopedic department. We enrolled the participants of the present study consecutively between 2015 and 2017.

2.2. Questionnaire Measures

Knee pain and function were assessed using the Western Ontario and McMaster Universities Osteoarthritis Index (WOMAC) pain and function subscales (WOMAC A and WOMAC C). Cronbachs α's of the WOMAC range from 0.8 to 0.96 and its psychometric properties are judged as being good [39]. The WOMAC used in this study was the Likert version in the format of a numerical rating scale ranging from 0 to 10.

The brief symptom inventory (BSI-18), a short version of the Symptom Check List 90, assesses symptoms of depression, anxiety, and somatization in three subscales. Internal consistency for the subscales ranges between 0.79 and 0.91, discriminant and convergent validity are deemed good, and the scale is useful as a screening for psychological distress in physically ill populations [40]. This distress is particularly marked prior to TKA and is also a predictor of a worse postoperative algofunction.

The Fragebogen zu dissoziativen Symptomen (FDS) [41] represents the German version of the Dissociative Experiences Scale, of which we used the short form (FDS-20). The FDS-20 is composed of the most sensitive items of the longer version on the condition they reach a Cronbachs α of at least 0.9. The total scale has a good internal consistency ($\alpha = 0.93$). Items are rated in terms of frequency on a scale ranging from never present (0%) to always present (100%). However, for the purpose of the exploratory factor analysis, we transformed the data into four categories reflecting the following ranges of values: 0%–25%, 26%–50%, 51%–75%, and 76%–100% (of the time), respectively. Rodewald et al. [42] determined the cut-off of the FDS-20 to be 13, allowing for differentiation between severe and non-severe dissociation. Means of the FDS-20 are reported to range from 5.0 in non-psychiatric samples to 25.43 in personality disorders [41]. The factorial structure of the Dissociative Experiences Scale does not apply to its short version, FDS-20.

The Pain-Catastrophizing Scale (PCS) is a 13-item rating-scale comprising the subscales rumination (PCS-Rumi), magnification (PCS-Magni), and helplessness (PCS-Help) [43]. It assesses thoughts and feelings about the pain experience on a 5 point Likert scale. The PCS has proven adequate to excellent internal consistency (Cronbachs α's: total score: 0.87, PCS-Rumi: 0.87, PCS-Magni: 0.66, PCS-Help: 0.78). The cut-off serving the distinction between severe and non-severe pain-catastrophizing was set at 30.

The Tampa Scale of Kinesiophobia (TSK) is a 13 item rating scale rated on a 4 point Likert scale. Assessing fear of movement and re-injury, it is a valid and reliable instrument with the Cronbach's α being 0.73 for its German version [44]. The TSK is divided into two subscales termed activity avoidance (AA) and somatic focus (SF). Kinesiophobia is essential to fear avoidance, which makes it a relevant construct also for pain-related psycho-traumatology.

The CTS is a five-item-self-report instrument assessing childhood emotional, physical, and sexual abuse, as well as childhood emotional and physical neglect. The CTS is derived from the Childhood

Trauma Questionnaire for use as a screening for childhood trauma. Cronbach's α of the CTS is 0.75, and it is judged to be reliable and valid for its purpose [45].

2.3. Statistical Analysis

We used t-testing to compare groups (e.g., male/female) and non-parametric correlations (Kendall's Tau) to explore the relationships between continuous variables. The latter choice corresponds to the skewed distribution of dissociative symptoms in non-psychiatric populations [41]. Principal axis factor analysis (PAF) [46] was applied for the 33 items of the FDS-20 and the PCS. We were advised to do so, because the factorial structure of the Dissociative Experiences Scale does not apply to its short version and, in addition, this chosen procedure suits our intention to identify the presumed latent structure of the two scales and their observed covariation [4]. The factors were based on the Kaiser-Guttman-Criterion (eigenvalue > 1) [47] and rotated using the promax method. After that, parallel analysis [48] was applied, which revealed three factors to extract. We discarded those items, which had their highest loading in the rotated loading matrices on a factor other than 1, 2, or 3.

The factor scores represent the criteria used in the linear regression analyses. We selected the corresponding independent variables according to their significance in the preceding non-parametric correlations. All regressions were controlled for age, gender, and the severity of dissociation or PC (according to the respective cut-off scores), respectively, each depending on their use as a predictor.

3. Results

3.1. Description of the Sample

The sample was comprised of 98 participants (53% female) with an average age of 64.64 (±10.55) years (males: 64.27 ± 9.87, females: 64.98 ± 11.22). Five patients refused to participate due to reluctance to fill in questionnaires. In case of missing data, the participants were contacted and the values recovered on the occasion of follow-up visits in the orthopedic university clinic. Table 1 displays the sociodemographic description of the sample with complete data (*n* = 93). The mean score (SD) and ranges of the WOMAC A and C scales were as follows: A = 5.3 (2.05) and 0.2 to 10.0, C = 4.88 (2.3) and 0.29 to 12.53.

Table 1. Sociodemographic description of the sample.

Variable	N	%
Marital Status		
single	5	5.4
married/in a relationship	61	65.6
divorced	10	10.8
widow	15	16.1
other	2	2.2
School		
no school degree	2	2.15
special school	2	2.15
8 classes	25	26.88
10 classes	43	46.24
12 classes	17	17.20
other	4	4.30
Education		
no profess-ion/untrained	24	25.81
completed apprenticeship	46	49.46
university	16	17.2
other	7	7.53

Table 1. Cont.

Variable	N	%
Accommodation		
own home	87	93.54
other	6	6.45
Occupation		
full-time	28	30.11
part time	8	8.60
at home (housewife)	4	4.30
jobless	1	1.08
pension	51	54.84
other	1	1.08

Mean (SD) of the FDS and the PCS total scores were 4.66 (7.94) and 17.75 (12.35), respectively.

Hence, the FDS-20 scores were skewed with most participants reporting only low levels of dissociation as expected in a non-psychiatric sample [41]. In total, 22 participants (23.66%) endorsed dissociation (FDS-total score) at 0% of the time. The mean (SD) of the TSK and the BSI were 21.09 (6.24) and 6.59 (7.14). The mean (SD) scores of the CTS-subscales were: EN: 1.70 (0.93); PA: 1.47 (0.9); EA: 1.32 (0.8); SA: 1.1 (0.39); and PN: 2.23 (1.27). There were significant (Pearson) correlations between the TSK and PCS (r = 0.35, $p < 0.01$), the GSI and pain-related anxieties (TSK: r = 0.21, $p < 0.01$; PCS: r = 0.43, $p < 0.01$), and between the FDS and the TSK (r = 0.22, $p < 0.01$). Table 2 shows the specific correlational matrix between the PCS and the FDS-20, respectively.

Table 2. Correlational matrix (Kendall's tau, p) between the Fragebogen zu dissoziativen Symptomern-20 (FDS-20) total score and the Pain Catastrophizing Scale (PCS) total and subscale scores.

	PCS-Rumination	PCS-Magnification	PCS Helplessness	PCS-Total
FDS-20 total score	0.44	0.36	0.47	0.45
	<0.01	<0.01	<0.01	<0.01

3.2. Common Factorization of the PCS and FDS-20:

Kaiser-Meyer-Olkin-statistics (KMO) for testing the usability of data for exploratory factor analysis revealed a very good result (0.901). Parallel analysis after PAF-analysis and promax-rotation revealed three factors.

Table 3 shows the latent factors at which the exploratory factor analysis arrived, the respective proportion of explained variance, and the wording and the mapping on the original scale. Items with the highest loadings on a factor represent that factor (bold face in Table 3). The loss of 13 (factors 4 to 7) of the 33 items, with which the PAF was fed, is due to the determination of three factors by parallel analysis. An item was allocated to a certain factor, on the condition that its highest loading was on that factor. The lowest loading on a factor was 0.38 (Table 3). The most influential factor reflects a compound of the subscales of the PCS, apparently reflecting the core affective and cognitive responses to pain typically displayed by patients with chronic pain. It is therefore referred to as the pain-catastrophizing factor (PC-factor). The second factor, termed absorptive detachment in reference to Allen, Console, and Lewis (49), contains items that map onto the subscales of amnesia and derealisation of the FDS. The third factor reflects the conversion subscale of the FDS and was named accordingly. Mean (SD) of the factor scores for low/high dissociators (in accordance to the respective cut-off point) were the following: Helplessness: −0.12 (0.9)/1.59 (0.71); absorptive detachment: −0.23 (0.32)/2.87 (2.15); conversion: −0.2 (0.62)/1.98 (1.81).

Table 3. Latent factors (F1-F7) of the PCS and the FDS-20, respectively, along with the respective factor loadings and wordings of the items. * The number of factors determined to be kept by parallel analysis was 3. Items with the highest loadings on a factor represent that factor (bold face).

Scale (Item nr.)	Factors Kept * (% Explained Variance)			Factors Lost * (% Explained Variance)				Wording
	F1 (44.7)	F2 (13.25)	F3 (5.41)	F4 (3.6)	F5 (3.45)	F6 (3.23)	F7 (3.1)	
PCS (2)	**0.94**						−0.13	Feeling one can't go on
PCS (1)	**0.92**		−0.18		−0.12			Worrying all the time about whether the pain will end
PCS (4)	**0.92**		0.25			−0.16	−0.10	Feeling overwhelmed
PCS (6)	**0.86**		−0.20	0.14				Being afraid of pain getting worse
PCS (3)	**0.85**		0.15			−0.10		Thinking it's never getting better
PCS (5)	**0.84**							Feeling one can't stand it anymore
PCS (8)	**0.70**		−0.17			−0.11	0.30	Anxiously wanting pain to go away
PCS (11)	**0.64**		−0.18		0.15		0.32	Badly wanting pain to go away
PCS (13)	**0.51**	0.12			−0.15	0.22	0.35	I wonder whether something serious might happen.
PCS (7)	**0.44**		0.25	0.17			0.19	Thinking of other painful events
FDS (19)		**0.89**			0.14			Being in a familiar place but finding it unfamiliar
FDS (20)		**0.86**	−0.18			0.19		Feeling as though one were different people
FDS (8)		**0.78**	0.30	0.12		−0.15		Hearing voices inside one's head
FDS (13)	−0.11	**0.59**		0.18	0.29		0.11	Other people and objects do not seem real
FDS (15)	0.16	**0.52**	0.21	−0.11	0.31			Abidance without movement, communication or reaction
FDS (4)		**0.38**	0.10	0.32	−0.23	0.33		Seeing oneself as if looking at another person
FDS (10)			**0.87**				0.10	Feeling one's extremities are weak, not being able to use them
FDS (9)			**0.68**	0.14				Paresthesia or not feeling parts of one's body
FDS (18)		0.33	**0.55**			0.16	0.12	Feeling uncertain when walking or standing
FDS (12)		0.39	**0.46**	−0.33	0.14	0.25		Unable to coordinate movements
FDS (2)		−0.16		**0.74**	0.26			Looking at the world through a fog
FDS (3)			0.13	**0.70**		0.12		Not recognizing one's reflection in a mirror
FDS (1)	0.15	0.15		**0.51**	0.20	−0.26		Feeling one's body is not one's own
FDS (16)	0.15	0.33	−0.11	**0.43**		0.13	−0.16	Remembering past so vividly one seems to be reliving it
FDS (17)					**0.68**	0.22		Staring into space
FDS (7)		0.23		0.13	**0.64**			So involved in phantasy that it seems real
FDS (11)				0.22	**0.50**	0.31	−0.11	Being accused of lying when telling the truth
FDS (6)	−0.11		0.20			**0.68**		Finding evidence of having done things one can't remember doing
FDS (5)		−0.16	0.11	0.29	0.26	**0.57**		Not sure if remembered event happened or was a dream
FDS (14)					0.38	**0.55**		Not sure whether one has done something or only thought about it
PCS (9)	0.49						**0.60**	Unable to stop thinking about pain
PCS (10)	0.48						**0.58**	Permanently thinking of how one wished pains to end
PCS (12)	0.29	−0.14	0.23			−0.15	**0.54**	Nothing one can do to relieve the pain

3.3. Factor Correlations and Interrelation

Table 4 shows the correlational matrix of these factors as well as their correlations with the clinical variables of interest. The PC-factor and the absorptive detachment factor were highly correlated with each other (cf. Table 4), but not with the factor conversion. The event of an item loading highly on two factors did not occur among factors 1 to 3, although the three items of factor 6 had their second highest loadings on factor 1. Regarding the BSI-18, the conversion factor was only linked to somatization, whereas the other two were linked to depression and anxiety, as well. The conversion factor—unlike its companions—lacked an association with TSK-subscales. Knee-pain and function were related to the PC-factor only, whereas childhood trauma solely showed correlations with dissociative factors. Based on the cut-off score of the FDS-20, six participants qualified as severe dissociators.

Table 4. Correlations (Kendall's Tau, first rows and *p* values, second rows) of the factors 1 to 3 with WOMAC and psychometric scores and interfactor-correlations. WOMAC A: knee-pain; WOMAC C: knee-function; TSK: Tampa scale of kinesiophobia; CEA: childhood emotional abuse; CPA: childhood physical abuse; CSA: childhood sexual abuse; CEN: childhood emotional neglect; CPN: childhood physical neglect; GSI: global severity index, -: no correlation could be computed.

	PC-Factor	Absorptive Detachment-Factor	Conversion-Factor
PC-factor	-	0.36 0.000	0.09 0.27
Absorptive detachment-factor	0.36 0.000	-	0.02 0.76
Conversion-factor	0.09 0.27	0.02 0.76	-
CEN	0.06 0.50	0.21 0.02	0.13 0.15
CPA	0.15 0.09	0.20 0.03	0.20 0.03
CEA	0.18 0.05	0.30 0.001	0.10 0.29
CSA	0.13 0.16	0.07 0.44	0.06 0.55
CPN	0.10 0.2	0.22 0.009	0.15 0.08
WOMAC A	0.28 0.001	0.12 0.1	0.02 0.8
WOMAC C	0.2 0.01	0.09 0.3	−0.03 0.7
TSK total score	0.36 0.000	0.31 0.000	0.09 0.23
-Somatic focus	0.33 0.000	0.28 0.001	0.07 0.38
-Activity avoidance	0.32 0.000	0.31 0.000	0.13 0.10
BSI-GSI	0.46 0.000	0.41 0.000	0.15 0.06
-Somatisation	0.4 0.000	0.34 0.000	0.27 0.002
-Depression	0.46 0.000	0.35 0.000	0.10 0.22
-Anxiety	0.41 0.000	0.41 0.000	0.11 0.19

Table 5 displays the results of the stepwise linear regression analyses, with the dependent variables being the factors 1, 2 and 3, and the predictors having been chosen based on the finding of a significant non-parametric correlation with the dependent variable in the previous step. The PC-factor was best predicted by the absorptive detachment-factor, but also by depression. The former was best predicted by activity avoidance, and the conversion factor by high PC. Hence, the two scales were separated by the factor analysis, but regression revealed their specific interactions in patients with imminent TKA.

Table 5. Linear regression analyses, dependent variables: factors PC-factor, absorptive detachment, and conversion. WOMAC A/C: knee-pain/-function; CEA: childhood emotional abuse; CPA: childhood physical abuse, CEN: childhood emotional neglect, CPN: childhood physical neglect, TSK-SF: subscale somatic focus (Tampa scale of kinesiophobia), TSK-AA: subscale activity avoidance (Tampa scale of kinesiophobia), BSI: brief symptom inventory, GSI: general severity index (summary score of the BSI).

Dependent Variable	Predictor	B	SE	β	t	p	CI Lower	CI Upper
PC-factor (total model: df = 12; F = 7.03; $p = 0.000$ $R^2 = 0.61$)	Gender	0.18	0.20	0.09	0.94	0.35	−0.21	0.58
	Age	−0.26	0.01	−0.26	−2.57	0.01	−0.05	0.01
	CEA	0.03	0.16	0.02	0.18	0.86	−0.30	0.36
	Absorptive detachment	0.35	0.15	0.38	2.37	0.02	0.05	0.65
	WomacA	0.05	0.08	0.10	0.61	0.55	−0.12	0.22
	WomacC	0.02	0.08	0.04	0.27	0.79	−0.14	0.18
	TSK-SF	0.02	0.05	0.05	0.40	0.69	−0.07	0.11
	TSK-AA	0.01	0.04	0.05	0.38	0.71	−0.06	0.09
	BSI-Somatisation	0.12	0.09	0.26	1.41	0.17	−0.05	0.29
	BSI-Depression	0.14	0.06	0.322	2.13	0.04	0.008	0.26
	BSI-anxiety	−0.01	−0.07	−0.01	−0.08	0.94	−0.14	0.13
	High dissociation	−0.93	0.64	−0.26	−1.45	0.15	−2.22	0.36
Factor absorptive detachment (df = 13; F = 3.25; $p = 0.001$ $R^2 = 0.41$)	Gender	0.28	0.24	0.13	1.14	0.26	−0.21	0.76
	Age	0.01	0.01	0.05	0.47	0.64	−0.02	0.03
	High pain-catastrophizing	0.57	0.50	0.22	1.13	0.26	−0.43	1.56
	CPA	−0.05	0.18	−0.04	−0.27	0.79	−0.40	0.31
	CEA	0.32	0.21	0.23	1.51	0.14	−0.10	0.74
	CEN	−0.26	0.20	−0.21	−1.31	0.19	−0.65	0.14
	CPN	0.21	0.11	0.24	1.93	0.06	−0.01	0.43
	PC-factor	0.06	0.23	0.06	0.28	0.78	−0.39	0.52
	TSK-SF	−0.06	0.06	−0.17	−1.16	0.25	−0.17	0.05
	TSK-AA	0.09	0.04	0.33	2.15	0.04	0.01	0.18
	BSI-Somatisation	0.10	0.10	−0.20	−0.96	0.34	−0.10	0.30
	BSI-depression	−0.09	0.08	−0.21	−1.19	0.24	−0.25	0.06
	BSI-anxiety	0.12	0.09	0.24	1.23	0.22	−0.07	0.30
conversion factor (df = 6; F = 7.09; $p = 0.000$ $R^2 = 0.39$)	Gender	0.18	0.19	0.09	0.92	0.36	−0.21	0.56
	Age	0.008	0.01	0.08	0.82	0.42	−0.01	0.03
	High pain-catastrophizing	0.79	0.28	0.33	2.78	0.007	0.22	1.35
	CPA	−0.012	0.11	−0.01	−0.10	0.92	−0.24	0.22
	GSI	−0.018	0.04	−0.12	−0.44	0.66	−0.10	0.06
	BSI-Somatisation	0.21	0.12	0.46	1.76	0.08	−0.03	0.44

B = unstandardized regression weights of predictors, SE = Standard errors of unstandardized regression weights, β = standardized regression weights, t = t-value of regression weights, p = p-value of regression weights, CI-lower = 95% confidence interval lower border of B, CI-upper = 95% confidence interval upper border of B.

4. Discussion

The present study explored the relationships between childhood trauma, PC, and dissociation in patients with end-stage knee osteoarthritis scheduled for TKA, based on the assumption of (1) a phenomenological overlap and clinical interaction [29], and (2) a hierarchical organization [3] between dissociation and PC [33]. Pain-related anxieties and negative affect (as represented by the global severity index of the BSI-18) proved highly intercorrelated, as did the FDS and pain-related anxieties, suggesting that negative affect, pain-related anxieties, and dissociation are nested. This prerequisite of the hierarchical model of pain-related anxieties aside, the factor analysis separated the FDS and the PCS, yielding one PCS-(catastrophizing) and two FDS-(dissociative) factors. The three factors together explained about 60% of the variance of the two scales and were subsequently correlated to knee-pain and function, as well as to psychopathological distress, including kinesiophobia, and to childhood trauma scores. All factors showed correlations with psychopathological distress and kinesiophobia, but the latter was more closely related to the PC-factor. Finally, linear regression showed that the latter (accounting for 44% of the variance of the two scales according to the factor analysis) was best predicted by the absorptive detachment factor. Contrarily, the conversion factor was predicted by high PC, and the absorptive detachment factor by activity avoidance. Thus, the factors apparently differ with regard to their elicitation as well as to their maintenance in patients with chronic pain undergoing TKA. Interestingly, the correlational patterns reveal specific associations between PC and knee-pain and function, and between dissociation and childhood trauma, respectively. On the contrary, all three factors showed close relationships with psychopathological distress, except for the conversion factor, which was not linked to kinesiophobia. Importantly, the regression analyses controlled for severe dissociation and severe PC, respectively, based on cut-offs, and the correlations were non-parametric, hence the present results do take the skewed distribution of dissociative symptoms in this non-psychiatric population into account.

4.1. A Topography of Specific Associations

The absorptive detachment factor is made up by a choice of dissociative symptoms, representing derealisation/depersonalisation (also referred to as detachment–dissociation) [15] on the one hand, and items, that are best described as relating to mal-integrated memory (amnesia) and the corresponding disruptions of identity, on the other. The latter result from the failure to properly contextualize and encode personal and (auto-) biographic memories constitutive of the self [49,50]. These specific dissociative experiences represent severe dissociation, as they are causing interruptions to the stream of consciousness, leading to gaps in identity and to ruminating, self-absorbed states (absorption) due to the preoccupation with, e.g., dissociative hallucinations [51] or other forms of compartmentalized traumatic memories. Likewise, jamais-vu (i.e., spurious non-familiarity) experiences are epiphenomena of severe dissociation [52], which could explain their high loading on the absorptive detachment-factor. Thus, this latent factor could be indicative of a dynamic interaction between states of detachment from the body, self, and/or environment, on the one hand, and the resulting lapses in memory formation, on the other. Moreover, the pain-specific construct of pain-related helplessness behaved as predicted by the hierarchical model and appears to be hierarchically nested within the generic (higher-order) construct of negative affect, which, as the present results suggest, does include detachment-dissociation.

4.2. Dissociative Coping: Legacy of Childhood Trauma in TKA and Beyond

This interaction is likely linear, dependent on the severity of dissociative symptoms and therefore possibly driven by the severe dissociators in the present study. Nevertheless, our results suggest a principal covariation of the two constructs, and are therefore in-line with [3], who incorporated alienation (i.e., detachment dissociation) in their concept of pain-related negative affect, although those authors do not lay their focus on dissociation. Comparable, specific interactions between the subtypes of dissociation, compartmentalization–dissociation, and detachment–dissociation, and different kinds of psychopathology, as well as their relation to childhood trauma have been described regarding psychiatric patients [53]. The respective differences pertain to the differential influence of detachment–dissociation and compartmentalization–dissociation, respectively, on the process of coping with psychic, and possibly also psychosomatic, as well as physical distress. While the population under study here is not psychiatric, it is facing TKA instantaneously and therefore under an enormous psychological strain. The latter includes a magnifying pain focus, which may initiate a dissociative response [29], possibly following a similar pattern as has been revealed in a psychiatric population, in principle. Dissociation is viewed as a means of coping with adversities, such as mental or physical harm, which makes it relevant to coping with, e.g., severe psychopathology or major surgery [54]. The latter may be viewed as an interpersonal act of violating the bodily integrity, especially based on the prior experience of interpersonal trauma.

Unlike other authors [30], we did not find an association between childhood trauma and PC. Rather, the present findings could suggest that those reports reflect the extent to which variances are being shared between measures of PC and dissociation. Accordingly, the type of trauma seemingly involved in the dynamics between PC and dissociation for the most part in the present study is childhood abuse, which Sansone et al. [30] also found to be linked to PC. Hence, the present findings suggest preoperative PC not only to be embedded in psychopathological distress, but also to be hierarchically nested within the more content-general construct of detachment–dissociation. Considering the trauma model of dissociation, which posits the causation of dissociative experiences by trauma [32], any cue reminiscent of an experienced trauma could therefore sensitize the individual by creating the expectation of another aggressive and hurtful encounter happening [30]. Regarding the dissociative factors, their prediction by activity avoidance and high pain catastrophizing surprises in that detachment was linked to kinesiophobia (or more precisely, activity avoidance). Kinesiophobia, apart from being correlated with catastrophizing, is obviously linked to self-absorbing inner experience and phantasies. That state possibly prevents the individual from being occupied with any activity other than that. Moreover, the link between the conversion factor and high PC underscores the relevance of phobic mechanisms for coping with major surgery [55]. Accordingly, joint function after TKA has been related to anxiety levels [56], a finding which possibly points to a subgroup of patients undergoing TKA, who are also suffering from trauma and dissociation.

Hence, in-line with the experimental data [29] indicating a dynamic relationship between dissociation and PC, the present results suggest dissociation severe enough to interfere with the consolidation of one's identity to maximize the psychopathological distress in traumatized individuals with TKA. This process seems to be driven by a lack of inner cohesion (that is, detachment from certain aspects of one's body, self, or environment) and by the systematic interactions between PC and trauma-related psychopathology. Accordingly, helplessness has been found to mediate the effect of catastrophizing on pain [57]. Inner cohesion is a reasonable prerequisite of effective self-regulation and competent mastery; consequently, unfavorable coping styles, such as rumination and self-blame, have been linked to detachment, a finding [58] possibly relevant to somato-psychic pathology, on a larger scale.

4.3. Synergism Between Pain-Catastrophizing and Dissociation

This notwithstanding, another effective way to induce dissociative symptoms, as well as PC in patients with TKA, apparently is to develop emotional distress, which—as many studies could demonstrate [26,28]—is especially pronounced in the face of imminent TKA. While affection with feelings of anxiety and depression may be a frequent reaction to facing invasive surgery for most people [59], the present study illustrates that it echoes the hierarchically structured interaction of detachment–dissociation and PC. As to the correlational conflation of the FDS-20 and the PCS in this study, it is consistent with a synergism rather than with the assumption of an antagonistic nature of their relationship [60]. This is also evident from studies reporting that the two forms of psychopathology converge to the effect of increasing the propensity for nocebo-like reactions [61], as one could call the events of impaired postoperative algofunction after TKA in the absence of medical causes. Moreover, from a theoretical point of view, the universal nature of the non-parametric correlation between the FDS-scale and the PCS, as well as the prediction of pain-related helplessness by detachment–dissociation correspond to the literature that conceives dissociation as being bound to cognitive failures. This stance [34], however, does not necessarily involve a functional hierarchy. Nevertheless, the latter could reconcile the controversy on the nature of dissociation at least in relation to pain-related cognitions. Moreover, the present results imply an overlap of PC, as assessed by the PCS, with various kinds of dissociative symptomatology.

4.4. Forced to the Knee: The Special Implications of Knee-Osteoarthritis

In accordance to this, several studies reported an association of PC either with amnesia or with depersonalization/derealisation, or both [29,62]. However, the cited studies are concerned with different samples and, most of all, different pain sites. In order to understand the psychological strain on patients awaiting TKA, the essentiality of the knee for our two-legged mobility ought to be considered: The respective patients with TKA are known to suffer markedly from functional problems as a result of malposition due to fear of pain and re-injury [63], to depend on help with their personal care and routine needs [64], and to experience a faster decline in gait speed, allowing for less participation to be reached as the disorder progresses compared to OA of the hip [65]. In conclusion, the present study, albeit retrospective and cross-sectional in nature, does encourage important clinical conclusions. A subgroup of patients with TKA may have specific difficulty coping with TKA as a result of childhood trauma and dissociative symptomatology and should therefore be offered psychosocial support based on psychological screenings. Moreover, the remarkable extent of psychopathological distress born by patients with imminent TKA may lead orthopedic surgeons to administer antidepressants peri-operatively in order to counterbalance the impact of psychopathological distress on the outcomes of TKA. As to the caveats of this study, the lack of psychiatric diagnostic interviews, which can hardly be implemented in an orthopedic setting, deserves mentioning. Moreover, the sample was limited in size and restricted to patients with OA scheduled for primary TKA and may therefore not be representative of other indications. Also, the five drop-outs in this study limit the interpretability of the results, especially since we cannot describe them due to a lack of sociodemographic information, which they did not provide. Furthermore, the common factorization deployed in the present work is a controversial procedure, although it offers the possibility of explaining the observed covariation of the variables under study by the identification of unobserved, latent factors [4] and is, in addition, a proven method in personality psychology [12]. However, since 13 items were excluded from the analysis by the parallel analysis, their covariation and latent contribution to the presumed hierarchical organization of pain-related anxieties and trauma-related symptoms remains obscure, although the contribution of factors 4 to 7 to the total variance of the two scales was comparatively small. The alternative price to pay would have been a reduced factor variance in connection with a heightened error variance as a result of a forceful allocation of the 13 omitted items on factors 1 to 3 based on secondary loadings. The latter procedure would have caused error correlations to occur, which would oppose the classical test theory [66]. Nevertheless, the present study is the first to suggest absorptive detachment as a latent factor crucial for the maladaptation to pain and its chronification. Moreover, the results reinforce the notion that childhood trauma and dissociation are relevant to coping with surgery and also deserve diagnostic attention in a surgical setting.

Author Contributions: M.V.: Conceptualization, writing, writing, and review editing L.F.: Data collection and curation, writing M.K.: Methodology, writing C.R.: Data collection and curation J.F.: Supervision C.L.: Writing S.I.: Supervision.

Funding: This study was funded by the Heigl-Evers-Stiftung (grant number: 472243/990099).

Conflicts of Interest: On behalf of all co-authors, I declare no conflict of interest regarding this submission.

References

1. Sullivan, M.J.L.; Thorn, B.; Keefe, F.J.; Martin, M.; Bradley, L.A.; Lefebvre, J.C. Theoretical perspectives on the relation between catastrophizing and pain. *Clin. J. Pain.* **2001**, *17*, 52–64. [CrossRef]
2. Keogh, E.; Asmundson, G.J. Negative affectivity, catastrophizing, and anxiety sensitivity. In *Understanding and Treating Fear of Pain*; Asmundson, G.J.G., Vlaeyen, J.W.S., Crombez, G., Eds.; University Press: New York, NY, USA, 2004; pp. 91–115.
3. Vancleef, L.M.; Vlaeyen, J.W.; Peters, M.L. Dimensional and componential structure of a hierarchical organization of pain-related anxiety constructs. *Psychol. Assess.* **2009**, *21*, 340–351. [CrossRef] [PubMed]
4. Lilienfeld, S.O.; Turner, S.M.; Jacob, R.G. Anxiety sensitivity: An examination of theoretical and methodological issues. *Adv. Behav. Res. Ther.* **1993**, *15*, 147–183. [CrossRef]
5. Krsmanovic, A.; Tripp, D.A.; Nickel, J.C.; Shoskes, D.A.; Pontari, M.; Litwin, M.S.; McNaughton-Collins, M.F. Psychosocial mechanisms of the pain and quality of life relationship for chronic prostatitis/chronic pelvic pain syndrome (CP/CPPS). *Can. Urol. Assoc.* **2014**, *8*, 403–408. [CrossRef]
6. Kleiman, V.; Clarke, H.; Katz, J. Sensitivity to pain traumatization: A higher-order factor underlying pain-related anxiety, pain catastrophizing and anxiety sensitivity among patients scheduled for major surgery. *Pain Res. Manag.* **2011**, *16*, 169–177. [CrossRef]

7. Ó Laoide, A.; Egan, J.; Osborn, K. What was once essential, may become detrimental: The mediating role of depersonalization in the relationship between childhood emotional maltreatment and psychological distress in adults. *J. Trauma. Dissociation* **2018**, *19*, 514–534. [CrossRef]
8. Watson, D.; Clark, L.A. Negative Affectivity: The disposition to Experience aversive emotional states. *Psychol. Bull.* **1984**, *96*, 465–490. [CrossRef]
9. Tellegen, A. *Multidimensional Personality Questionnaire*; University of Minnesota Press: Minneapolis, MN, USA, 2003.
10. Patrick, C.J.; Kramer, M.D. Multidimensional Personality Questionnaire. In *Enzyklopedia of Personality MD and Individual Differences*; Shekkelford, T.K., Virgilo-Zeigler, H., Eds.; Springer: New York, NY, USA, 2017.
11. Miller, M.W.; Greif, J.L.; Smith, A.A. Multi-dimensional Personality Questionnaire profiles of vet-erans with traumatic combat exposure: Externalizingand internalizing subtypes. *Psychol. Assess.* **2003**, *15*, 205–215. [CrossRef] [PubMed]
12. Wright, A.G.C. The current state and future of factor analysis in personality disorder research. *Pers. Disord.* **2017**, *8*, 14–25. [CrossRef] [PubMed]
13. Vogel, M.; Riediger, C.; Illiger, S.; Frommer, J.; Lohmann, C.H. Übersicht zu psychosomatischen Aspekten des Kniegelenksersatzes. [A review on psychosomatic factors affecting the outcome after total knee-arthroplasty (TKA)]. *Z. Psychosom. Med. Psychother.* **2017**, *63*, 370–387.
14. American Psychiatric Association. *Diagnostic and Statistical Manual of Mental Disorders–DSM-5*, 5th ed.; American Psychiatric Publishing: Arlington, TX, USA, 2013.
15. Schauer, M.; Elbert, T. Dissociation following traumatic stress. Etiology and treatment. *J. Psychol.* **2010**, *218*, 109–127.
16. Holmes, E.A.; Brown, R.J.; Mansell, W.; Fearon, R.P.; Hunter, E.C.M.; Frasquilho, F.; Oakley, D.A. Are there two distinct forms of dissociation? A review and some clinical implications. *Clin. Psychol. Rev.* **2005**, *25*, 1–23. [CrossRef]
17. Brown, R.J. The cognitive psychology of dissociative states. *Cognit. Neuropsychiat.* **2002**, *7*, 221–235. [CrossRef]
18. Duckworth, M.P.; Iezzi, T.; Archibald, Y.; Haertlein, P.; Klinck, A. Dissociation and posttraumatic stress symptoms in patients with chronic pain. *Int. J. Rehabil. Health* **2000**, *5*, 129–139. [CrossRef]
19. Gast, U.; Rodewald, F.; Nickel, V.; Emrich, H.M. Prevalence of dissociative disorders among psychiatric inpatients in a German university clinic. *J. Nerv. Ment. Dis.* **2001**, *189*, 249–257. [CrossRef]
20. Fuller-Thomson, E.; Stefanyk, M.; Brennenstuhl, S. The robust Association between childhood physical abuse and osteoarthritis in adulthood: Findings from a representative community sample. *Arthritis Rheum.* **2009**, *61*, 1554–1562. [CrossRef] [PubMed]
21. Burns, L.C.; Ritvo, S.E.; Ferguson, M.K.; Clarke, H.; Seltzer, Z.; Katz, J. Pain catastrophizing as a risk factor for chronic pain after total knee arthroplasty: A systematic review. *J. Pain Res.* **2015**, *5*, 21–32.
22. Crombez, G.; Viane, I.; Eccleston, C.; Devulder, J.; Goubert, L. Attention to Pain and fear of pain in patients with chronic pain. *J. Behav. Med.* **2013**, *36*, 371–378. [CrossRef] [PubMed]
23. Rakel, B.A.; Blodgett, N.P.; Bridget Zimmerman, M.; Logsden-Sackett, N.; Clark, C.; Noiseux, N.; Callaghan, J.; Herr, K.; Geasland, K.; Yang, X.; et al. Predictors of postoperative movement and resting pain following total knee replacement. *Pain* **2012**, *153*, 2192–2203. [CrossRef]
24. Glyn-Jones, S.; Palmer, A.J.; Agricola, R.; Price, A.J.; Vincent, T.L.; Weinans, H.; Carr, A.J. Osteoarthritis. *Lancet* **2015**, *386*, 376–387. [CrossRef]
25. Neogi, T. The Epidemiology and Impact of Pain in Osteoarthritis. *OARS* **2013**, *21*, 1145–1153. [CrossRef] [PubMed]
26. Riddle, D.L.; Wade, J.B.; Jiranek, W.A.; Kong, X. Preoperative Pain Catastrophizing Predicts Pain Outcome after Knee Arthroplasty. *Clin. Orthop. Relat. Res.* **2010**, *468*, 798–806. [CrossRef]
27. Hirschmann, M.T.; Testa, E.; Amsler, F.; Friederich, N.F. The unhappy Knee arthroplasty patient: Higher WOMAC and lower KSS in depressed patients prior and after TKA. *Knee Surg. Sports Traumatol. Arthrosc.* **2013**, *21*, 93–100. [CrossRef] [PubMed]
28. Wong, W.S.; Lam, H.M.; Chen, P.P.; Chow, Y.F.; Wong, S.; Lim, H.S.; Jensen, M.P.; Fielding, R. The fear-avoidance model of chronic pain: Assessing the role of neuroticism and negative affect in pain catastrophizing using structural equation modeling. *Int. J. Behav. Med.* **2015**, *22*, 118–131. [CrossRef]

29. Gómez-Pérez, L.; López-Martínez, A.E.; Asmundson, G.J. Predictors of Trait dissociation and peritraumatic dissociation induced via cold pressor. *Psychiat. Res.* **2013**, *210*, 274–280. [CrossRef] [PubMed]
30. Ehlers, A.; Steil, R. Maintenance of intrusive memories in posttraumatic Stress disorder: A cognitive approach. *Behav. Cogn. Psychother.* **1995**, *23*, 217–249. [CrossRef]
31. Sansone, R.A.; Watts, D.A.; Wiederman, M.W. Childhood trauma and Pain catastrophizing in adulthood: A cross-sectional survey study. *Prim. Care Companion CNS Disord.* **2013**, *15*. [CrossRef]
32. Bremner, J.D. Cognitive processes in dissociation: Comment on Giesbrecht et al. (2008). *Psychol. Bull.* **2010**, *136*, 1–6. [CrossRef] [PubMed]
33. Lynn, S.J.; Lilienfeld, S.O.; Merckelbach, H.; Giesbrecht, T.; van der Kloet, D. Dissociation and Dissociative disorders: Challenging conventional wisdom. *Curr. Dir. Psychol. Sci.* **2012**, *21*, 48–53. [CrossRef]
34. Giesbrecht, T.; Lilienfeld, S.O.; Lynn, S.J.; Merckelbach, H. Cognitive processes in dissociation: An analysis of core theortical assumptions. *Psychol. Bull.* **2008**, *134*, 617–647. [CrossRef]
35. Merckelbach, H.; Muris, P.; Rassin, E. Fantasy proneness and cognitive failures as correlates of dissociative experiences. *Pers. Individ. Differ.* **1999**, *26*, 961–967. [CrossRef]
36. Bernstein, E.M.; Putnam, F.W. Development, reliability, and validity of a dissociation scale. *J. Nerv. Ment. Dis.* **1986**, *174*, 727–735. [CrossRef] [PubMed]
37. Broadbent, D.E.; Cooper, P.F.; Fitzgerald, P.; Parkes, K.R. The Cognitive Failures Questionnaire (CFQ) and its correlates. *Brit. J. Clin. Psychol.* **1982**, *21*, 1–16. [CrossRef]
38. Faul, F.; Erdfelder, E.; Lang, A.-G.; Buchner, A. G*Power 3: A flexible statistical power analysis program for the social, behavioral, and biomedical sciences. *Behav. Res. Methods* **2007**, *39*, 175–191. [CrossRef] [PubMed]
39. Bellamy, N.; Buchanan, W.W.; Goldsmith, C.H.; Campbell, J.; Stitt, L.W. Validation study of WOMAC: A health status instrument for measuring clinically important patient relevant outcomes to antirheumatic drug therapy in patients with osteoarthritis of the hip or knee. *J. Rheumatol.* **1998**, *15*, 1833–1840.
40. Franke, G.H.; Jäger, S.; Morfeld, M.; Salewski, C.; Reimer, J.; Rensing, A.; Witzke, O.; Türk, T. Is the BSI-18 useful for screening for psychological distress in kidney transplanted patients? *Z. Med. Psychol.* **2010**, *19*, 30–37.
41. Spitzer, C.; Michels, F.; Siebel, U.; Gänsicke, M.; Freyberger, H. Veränderungsmessung dissoziativer Psychopathologie: Die Kurzform des Fragebogens zu dissoziativen Symptomen (FDS-20). *Fortschr. Neurol. Psychiat.* **1999**, *67*, 36.
42. Rodewald, F.; Gast, U.; Emrich, H.M. Screening for major dissociative Disorders with the FDS, the German version of the Dissociative Experience Scale. *Psychother. Psychosom. Med. Psychol.* **2006**, *56*, 249–258. [CrossRef]
43. Sullivan, M.J.L. *The Pain Catastrophizing Scale. User Manual*; Department of Psychology, Medicine and Neurology, School of Physical and Occupational Therapy, McGill University: Montreal, QC, Canada, 2009.
44. Rusu, A.C.; Kreddig, N.; Hallner, D.; Hülsebusch, J.; Hasenbring, M.I. Fear of movement/(Re)injury in low back pain: Confirmatory validation of a German version of the Tampa Scale for Kinesiophobia. *BMC Musculoskelet Disord.* **2014**, *15*, 280. [CrossRef]
45. Grabe, H.J.; Schulz, A.; Schmidt, C.O.; Appel, K.; Driessen, M.; Wingenfeld, K.; Barnow, S.; Spitzer, C.; John, U.; Berger, K.; Wersching, H.; Freyberger, H.J. A brief instrument for the assessment of childhood abuse and neglect: The childhood trauma screener (CTS). *Psychiat. Prax.* **2012**, *39*, 109–115.
46. Mulaik, S.A. *The Foundations of Factor Analysis*; McGraw-Hill: New York, NY, USA, 1972.
47. Kaiser, H.F.; Dickman, K.W. Analytic determination of common factors. *Am. Psychol.* **1959**, *14*, 425.
48. Horn, J.L. A rationale and test for the number of factors in factor analysis. *Psychometrika* **1965**, *30*, 179–185. [CrossRef]
49. Allen, J.G.; Console, D.A.; Lewis, L. Dissociative detachment and memory impairment: Reversible amnesia or encoding failure. *Compr. Psychiat.* **1999**, *40*, 160–171. [CrossRef]
50. Van der Kolk, B.; Van der Hart, O.; Marmar, C. Dissociation and information processing in Posttraumatic Stress Disorder (PTSD). In *Traumatic Stress: The Effects of Overwhelming Experience on Mind, Body, and Society*; van der Kolk, B., McFarlane, A., Weisaeth, L., Eds.; Guilford Press: New York, NY, USA, 1996; pp. 303–327.
51. Anketell, C.; Dorahy, M.J.; Curran, D. A preliminary qualitative investigation of voice hearing and its association with dissociation in chronic PTSD. *J. Trauma Dissociation* **2011**, *12*, 88–101. [CrossRef] [PubMed]
52. Adachi, N.; Akanuma, N.; Adachi, T.; Takekawa, Y.; Adachi, Y.; Ito, M.; Ikeda, H. Déjà vu experiences are rarely associated with pathological dissociation. *J. Nerv. Ment. Dis.* **2008**, *196*, 417–419. [CrossRef] [PubMed]

53. Vogel, M.; Braungardt, T.; Grabe, H.J.; Schneider, W.; Klauer, T. Detachment, Compartmentalization, and Schizophrenia: Linking Dissociation and Psychosis by Subtype. *J. Trauma Dissociation* **2013**, *14*, 273–287. [CrossRef]
54. Thomson, P.; Jaque, S.V. Depersonalization, adversity, emotionality, and coping with stressful situations. *J. Trauma Dissociation* **2018**, *19*, 143–161. [CrossRef] [PubMed]
55. Doménech, J.; Sanchis-Alfonso, V.; Espejo, B. Changes in catastrophizing and kinesiophobia are predictive of changes in disability and pain after treatment in patients with anterior knee pain. *Knee Surg. Sports Traumatol. Arthrosc.* **2014**, *22*, 2295–2300. [CrossRef] [PubMed]
56. Herbert, J.D.; Sageman, M. "First do no harm:" Emerging guidelines in the treatment of posttraumatic reactions. In *Posttraumatic Stress Disorder: Issues and Controversies*; Rosen, G.M., Ed.; John Wiley & Sons: Chichester, UK, 2002.
57. Hülsebusch, J.; Hasenbring, M.I.; Rusu, A.C. Understanding Pain and Depression in back pain: The role of catastrophizing, Help-/Hopelessness, and thought suppression as potential mediators. *Int. J. Behav. Med.* **2013**, *23*, 251–259. [CrossRef]
58. Wolfradt, U.; Engelmann, S. Depersonalization, fantasies, and coping behavior in clinical context. *J. Clin. Psychol.* **1999**, *55*, 225–232. [CrossRef]
59. Yilmaz, M.; Sezer, H.; Gürler, H.; Bekar, M. Predictors of preoperative Anxiety In surgical inpatients. *J. Clin. Nurs.* **2011**, *21*, 956–964. [CrossRef]
60. Defrin, R.; Schreiber, S.; Ginzburg, K. Paradoxical Pain Perception in Posttraumatic Stress Disorder: The Unique Role of Anxiety and Dissociation. *J. Pain.* **2015**, *16*, 961–970. [CrossRef] [PubMed]
61. Fillingim, R.B.; Hastie, B.A.; Ness, T.J.; Glover, T.L.; Campbell, C.M.; Staud, R. Sex-related psychological predictors of baseline pain perception and analgesic responses to pentazocine. *Biol. Psychol.* **2005**, *69*, 97–112. [CrossRef]
62. Michal, M.; Wiltink, J.; Subic-Wrana, C.; Zwerenz, R.; Tuin, I.; Lichy, M.; Brähler, E.; Beutel, M.E. Prevalence, correlates, and predictors of depersonalization experiences in the German general population. *J. Nerv. Ment. Dis.* **2009**, *197*, 499–506. [CrossRef]
63. Bushnell, M.C.; Ceko, M.; Low, L.A. Cognitive and emotional control of pain and its disruption in chronic pain. *Nat. Rev. Neurosci.* **2013**, *14*, 502–511. [CrossRef] [PubMed]
64. White, D.K.; Niu, J.; Zhang, Y. Is symptomatic knee osteoarthritis a risk factor for a fast decline in gait speed? Results from the Osteoarthritis Initiative. *Arthritis Care Res.* **2013**, *65*, 187–194. [CrossRef] [PubMed]
65. Creamer, P.; Lethbridge-Cejku, M.; Hochberg, M.C. Determinants of pain severity in knee osteoarthritis: Effect of demographic and psychosocial variables using 3 pain measures. *J. Rheumatol.* **1999**, *26*, 1785–1792.
66. Bühner, M. *Einführung in die Test- und Fragebogenkonstruktion*; Pearson Education: Munich, Germany, 2010.

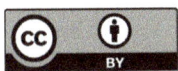

© 2019 by the authors. Licensee MDPI, Basel, Switzerland. This article is an open access article distributed under the terms and conditions of the Creative Commons Attribution (CC BY) license (http://creativecommons.org/licenses/by/4.0/).

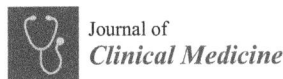

Article

Effectiveness of an Attachment-Informed Working Alliance in Interdisciplinary Pain Therapy

Ann-Christin Pfeifer [1,2,*], Pamela Meredith [3,4], Paul Schröder-Pfeifer [5], Juan Martin Gomez Penedo [6], Johannes C. Ehrenthal [2], Corinna Schroeter [1], Eva Neubauer [1] and Marcus Schiltenwolf [1]

1. Department of Orthopedics, Trauma Surgery and Paraplegiology, Heidelberg University Hospital, Schlierbacher Landstr. 200a, 69118 Heidelberg, Germany; corinna_schroeter@t-online.de (C.S.); eva.neubauer@med.uni-heidelberg.de (E.N.); marcus.schiltenwolf@med.uni-heidelberg.de (M.S.)
2. Institute of Medical Psychology, Center for Psychosocial Medicine, University Hospital Heidelberg, Bergheimer Str. 20, 69115 Heidelberg, Germany; Johannes.Ehrenthal@med.uni-heidelberg.de
3. School of Health and Rehabilitation Sciences, The University of Queensland, St. Lucia, QLD 4072, Australia; p.meredith@cqu.edu.au
4. School of Health, Medical and Applied Sciences, Central Queensland University, North Rockhampton, QLD 4701, Australia
5. Institute of Psychosocial Prevention at the Center for Psychosocial Medicine, University Hospital Heidelberg, Bergheimer Str. 54, 69115 Heidelberg, Germany; paul.schroeder-pfeifer@med.uni-heidelberg.de
6. CONICET and Universidad de Buenos Aires, C1053 CABA, Buenos Aires, Argentina; jmgomezpenedo@gmail.com
* Correspondence: ann-christin.pfeifer@med.uni-heidelberg.de; Tel.: +49-0-6221-5635492

Received: 7 February 2019; Accepted: 5 March 2019; Published: 14 March 2019

Abstract: Attachment theory provides a useful framework for understanding individual differences in pain patients, especially with insecure attachment shown to be more prevalent in chronic pain patients compared to the general population. Nevertheless, there is little evidence of attachment-informed treatment approaches for this population. The present study compares outcomes from two different attachment-informed treatment modalities for clinicians, with outcomes from treatment as usual (TAU). In both intervention groups (IG1 and IG2), clinicians received bi-monthly training sessions on attachment. Additionally, clinicians in IG1 had access to the attachment diagnostics of their patients. All treatments lasted for four weeks and included a 6-month follow up. A total of 374 chronic pain patients were recruited to participate in this study (TAU = 159/IG1 = 163/IG2 = 52). Analyses were carried out using multilevel modeling with pain intensity as the outcome variable. Additionally, working alliance was tested as a mediator of treatment efficacy. The study was registered under the trial number DRKS00008715 on the German Clinical Trials Register (DRKS). Findings show that while IG2 was efficient in enhancing treatment outcomes, IG1 did not outperform TAU. In IG2, working alliance was a mediator of outcome. Results of the present study indicate that attachment-informed treatment of chronic pain can enhance existing interdisciplinary pain therapies; however, caveats are discussed.

Keywords: chronic pain; attachment theory; attachment-informed intervention

1. Introduction

Chronic pain syndromes are a result of complex interactions between biological, psychological, and social influences, including patients' beliefs about their self-efficacy, hypervigilant monitoring of bodily sensations, and familial conflict or social support [1–3]. Due to maladaptive behavior or cognitive responses to acute episodes of pain stemming from these interactions, the pain may become chronic, affecting the long-term course [4].

Attachment theory provides a useful framework to classify patients' relatively stable cognitive, emotional, and behavioral response styles to stressors (such as pain). These attachment-related response styles, or attachment patterns, have been linked to disease processes in general [5–8] and to pain-related diagnoses and processes in particular [9,10]. Hence, the individual attachment pattern can provide some indications regarding how chronically ill patients behave in treatment; for instance, with regards to health-care utilization, trust, and compliance with the treatment [6,7] as well as self-management [11] and coping strategies used [8].

Based on their dominant response patterns, adults can be classified into one of four attachment styles—one secure style, and the three insecure styles: dismissing, preoccupied, and fearful [12,13] (see Figure 1). Attachment can also be operationalized as dimensions, with low scores on both attachment anxiety and avoidance representing secure attachment, and high scores in either attachment anxiety or avoidance (or both) representing insecure attachment [14].

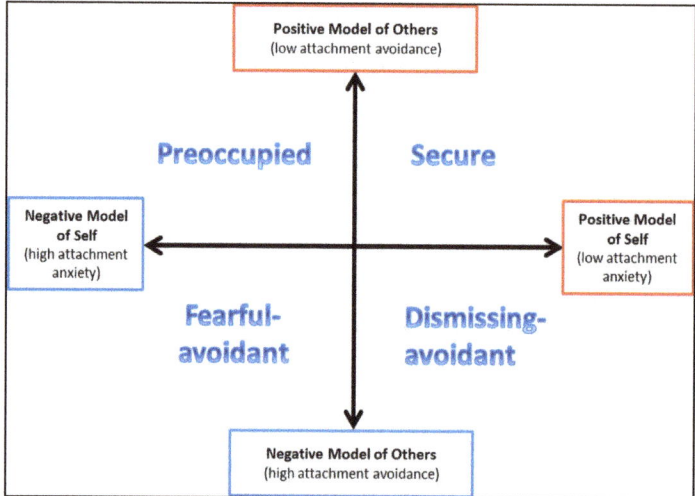

Figure 1. Different attachment styles described by Griffin and Bartholomew [15].

Evidence in the pain literature suggests that these attachment styles relate to patients' stress response, beliefs about their ability to cope with the experience of pain, perceptions of the pain as threatening, and specific interaction patterns with partners and health care personnel [16,17]. In general, patients with insecure attachment patterns report higher levels of pain [18–20], higher burden of disability [21], lower levels of pain self-efficacy [17], less functional and more dysfunctional coping strategies such as catastrophizing [22], and greater levels of depression and anxiety [23,24]. These findings are especially relevant given that insecure attachment styles are overrepresented in patients with chronic pain [20,21,25,26].

Given available evidence, it is likely that insecurely attached patients have different needs in terms of both their relationship with the clinician and the treatment [27]. Examples of attachment-informed therapies can be found within family therapy [28,29], psychoanalytic therapy [30], therapy for personality disorders [31], and within psychotherapy in general [32]. Traditional interdisciplinary pain therapy includes physical activation, improvement of mobility, the ability to relax, occupational therapy, psychological pain management, reduction of pain killer intake, and coping-related interventions. An attachment-informed treatment approach for people in pain may assist clinicians to deepen their understanding of the individual patient, individualize treatment, and develop therapy as a safe place, potentially improving outcomes; however, no evidence in the pain field exists to support this proposition.

In the present study, clinicians in a four-week interdisciplinary multimodal pain treatment program at the Heidelberg Orthopedic Hospital, Heidelberg University Clinic, were trained in: attachment theory, attachment-related individual differences, related clinical implications, and suggestions for building a meaningful working alliance. This training was expected to facilitate the attainment of the program's aims by enhancing the working alliance, the therapists' ability to provide a secure base for patients, and the therapists' understanding and support of their patients' individual attachment-based motivations and needs. The aims of this study were to examine whether: (a) there is a main effect of group (two attachment-informed groups (IG1 and IG2) versus treatment as usual (TAU)) on treatment outcome; (b) group effect is mediated by working alliance; and (c) working alliance is moderated by insecure attachment. The main hypotheses are that:

(1) Patients in IG1 and IG2, who both receive an attachment-informed multidisciplinary treatment, will report a larger mean reduction in pain intensity between pre-treatment, post-treatment, and follow-up assessments than patients in the TAU group who receive state-of-the-art multidisciplinary treatment.
(2) As the interventions (IG1 and IG2) are specifically designed to improve the working alliance, we expect higher ratings for the working alliance in IG1 and IG2 compared to TAU.
(3) The quality of the working alliance will be the core mechanism of change in IG1 and IG2; that is, it will be the mediating variable between intervention and outcome.
(4) As patients with higher levels of insecure attachment might not profit from the alliance in the same way as securely attached patients, we expect this mediation effect to be moderated by insecure attachment.

2. Materials and Methods

2.1. Participants

Of the 545 patients attending the Heidelberg Orthopedic Hospital, University Clinic Heidelberg, between March 2012 and January 2016, 127 patients did not meet the inclusion criteria to be treated in the clinic (see below) and another 44 patients declined to participate. Therefore, a total of 374 (68.6%) were recruited to this study. As seen in the flow chart in Figure 2, 159 of these participants were assigned to the TAU group, 163 to the IG1 group, and 52 to the IG2 group. Table 1 displays descriptive details for the demographic variables of the patient population.

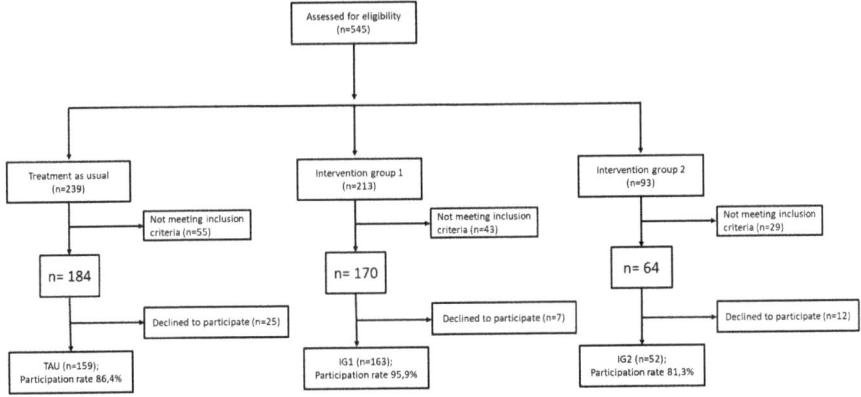

Figure 2. Trial flow chart describing the recruitment process of all three study arms.

Table 1. Descriptive details for demographic variables for the patient population and comparisons across treatment groups, $n = 374$.

Variable		TAU $n = 159$		IG1 $n = 163$		IG2 $n = 52$		Statistical Test	p Value
		M/%	SD	M/%	SD	M/%	SD		
Age		66.67	12.04	58.90	13.01	67.31	12.90	$F_{(2,367)} = 0.81$	0.45
Gender	Female	54%	-	54%	-	52%	-	$\chi^2_{(2)} = 2.50$	0.29
Marital status	Married	61%	-	58%	-	58%	-	$\chi^2_{(2)} = 0.32$	0.85
	Divorced	18%	-	15%	-	21%	-	$\chi^2_{(2)} = 0.99$	0.61
	Single	15%	-	21%	-	19%	-	$\chi^2_{(2)} = 1.84$	0.40
	Widowed	6%	-	6%	-	2%	-	$\chi^2_{(2)} = 1.49$	0.47
Employment	Currently working	47%	-	45%	-	67%	-	$\chi^2_{(2)} = 9.88$	0.01*
	Unemployed	53%	-	55%	-	33%	-	$\chi^2_{(2)} = 9.88$	0.01*
	Old-age pension	71%	-	70%	-	58%	-	$\chi^2_{(2)} = 3.46$	0.17
	Disability pension	15%	-	18%	-	27%	-	$\chi^2_{(2)} = 370$	0.16
Education	Lower/middle secondary	81%	-	86%	-	77%	-	$\chi^2_{(2)} = 2.34$	0.27
	College/university	19%	-	14%	-	23%	-	$\chi^2_{(2)} = 2.34$	0.27

Note: TAU = Treatment as usual, IG1 = Intervention group 1, IG2 = Intervention group 2, M = Mean, SD = Standard deviation, * $p \leq 0.05$.

2.2. Inclusion and Exclusion Criteria

All participants were enrolled as day-clinic patients in the orthopedic clinic of the Heidelberg University Hospital, and participated in a four-week outpatient multidisciplinary pain treatment program, including physiotherapy, occupational therapy, music and dance therapy, and individual and group psychotherapy. To attend this clinic they must: (1) have experienced chronic pain for at least six months, for which pain intensity, location, and spreading was not fully explained by specific somatic pathology; (2) be between 18 and 80 years of age; (3) have previously received standard treatment consisting of at least one rehabilitation program or two inpatient treatments, which did not yield lasting effects; and (4) have a diagnosis of somatoform disorder according to DSM-IV. In order to check whether or not these inclusion criteria were fulfilled, comprehensive diagnostic imaging and examination by an orthopedic specialist was conducted, as well as an interview with the structured clinical interview for DSM-IV (SCID) by a trained psychologist.

Exclusion criteria were:

- High C-Reactive Protein (CRP) levels as an indicator of rheumatoid arthritis;
- Acute inflammation of the spine;
- A tumor;
- A diagnosis of psychosis;
- A diagnosis of a bipolar or neurological disorder;
- Insufficient ability to communicate in German.

Use of medication was discouraged throughout the treatment, and the number of patients taking opioids or equivalent drugs in the outpatient clinic was very low (only 8.6%). While information regarding medication usage (including antidepressants and antiepileptics) was gathered at all time-points, it was not part of the exclusion criteria.

2.3. Design

All study procedures were approved by the Institutional Ethics Review Board of the Medical Faculty, University of Heidelberg. All procedures were in accord with the newest version of the Declaration of Helsinki [33], as well as with the guidelines for good clinical practice.

After a briefing about the study procedures and aims, all participating patients provided written consent. The study was conducted in a block design with three patient groups (TAU, IG1, and IG2) and three assessments times (before treatment = T1, post-treatment = T2, and 6-months follow-up=T3; see Figure 3). Patients who were registered between March 2012 and September 2013 were assigned to the TAU group, patients who were registered between March 2014 and June 2015 were assigned to IG1, and patients who were registered between June 2015 and January 2016 were assigned to IG2. All measures were given in paper pencil format and completed in the clinic for T1 and T2. For T3, the questionnaires were mailed to the participating patients. A randomized controlled trial was not suitable for this study because of ethical concerns that patients would be put on a waiting list for several months. A block design increases the chance that the key influence on outcomes is the intervention used, and was approved by the Institutional Review Board.

After data collection for the TAU group was complete for all time points, the health care personnel of the outpatient pain clinic received two initial 90-min training sessions on attachment theory and its use in the therapeutic context. The intervention training offered to the healthcare professionals working at the outpatient pain clinic included both (a) general directions for building a meaningful working alliance; and (b) guidelines for the clinicians to enable them to tailor treatment to the specific needs of individual patient attachment styles and behaviors. More attachment-related training sessions, alternating with supervision meetings, were held on a monthly basis to assist clinicians in the practical application of this approach during interventions for the second (IG1) and third (IG2) study samples. Further, "situations" (e.g., instances in which the patient misses entire therapeutic sessions or appears too late to them on a regular basis), which are perceived to be critical for forming a working alliance, were discussed at the weekly meetings. These situations were subsequently used to structure case discussions in the bi-monthly 90-min training sessions.

The only difference between the IG1 and IG2 interventions was that, in IG1 only, weekly team meetings incorporated case reviews with discussion regarding the attachment diagnostics (i.e., individual attachment styles) of each patient. The IG2 group also had weekly team meetings, but the clinicians were not informed about the specific attachment style of each patient. Instead, it was expected that after receiving the attachment-based training sessions, the team would be more sensitive to the individual attachment behavior of patients without knowing the specific attachment style.

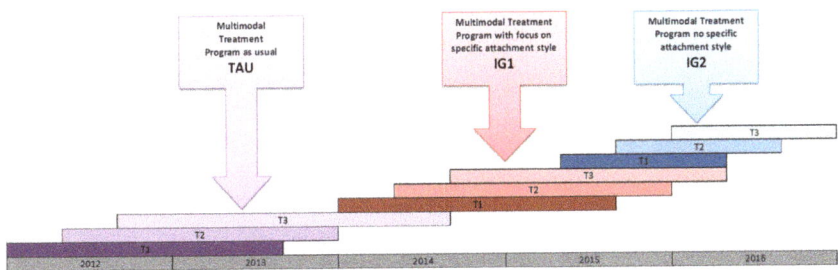

Figure 3. Study design.

2.4. Interdisciplinary Multimodal Pain Treatment

The interdisciplinary multimodal pain therapy provided to the patients in the TAU group consisted of an intensive, structured interdisciplinary program provided in an outpatient setting with five hours of treatment per day, five days per week, for four weeks. The treatment included physiotherapy, occupational therapy, psychotherapy, and medical treatments in both individual and group modalities. Additionally, patients could participate in Nordic walking and dance and music therapy, as well as relaxation training and guided physical activity supervised by physiotherapists.

2.5. Attachment-Informed Training

In the attachment-informed approach, the same clinicians received training about attachment theory and attachment-informed treatment principles [34]. The primary aim was to improve the working alliance by improving the therapists' ability to: (a) provide a secure base for patients; and (b) understand and deal with patients' individual attachment-focused motivations and needs.

They then sought to integrate these attachment approaches and techniques within the treatment as usual approach. The usual aims of the multimodal pain treatment were retained. Importantly, the approach did *not* aim to modify underlying insecure attachment patterns, which would have been unrealistic within four weeks in this setting.

The motive-orientated working alliance (former known as complementary therapeutic relationship) [35] informed the development of general guidelines for an improved working alliance. This approach emphasizes the underlying motives (such as attachment motives) of patients. Using existing literature on the application of attachment ideas to specific therapeutic settings (e.g., borderline personality disorder, depression, medically unexplained symptoms, and family and couple therapy [30,36–38]) as a starting point, specific guidelines were created for developing a working alliance for each attachment style. As an example, patients with anxious attachment styles might benefit more from an initially concordant approach that emphasizes the therapist's role as a secure base. These patients might feel overwhelmed by a program which is too quick to emphasize autonomy, possibly reinforcing existing fears of rejection and abandonment. On the other hand, avoidantly attached patients might feel uncomfortable with high levels of proximity or intimacy, and the amount of guidance and care favored by anxiously attached patients [39,40].

In the interdisciplinary setting, it was necessary that the attachment-based approach be readily employed by healthcare professionals with diverse professional backgrounds (e.g., doctors, physiotherapists, occupational therapists, and music and dance therapists); therefore, all guidelines needed to be easily incorporated into all professional approaches.

2.6. Outcome Measures

2.6.1. Pain Visual Analogue Scale (VAS)

Current pain was assessed by a VAS, asking the patients to rate their acute pain during the present day on a scale ranging from 0 to 100. Similarly, average pain over the previous week was assessed using a visual analogue scale ranging from 0 to 100. For rating purposes these scales were collapsed to indicate values between 0 and 10. Visual analogue scales have been proven to provide a valid and reliable way of measuring chronic and acute pain [41,42]. VAS were assessed at each time point.

2.6.2. Oswestry Low Back Pain Disability Questionnaire [43]

The Oswestry Low Back Pain Disability Questionnaire is a self-report measure of the functional disability of the patients and consists of 10 items assessing pain and disability in specific contexts of life to measure functional disability due to pain [44]. The items are scored on a 6-point Likert scale ranging from "no functional disability" (0) to "complete functional disability" (5). The original measure is considered the gold standard in assessing functional disability due to back pain [45]. The present study used the German version of this questionnaire, which has shown very good internal consistency ($\alpha = 0.94$) [43]. The original questionnaire (in English) has also shown good construct validity and test-retest reliability over a span of two weeks ($r = 0.82$; [46]). In the present study, the Oswestry Low Back Pain Disability Questionnaire showed good internal consistency, with Cronbach's α values ranging from 0.80 at T1 to 0.88 at T3. The Oswestry Low Back Pain Disability Questionnaire was assessed at each time point.

2.6.3. Experiences in Close Relationships Scale Revised 12—German Version (ECR-RD12) [47]

The ECR-RD12 is a German short version of the ECR-RD scale, which has previously revealed very good internal consistency ($\alpha = 0.91$–0.92; [48]). The ECR-RD12 is a self-report measure of attachment, with questions referring to participants' behavior in romantic relationships. The ECR-RD12 consists of 12 items, with 6 items loading on two scales: avoidant attachment and anxious attachment. Items are scored on a 7-point Likert scale ranging from "disagree strongly" (1) to "agree strongly" (7) [47]. The original English instrument has a stable factor structure, as well as good test-retest reliability ($r = 0.80$–0.83) and construct validity [49]. The attachment patterns measured by the

ECR-RD12 were treated as continuous variables with mean values computed. Additionally, attachment insecurity was derived from the ECR-RD12 as a sum score of both scales, with high values representing attachment insecurity and low scores representing attachment security. In the present study, the ECR-RD12 showed good internal consistency, with Cronbach's α values of 0.78 for anxious attachment and 0.82 for avoidant attachment. The ECR-RD12 was assessed at T1 only.

2.6.4. Inpatient and Day-Clinic Experience Scale—German Version (German TSEB/English IDES) [50]

The TSEB is a self-report questionnaire with 35 items, which assesses various facets of the working alliance specifically designed for day-clinic patients [50]. Seven scales are calculated: bond with individual therapist, bond with therapeutic team, agreement on tasks and goals, cohesion with the patient group, self-disclosure, critical attitude, and positive self-view. Items are scored on a 6-point Likert scale ranging from "not at all true" (1) to "completely true" (6). The authors have reported mixed internal consistency, ranging from α = 0.53 for critical attitude to α = 0.89 for positive self-view, while they found evidence of construct validity with good confirmatory factor analysis model fit. In the present study, the TSEB showed varying internal consistency ranging from poor to high (from α = 0.58 for critical attitude to α = 0.89 for bond with individual therapist), congruent with the results of the validation study. The bond with therapeutic team subscale was primarily used, as this was deemed best fitting for the day-clinic setting. The TSEB was assessed at T2.

2.7. Statistical Analyses

SPSS 22 [51] was used for descriptive analysis and data management, while R [52] was used for missing data analysis and handling of outliers. Power was computed analytically via the R package "powerlmm". Assuming a small to medium effect of the treatment of Cohens $d = 0.5$, a power analysis was computed for an ICC of 0.2 for three time-points. According to the power analysis, 95% power was achieved at a group size of $n = 160$. Unfortunately, due to the nature of the block design and complications in recruitment, IG2 had only $n = 52$ willing participants. Thus, IG2 was underpowered at only 51% power.

The data contained 9.82% missing values. The group of complete cases did not differ from the group with missing values on one or more variables in mean or standard deviation on any variable of interest. All analyses were conducted assuming the data was missing at random (MAR). Under MAR, observation missingness is assumed to be unrelated to the dependent variable at dropout [53]. Multiple imputations by chained equations (MICE) [54] with 20 iterations were used to impute missing values for available time points. MICE produces asymptotically unbiased estimations of the data under MAR assumptions [55]. Using $p > 0.001$ for the χ^2 value of the Mahalanobis distance as a measure of multivariate outliers, no outliers were identified.

HLM7 software was used for multilevel modeling [56]. We used longitudinal multilevel models with measurements over time (level 1) nested in patients (level 2), since it can be expected that measurements within patients over time are non-independent [57]. Multilevel models offer a good way of handling unbalanced designs, accounting naturally for the different number of measurements per person [58,59]. To answer the questions regarding whether or not there were significant differences in level of the outcome variable (pain intensity) at six months follow-up and weekly rate of change during treatment and follow-up period, dependent on treatment group (IG1 vs. IG2 vs. TAU) we tested several models. For each outcome variable, we tested a two-level conditional model with time in weeks (centered at the end of the 6-month follow-up) as the only level-1 predictor. At level two, we included the treatment conditions as well as attachment anxiety as predictors both of the intercept and the slope of the model. As patients were nested with therapists, but only four therapists participated in the study, instead of conducting three-levels to control for therapist effects, we decided to include the therapist as a covariate (dummy coded) in all models.

Since there was prior evidence from another study conducted at the Orthopedic Hospital that patient trajectories would be markedly different during treatment as opposed to during follow up, we decided to use a piecewise modeling approach. In the earlier study, symptoms declined steeply during treatment, and started increasing again during follow up. Change in each piece of the model was estimated using the technique outlined by Smith and colleagues [60] by providing the estimated error variance at level 1 for the outcomes in the model [60,61]. The level-1 error variance of each outcome measure was estimated as the product of its measurement error (1-Cronbach's α) and the variance of the measure at each time-point.

Full maximum likelihood was used as the estimator in all models. Significance values and standard errors for fixed effects were computed using Kenward-Roger approximation [62]. Plotting the fitted against the residual values did not indicate non-constant error variance for any of the models and visual inspections of Q-Q plots did not reveal marked non-normality for any of the models.

To test mediation and moderated mediation effects, we used PROCESS macro version 2.11 for SPSS version 22.0 [63]. For these models, the Empirical Bayes estimates of patient's scores at the end of follow-up and of the weekly rated of change, estimated in the above-mentioned two-level models, were used as the outcome variables [57]. Hayes's models 1 and 14 were used to test mediation and moderated mediation effects.

3. Results

In terms of descriptive statistics, there were no significant differences between the three groups in terms of the core study variables (see Table 2).

Table 2. Descriptive details of the core study variables and differences between the three treatment groups, $n = 374$.

Variable	TAU		IG1		IG2		Statistical Test	p Value
	M/%	SD	M/%	SD	M/%	SD		
Age	53.56	12.04	54.45	13.01	51.92	12.90	$F_{(2,367)} = 0.81$	0.45
Female	66.7%	-	58.9%	-	67.31	-	$\chi^2_{(2)} = 2.50$	0.29
Average Pain	6.44	1.80	6.74	1.79	6.29	1.75	$F_{(2,371)} = 1.80$	0.17
Current Pain	5.97	2.08	6.04	2.26	5.38	2.22	$F_{(2,364)} = 1.83$	0.16
ECR-RD12 Anxiety	2.30	1.39	2.40	1.39	2.37	1.38	$F_{(2,338)} = 0.21$	0.81
ECR-RD12 Avoidance	2.46	1.22	2.54	1.17	2.43	1.19	$F_{(2,340)} = 0.22$	0.81

Note: ECR-RD12 Anxiety= Anxious attachment subscale of the Experiences in Close Relationships Scale Revised 12—German Version, ECR-RD12 Avoidance= Avoidant attachment subscale of the Experiences in Close Relationships Scale Revised 12—German Version.

Table 3 summarizes correlations among core study variables at intake using Pearson's correlation for continuous variables and Spearman-rank coefficients for non-continuous variables. Alpha levels were adjusted using Bonferroni correction.

Table 3. Correlations among core study variables, $n = 374$.

I	Gender	Average Pain	Current Pain	Physical Functioning	ECR-RD12 Anxiety	ECR-RD12 Avoidance
Age	0.12 *	0.15 **	0.12 *	0.25 ***	−0.06	0.19 ***
Gender		0.05	0.06	0.09	0.01	0.08
Average Pain			0.70 ***	0.42 ***	0.01	0.02
Current Pain				0.44 ***	0	0.05
Physical Functioning					0.05	0.1
ECR-RD12 Anxiety						0.22 ***

Note: * $p \leq 0.05$; ** $p \leq 0.01$; *** $p \leq 0.001$.

3.1. Treatment's Main Effects Analysis

Concerning Hypothesis 1, the conditional model including average pain as the outcome variable showed no difference between either IG1 or IG2 to TAU at post-treatment (see Figure 4) but a significant difference at 6-month follow-up in average pain for IG1 compared to IG2 ($\gamma 01 = -0.92$, SE = 0.45, t(358)

= −2.027, p < 0.05), in favor of IG2 (see Table 4). Additionally, IG2 worked markedly better in the long run for patients with high attachment anxiety (see Figure 4). While having significantly worse pain intensity scores in IG2 after treatment compared to TAU and IG1 ($\gamma 03$ = −0.52, SE = 0.22, t(358) = 2.32, p < 0.05), patients with high attachment anxiety achieved the lowest scores of pain at follow-up ($\gamma 23$ = −0.02, SE = 0.01, t(358) = −1.78, p = 0.08), although this effect did not reach significance.

Figure 4 shows the effect of insecure attachment across the three treatment groups over time. Gray shaded areas indicate 95% confidence intervals around the parameter estimates, with darker areas indicating overlapping confidence intervals.

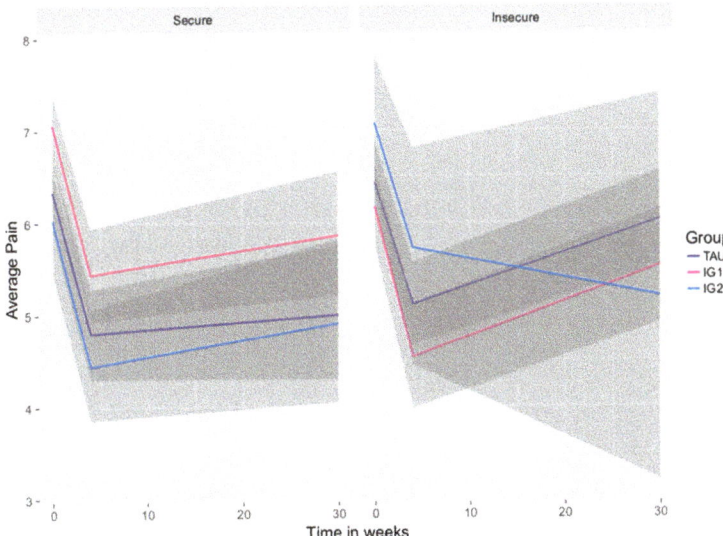

Figure 4. Effect of attachment on average pain across treatment groups.

Table 4. Results of multilevel model with average pain intensity as outcome, n = 374.

Fixed Effect	Coefficient	Standard Error	t-Ratio	Approx. df	p
For Intercept, β_0					
Intercept	4.823	0.116	41.556	358	<0.001
IG1 vs. IG2	−0.923	0.269	−2.11	358	0.058
ECR-RD12 Anxiety	−0.132	0.092	−1.429	358	0.154
IG2 × ECR-RD12 Anxiety	0.522	0.224	2.322	358	0.021
For Piece 1 slope, β_1					
Intercept	−0.364	0.026	−13.529	358	<0.001
IG1 vs. IG2	0.028	0.073	0.396	358	0.693
ECR-RD12 Anxiety	0.013	0.020	0.660	358	0.510
IG2 × ECR-RD12 Anxiety	−0.052	0.064	−0.812	358	0.417
For Piece 2 slope, β_2					
Intercept	0.018	0.005	3.332	358	<0.001
IG1 vs. IG2	−0.024	0.016	−1.498	358	0.135
ECR-RD12 Anxiety	0.001	0.004	0.023	358	0.981
IG2 × ECR-RD12 Anxiety	−0.021	0.011	−1.774	358	0.077

Note: Approx. df = Approximate degrees of freedom, * $p \leq 0.05$; ** $p \leq 0.01$; *** $p \leq 0.001$.

3.2. Mediational Effects Analysis

Although there was no significant difference between TAU and the two intervention conditions, mediational analyses were conducted to see if there was an indirect effect of treatment condition on outcome by working alliance, as specified in Hypotheses 2 and 3. For these models we used a dummy variable as the independent variable comparing IG2 with TAU (i.e., IG2 = 1, TAU = 0). IG2 was compared to TAU, since previous analysis hinted that these groups provided the greatest potential to explore this mediation effect by way of being conceptually different and also boasting bigger outcome differences than IG1 vs. TAU. The working alliance with team score provided by the TSEB was introduced as the mediator. For outcome variables we used the estimated score at post-treatment and at follow-up, as well as the slope (weekly rate of change) of pain intensity, leading to a total of six mediation analyses.

Regardless of the model, the treatment condition was significantly related to scores at TSEB (B = 0.23, SE = 0.12, t(179) = 2.003, $p < 0.01$). Patients in IG2 revealed a TSEB score of an estimated 0.23 units higher than patients in the control group. Furthermore, TSEB scores were significantly related with average pain at follow-up (B = −0.21, SE = 0.10, t(178) = −2.183, $p = 0.03$) and the weekly rate of change in average pain (B = −0.002, SE = 0.001, t(178) = −2.227, $p = 0.03$). Overall, the indirect effect of treatment condition by TSEB scores was significant for average pain at the end of follow-up, but not for the weekly rate of change in average pain.

In the mediational models for current pain, we again found that TSEB scores were significantly related with current pain at the end of follow-up (B = −0.27, SE = 0.14, t(178) = −1.986, $p < 0.05$) and the weekly rate of change in current pain (B = −0.002, SE = 0.001, t(178) = −2.075, $p = 0.04$). There was a significant indirect effect of treatment by TSEB scores on current pain at the end of follow-up; however, the indirect effect of treatment by TSEB scores on weekly change in current pain was not significant. On the other hand, there was no significant direct effect of treatment on current pain at follow-up (B = −0.13, SE = 0.21, t(178) = −0.616, $p = 0.54$) or in current pain weekly change (B = −0.001, SE = 0.001, t(178) = −0.596, $p = 0.55$).

3.3. Moderated Mediational Effects Analysis

We conducted moderated mediational effects analysis to check if the mediational effects reported (indirect effect of treatment by TSEB scores) were, in turn, moderated by patient attachment pattern (Hypothesis 4). As presented in Figure 5, attachment anxiety significantly moderated the mediational effect of treatment by TSEB scores on average pain at the end of follow-up (B = 0.23, SE = 0.09, t(155) = 2.628, $p < 0.01$) and the weekly change in average pain (B= 0.003, SE = 0.001, t(155) = 2.650, $p < 0.01$).

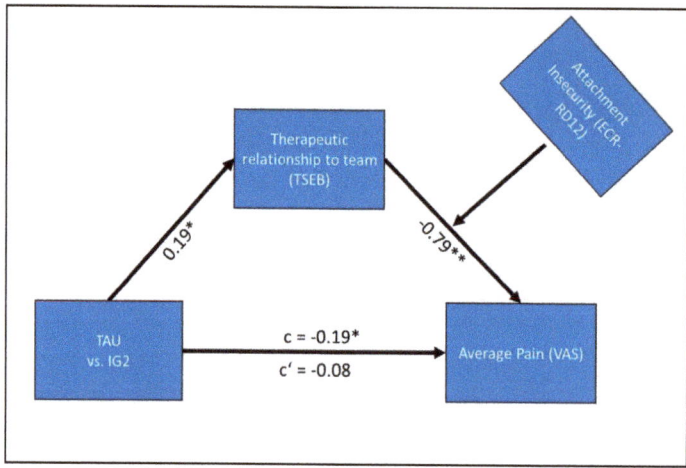

Figure 5. Summary of results for moderated mediation analysis. Note: $p < 0.05 = *$, $p < 0.01 = **$, c = direct effect before mediation, c' = direct effect after mediation.

In summary, the mediation analysis indicated a difference in pain reduction between IG2 and TAU that is mediated by working alliance, measured by the TSEB. This effect, in turn, is dependent on attachment insecurity, as shown in Figure 6. High values of attachment insecurity negate the positive effect of the working alliance, while low values reinforce it. This moderating effect extends to both the average level of pain at follow-up (-1 SD ECR-RD12 Insecurity B = -0.11, SE = 0.7; $+1$ SD ECR-RD12 Insecurity B = 0.01, SE = 0.03), and rate of change during therapy (-1 SD ECR-RD12 Insecurity B = -0.0012, SE = 0.0008; $+1$ SD ECR Insecurity B = 0.0001, SE = 0.0003).

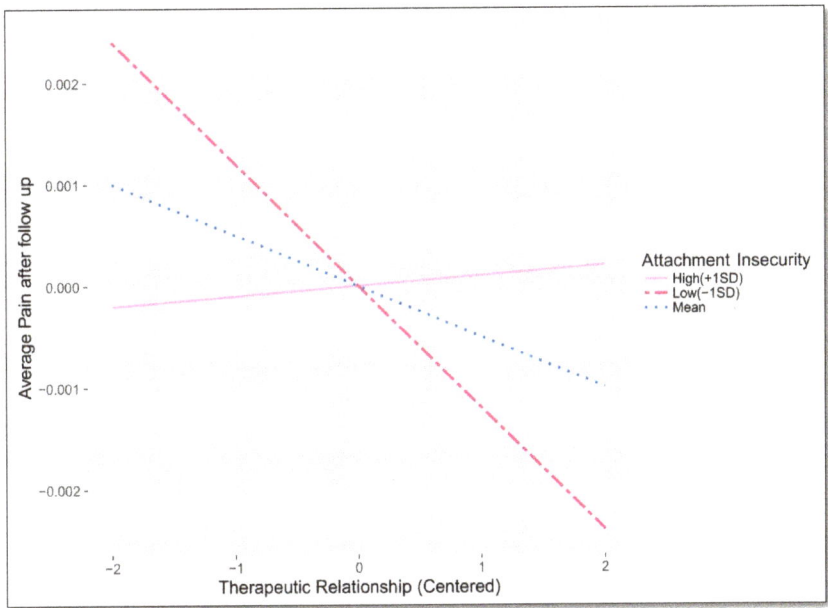

Figure 6. Moderated effect of attachment insecurity on the relationship between working alliance and average pain after follow up.

4. Discussion

The primary aim of this study was to examine whether providing attachment-informed training to clinicians in an interdisciplinary pain program could influence pain outcomes compared to treatment as usual (TAU). According to Hypothesis 1, it was anticipated that this would be the case. Results only partially supported this hypothesis, however. Patients in IG2 reported a larger mean reduction in average pain intensity between pre-treatment and post-treatment assessments compared to patients in both IG1 and TAU groups. Perhaps surprisingly, IG2, in which therapists were *not* informed of patient attachment style, outperformed IG1, where therapists knew the attachment styles. Thus, this additional knowledge seemed to have had an adverse effect. There are a number of possible explanations for this phenomenon. Most likely, with therapists at the IG1 stage being new to attachment theory, they will have been consolidating information and gaining new perspectives throughout the IG1 stage, which would presumably support practice during IG2. The clinicians in IG1 may have felt overwhelmed, having access to a large amount of new information and to the patients' attachment style, and trying to integrate these components "on the job". The changed role of the therapist, in which they serve as a form of substitute attachment figure for the patients that has to attune to each individual attachment pattern by addressing the specifically related needs [64], also takes time to develop. These considerations are particularly relevant given the short length of the treatment (four weeks). It may also be that knowing a patient's attachment style might evoke a form of unconscious stigma on the part of the therapist, which may impact on the therapeutic relationship. Another possible explanation is that attachment, as measured by the ECR-RD12, is not representative of the attachment behavior exhibited during therapy, therefore misleading clinicians in IG1. Finally, the smaller number of participants in IG2, and reduced power, may have impacted on results. Further research is needed to gain clarity about these possible explanations.

The interdisciplinary pain therapy includes physical activation, improvement of mobility, the ability to relax, occupational therapy, psychological pain management, reduction of pain killer intake, and coping-related interventions. An ordinary treatment can last up to 4 weeks for a full-time intensive outpatient treatment. Due to the limited time available, it is generally very difficult to build a stable and trusting work-alliance between the therapist and the patient to allow the patient to properly take in the content of the therapy. Even though it is much harder for insecure patients to establish and maintain a stable and trusting working alliance [21,65], the development of trust is essential for the success of therapy [40,66]. One therapeutic approach that already includes these relationship related aspects is the psychodynamic interactional group therapy by Nickel and Egle [67] that already works with these relationship aspects in a clinical setting, with a focus on the working alliance and conflict management during 40 sessions.

The second hypothesis was that the intervention groups (IG1 and IG2) would produce stronger average working alliances compared to TAU. This was partly supported, with patients in IG2 reporting significantly better working alliances compared to those in TAU. Working alliances for patients in IG1 did not differ from those in TAU.

The third hypothesis suggested that the quality of the working alliance would be the core mechanism of change in IG1 and IG2 (i.e., the mediating variable between intervention and outcome). As expected, working alliance was found to be a strong mediator between the intervention effect and treatment outcome, suggesting that training staff in attachment theory and its implications for people in pain can help to improve the working alliance, and therefore strengthen outcomes. This is consistent with expectations based on parent-infant attachment-based interventions, where training in attachment theory enhanced maternal-sensitivity and infant-security [68]. Literature and some empirical evidence point to the importance of the working alliance for the course of the treatment and its outcomes, as well as for the maintenance of positive treatment outcomes after therapy ends [69,70]. The results of this study correspond to attachment theoretical assumptions [7,71] as well as to the impact of the working alliance [72]. This is one of first studies to consider these assumptions in a clinical setting with a longitudinal design, and the first to do so with chronic pain samples.

As expected in Hypothesis 4, the link between working alliance and pain outcome was moderated by insecure attachment. Patients with higher levels of insecure attachment reported poorer working alliances compared to securely attached patients, with implications for pain outcome. This finding was evident despite attachment-informed intervention provided in this study, suggesting that this intervention did not counter the effects of attachment insecurity on pain outcome. While anticipated, based on previous research, this finding suggests the need for attachment-informed modifications to treatment that extends beyond the therapeutic alliance. The mentalization-based approach [73] has been successfully utilized with mostly insecure attached patient groups before (e.g., [74,75]) and could provide a useful addition in working with chronic pain patients. In contrast to the focus of present study on how to establish a good therapeutic alliance with insecure patients, the mentalization-based approach could aid in understanding how the communication in these therapeutic alliances works and how the patient mentalizes the relationship. This might help explain why the insecure patients were not able to profit from the therapeutic alliance in the same way as did secure patients.

Findings support working alliance as a mechanism of change linked to patient attachment. Nevertheless, the path model also indicated that the insecure patients in IG2 were the only insecure patients who did not experience deteriorations in pain during the post-treatment phase. Although the mean difference in pain at the 30-week follow-up was non-significant, this trend hints at the attachment-specific training having a positive effect on post-treatment adjustment to pain [76,77].

The results from TAU, on the other hand, replicate the evidence from the empirical literature stating that insecurely attached patients have, on average, poorer treatment compliance [7,71] and adjustment to pain [4,9,78].

Limitations

The primary limitation for this study can be found in the study design. The block design was chosen even though the optimal design for the study would have been a randomized controlled trial (RCT), with patients being randomly assigned to one of the treatment arms with separate groups of treating clinicians. However, this was not feasible in this orthopedic hospital setting. The very limited number of clinicians working at the outpatient department would have made it impossible to divide the clinicians into more than one interdisciplinary pain treatment at a time. A future study replicating the results of the current study might use a multicenter trial in order to control for spillover effects, while providing an adequate number of clinicians for an RCT design.

Another limitation is the failure to control for therapist adherence to the treatment guidelines. While the clinicians were regularly asked during the weekly team meeting whether or not they implemented the training contents into their treatment routine, no adherence data is available. Future studies might profit from development of an intervention manual with clearly defined treatment characteristics and working mechanisms to support development of systematic adherence ratings. These might then be ascertained either from expert rated videos of therapy sessions, or a comparable approach, such as a manualized adherence rating. This information could be used as a control variable or descriptively to support interpretation of findings.

While the main objective of the present study was to compare the three treatments, i.e., investigating between-person effects, we were also interested in the trajectories of treatment over time in our treatment groups. The short duration of the treatment combined with relatively long assessments at each measurement point has resulted in having only the minimum number of time points needed for longitudinal modeling. This, combined with large standard errors for our estimates of within-person effects, render low levels of certainty in those estimates. For future studies of multimodal pain therapies with attachment focus, a shorter assessment battery with more time points is needed to properly investigate the trajectories in patients' symptoms over time.

A further methodological issue is the sample size of IG2 and the high dropout rate at follow-up across all treatment arms. While the non-significant *t*-tests across dropouts and non-dropouts suggest that dropout is not systematically related to outcome, the question remains why the dropout at T3 was so high. Although significant effects between treatments were found, the results of the present study need to be replicated in a future study with all treatment arms being powered equally.

Finally, the intervention was provided over only a four-week period. If adapted for longer outpatient settings, more pronounced differences may be seen over time as, hypothetically, attachment patterns might slowly alter over the course of therapy, increasing the positive effect of the working alliance on pain over time.

5. Conclusions

The results of the present study provide preliminary support for the utility of incorporating attachment-informed interventions with existing multimodal pain therapies in short-term outpatient settings. Although the clinicians trained in the attachment-informed treatment only had four weeks to implement the treatment, this approach was more effective in reducing perceived pain intensity in IG2 relative to TAU. Findings suggest that one reason for this was the facilitation of a more stable working alliance between the therapist and the patient in the attachment-informed treatment. Findings also suggest that classifying patients into one of the four attachment categories prior to treatment may not be needed to build a stable working alliance. As a result of this study, a number of needs are identified. First, there is a need for a written manual with a detailed description of the intervention to support clinicians to adhere to and integrate the new techniques of the intervention into their daily treatment routine. Second, based on this manual, measures of treatment adherence by clinicians should be developed. Finally, more in-depth attachment-informed treatments should be developed, manualized, and evaluated. It is anticipated that these steps will contribute to even greater and more lasting clinical improvements, especially for those with insecure attachment patterns.

Author Contributions: Study concept and design, A.-C.P., C.S., and J.C.E.; collection of data, A.-C.P. and C.S.; analysis and interpretation of data, A.-C.P., P.S.-P., and J.M.G.P.; statistical analysis, A.-C.P., P.S.-P., and J.M.G.P.; writing, original draft, A.-C.P.; writing, review and editing, A.-C.P., P.M., P.S.-P., and J.C.E.; visualization, A.-C.P. and P.S.-P.; supervision, P.M., J.C.E., E.N., and M.S.; access to data, all authors.

Funding: This research was funded by the private foundation "Psychosomatik der Wirbelsäulenerkrankungen" ("Psychosomatics of spine disorders"), as well as the Federal Ministry of Education and Research, grant number 01DR17021.

Acknowledgments: The authors gratefully acknowledge the support of the staff and clients of the Department of Orthopedics, Trauma Surgery, and Paraplegiology at Heidelberg University Hospital. We would like to thank the private foundation "Psychosomatik der Wirbelsäulenerkrankungen" ("Psychosomatics of spine disorders"), as well as the Federal Ministry of Education and Research for funding this work. The authors would also like to acknowledge the support of Prof. Jenny Strong at the end of the manuscript.

Conflicts of Interest: The authors declare no conflict of interest.

References

1. Gatchel, R.J.; Turk, D.C. *Psychosocial Factors in Pain: Critical Perspectives*; Guilford Press: New York, NY, USA, 1999.
2. Flor, H.; Hermann, C. Biopsychosocial models of pain. *Prog. Pain Res. Manag.* **2004**, *27*, 47–78.
3. Gatchel, R.J.; Peng, Y.B.; Peters, M.L.; Fuchs, P.N.; Turk, D.C. The biopsychosocial approach to chronic pain: Scientific advances and future directions. *Psychol. Bull.* **2007**, *133*, 581. [CrossRef]
4. Meredith, P.; Ownsworth, T.; Strong, J. A review of the evidence linking adult attachment theory and chronic pain: Presenting a conceptual model. *Clin. Psychol. Rev.* **2008**, *28*, 407–429. [CrossRef] [PubMed]
5. Maunder, R.; Hunter, J. An integrated approach to the formulation and psychotherapy of medically unexplained symptoms: Meaning-and attachment-based intervention. *Am. J. Psychother.* **2004**, *58*, 17. [CrossRef]
6. Graetz, C.; Ehrenthal, J.C.; Senf, D.; Semar, K.; Herzog, W.; Dörfer, C.E. Influence of psychological attachment patterns on periodontal disease—A pilot study with 310 compliant patients. *J. Clin. Periodontol.* **2013**, *40*, 1087–1094. [CrossRef]
7. Ciechanowski, P.S.; Katon, W.J.; Russo, J.E.; Walker, E.A. The patient-provider relationship: Attachment theory and adherence to treatment in diabetes. *Am. J. Psychiatry* **2001**, *158*, 29–35. [CrossRef] [PubMed]
8. Ciechanowski, P.; Russo, J.; Katon, W.; Von Korff, M.; Ludman, E.; Lin, E.; Simon, G.; Bush, T. Influence of patient attachment style on self-care and outcomes in diabetes. *Psychosom. Med.* **2004**, *66*, 720–728. [CrossRef]
9. Porter, L.S.; Davis, D.; Keefe, F.J. Attachment and pain: Recent findings and future directions. *Pain* **2007**, *128*, 195–198. [CrossRef] [PubMed]
10. McWilliams, L.A.; Murphy, P.D.; Bailey, S.J. Associations between adult attachment dimensions and attitudes toward pain behaviour. *Pain Res. Manag.* **2010**, *15*, 378–384. [CrossRef]
11. Schmidt, S.; Nachtigall, C.; Wuethrich-Martone, O.; Strauss, B. Attachment and coping with chronic disease. *J. Psychosom. Res.* **2002**, *53*, 763–773. [CrossRef]
12. Bartholomew, K.; Horowitz, L.M. Attachment styles among young adults: A test of a four-category model. *J. Pers. Soc. Psychol.* **1991**, *61*, 226–244. [CrossRef] [PubMed]
13. Mikulincer, M.; Shaver, P.R. *Attachment in Adulthood: Structure, Dynamics, and Change*; Guilford Press: New York, NY, USA, 2007.
14. Fraley, R.C.; Waller, N.G.; Brennan, K.A. An item response theory analysis of self-report measures of adult attachment. *J. Pers. Soc. Psychol.* **2000**, *78*, 350. [CrossRef] [PubMed]
15. Griffin, D.W.; Bartholomew, K. Models of the self and other: Fundamental dimensions underlying measures of adult attachment. *J. Pers. Soc. Psychol.* **1994**, *67*, 430. [CrossRef]
16. Ditzen, B.; Schmidt, S.; Strauss, B.; Nater, U.M.; Ehlert, U.; Heinrichs, M. Adult attachment and social support interact to reduce psychological but not cortisol responses to stress. *J. Psychosom. Res.* **2008**, *64*, 479–486. [CrossRef] [PubMed]

17. Meredith, P.; Strong, J.; Feeney, J.A. Adult attachment, anxiety, and pain self-efficacy as predictors of pain intensity and disability. *Pain* **2006**, *123*, 146–154. [CrossRef]
18. McWilliams, L.A.; Cox, B.J.; Enns, M.W. Impact of adult attachment styles on pain and disability associated with arthritis in a nationally representative sample. *Clin. J. Pain* **2000**, *16*, 360–364. [CrossRef] [PubMed]
19. Tremblay, I.; Sullivan, M.J. Attachment and pain outcomes in adolescents: The mediating role of pain catastrophizing and anxiety. *J. Pain* **2010**, *11*, 160–171. [CrossRef]
20. Pfeifer, A.-C.; Penedo, J.M.G.; Ehrenthal, J.C.; Neubauer, E.; Amelung, D.; Schroeter, C.; Schiltenwolf, M. Impact of attachment behavior on the treatment process of chronic pain patients. *J. Pain Res.* **2018**, *11*, 2653. [CrossRef] [PubMed]
21. Davies, K.A.; Macfarlane, G.J.; McBeth, J.; Morriss, R.; Dickens, C. Insecure attachment style is associated with chronic widespread pain. *Pain* **2009**, *143*, 200–205. [CrossRef]
22. Ciechanowski, P.; Sullivan, M.; Jensen, M.; Romano, J.; Summers, H. The relationship of attachment style to depression, catastrophizing and health care utilization in patients with chronic pain. *Pain* **2003**, *104*, 627–637. [CrossRef]
23. Andersen, T.E. Does attachment insecurity affect the outcomes of a multidisciplinary pain management program? The association between attachment insecurity, pain, disability, distress, and the use of opioids. *Soc. Sci. Med.* **2012**, *74*, 1461–1468. [CrossRef] [PubMed]
24. Meredith, P.J.; Strong, J.; Feeney, J.A. Adult attachment variables predict depression before and after treatment for chronic pain. *Eur. J. Pain* **2007**, *11*, 164–170. [CrossRef]
25. Pfeifer, A.-C.; Ehrenthal, J.; Neubauer, E.; Gerigk, C.; Schiltenwolf, M. Einfluss des Bindungsverhaltens auf chronischen und somatoformen SchmerzImpact of attachment behavior on chronic and somatoform pain. *Der Schmerz* **2016**, *30*, 444–456. [CrossRef] [PubMed]
26. Kowal, J.; McWilliams, L.A.; Péloquin, K.; Wilson, K.G.; Henderson, P.R.; Fergusson, D.A. Attachment insecurity predicts responses to an interdisciplinary chronic pain rehabilitation program. *J. Behav. Med.* **2015**, *38*, 518–526. [CrossRef]
27. Gillath, O.; Karantzas, G.C.; Fraley, R.C. *Adult Attachment: A Concise Introduction to Theory and Research*; Academic Press: Cambridge, MA, USA, 2016.
28. Byng-Hall, J. Evolving Ideas about Narrative: Re-editing the Re-editing of Family Mythology. *J. Fam. Ther.* **1998**, *20*, 133–142. [CrossRef]
29. Slade, A. The move from categories to process: Attachment phenomena and clinical evaluation. *Infant Ment. Health J.* **2004**, *25*, 269–283. [CrossRef]
30. Harris, T. Implications of attachment theory for working in psychoanalytic psychotherapy. *Int. Forum Psychoanal.* **2004**, *13*, 147–156. [CrossRef]
31. Meyer, B.; Pilkonis, P.A. An attachment model of personality disorders. *Major Theories Pers. Disord.* **2005**, *2*, 231–281.
32. Wallin, D.J. *Attachment in Psychotherapy*; Guilford Press: New York, NY, USA, 2007.
33. World Medical Association. World medical association declaration of Helsinki: Ethical principles for medical research involving human subjects. *JAMA* **2013**, *310*, 2191–2194. [CrossRef] [PubMed]
34. Obegi, J.H.; Berant, E. *Attachment Theory and Research in Clinical Work with Adults*; Guilford press: New York, NY, USA, 2010.
35. Caspar, F.; Grossmann, C.; Unmüssig, C.; Schramm, E. Complementary therapeutic relationship: Therapist behavior, interpersonal patterns, and therapeutic effects. *Psychother. Res.* **2005**, *15*, 91–102. [CrossRef]
36. Diamond, G.S.; Reis, B.F.; Diamond, G.M.; Siqueland, L.; Isaacs, L. Attachment-based family therapy for depressed adolescents: A treatment development study. *J. Am. Acad. Child Adolesc. Psychiatry* **2002**, *41*, 1190–1196. [CrossRef] [PubMed]
37. Bateman, A.W.; Fonagy, P. The development of an attachment-based treatment program for borderline personality disorder. *Bull. Menninger Clin.* **2003**, *67*, 187. [CrossRef] [PubMed]
38. Johnson, S.M.; Whiffen, V.E. *Attachment Processes in Couple and Family Therapy*; Guilford Press: New York, NY, USA, 2003.
39. Geller, J.D.; Farber, B.A. Attachment style, representations of psychotherapy, and clinical interventions with insecurely attached clients. *J. Clin. Psychol.* **2015**, *71*, 457–468. [CrossRef] [PubMed]
40. Levy, K.N.; Ellison, W.D.; Scott, L.N.; Bernecker, S.L. Attachment style. *J. Clin. Psychol.* **2011**, *67*, 193–203. [CrossRef]

41. Carlsson, A.M. Assessment of chronic pain. I. Aspects of the reliability and validity of the visual analogue scale. *Pain* **1983**, *16*, 87–101. [CrossRef]
42. Bijur, P.E.; Silver, W.; Gallagher, E.J. Reliability of the visual analog scale for measurement of acute pain. *Acad. Emerg. Med.* **2001**, *8*, 1153–1157. [CrossRef] [PubMed]
43. Gaul, C.; Mette, E.; Schmidt, T.; Grond, S. Practicability of a German version of the "Oswestry Low Back Pain Disability Questionnaire". A questionnaire to assess disability caused by back pain. *Schmerz* **2008**, *22*, 51–58. [CrossRef]
44. Fairbank, J.C.; Pynsent, P.B. The Oswestry disability index. *Spine* **2000**, *25*, 2940–2953. [CrossRef]
45. Davidson, M.; Keating, J. Oswestry disability questionnaire (ODQ). *Aust. J. Physiother.* **2005**, *51*, 270. [CrossRef]
46. Firch, E.; Brooks, D.; Stratford, P.; Mayo, N. *Physical Rehabilitation Outcome Measures*; BC Decker Inc.: Hamilton, ON, Canada, 2002.
47. Brenk-Franz, K.; Ehrenthal, J.; Freund, T.; Schneider, N.; Strauß, B.; Tiesler, F.; Schauenburg, H.; Gensichen, J. Evaluation of the short form of "Experience in Close Relationships" (Revised, German Version "ECR-RD12")-A tool to measure adult attachment in primary care. *PLoS ONE* **2018**, *13*, e0191254. [CrossRef]
48. Ehrenthal, J.C.; Dinger, U.; Lamla, A.; Funken, B.; Schauenburg, H. Evaluation der deutschsprachigen Version des Bindungsfragebogens „Experiences in Close Relationships—Revised"(ECR-RD). *PPmP-Psychother. Psychosom. Med. Psychol.* **2009**, *59*, 215–223. [CrossRef]
49. Wei, M.; Russell, D.W.; Mallinckrodt, B.; Vogel, D.L. The Experiences in Close Relationship Scale (ECR)-short form: Reliability, validity, and factor structure. *J. Pers. Assess.* **2007**, *88*, 187–204. [CrossRef] [PubMed]
50. Dinger, U.; Schauenburg, H.; Ehrenthal, J.C.; Nicolai, J.; Mander, J.; Sammet, I. Inpatient and Day-Clinic Experience Scale (IDES)-a Psychometric Evaluation/Tageskliniks-und Stationserfahrungsbogen–eine psychometrische Evaluation. *Z. Psychosom. Med. Psychother.* **2015**, *61*, 327–341. [CrossRef] [PubMed]
51. Corp, I. *IBM SPSS Statistics for Windows*; Version 22.0; IBM Corp.: Armonk, NY, USA, 2013.
52. Team, R.C. R: A language and environment for statistical computing. 2013.
53. Enders, C.K. *Applied Missing Data Analysis*; Guilford Press: New York, NY, USA, 2010.
54. Buuren, S.V.; Groothuis-Oudshoorn, K. Mice: Multivariate imputation by chained equations in R. *J. Stat. Softw.* **2010**, *45*, 1–68. [CrossRef]
55. White, I.R.; Royston, P.; Wood, A.M. Multiple imputation using chained equations: Issues and guidance for practice. *Stat. Med.* **2011**, *30*, 377–399. [CrossRef] [PubMed]
56. Raudenbush, S.W. *HLM 6: Hierarchical Linear and Nonlinear Modeling*; Scientific Software International: Skokie, IL, USA, 2004.
57. Raudenbush, S.W.; Bryk, A.S. *Hierarchical Linear Models: Applications and Data Analysis Methods*; Sage: Thousand Oaks, CA, USA, 2002; Volume 1.
58. Fitzmaurice, G.M.; Laird, N.M.; Ware, J.H. *Applied Longitudinal Analysis*; John Wiley & Sons: Hoboken, NJ, USA, 2012; Volume 998.
59. Singer, J.D.; Willett, J.B. *Applied longitudinal Data Analysis: Modeling Change and Event Occurrence*; Oxford University Press: Oxford, UK, 2003.
60. Smith, J.Z.; Sayer, A.G.; Goldberg, A.E. Multilevel modeling approaches to the study of LGBT-parent families: Methods for dyadic data analysis. In *LGBT-Parent Families*; Springer: Berlin/Heidelberg, Germany, 2013; pp. 307–323.
61. Barnett, R.C.; Marshall, N.L.; Raudenbush, S.W.; Brennan, R.T. Gender and the relationship between job experiences and psychological distress: A study of dual-earner couples. *J. Pers. Soc. Psychol.* **1993**, *64*, 794. [CrossRef]
62. Kenward, M.G.; Roger, J.H. Small sample inference for fixed effects from restricted maximum likelihood. *Biometrics* **1997**, *53*, 983–997. [CrossRef]
63. Hayes, A.F. *Introduction to Mediation, Moderation, and Conditional Process Analysis: A Regression-Based Approach*; The Guilford Press: New York, NY, USA, 2017.
64. Kolb, L.C. Attachment behavior and pain complaints. *Psychosomatics* **1982**, *23*, 413–425. [CrossRef]
65. Smith, A.E.; Msetfi, R.M.; Golding, L. Client self rated adult attachment patterns and the therapeutic alliance: A systematic review. *Clin. Psychol. Rev.* **2010**, *30*, 326–337. [CrossRef]
66. Damasio, A. Human behaviour: Brain trust. *Nature* **2005**, *435*, 571–572. [CrossRef]

67. Nickel, R.; Egle, U.T. Manualisierte psycho-dynamisch-interaktionelle Gruppentherapie. *Psychotherapeut* **2001**, *46*, 11–19. [CrossRef]
68. van IJzendoorn, M.H.; Juffer, F.; Duyvesteyn, M.G. Breaking the intergenerational cycle of insecure attachment: A review of the effects of attachment-based interventions on maternal sensitivity and infant security. *J. Child Psychol. Psychiatry* **1995**, *36*, 225–248. [CrossRef] [PubMed]
69. Blatt, S.J.; Zuroff, D.C.; Hawley, L.L.; Auerbach, J.S. Predictors of sustained therapeutic change. *Psychother. Res.* **2010**, *20*, 37–54. [CrossRef] [PubMed]
70. Barber, J.P.; Luborsky, L.; Gallop, R.; Crits-Christoph, P.; Frank, A.; Weiss, R.D.; Thase, M.E.; Connolly, M.B.; Gladis, M.; Foltz, C. Therapeutic alliance as a predictor of outcome and retention in the National Institute on Drug Abuse Collaborative Cocaine Treatment Study. *J. Consult. Clin. Psychol.* **2001**, *69*, 119. [CrossRef] [PubMed]
71. Bennett, J.K.; Fuertes, J.N.; Keitel, M.; Phillips, R. The role of patient attachment and working alliance on patient adherence, satisfaction, and health-related quality of life in lupus treatment. *Patient Educ. Couns.* **2011**, *85*, 53–59. [CrossRef] [PubMed]
72. Horvath, A.O.; Del Re, A.; Flückiger, C.; Symonds, D. Alliance in Individual Psychotherapy. *Psychotherapy* **2011**, *48*, 9–16. [CrossRef] [PubMed]
73. Bateman, A.; Fonagy, P. *Mentalization-Based Treatment for Personality Disorders: A Practical Guide*; Oxford University Press: Oxford, UK, 2016.
74. Bateman, A.; Fonagy, P. 8-Year follow-up of patients treated for borderline personality disorder: Mentalization- based treatment versus treatment as usual. *Am. J. Psychiatry* **2008**, *165*, 631–638. [CrossRef]
75. Jørgensen, C.R.; Freund, C.; Bøye, R.; Jordet, H.; Andersen, D.; Kjølbye, M. Outcome of mentalization-based and supportive psychotherapy in patients with borderline personality disorder: A randomized trial. *Acta Psychiatr. Scand.* **2013**, *127*, 305–317. [CrossRef]
76. Simpson, S.H.; Eurich, D.T.; Majumdar, S.R.; Padwal, R.S.; Tsuyuki, R.T.; Varney, J.; Johnson, J.A. A meta-analysis of the association between adherence to drug therapy and mortality. *BMJ* **2006**, *333*, 15. [CrossRef]
77. Simpson, R.J. Challenges for improving medication adherence. *JAMA* **2006**, *296*, 2614–2616. [CrossRef]
78. Mikail, S.F.; Henderson, P.R.; Tasca, G.A. An interpersonally based model of chronic pain: An application of attachment theory. *Clin. Psychol. Rev.* **1994**, *14*, 1–16. [CrossRef]

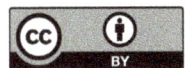

© 2019 by the authors. Licensee MDPI, Basel, Switzerland. This article is an open access article distributed under the terms and conditions of the Creative Commons Attribution (CC BY) license (http://creativecommons.org/licenses/by/4.0/).

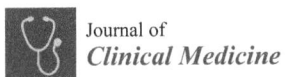

Article

Effects of Adding Interferential Therapy Electro-Massage to Usual Care after Surgery in Subacromial Pain Syndrome: A Randomized Clinical Trial

Manuel Albornoz-Cabello [1], Jose Antonio Sanchez-Santos [2], Rocio Melero-Suarez [3], Alberto Marcos Heredia-Rizo [1,*] and Luis Espejo-Antunez [4]

[1] Department of Physiotherapy, Faculty of Nursing, Physiotherapy and Podiatry, University of Seville, 41009 Seville, Spain; malbornoz@us.es
[2] High Resolution Hospital, Andalusian Health Service, Utrera, 41710 Sevilla, Spain; jossansan@alum.us.es
[3] Department of Podiatry, Faculty of Nursing, Physiotherapy and Podiatry, University of Seville, 41009 Seville, Spain; rms-1000@hotmail.com
[4] Department of Medical-Surgical Therapeutics, Faculty of Medicine, University of Extremadura, 06006 Badajoz, Spain; luisea@unex.es
* Correspondence: amheredia@us.es; Tel.: +34-954486507

Received: 13 January 2019; Accepted: 30 January 2019; Published: 2 February 2019

Abstract: Subacromial pain syndrome (SAPS) is a prevalent condition that results in loss of function. Surgery is indicated when pain and functional limitations persist after conservative measures, with scarce evidence about the most-appropriate post-operative approach. Interferential therapy (IFT), as a supplement to other interventions, has shown to relieve musculoskeletal pain. The study aim was to investigate the effects of adding IFT electro-massage to usual care after surgery in adults with SAPS. A randomized, single-blinded, controlled trial was carried out. Fifty-six adults with SAPS, who underwent acromioplasty in the previous 12 weeks, were equally distributed into an IFT electro-massage group or a control group. All participants underwent a two-week intervention (three times per week). The control group received usual care (thermotherapy, therapeutic exercise, manual therapy, and ultrasound). For participants in the IFT electro-massage group, a 15-min IFT electro-massage was added to usual care in every session. Shoulder pain intensity was assessed with a 100-mm visual analogue scale. Secondary measures included upper limb functionality (Constant-Murley score), and pain-free passive range of movement. A blinded evaluator collected outcomes at baseline and after the last treatment session. The ANOVA revealed a significant group effect, for those who received IFT electro-massage, for improvements in pain intensity, upper limb function, and shoulder flexion, abduction, internal and external rotation (all, $p < 0.01$). There were no between-group differences for shoulder extension ($p = 0.531$) and adduction ($p = 0.340$). Adding IFT electro-massage to usual care, including manual therapy and exercises, revealed greater positive effects on pain, upper limb function, and mobility in adults with SAPS after acromioplasty.

Keywords: electric stimulation therapy; manual therapies; musculoskeletal pain; pain assessment; range of motion; shoulder pain

1. Introduction

Shoulder complaints are a common musculoskeletal disorder. The one-year prevalence of shoulder pain in the general population ranges from 5% to 47%, while the lifetime prevalence has been estimated up to 67% [1]. Work-related physical and psychosocial factors may be associated with onset and/or worsening of shoulder pain within the working-age population [2]. Among shoulder complaints, subacromial pain syndrome (SAPS) is the most common disorder that result in loss of function, increased pain sensitivity [3], and impaired quality of life, accounting for up to 70% of consultations in primary care [4]. SAPS is characterized by persistent pain around the acromion, which usually worsens during or after lifting the upper extremity [5], and embraces clinical diagnosis such as subacromial impingement and rotator cuff tears [6]. The clinical course of SAPS remains unclear, and previous evidence suggests that 50% of adults with chronic SAPS may only recover after 10 to 18 months of initial onset [7]. This leads to a considerable economic burden [8], due to absenteeism from work, productivity loss, and high expenditure for health care services [9].

A great diversity of conservative interventions, combining pharmacological and physical therapy treatments, is often used to decrease pain and enhance function in SAPS [5]. There exists; however, very limited evidence about the effectiveness of existing treatments to improve the functional limitations associated with this condition [10]. Amongst them, exercise therapy has been suggested as the core conservative treatment [11]. Likewise, the use of deep dry needling has shown to relieve shoulder pain [12], and ultrasound-guided injection therapy is widely used before surgery, with good outcomes in the short-term [13,14]. Surgical intervention is mainly indicated when pain and functional limitations persist after conservative measures, and for patients with clearly distinguished clinical signs [11,15]. Indeed, there is conflicting evidence about the efficacy of surgery compared to conservative approaches [16,17], or no treatment [15]. Despite that, the frequency of acromioplasty has dramatically increased in the last decades [18,19]. There is; however, scarce evidence about the most-appropriate post-operative intervention for SAPS, with exercise therapy showing good results [20,21].

Interferential therapy (IFT) is a highly popular treatment modality in the clinical setting, which involves crossing two medium frequency currents to generate a low-frequency beating effect in the deep tissues [22], and can be used alone or combined with massage [23]. Although IFT is purported to provide pain relief and increased blood flow to the tissues [24], there is still inadequate evidence to support its use as a sole intervention for pain management in musculoskeletal disorders in general [22], and in shoulder pain in particular [25,26]. Nevertheless, IFT as a supplement to other interventions has demonstrated advantages over placebo and control treatments for reducing musculoskeletal pain [27], although there are conflicting findings on this issue [28]. Current research also highlights the need for high quality clinical trials assessing the effectiveness of multimodal approaches for SAPS [29].

The study aim was to investigate the effects of adding IFT electro-massage to a two-week usual care protocol, compared with the usual care protocol alone, on pain intensity, upper limb functionality, and shoulder passive range of motion in adults with SAPS who underwent acromioplasty. It was hypothesized that adding IFT electro-massage to the usual care intervention would achieve higher effectiveness than the sole use of the usual care regime.

2. Methods

2.1. Study Design

A single-blinded (the evaluator assessing the outcome measures remained blinded to the participants' allocation group) randomized controlled trial was carried out. The Consolidated Standards of Reporting Trials (CONSORT) statement and checklist were followed. The research protocol was conducted in accordance with the Declaration of Helsinki statement of ethical, legal, and regulatory principals to provide guidance for health-related research involving human subjects. The study was approved by the Ethical Research Committee of the Hospital Universitario Virgen del Rocío, Sevilla, Spain (project code CEI 2012PI/172, approval date: September 26th 2012), and prospectively registered (Clinical Trials.gov, Identifier NCT03338283). All participants provided written informed consent.

2.2. Participants

Adult patients with shoulder pain, who underwent acromioplasty in the 12 weeks before data collection, were referred by an orthopedic surgeon at a large public hospital in Southern Spain. Before surgery, SAPS was diagnosed following a positive response to clinical examination (Hawkins–Kennedy test, drop-arm test, external rotation lag sign, and empty can test) and radiologic diagnostic criteria to differentiate SAPS from other conditions (e.g., bone or joint abnormalities) [30]. A detailed description of the clinical tests can be found elsewhere [31]. For the diagnostic accuracy of clinical examination, a negative response to the Hawkins–Kennedy test appears to rule out SAPS (pooled sensitivity and specificity, 79% and 59%, respectively) [32]. The drop-arm test or the external rotation lag sign (specificity, 90–97%) are likely to rule in SAPS when positive [30], and the empty can test is a reliable and helpful tool to confirm subacromial impingement syndrome (87% specificity) [33]. Overall, the combination of imaging features and clinical tests can help to confirm the presence of SAPS [30]. Acromioplasty was considered a feasible intervention for patients between 20 and 80 years, with anterior shoulder pain lasting more than three months [34], and who received previous conservative treatment (manual therapy, pharmacological treatment, and use of corticosteroid injections) with no satisfactory results [35]. Those participants with a self-reported pain intensity $\geq$30mm in the visual analogue scale (VAS), and a score <45 points on the personal psychological apprehension scale (PPAS) [36], were invited to participate. The PPAS is a valid, reliable, and simple-to-handle tool to assess the subjects' apprehension to receive electrical stimulation therapy [37]. The exclusion criteria were as follows: Any contraindication to the use of IFT (Table 1) [38,39]; previous cervical spine or shoulder surgery; a history of neurological or mental illnesses; diagnosed central or peripheral nervous system diseases [23]; concomitant fracture in the neck/shoulder; altered sensitivity to tactile stimuli or loss of sensation in the neck/shoulder or upper extremity [6]; concomitant radiological diagnosis of osteoarthritis of the glenohumeral or acromioclavicular joints; fibromyalgia or rheumatoid arthritis [23]; having received injections of corticoids or hyaluronic acid following surgery; symptoms of frozen shoulder [40]; impaired cognition or communication; and being involved in an on-going medico-legal dispute.

Table 1. List of contraindications to the use of interferential therapy.

Contraindications
• Acute inflammation
• Pregnancy
• Use of electronic devices, including cardiac pacemakers
• Active deep vein thrombosis or thrombophlebitis
• Tumoral diseases
• Use of metal implants when the subject refers unpleasant sensations
• Untreated hemorrhagic conditions or active bleeding tissues
• Recently radiated tissues
• Active tuberculosis, infected tissues, or wounds with underlying osteomyelitis
• To the neck or head in individuals with previous seizures
• To anterior neck, carotid sinus, over the eyes, or reproductive organs

2.3. Study Protocol

An external website (http://www.randomization.com) was used to complete the randomization schedule for treatment order, considering a 1:1 ratio distribution of participants in the study groups (IFT electro-massage and control group). An external assistant safeguarded the randomization sequence and prepared sealed opaque envelopes concealing the treatment order allocation. Following baseline allocation, demographic and clinical data were initially collected. A blinded evaluator collected all measurements at baseline and immediately after the last treatment session. The treatment protocol consisted of a two-week intervention regime. Three treatment sessions, each lasting around 70–85 min, were made per week and supervised by a physiotherapist with more than 15 years of clinical experience.

2.4. Outcome Measures

Participants were asked to rate their worst shoulder pain intensity during the last 24 h using a 100-mm VAS, with 0 denoting "no pain" and 100 denoting "extreme and unbearable pain" [41]. Minimal clinically-important differences for the VAS are based on a 15–20% change [42], or a decrease above 14 mm [43], following intervention.

The upper limb functionality was evaluated using the Constant-Murley score, which consists of a 100-point scale, with final values representing different functional levels: excellent (>80), good (65–79), medium (50–64), and bad (<50) [44]. The minimal detectable change for the Constant-Murley score has been set at 17 points for individuals with subacromial impingement syndrome [45].

The Simple Goniometer iPhone®app (version 1.1, Ockendon.net, Oswestry, England) was used to assess the shoulder pain-free passive range of movement. An iPhone®3GS, iOS 4.3.5 (Apple, Cupertino, CA, USA) was fixed to the participants' arm with an armband bracelet (Kalenji, Villeneuve d'Ascq, France). The recordings of shoulder range of motion were made twice (2-min break between assessments), using the average value of the two measures for further analysis. Before assessments, participants were asked to stop the evaluator when they started to feel low-intensity pain during movement (below 20 mm in the VAS). To evaluate shoulder flexion and extension, participants were seated with back support and no armrests, and the iPhone®was fixed on the lateral side of the arm (2 cm proximal to the glenohumeral joint). For shoulder abduction, participants kept the same position, and the iPhone®was placed on the ventral side of the arm (2 cm proximal to the glenohumeral joint). Shoulder adduction was assessed with the participant lying supine, with 90 degrees of shoulder flexion (or the maximum possible pain-free flexion), and with the iPhone®placed on the ventral side of the arm. Internal and external rotation were evaluated with participants in supine, with 90 degrees of shoulder abduction (or the maximum possible pain-free abduction), 90 degrees of elbow flexion, forearm in neutral position, and the iPhone®was placed in the ventral side of the arm (2 cm proximal to the glenohumeral joint). During all assessments, the evaluator applied gentle pressure to the arm or forearm until the edge of movement was reached [46], and maximum caution was taken to minimize the scapular motion by keeping the shoulder and back in contact with the back support. A smartphone inclinometer or virtual goniometer is an easy-to-use, valid, and reliable tool, comparable to other clinical methods, to assess shoulder range of motion in healthy subjects and in individuals with shoulder disorders [46–48]. The Simple Goniometer iPhone®app has shown to be reliable and possesses concurrent validity [49].

2.5. Interventions

Participants in the control group underwent an usual care protocol involving: Fifteen minutes of transcutaneous infrared thermotherapy (INFRA-2000, Enraf-Nonius BV, Rotterdam, The Netherlands) [50]; 35 min of active, self-assisted, and isometric exercise therapy [51,52]; 20 min of manual therapy to retrain scapulohumeral movement and to provide soft and pain-free shoulder traction [51]; and 5 min of pulsatile ultrasound (Sonopuls 490®, Enraf-Nonius BV, Rotterdam, The Netherlands) over the acromium and scapulohumeral area, with a 5 cm^2 head, and using a frequency of 3 Mhz and a power of 1.2 w/cm^2. For participants in the IFT electro-massage group, a 15-min IFT electro-massage over the neck-shoulder and the glenohumeral joint was added in every treatment session to the usual care treatment previously described. A bipolar application, using a carrier frequency of 4000 Hz at constant voltage and an amplitude-modulated frequency of 100 Hz, was administered. The current intensity was set at a medium-high level, but always adapted to individual tolerance, to achieve a "strong but comfortable tingling" without evoking visible muscle twitches [28]. Two rubber electrodes (6 × 8 cm) were fitted inside sponges of equal size. The sponges were dampened with hot water to avoid unpleasant sensations and to allow a normal sliding over the skin during the electro-massage [23]. Some needles with hot water were prepared to dampen the sponges during the procedure, if required. The physiotherapist wore vinyl gloves and moved the sponges over the neck, shoulder and scapular areas. Occasionally, the therapist performed slight traction of the glenohumeral joint, and stretching of the neck-shoulder muscles (e.g., upper trapezius and levator scapulae) while administering the IFT (Figure 1).

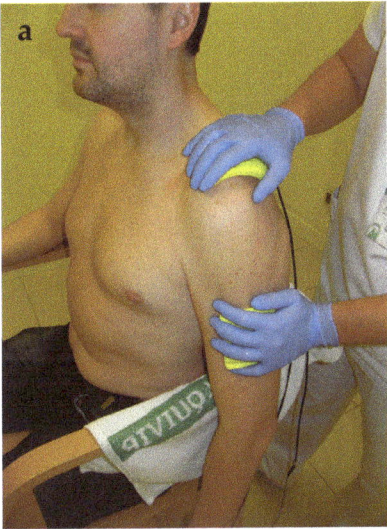 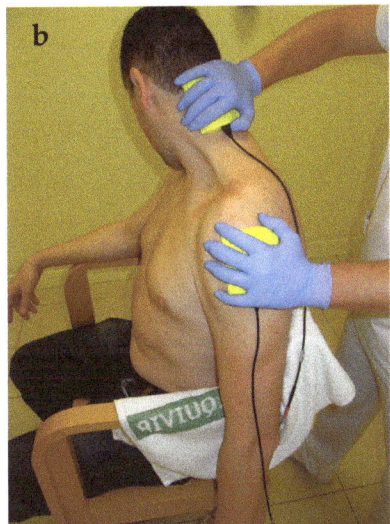

Figure 1. Interferential therapy electro-massage alone (**a**) or combined with stretching (**b**).

2.6. Statistical Analysis

The sample size calculation was based on detecting: (1) a 15% change in self-reported pain intensity [42]; and (2) a 17-points difference in the Constant-Murley score in the comparison between groups after intervention [45]. Taking into account a one-tailed hypothesis, an alpha value of 0.05, a desired power of 90%, and a high effect size (d = 0.8), 28 participants were required per study group (G*Power, version 3.1.9.2, Heinrich Heine University, Düsseldorf, Germany).

Statistical processing of the data was carried out using the PASW Advanced Statistics (SPSS Inc, Chicago, IL, USA), version 24.0. Data were reported as mean (standard deviation), and confidence intervals (95% CI). The Shapiro–Wilk test was used to test the normal distribution of the study variables. Differences in the outcome measures were detected using a repeated measures analysis of variance (ANOVA), with the group (IFT electro-massage or control) as the between-subjects factor, and time (baseline or immediately after intervention) as the within-subjects factor. Post-hoc comparisons (Bonferroni) were performed for significant effects. Eta-squared (η^2) was used to calculate the effect size (small, $0.01 \leq \eta^2 < 0.06$; medium, $0.06 \leq \eta^2 < 0.14$; and large, $\eta^2 > 0.14$). Statistical significance was set at a *p* value < 0.05.

3. Results

Sixty-six individuals who underwent acromioplasty were assessed for eligibility between December 2017 to April 2018. Finally, fifty-six participants (30 females, 53.6%), aged between 23 to 76 years (mean age ± SD, 49.6 ± 12.4), met the eligibility criteria and were recruited. There were no adverse reactions or dropouts during the study protocol (Figure 2).

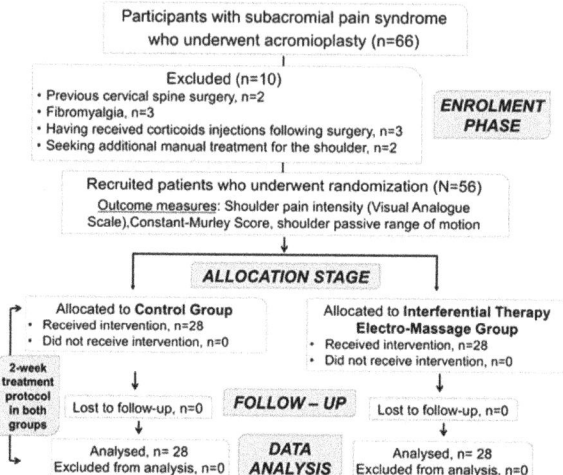

Figure 2. CONSORT flowchart diagram of study participants.

Table 2 lists the baseline characteristics of participants in the study groups. At baseline, there were no between-group differences for any study variable (all, $p > 0.05$), except for participants' height ($p = 0.029$).

Table 2. Baseline characteristics of participants in the study groups (mean ± standard deviation, or in frequency percentages).

Variable	Intereferential Therapy Electro-Massage Group ($n = 28$)	Control Group ($n = 28$)	p Value
Mean age (years)	47.2 ± 11.6	51.9 ± 13.1	0.159
Sex (female) % (n)	42.9% (12)	64.3% (18)	0.111
Height (cm)	170.18 ± 9.21	164.64 ± 9.27	0.029
Weight (kg)	80.53 ± 12.72	75.71 ± 15.44	0.208
Body mass index (kg/m^2)	27.76 ± 3.37	27.93 ± 5.08	0.884
Arthroscopy surgery % (n)	85.7% (24)	89.3% (25)	0.689
Days after surgery *	42 (21–58)	51 (18–62)	0.221
Affected shoulder; right % (n)	50% (14)	57.1% (16)	0.595
PPAS	34.21 ± 4.74	33.54 ± 9.78	0.743
Visual analogue scale (mm)	69.82 ± 16.74	65.71 ± 20.75	0.419
Constant-Murley score (0–100)	29.68 ± 10.4	29.71 ± 12.24	0.991
Shoulder flexion (°)	103.61 ± 30.89	107.07 ± 32.53	0.684
Shoulder extension (°)	40 ± 10.79	40.18 ± 13.3	0.956
Shoulder abduction (°)	84.43 ± 27.5	84.25 ± 29.56	0.981
Shoulder abduction (°)	34.5 ± 12.08	30.86 ± 9.78	0.221
Shoulder internal rotation (°)	29.32 ± 14.75	32.21 ± 8.86	0.440
Shoulder external rotation (°)	59 ± 17.22	62.96 ± 20.74	0.378

* Median and interquartile range. PPAS—personal psychological apprehension scale.

Table 3 includes the baseline, post-intervention scores, and the mean differences in the within-group and between-group comparisons for all outcome measures. Both interventions significantly improved pain perception, upper limb functionality and shoulder passive range of motion in all directions (all, $p < 0.001$). For the between-group analysis of the mean score changes after intervention, the ANOVA revealed a significant group effect, for those included in the IFT electro-massage group, for the decrease in shoulder pain intensity (F = 29.82; $p < 0.001$; $\eta^2 = 0.35$), the improvement in the Constant-Murley score (F = 29.45; $p < 0.001$; $\eta^2 = 0.35$), and the increase in pain-free passive shoulder flexion (F = 21.51; $p < 0.001$; $\eta^2 = 0.28$), abduction (F = 7.77; $p = 0.007$; $\eta^2 = 0.12$), internal rotation (F = 31.97; $p < 0.001$; $\eta^2 = 0.37$), and external rotation (F = 8.26; $p = 0.006$; $\eta^2 = 0.13$). There were no differences between groups for shoulder extension (F = 0.39; $p = 0.531$; $\eta^2 = 0.007$) and adduction (F = 0.92; $p = 0.340$; $\eta^2 = 0.017$).

Table 3. Baseline, post-intervention values, and mean score changes after intervention of the outcome measures; mean ± standard deviation (95% confidence interval).

	Baseline	After the Two-Week Intervention	Within-Group Changes after Intervention	Between-Group Mean Changes
Visual Analogue Scale (mm)				
IFT Electro-Massage Group	69.82 ± 16.74	32.68 ± 13.64	−37.14 ± 13.22 (−42.27 to −32.01) *	−18.92 ± 3.46 (−25.8 to −11.97) †
Control Group	65.71 ± 20.75	47.5 ± 22.95	−18.21 ± 12.71 (−23.14 to −13.28) *	
Constant-Murley Score (0–100)				
IFT Electro-Massage Group	29.68 ± 10.41	56.07 ± 10.96	26.39 ± 5.9 (24.1 to 28.68) *	10.71 ± 1.97 (6.74 to 14.68) †
Control Group	29.71 ± 12.24	45.39 ± 13.82	15.67 ± 8.61 (12.33 to 19.01) *	
Shoulder Flexion (°)				
IFT Electro-Massage Group	103.61 ± 30.89	146.86 ± 22.1	43.25 ± 16.75 (36.75 to 49.74) *	19.32 ± 4.16 (10.96 to 27.67) †
Control Group	107.07 ± 32.53	131 ± 25.93	23.92 ± 14.32 (18.37 to 29.4) *	
Shoulder Extension (°)				
IFT Electro-Massage Group	40 ± 10.79	52 ± 9.86	12 ± 7.21 (9.2 to 14.79) *	1.21 ± 0.92 (−2.64 to 5.07)
Control Group	40.18 ± 13.3	50.96 ± 10.38	10.78 ± 7.21 (7.99 to 13.57) *	
Shoulder Abduction (°)				
IFT Electro-Massage Group	84.43 ± 27.5	112.18 ± 29.1	37.75 ± 15.86 (31.6 to 43.9) *	12.25 ± 4.39 (3.43 to 21.06) †
Control Group	84.25 ± 29.56	109.75 ± 30.1	25.5 ± 17.01 (18.9 to 32.09) *	
Shoulder Adduction (°)				
IFT Electro-Massage Group	34.5 ± 12.08	45.54 ± 10.87	11.03 ± 7.27 (8.21 to 13.85) *	−2.25 ± 2.33 (−6.93 to 2.43)
Control Group	30.86 ± 9.78	44.14 ± 12.94	13.28 ± 10 (9.4 to 17.16) *	
Shoulder Internal Rotation (°)				
IFT Electro-Massage Group	29.32 ± 14.75	50.61 ± 13.31	21.28 ± 7.71 (18.29 to 24.27) *	10.5 ± 1.85 (6.77 to 14.22) †
Control Group	32.21 ± 8.86	43 ± 11.2	10.78 ± 6.09 (8.42 to 13.14) *	
Shoulder External Rotation (°)				
IFT Electro-Massage Group	59 ± 17.22	82.5 ± 10.94	23.5 ± 13.82 (18.14 to 28.86) *	9.46 ± 3.2 (2.86 to 16.06) †
Control Group	62.96 ± 20.74	77 ± 16.63	14.03 ± 10.61 (9.92 to 18.15) *	

* Indicates significant differences in the within-group comparisons (all, $p < 0.001$). † Indicates significant differences in the between-group comparisons. IFT—interferential therapy.

4. Discussion

The present findings demonstrated that including IFT electro-massage in a two-week usual care protocol, combining manual therapy, exercises, thermotherapy, and ultrasound, achieved better immediate results on shoulder pain intensity, upper limb function, and pain-free passive range of movement (except for shoulder extension and adduction), compared with the sole use of the usual care regime, in adults with SAPS who underwent recent shoulder surgery.

The decrease in shoulder pain intensity and the improvement in upper limb functionality was significantly higher, with a high effect size, for participants who received IFT electro-massage, although individuals in both groups reduced their shoulder pain after the two-week protocol above the minimum clinically important difference for the VAS [42,43]. On the contrary, changes in the Constant-Murley score surpassed the 17-point clinically relevant threshold [45] only for those in the IFT electro-massage group. The passive shoulder range of movement increased by 20–40% in the control group, and by 30–70% in the IFT electro-massage group. The differences between groups for shoulder pain-free passive mobility achieved a high effect size for shoulder flexion and internal rotation and a medium effect size for shoulder abduction and external rotation. To date, there has been a single previous study investigating the effects of IFT electro-massage [23]. This former trial used IFT as a sole intervention in individuals with chronic low-back pain and concluded greater improvements on pain, disability, and quality of life, compared to the use of superficial massage. These positive effects were explained based on the purported capacity of IFT to stimulate cutaneous sensory nerves and evoke mild vasodilation [23]. To the author's knowledge, this is the first study assessing the effectiveness of a multimodal intervention including IFT electro-massage in adults with post-operative shoulder pain after acromioplasty.

There is a huge debate about the clinical impact of including IFT and other electrotherapeutic modalities for the management of chronic shoulder pain. Conflicting to the current results, the addition of IFT to exercise and/or manual therapy did not demonstrate greater clinical effects on shoulder pain and disability, compared to the use of exercise and/or manual therapy alone, in individuals with non-specific soft-tissue shoulder disorders [53], or with unilateral shoulder impingement syndrome [54]. Similarly, Nazligul et al. [28] recently concluded that IFT does not provide additional effect to a multimodal approach including cryotherapy, exercise, and non-steroidal anti-inflammatory drugs for patients with SAPS. On the contrary, it has been demonstrated that the combination of IFT with shoulder exercises [55], ultrasound, thermotherapy, and stretching [56] is effective in the management of frozen shoulders. Likewise, the use of IFT alone has shown to be clinically effective to relieve pain during movement and to increase pain-free passive shoulder mobility in hemiplegic shoulder pain [57] and, when combined with exercise therapy, seems to improve pain, function, and quality of life in individuals with shoulder impingement syndrome [58]. In the latter study, the effect of combining IFT with exercise therapy was; however, similar to that of including ultrasound or transcutaneous electrical nerve stimulation instead, in the intervention protocol [58]. Indeed, IFT seems to be a potential, although modest, effective supplement to other interventions to decrease pain, compared to control or placebo treatments, in musculoskeletal pain disorders [27]. There are; however, many controversies on this issue [25,26], and the heterogeneity and methodological problems across studies make it difficult to reach conclusive statements.

This inconclusive evidence about the impact of using IFT, alone or in addition to other conservative approaches, persists when considering other chronic musculoskeletal pain conditions, such as neck or low-back pain [59]. There are some plausible explanations to account for this issue. First, the carrier frequency of the IFT current differs among studies, and this may influence the hypoalgesic response after stimulation [60]. Second, the use of electrotherapy may evoke a long sustained placebo-induced pain relief effect [61]. In this sense, most of the previous studies investigating the role of IFT on shoulder pain have not included sham IFT as a control intervention [54–56,58]. Third, the clinical context and the social connection between patient and therapist seem to modulate the effect of IFT [62,63], although these aspects have been scarcely controlled in the existing literature. Finally, only one previous trial has evaluated the effects of IFT, compared to sham IFT, on post-operative pain, and range of motion in patients undergoing knee surgery [64]. Even though IFT showed positive findings on increasing range of motion, and reducing pain, medication intake, and swelling [64], more definite conclusions need to be built upon more high-quality evidence [27].

Some potential study limitations should be mentioned. First, the study did not include a sham IFT electro-massage group. Second, only immediate results after the last session of the two-week intervention protocol were collected, thus it would be highly relevant to investigate the medium and long-term follow-up effects of IFT on post-operative pain in further studies. Third, the therapist in charge of the interventions was not blinded to participants allocation group. Finally, further research is warranted to investigate if different results could be expected using different current parameters.

5. Conclusions

Adding IFT electro-massage to a two-week supervised usual care protocol combining manual therapy, exercises, ultrasound, and infrared thermotherapy achieved better results on decreasing shoulder pain, and improving upper limb functionality and shoulder pain-free passive range of motion, compared to usual care alone, in adults with SAPS who underwent recent acromioplasty.

Author Contributions: Conceptualization, M.A.-C. and J.A.S.-S.; Methodology, M.A.-C., J.A.S.-S., R.M.-S., A.M.H.-R., and L.E.-A.; Formal analysis, M.A.-C., J.A.S.-S., R.M.-S., and A.M.H.-R.; Investigation, M.A.-C., J.A.S.-S., R.M.-S., A.M.H.-R., and L.E.-A.; Resources, M.A.-C., J.A.S.-S., and R.M.-S.; Data curation, M.A.-C., J.A.S.-S., R.M.-S., and A.M.H.-R.; Writing—Original draft preparation, M.A.-C., J.A.S.-S., R.M.-S., A.M.H.-R., and L.E.-A.; Writing—Review and editing, M.A.-C., J.A.S.-S., R.M.-S., A.M.H.-R., and L.E.-A.; Visualization, M.A.-C., J.A.S.-S., and A.M.H.-R.; Supervision, M.A.-C., J.A.S.-S., A.M.H.-R., and L.E.-A.; Project administration, M.A.-C., J.A.S.-S., and L.E.-A.

Acknowledgments: The authors of this manuscript certify that they have no financial or non-financial interest (including research funding) or involvement with any commercial organization that has a direct financial interest in any matter included in this manuscript.

Conflicts of Interest: The authors declare no conflicts of interest.

References

1. Luime, J.J.; Koes, B.W.; Hendriksen, I.J.; Burdorf, A.; Verhagen, A.P.; Miedema, H.S.; Verhaar, J.A. Prevalence and incidence of shoulder pain in the general population; a systematic review. *Scand. J. Rheumatol.* **2004**, *33*, 73–81. [CrossRef]
2. Van der Windt, D.A.; Thomas, E.; Pope, D.P.; de Winter, A.F.; Macfarlane, G.J.; Bouter, L.M.; Silman, A.J. Occupational risk factors for shoulder pain: A systematic review. *Occup. Environ. Med.* **2000**, *57*, 433–442. [CrossRef]
3. Calvo Lobo, C.; Romero Morales, C.; Rodríguez Sanz, D.; Sanz Corbalán, I.; Sánchez Romero, E.A.; Fernández Carnero, J.; López López, D. Comparison of hand grip strength and upper limb pressure pain threshold between older adults with or without non-specific shoulder pain. *PeerJ* **2017**, *5*, e2995. [CrossRef] [PubMed]
4. Mitchell, C.; Adebajo, A.; Hay, E.; Carr, A. Shoulder pain: Diagnosis and management in primary care. *BMJ* **2005**, *331*, 1124–1128. [CrossRef] [PubMed]
5. Diercks, R.; Bron, C.; Dorrestijn, O.; Meskers, C.; Naber, R.; de Ruiter, T.; Willems, J.; Winters, J.; van der Woude, H.J.; Association, D.O. Guideline for diagnosis and treatment of subacromial pain syndrome: A multidisciplinary review by the Dutch Orthopaedic Association. *Acta Orthop.* **2014**, *85*, 314–322. [CrossRef]
6. Lewis, J.; Sim, J.; Barlas, P. Acupuncture and electro-acupuncture for people diagnosed with subacromial pain syndrome: A multicentre randomized trial. *Eur. J. Pain* **2017**, *21*, 1007–1019. [CrossRef] [PubMed]
7. Tangrood, Z.J.; Gisselman, A.S.; Sole, G.; Ribeiro, D.C. Clinical course of pain and disability in patients with subacromial shoulder pain: A systematic review protocol. *BMJ Open* **2018**, *8*, e019393. [CrossRef]
8. Virta, L.; Joranger, P.; Brox, J.I.; Eriksson, R. Costs of shoulder pain and resource use in primary health care: A cost-of-illness study in Sweden. *BMC Musculoskelet. Disord.* **2012**, *13*, 17. [CrossRef] [PubMed]
9. Desmeules, F.; Braën, C.; Lamontagne, M.; Dionne, C.E.; Roy, J.S. Determinants and predictors of absenteeism and return-to-work in workers with shoulder disorders. *Work* **2016**, *55*, 101–113. [CrossRef] [PubMed]
10. Faber, E.; Kuiper, J.I.; Burdorf, A.; Miedema, H.S.; Verhaar, J.A. Treatment of impingement syndrome: A systematic review of the effects on functional limitations and return to work. *J. Occup. Rehabil.* **2006**, *16*, 7–25. [CrossRef] [PubMed]

11. Steuri, R.; Sattelmayer, M.; Elsig, S.; Kolly, C.; Tal, A.; Taeymans, J.; Hilfiker, R. Effectiveness of conservative interventions including exercise, manual therapy and medical management in adults with shoulder impingement: A systematic review and meta-analysis of RCTs. *Br. J. Sports Med.* **2017**, *51*, 1340–1347. [CrossRef] [PubMed]
12. Calvo-Lobo, C.; Pacheco-da-Costa, S.; Hita-Herranz, E. Efficacy of deep dry needling on latent myofascial trigger points in older adults with nonspecific shoulder pain: A randomized, controlled clinical trial pilot study. *J. Geriatr. Phys. Ther.* **2017**, *40*, 63–73. [CrossRef] [PubMed]
13. Chang, K.V.; Wu, W.T.; Han, D.S.; Özçakar, L. Static and dynamic shoulder imaging to predict initial effectiveness and recurrence after ultrasound-guided subacromial corticosteroid injections. *Arch. Phys. Med. Rehabil.* **2017**, *98*, 1984–1994. [CrossRef] [PubMed]
14. Chang, K.V.; Mezian, K.; Naňka, O.; Wu, W.T.; Lin, C.P.; Özçakar, L. Ultrasound-guided interventions for painful shoulder: From anatomy to evidence. *J. Pain Res.* **2018**, *11*, 2311–2322. [CrossRef] [PubMed]
15. Beard, D.J.; Rees, J.L.; Cook, J.A.; Rombach, I.; Cooper, C.; Merritt, N.; Shirkey, B.A.; Donovan, J.L.; Gwilym, S.; Savulescu, J.; et al. Arthroscopic subacromial decompression for subacromial shoulder pain (CSAW): A multicentre, pragmatic, parallel group, placebo-controlled, three-group, randomised surgical trial. *Lancet* **2018**, *391*, 329–338. [CrossRef]
16. Dong, W.; Goost, H.; Lin, X.B.; Burger, C.; Paul, C.; Wang, Z.L.; Zhang, T.Y.; Jiang, Z.C.; Welle, K.; Kabir, K. Treatments for shoulder impingement syndrome: A PRISMA systematic review and network meta-analysis. *Medicine* **2015**, *94*, e510. [CrossRef] [PubMed]
17. Dorrestijn, O.; Stevens, M.; Winters, J.C.; van der Meer, K.; Diercks, R.L. Conservative or surgical treatment for subacromial impingement syndrome? A systematic review. *J. Should. Elb. Surg.* **2009**, *18*, 652–660. [CrossRef] [PubMed]
18. Yu, E.; Cil, A.; Harmsen, W.S.; Schleck, C.; Sperling, J.W.; Cofield, R.H. Arthroscopy and the dramatic increase in frequency of anterior acromioplasty from 1980 to 2005: An epidemiologic study. *Arthroscopy* **2010**, *26*, S142–S147. [CrossRef]
19. Vitale, M.A.; Arons, R.R.; Hurwitz, S.; Ahmad, C.S.; Levine, W.N. The rising incidence of acromioplasty. *J. Bone Jt. Surg. Am.* **2010**, *92*, 1842–1850. [CrossRef]
20. Christiansen, D.H.; Frost, P.; Falla, D.; Haahr, J.P.; Frich, L.H.; Andrea, L.C.; Svendsen, S.W. Effectiveness of standardized physical therapy exercises for patients with difficulty returning to usual activities after decompression surgery for subacromial impingement syndrome: Randomized controlled trial. *Phys. Ther.* **2016**, *96*, 787–796. [CrossRef]
21. Pastora-Bernal, J.M.; Martín-Valero, R.; Barón-López, F.J.; Moyano, N.G.; Estebanez-Pérez, M.J. Telerehabilitation after arthroscopic subacromial decompression is effective and not inferior to standard practice: Preliminary results. *J. Telemed. Telecare* **2018**, *24*, 428–433. [CrossRef]
22. Beatti, A.; Raynor, A.; Souvlis, T.; Chipchase, L. The analgesic effect of interferential therapy on clinical and experimentally induced pain. *Phys. Ther. Rev.* **2010**, *15*, 243–252. [CrossRef]
23. Lara-Palomo, I.C.; Aguilar-Ferrándiz, M.E.; Matarán-Peñarrocha, G.A.; Saavedra-Hernández, M.; Granero-Molina, J.; Fernández-Sola, C.; Castro-Sánchez, A.M. Short-term effects of interferential current electro-massage in adults with chronic non-specific low back pain: A randomized controlled trial. *Clin. Rehabil.* **2013**, *27*, 439–449. [CrossRef] [PubMed]
24. Airaksinen, O.; Brox, J.I.; Cedraschi, C.; Hildebrandt, J.; Klaber-Moffett, J.; Kovacs, F.; Mannion, A.F.; Reis, S.; Staal, J.B.; Ursin, H.; et al. Chapter 4. European guidelines for the management of chronic nonspecific low back pain. *Eur. Spine J.* **2006**, *15* (Suppl. 2), S192–S300. [CrossRef]
25. Yu, H.; Côté, P.; Shearer, H.M.; Wong, J.J.; Sutton, D.A.; Randhawa, K.A.; Varatharajan, S.; Southerst, D.; Mior, S.A.; Ameis, A.; et al. Effectiveness of passive physical modalities for shoulder pain: Systematic review by the Ontario protocol for traffic injury management collaboration. *Phys. Ther.* **2015**, *95*, 306–318. [CrossRef] [PubMed]
26. Page, M.J.; Green, S.; Mrocki, M.A.; Surace, S.J.; Deitch, J.; McBain, B.; Lyttle, N.; Buchbinder, R. Electrotherapy modalities for rotator cuff disease. *Cochrane Database Syst. Rev.* **2016**, *6*, CD012225. [CrossRef] [PubMed]
27. Fuentes, J.P.; Armijo Olivo, S.; Magee, D.J.; Gross, D.P. Effectiveness of interferential current therapy in the management of musculoskeletal pain: A systematic review and meta-analysis. *Phys. Ther.* **2010**, *90*, 1219–1238. [CrossRef]

28. Nazligul, T.; Akpinar, P.; Aktas, I.; Unlu Ozkan, F.; Cagliyan Hartevioglu, H. The effect of interferential current therapy on patients with subacromial impingement syndrome: A randomized, double-blind, sham-controlled study. *Eur. J. Phys. Rehabil. Med.* **2018**, *54*, 351–357. [CrossRef]
29. Kelly, S.M.; Wrightson, P.A.; Meads, C.A. Clinical outcomes of exercise in the management of subacromial impingement syndrome: A systematic review. *Clin. Rehabil.* **2010**, *24*, 99–109. [CrossRef]
30. Cadogan, A.; McNair, P.J.; Laslett, M.; Hing, W.A. Diagnostic accuracy of clinical examination and imaging findings for identifying subacromial pain. *PLoS ONE* **2016**, *11*, e0167738. [CrossRef]
31. Van Kampen, D.A.; van den Berg, T.; van der Woude, H.J.; Castelein, R.M.; Scholtes, V.A.; Terwee, C.B.; Willems, W.J. The diagnostic value of the combination of patient characteristics, history, and clinical shoulder tests for the diagnosis of rotator cuff tear. *J. Orthop. Surg. Res.* **2014**, *9*, 70. [CrossRef] [PubMed]
32. Hegedus, E.J.; Goode, A.P.; Cook, C.E.; Michener, L.; Myer, C.A.; Myer, D.M.; Wright, A.A. Which physical examination tests provide clinicians with the most value when examining the shoulder? Update of a systematic review with meta-analysis of individual tests. *Br. J. Sports Med.* **2012**, *46*, 964–978. [CrossRef] [PubMed]
33. Michener, L.A.; Walsworth, M.K.; Doukas, W.C.; Murphy, K.P. Reliability and diagnostic accuracy of 5 physical examination tests and combination of tests for subacromial impingement. *Arch. Phys. Med. Rehabil.* **2009**, *90*, 1898–1903. [CrossRef] [PubMed]
34. Kvalvaag, E.; Røe, C.; Engebretsen, K.B.; Soberg, H.L.; Juel, N.G.; Bautz-Holter, E.; Sandvik, L.; Brox, J.I. One year results of a randomized controlled trial on radial extracorporeal shock wave treatment, with predictors of pain, disability and return to work in patients with subacromial pain syndrome. *Eur. J. Phys. Rehabil. Med.* **2018**, *54*, 341–350. [CrossRef] [PubMed]
35. Paavola, M.; Malmivaara, A.; Taimela, S.; Kanto, K.; Järvinen, T.L.; Investigators, F. Finnish Subacromial Impingement Arthroscopy Controlled Trial (FIMPACT): A protocol for a randomised trial comparing arthroscopic subacromial decompression and diagnostic arthroscopy (placebo control), with an exercise therapy control, in the treatment of shoulder impingement syndrome. *BMJ Open* **2017**, *7*, e014087. [CrossRef] [PubMed]
36. Albornoz-Cabello, M.; Maya-Martín, J.; Domínguez-Maldonado, G.; Espejo-Antúnez, L.; Heredia-Rizo, A.M. Effect of interferential current therapy on pain perception and disability level in subjects with chronic low back pain: A randomized controlled trial. *Clin. Rehabil.* **2017**, *31*, 242–249. [CrossRef] [PubMed]
37. Albornoz-Cabello, M.; Rebollo, J.; García, R. Personal Psychological Apprehension Scale (EAPP) in physical therapy. *Rev. Iberoam. Fisioter. Kinesiol.* **2005**, *8*, 77–87. [CrossRef]
38. Houghton, P.E.; Nussbaum, E.L.; Hoens, A.M. Electrophysical agents—Contraindications and precautions: An evidence-based approach to clinical decision making in physical therapy. *Physiother. Can.* **2010**, *62*, 1–80. [CrossRef]
39. Albornoz-Cabello, M.; Maya-Martin, J.; Toledo-Marhuenda, J.V. *Electroterapia practica. Avances en Investigación Clínica*; Elsevier: Barcelona, Spain, 2016.
40. Holmgren, T.; Oberg, B.; Sjöberg, I.; Johansson, K. Supervised strengthening exercises versus home-based movement exercises after arthroscopic acromioplasty: A randomized clinical trial. *J. Rehabil. Med.* **2012**, *44*, 12–18. [CrossRef]
41. Hawker, G.A.; Mian, S.; Kendzerska, T.; French, M. Measures of adult pain: Visual Analog Scale for Pain (VAS Pain), Numeric Rating Scale for Pain (NRS Pain), McGill Pain Questionnaire (MPQ), Short-Form McGill Pain Questionnaire (SF-MPQ), Chronic Pain Grade Scale (CPGS), Short Form-36 Bodily Pain Scale (SF-36 BPS), and Measure of Intermittent and Constant Osteoarthritis Pain (ICOAP). *Arthritis Care Res.* **2011**, *63* (Suppl. 11), S240–S252. [CrossRef]
42. Dworkin, R.H.; Turk, D.C.; Wyrwich, K.W.; Beaton, D.; Cleeland, C.S.; Farrar, J.T.; Haythornthwaite, J.A.; Jensen, M.P.; Kerns, R.D.; Ader, D.N.; et al. Interpreting the clinical importance of treatment outcomes in chronic pain clinical trials: IMMPACT recommendations. *J. Pain* **2008**, *9*, 105–121. [CrossRef] [PubMed]
43. Tashjian, R.Z.; Deloach, J.; Porucznik, C.A.; Powell, A.P. Minimal clinically important differences (MCID) and patient acceptable symptomatic state (PASS) for visual analog scales (VAS) measuring pain in patients treated for rotator cuff disease. *J. Should. Elb. Surg.* **2009**, *18*, 927–932. [CrossRef] [PubMed]
44. Romeo, A.A.; Mazzocca, A.; Hang, D.W.; Shott, S.; Bach, B.R. Shoulder scoring scales for the evaluation of rotator cuff repair. *Clin. Orthop. Relat. Res.* **2004**, *427*, 107–114. [CrossRef]

45. Henseler, J.F.; Kolk, A.; van der Zwaal, P.; Nagels, J.; Vliet Vlieland, T.P.; Nelissen, R.G. The minimal detectable change of the Constant score in impingement, full-thickness tears, and massive rotator cuff tears. *J. Should. Elb. Surg.* **2015**, *24*, 376–381. [CrossRef] [PubMed]
46. Werner, B.C.; Holzgrefe, R.E.; Griffin, J.W.; Lyons, M.L.; Cosgrove, C.T.; Hart, J.M.; Brockmeier, S.F. Validation of an innovative method of shoulder range-of-motion measurement using a smartphone clinometer application. *J. Should. Elb. Surg.* **2014**, *23*, e275–e282. [CrossRef] [PubMed]
47. Cuesta-Vargas, A.I.; Roldán-Jiménez, C. Validity and reliability of arm abduction angle measured on smartphone: A cross-sectional study. *BMC Musculoskelet. Disord.* **2016**, *17*, 93. [CrossRef]
48. Mejia-Hernandez, K.; Chang, A.; Eardley-Harris, N.; Jaarsma, R.; Gill, T.K.; McLean, J.M. Smartphone applications for the evaluation of pathologic shoulder range of motion and shoulder scores-a comparative study. *JSES Open Access* **2018**, *2*, 109–114. [CrossRef]
49. Jones, A.; Sealey, R.; Crowe, M.; Gordon, S. Concurrent validity and reliability of the Simple Goniometer iPhone app compared with the Universal Goniometer. *Physiother. Theory Pract.* **2014**, *30*, 512–516. [CrossRef]
50. Koh, P.S.; Seo, B.K.; Cho, N.S.; Park, H.S.; Park, D.S.; Baek, Y.H. Clinical effectiveness of bee venom acupuncture and physiotherapy in the treatment of adhesive capsulitis: A randomized controlled trial. *J. Should. Elb. Surg.* **2013**, *22*, 1053–1062. [CrossRef]
51. Kuhn, J.E. Exercise in the treatment of rotator cuff impingement: A systematic review and a synthesized evidence-based rehabilitation protocol. *J. Should. Elb. Surg.* **2009**, *18*, 138–160. [CrossRef]
52. Karel, Y.H.J.M.; Scholten-Peeters, G.G.M.; Thoomes-de Graaf, M.; Duijn, E.; van Broekhoven, J.B.; Koes, B.W.; Verhagen, A.P. Physiotherapy for patients with shoulder pain in primary care: A descriptive study of diagnostic- and therapeutic management. *Physiotherapy* **2017**, *103*, 369–378. [CrossRef] [PubMed]
53. Van Der Heijden, G.J.; Leffers, P.; Wolters, P.J.; Verheijden, J.J.; van Mameren, H.; Houben, J.P.; Bouter, L.M.; Knipschild, P.G. No effect of bipolar interferential electrotherapy and pulsed ultrasound for soft tissue shoulder disorders: A randomised controlled trial. *Ann. Rheum. Dis.* **1999**, *58*, 530–540. [CrossRef] [PubMed]
54. Gomes, C.A.F.P.; Dibai-Filho, A.V.; Moreira, W.A.; Rivas, S.Q.; Silva, E.D.S.; Garrido, A.C.B. Effect of adding interferential current in an exercise and manual therapy program for patients with unilateral shoulder impingement syndrome: A randomized clinical trial. *J. Manip. Physiol. Ther.* **2018**, *41*, 218–226. [CrossRef]
55. Cheing, G.L.; So, E.M.; Chao, C.Y. Effectiveness of electroacupuncture and interferential eloctrotherapy in the management of frozen shoulder. *J. Rehabil. Med.* **2008**, *40*, 166–170. [CrossRef]
56. Alptekin, H.K.; Aydın, T.; İflazoğlu, E.S.; Alkan, M. Evaluating the effectiveness of frozen shoulder treatment on the right and left sides. *J. Phys. Ther. Sci.* **2016**, *28*, 207–212. [CrossRef]
57. Suriya-amarit, D.; Gaogasigam, C.; Siriphorn, A.; Boonyong, S. Effect of interferential current stimulation in management of hemiplegic shoulder pain. *Arch. Phys. Med. Rehabil.* **2014**, *95*, 1441–1446. [CrossRef]
58. Gunay Ucurum, S.; Kaya, D.O.; Kayali, Y.; Askin, A.; Tekindal, M.A. Comparison of different electrotherapy methods and exercise therapy in shoulder impingement syndrome: A prospective randomized controlled trial. *Acta Orthop. Traumatol. Turc.* **2018**, *52*, 249–255. [CrossRef] [PubMed]
59. Resende, L.; Merriwether, E.; Rampazo, É.; Dailey, D.; Embree, J.; Deberg, J.; Liebano, R.E.; Sluka, K.A. Meta-analysis of transcutaneous electrical nerve stimulation for relief of spinal pain. *Eur. J. Pain* **2018**, *22*, 663–678. [CrossRef] [PubMed]
60. Venancio, R.C.; Pelegrini, S.; Gomes, D.Q.; Nakano, E.Y.; Liebano, R.E. Effects of carrier frequency of interferential current on pressure pain threshold and sensory comfort in humans. *Arch. Phys. Med. Rehabil.* **2013**, *94*, 95–102. [CrossRef] [PubMed]
61. Oosterhof, J.; Wilder-Smith, O.H.; de Boo, T.; Oostendorp, R.A.; Crul, B.J. The long-term outcome of transcutaneous electrical nerve stimulation in the treatment for patients with chronic pain: A randomized, placebo-controlled trial. *Pain Pract.* **2012**, *12*, 513–522. [CrossRef] [PubMed]
62. Fuentes, J.; Armijo-Olivo, S.; Funabashi, M.; Miciak, M.; Dick, B.; Warren, S.; Rashiq, S.; Magee, D.J.; Gross, D.P. Enhanced therapeutic alliance modulates pain intensity and muscle pain sensitivity in patients with chronic low back pain: An experimental controlled study. *Phys. Ther.* **2014**, *94*, 477–489. [CrossRef] [PubMed]

63. Fuentes-Contreras, J.; Armijo-Olivo, S.; Magee, D.J.; Gross, D.P. A preliminary investigation into the effects of active interferential current therapy and placebo on pressure pain sensitivity: A random crossover placebo controlled study. *Physiotherapy* **2011**, *97*, 291–301. [CrossRef] [PubMed]
64. Jarit, G.J.; Mohr, K.J.; Waller, R.; Glousman, R.E. The effects of home interferential therapy on post-operative pain, edema, and range of motion of the knee. *Clin. J. Sport Med.* **2003**, *13*, 16–20. [CrossRef] [PubMed]

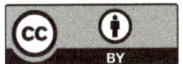
© 2019 by the authors. Licensee MDPI, Basel, Switzerland. This article is an open access article distributed under the terms and conditions of the Creative Commons Attribution (CC BY) license (http://creativecommons.org/licenses/by/4.0/).

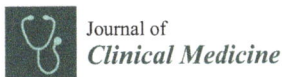

Article

Eye Gaze Markers Indicate Visual Attention to Threatening Images in Individuals with Chronic Back Pain

Zoë C. Franklin [1,*], Paul S. Holmes [1] and Neil E. Fowler [2]

1. Musculoskeletal Science and Sports Medicine Research Centre, Manchester Metropolitan University, Manchester M15 6BH, UK; p.s.holmes@mmu.ac.uk
2. Vice Chancellor's Office, University of Salford, Salford M5 4WT, UK; n.fowler1@salford.ac.uk
* Correspondence: z.franklin@mmu.ac.uk; Tel.: +44-161-247-5528

Received: 20 November 2018; Accepted: 27 December 2018; Published: 31 December 2018

Abstract: Research into attentional biases and threatening, pain-related information has primarily been investigated using reaction time as the dependent variable. This study aimed to extend previous research to provide a more in depth investigation of chronic back pain and individuals' attention to emotional stimuli by recording eye movement behavior. Individuals with chronic back pain (n = 18) were recruited from a back rehabilitation program and age and sex matched against 17 non-symptomatic controls. Participants' eye movements were recorded whilst they completed a dot probe task, which included back pain specific threatening images and neutral images. There were no significant differences between chronic pain and control participants in attentional biases recorded using reaction time from the dot probe task. Chronic pain participants, however, demonstrated a significantly higher percentage of fixations, larger pupil diameter, a longer average fixation duration and faster first fixation to threatening compared to neutral images. They also had a significantly longer average fixation duration and larger pupil diameter to threatening images compared to control participants. The findings of this study suggest eye gaze metrics may provide a more sensitive measure of attentional biases in chronic pain populations. These findings may have important therapeutic implications for the patient and therapist.

Keywords: chronic pain; attentional biases; eye gaze

1. Introduction

Attentional biases are a selective attention towards or away from a stimulus, which is both specific and salient to an individual's current environment and situation [1] and can result in a variety of cognitive, behavioral and physiological responses. Excessive attentional biases towards pain have been hypothesized to contribute towards the promotion of pain-related anxiety, fear of pain-related activity, physical disability and exacerbations in the pain experience [2]. Attentional biases towards pain-related stimuli have been proposed in theories of attention and pain [3,4]. The pain-specific models explain an individual's attentional response to the presence of pain-related stimuli. Todd et al. [5] proposed the threat interpretation model of attentional biases, suggesting that there is a relationship between an individual's interpretation of threat, which then influences their attentional bias towards it. As threat interpretation increases, initial vigilance towards pain-related stimuli increases; the level of the threat then influences whether the individual is able to disengage from the threat or avoid the threat.

Meta-analyses [6–8] have reported that pain participants have an attentional bias towards threat related information compared to controls, although with low effect sizes of 0.1–0.3 which may be due, in part, to the lack of consistency with the type of pain-related stimuli (e.g., words or pictures; sensory or affective pain). Within the most recent review [8], the majority of studies used word-based stimuli or pain-related faces, rather than pictures associated with movement. Kourtzi and Kanwasher [9] have identified that pictures which have implied physical movement lead to greater activation of the extended motor system, compared to images without implied movement. Therefore, it could be suggested that the increased motor activity associated with movement-related images might represent a marker of a more valid cognitive response to movement-related emotional stimuli.

Attentional biases have been assessed, traditionally, using the dot probe paradigm [10]. This technique captures a momentary cross-section of attention at the stimulus offset. Therefore, the method does not indicate duration of attention or attentional exertion to stimuli [11]. The use of eye-tracking equipment, however, can address some of these limitations and allows researchers to record location and duration of gaze fixations. In addition, eye-tracking also provides the opportunity to measure pupil diameter as an index of attentional effort [12]. Eye gaze markers can, therefore, provide researchers with a range of additional metrics to improve the understanding of attentional biases in chronic pain patients.

Several studies have utilised the dot probe method in conjunction with eye tracking and identified a bias towards pain-related information. Unfortunately, however, these studies were all conducted with pain-free undergraduate students, using pain-related words [13,14] or faces [15–17]. While these studies do provide some insight into the mechanisms associated with attention to pain-related information, further research is needed to be conducted in patients suffering from chronic pain. To our knowledge, only three studies have used eye movements to examine attentional biases to pictorial stimuli, and these were with chronic headache populations [18,19] and mixed chronic pain groups [20]. Both Liossi et al. [18] and Schoth et al. [19] used a visual search task to assess the attentional biases of chronic headache patients. Participants were shown four facial expressions (pain, angry, happy and neutral). Both studies [18,19] identified that the pain group demonstrated a significantly higher proportion of initial fixations on the pain face, compared to the other facial expressions. Furthermore, Liossi et al. [18] found that patients had an initial shift in their attention towards pain stimuli, but then maintained their gaze on happy" images. There was no evidence that pain patients maintained their gaze on pain related images. These findings support the theoretical models of pain and attentional biases [3–5] and propose that attentional biases may play an important role in the maintenance of chronic headache. Fashler and Katz [20] investigated the attentional biases of undergraduate students who were experiencing a variety of chronic pain conditions (e.g., neck/back, migraine, ankle/knee, stomach, hip, arm, eye and jaw pain). Participants completed a dot probe task using injury related (e.g., needle being inserted into the skin, black eye, open wound, burned skin) and neutral images while their eye movements were recorded. Reaction time results revealed that chronic pain individuals responded faster to neutral stimuli in contrast to the injury related images. In contrast, the eye tracking data demonstrated that chronic pain individuals maintained attention towards injury related pictures. Supporting Todd et al.'s [5] theory that as the interpretation of threat increases, vigilance towards the threat also increases. To date, however, no study has investigated the attentional biases of a chronic back pain patient population using both the dot probe paradigm and eye tracking approaches.

The aim of this study, therefore, was to provide a more in depth investigation of chronic back pain patients' attention to pain-related images in comparison to non-symptomatic controls by recording eye movement behavior whilst participants also completed a dot probe task. We hypothesized that chronic back pain participants would have: (i) a significantly higher percentage of fixations to threatening stimuli compared to controls; (ii) a longer average fixation duration to threatening images; and (iii) exhibit a faster reaction time to threatening images in the dot probe task.

2. Method

2.1. Participants

Participants were recruited from a back rehabilitation program at a UK NHS trust ($n = 18$) and an age and sex matched non-symptomatic control group was recruited from the university and local area (n = 17). Chronic pain participants had been suffering from back pain for a minimum of three months. Non-symptomatic controls were recruited through advertisements through unsolicited noticeboards and electronic advertising. Ethical approval was granted by NRES Committee North West Greater Manchester Central and by Manchester Metropolitan University Ethics Committee. All participants provided written informed consent to take part in this study. Inclusion criteria for the back pain group were: (i) over 18 years of age; (ii) a referral to a hospital-based back pain management program for non-specific musculoskeletal pain; (iii) pain duration of >3 months; and (iv) normal or corrected to normal vision. Inclusion criteria for the control group were: (i) over 18 years of age; and (ii) normal or corrected to normal vision. Exclusion criteria for the control group were: (i) any form of current or recent chronic or recurrent pain; and (ii) regular (daily or near daily) use of any form of analgesic medication.

2.2. Materials

2.2.1. Dot Probe Paradigm

All participants completed a dot probe task comprising 20 practice trials and 150 experimental trials (100 threat-neutral, 50 neutral-neutral). The threat images were taken from the Photograph Series of Daily Activities (PHODA) image bank [21] (back pain specific and showing movements known to be associated as threatening and evoking pain or pain-related fear, for example lifting or bending tasks). The neutral images were taken from the International Affective Picture System (IAPS) [22] and included images of neutral activities, faces and inanimate objects. The presentation of images were randomized for each participant. Dot probe stimuli were presented on a 23-inch screen (HP EliteDisplay E231, Hewlett-Packard Company, Palo Alto, CA, USA) with a 1920 × 1080-pixel resolution and a 100 Hz refresh rate. Participants were told to engage actively with the pictures that were presented to them on the screen. Each trial began with a central fixation cross presented for 500 ms, followed by an image pair on the left and right side of the screen, either threat-neutral or neutral-neutral pairs presented for 500 ms. Following presentation of the image pair, a probe stimulus (a pair of dots either vertical or horizontal) was presented in the location of either the emotional or the neutral image and remained displayed until the patient/participant responded (see Figure 1). Participants were instructed to press, as quickly and accurately as possible, one of two keys to identify the probe presented. The inter-trial interval varied randomly between 500 and 1250 ms. Response times shorter than 200 ms or longer than 1200 ms were removed from the data. Incorrect responses were also excluded from the analysis. Errors and outliers accounted for 2.5% of the data.

Congruent (e.g., the target followed the emotional picture) and incongruent (e.g., the target followed the neutral picture) attentional bias scores for threatening images relative to neutral were calculated for each participant from the response time data using the formula:

$$\text{Congruent} = ((T_{rpr} + T_{lpl})/2) - ((N_{rpr} + N_{lpr} + N_{rpl} + N_{lpl})/4) \qquad (1)$$

$$\text{Incongruent} = ((T_{lpr} + T_{rpl})/2) - ((N_{rpr} + N_{lpr} + N_{rpl} + N_{lpl})/4) \qquad (2)$$

T = threat, N = neutral, p = probe, r = right position, l = left position.

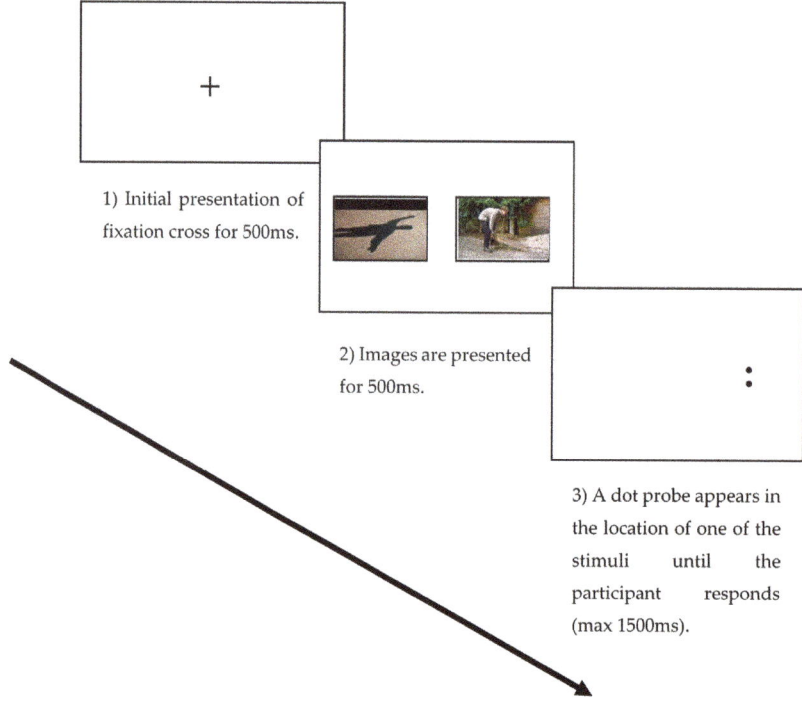

Figure 1. An example of the three stages of the dot probe task in the neutral threat condition.

2.2.2. Eye-Gaze

While participants completed the dot probe paradigm, their eye movements were also recorded. Eye movement data were recorded with an Applied Science Laboratories Mobile Eye System (ASL; Bedford, MA, USA) using a dark pupil tracking technique throughout the dot probe paradigm. This method uses the relationship between the pupil and a reflection from the cornea to calculate the point of gaze in relation to an external scene camera. The ASL software computes the relationship between the pupil and cornea to locate gaze within a scene at a sampling rate of 30 Hz. The system has an accuracy of 0.5° of visual angle, a resolution of 0.10° of visual angle, and a visual range of 50° horizontal and 40° vertical.

Previous eye gaze research has assessed: (i) percentage of fixations on the threat or neutral stimuli; (ii) average pupil diameter when fixating on the threat and neutral stimuli; (iii) average time spent fixating on the threat or neutral stimuli; and (iv) first fixation time on either the threat or the neutral stimuli. In this study, visual fixations were defined as maintaining gaze on a specific location on the screen for at least 100ms and a maximum fixation radius of 1°, as employed in previous studies [13,16].

2.3. Procedures

Participants were asked to sit at a desk in a black booth and facing the screen approximately 60 cm in front of them and at eye level. A desk mounted chin rest was used to reduce participants' head movements ensuring that participants' eyes were level with the middle of the monitor on which the stimuli were presented. This ensured that each participant's eyes were in the same location relative to the camera and monitor. A 9-point calibration check was used prior to the start of testing. A drift check was conducted before each trial and recalibration performed when necessary. Participants were instructed to look at the fixation cross before each trial to standardize the starting location of their eye gaze and were told to engage actively with the pictures that were presented to them on the screen. Participants provided demographic information after testing was completed to allow for age and sex matching.

2.4. Preparation of Eye Gaze Data

Eye gaze data were analyzed using ASL Results Plus (Applied Science Laboratories, Bedford, MA, USA). Each trial was parsed into 150 (100 threat-neutral, 50 neutral-neutral) separate trials. Individual trials were then analyzed by drawing two separate areas of interest (AOIs) around the threatening and neutral images. From this, the number of fixations, average fixation duration, and pupil diameter when fixating in each AOI were calculated. A fixation was defined as any gaze that remained stable (within 1 degree of visual angle) for a duration of over 100 ms. In accordance with previous studies [23], participants with missing data of more than 15% over the 150 trials were excluded from the study. Based on this criterion, no participants were excluded from the study. Due to technical difficulties with the eye tracking equipment, no eye movement data were recorded for one of the non-symptomatic control participants and this participant was excluded from further analysis.

2.5. Data Analysis

A series of 2 × 2 analysis of variances (ANOVA) were conducted on the eye gaze data (percentage fixation, average pupil diameter, average fixation duration, first fixation time), with group (patient, control) as a between participants independent variable, and image type (threat or neutral image) as a within participants variable. A 2 × 2 ANOVA of the probe response time data with group (patient, controls) as the between variable, and probe position (probe in same versus different location to threatening image) as the within participants variable. Bonferroni *post hoc* analyses were used where needed to clarify significant main effects and interactions. Alpha was set at $p < 0.05$ and effect sizes were calculated using Cohen's *d*.

3. Results

3.1. Group Characteristics

The chronic pain and control groups did not differ significantly in sex ratio (chronic pain: 12 (66%) female, control group 11 (64%) female, $\chi^2 = 0.15$, $p = 0.90$) or age (chronic pain group: M = 46.72, SD ± 9.97 years; control group: M = 40.47, SD ± 9.23 years, $t(33) = -1.92$, $p = 0.07$).

3.2. Power Analysis

Post-hoc power analyses [24] were conducted for the dot probe and eye movement data. The power analysis results for the dot probe data were: power = 0.64 ($\alpha = 0.05$; $\beta = 0.36$) $d = 0.6$, for number of fixations to threat; power = 0.82 ($\alpha = 0.05$; $\beta = 0.18$) $d = 0.8$, and neutral images; power = 0.83 ($\alpha = 0.05$; $\beta = 0.17$) $d = 0.9$. The power analysis results for the average pupil diameter; power = 0.76 ($\alpha = 0.05$; $\beta = 0.24$) $d = 0.8$; average fixation duration; power = 0.86 ($\alpha = 0.05$; $\beta = 0.14$) $d = 0.9$; and for total fixation duration; power = 0.99 ($\alpha = 0.05$; $\beta = 0.01$) $d = 1.6$. Therefore, despite the relatively modest sample size there was sufficient power to have confidence in the findings from the study.

3.3. Eye Gaze Reliability Analysis

Internal consistency, reflecting the interrelatedness of items on a test was calculated using Cronbach's alpha for both the control group and the patient group for each outcome variable. For both patient and control groups there was high reliability for percentage fixation count, pupil diameter and first fixation time (Cronbach's $\alpha = 0.73$–0.93). Average fixation duration subscale, however, had a relatively low reliability, Cronbach's $\alpha = 0.62$–0.64 (see Table 1).

Table 1. Internal consistency measured with Cronbach's alpha for each outcome variable in the patient and control group.

Group	Outcome Measure	Cronbach's α
Patient	Percentage fixation count	0.750
	Pupil diameter	0.802
	Average fixation duration	0.644
	First fixation time	0.722
Control	Percentage fixation count	0.927
	Pupil diameter	0.743
	Average fixation duration	0.616
	First fixation time	0.725

3.4. Percentage Fixation Count

The results of the two way mixed ANOVA showed a significant interaction between participant group and image type, (F (1, 33) = 32.01, $p < 0.001$) and a significant main effect of stimuli type, (F (1, 33) = 11.05, $p = 0.002$). Pairwise comparisons indicated that chronic pain individuals attended to threat images (M = 34.07, SD ± 10.58) significantly more than neutral stimuli (M = 18.27, SD ± 9.32); $t(17) = 6.25, p < 0.001, d = 1.57$, 95% CI [0.80, 2.29] (see Figure 2). For the control group, there was no significant difference between the percentage fixation count to threat (M = 21.61, SD = 5.97) or neutral (M = 25.72, SD ± 8.39) stimuli; $t(16) = -1.69, p = 0.11, d = 0.5$, 95% CI [−1.24, 0.13].

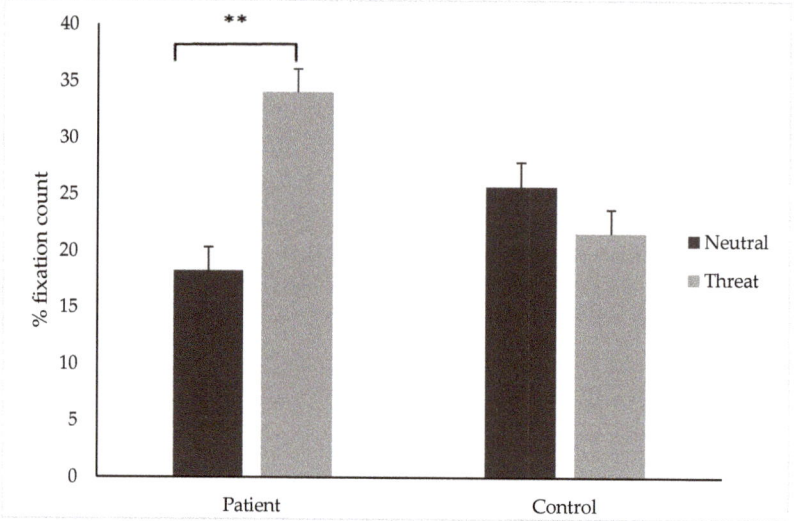

Figure 2. The percentage of fixations (±SE) on threatening or neutral stimuli in the patient and control group. ** indicates $p < 0.01$.

3.5. Average Pupil Diameter

A significant main effect of group was found (F (1,33) = 23.71, $p = 0.0001$); t-tests revealed that individuals in the pain group (M = 5.69, SD ± 0.18 mm) had a significantly larger pupil diameter compared to controls (M = 4.62, SD ± 0.18 mm), $d = 0.5$, 95% CI [4.29, 7.32]. A significant main effect for stimuli type was found (F (1, 33) = 11.65, $p = 0.002$); t-tests showed that participants had a significantly larger pupil diameter when attending to threatening (M = 5.30, SD ± 1.33 mm) compared to neutral (M = 4.64, SD ± 1.23mm) stimuli, $t(34) = 2.71, p = 0.01, d = 0.9$, 95% CI [−0.16, 1.17] (Figure 3). There was no significant interaction effect found (F (1,33) = 0.10, $p = 0.749$).

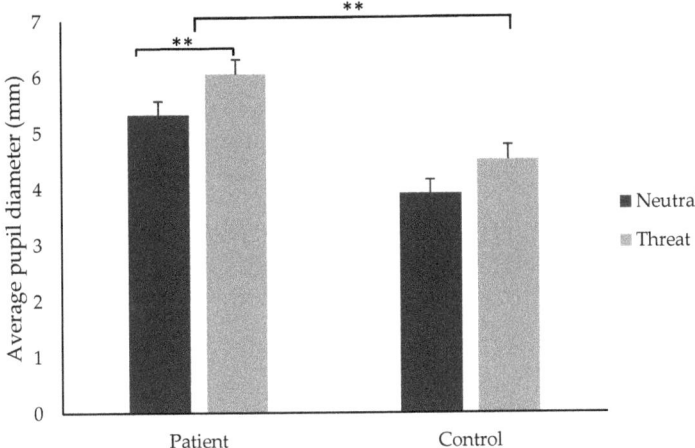

Figure 3. The average pupil diameter (mm) (±SE) for the patient and control groups when attending to threatening and neutral stimuli. ** indicates $p < 0.01$.

3.6. Average Fixation Duration

A significant group × image type interaction $F(1, 33) = 10.90$, $p = 0.02$, and a significant main effect of group $F(1, 33) = 4.72$, $p = 0.03$ was found. T-tests revealed that pain participants demonstrated a significantly higher average fixation duration on threatening (M = 219.18, SD ± 53.06 ms) compared to neutral stimuli (M = 185.04, SD ± 38.68 ms); $t(34) = -2.16$, $p = 0.03$, $d = 0.8$, 95% CI [−0.06, −0.001] (Figure 4). There was no significant difference between the control group's average fixation duration towards threatening or neutral stimuli. T-tests revealed that the pain group (M = 219.18, SD ± 53.06 ms) had a significantly longer average fixation duration to threatening stimuli compared to controls (M = 174.88, SD ± 17.36 ms); $t(68) = -3.35$, $p = 0.03$, $d = 0.9$, 95% CI [−0.04, −0.004].

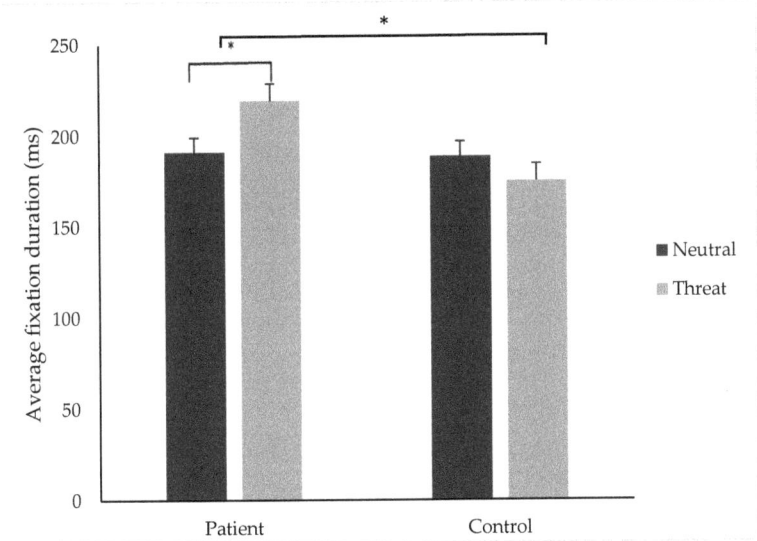

Figure 4. The average fixation (ms) duration (±SE) to threatening and neutral stimuli for the patient and control group. * indicates $p < 0.05$.

3.7. First Fixation Time

There was a significant interaction of group x first fixation time ($F (1,33) = 35.21, p = 0.0001$), and a significant main effect of group ($F (1,33) = 27.00, p = 0.0001$). Pairwise comparisons indicated that patients made significantly faster first fixations to threatening images, ($t(33) = 8.90, p = 0.0001, d = 0.7$, 95% CI [−3.59, −1.76] compared to controls (patient M = 124.98 ms, SD = 65.67; control M = 210.24, SD = 28.21) (Figure 5). The control group made significantly faster first fixations to the neutral stimuli compared to the threatening, ($t(16) = 3.97, p = 0.001, d = 1.02$, 95% CI [0.28, 1.71]). In contrast, the pain patients made significantly faster first fixations to the threatening image type compared to the neutral image type ($t(17) = 4.44, p = 0.0001, d = 0.9$, 95% CI [−1.47, −0.27]). There was no significant main effect of image type ($F (1,33) = 5.36, p = 0.469$).

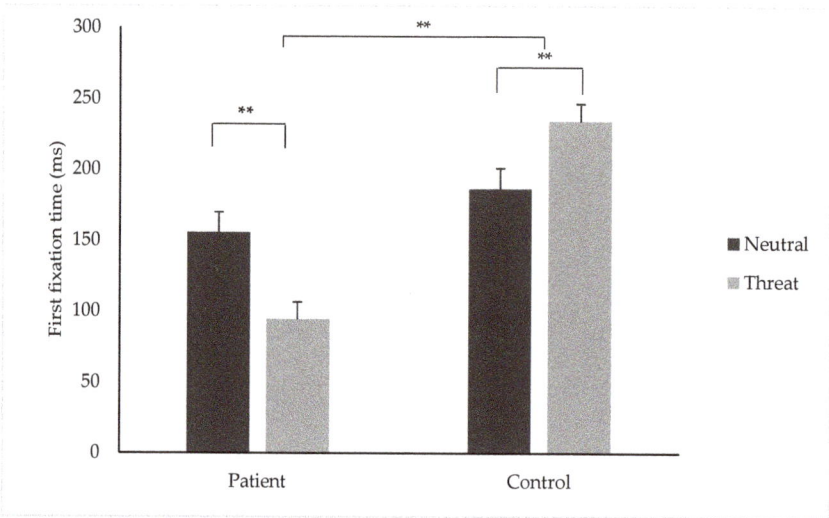

Figure 5. First fixation time (ms) (±SE) to threatening and neutral stimuli for the patient and control group. ** indicates $p < 0.01$.

3.8. Dot Probe Response Time Measures

There was no significant interaction of group x attentional bias ($F (1,33) = 3.17, p = 0.08$), and no significant main effect of group ($F (1, 33) = 1.69, p = 0.20$) or probe position ($F (1, 33) = 4.60, p = 0.12$). There was no significant difference between attentional bias to threatening images for either congruent ($t(33) = 1.79, p = 0.08, d = 0.6$, 95% CI [−3.35, 51.14]) or incongruent ($t(33) = 0.47, p = 0.64, d = 0.6$, 95% CI [−17.61, 28.29]) trials for the pain group (congruent, M= −14.23, SD ± 48.50 ms; incongruent, M = 6.22, SD ± 39.46 ms) and controls (congruent, M = 9.66, SD ± 27.09 ms; incongruent, M = 11.56, SD ± 25.32 ms). Table 2 shows the mean response times for the congruent, incongruent and neutral trials for the chronic pain and control groups.

Table 2. Mean reaction times of congruent and incongruent trials (in ms; standard deviations in brackets) for the threat and neutral images in the dot probe task for participants with chronic low back pain and the non-symptomatic control group.

	Stimuli	Chronic Pain Group	Non-Symptomatic Control Group
Congruent	Threat (ms)	595.79 (59.40)	548.74 (49.08)
	Neutral (ms)	591.32 (65.10)	540.44 (49.65)
Incongruent	Threat (ms)	597.31 (59.64)	552.69 (48.36)
	Neutral (ms)	591.32 (65.10)	540.44 (49.65)

4. Discussion

This study used an eye gaze protocol to consider the attentional biases of individuals with chronic back pain to threatening and neutral images using a modified dot probe paradigm. The eye gaze data highlight important new findings about the differences in attentional bias to threatening and neutral images between individuals with chronic pain and non-symptomatic controls that cannot be identified by using the standard dot probe paradigm.

Within-group analysis demonstrated that the chronic pain individuals had a significantly higher percentage of fixations, larger pupil diameter and longer average fixation duration on threatening compared to neutral images. There were no significant differences in eye gaze metrics to threatening or neutral images in non-symptomatic controls; the absence of attentional bias suggesting that the back pain specific images were not perceived as threatening for the non-symptomatic controls. Between-group analysis revealed that chronic pain participants also had a longer average fixation duration and larger pupil diameter to threatening images compared to the non-symptomatic controls. Chronic pain patients also had a faster initial fixation to the pain related image compared to the neutral image; the opposite pattern was found for the non-symptomatic controls. In contrast, and of concern to the validity of the standard dot probe procedure, there were no significant differences in attentional biases for the dot probe task between the chronic pain group and non-symptomatic controls. Taken together, the findings of this study suggest that eye gaze metrics may provide a more sensitive measure of attentional bias compared to the dot probe response time.

The majority of previous research investigating pain-related attentional biases using eye gaze has been within a non-symptomatic population and used word-based stimuli or pain-related faces [13–16]. To our knowledge, only three studies have previously used back pain-specific images in a dot probe task [25–27], but none have used eye-tracking markers concurrent with the dot probe test with pain-related physical activity movements. Consistent with the findings of Roelofs et al. [25] the dot probe data indicated that there was no difference between chronic pain participants and non-symptomatic controls for attention to threatening images in congruent trials. Whereas, the eye gaze behavior in this study demonstrated that chronic pain participants attended to the pain-related images significantly faster, more often and for a significantly longer average duration than neutral images compared to non-symptomatic controls. The attentional bias to threatening stimuli in the pain group may have been due to the implied motion cues within the image. Kourtzi et al. [9] found greater activation of the medial temporal/medial superior temporal cortex (MT/MST) when viewing photographs with implied movement and imaging studies have supported the role of these brain areas in the analysis of movement, but not object, recognition [28]. Action understanding depends, in part, on prior knowledge about the movement's goal and intention with predictions about an object's (or body's) future position being made from the motion implied in the static image [29]. Participant's memorial biases modulate the increase in attentional bias to threatening information and, therefore, they perceive implied painful motion in the image (e.g., rotation of the back, which causes them pain); the dynamic images accessing a more meaningful motor representation that is presented for analysis through the variety of eye gaze metrics employed in this study.

Eye tracking studies within healthy populations have identified vigilance towards pain-related words and faces [14,15]. In line with previous research [18,19], we identified that chronic pain patients attended to pain related images significantly faster than neutral images and in contrast to the profiles of non-symptomatic controls. Todd et al. [5] have proposed the Threat Interpretation Model of pain that can be used to consider some of the study's findings. Specifically, there is an initial vigilance towards the threat-related stimuli; as the threat continues, there is an avoidance of the threatening cues. Further, Fashler and Katz [20] identified that both pain and control participants responded faster to neutral images in the dot probe task, whereas the eye movement data demonstrated that in the early phase of the trial, participants attended to the neutral images, then in the later phases, gaze duration was maintained on the injury-related images. These findings are in contrast to those presented here; there were no differences found for reaction time data and chronic pain patients only made faster first fixations to pain related images. Due to the short presentation time used in this study, we were unable to assess whether participants would maintain their gaze on the pain stimuli or, in line with Todd et al., [5] the patients showed an active avoidance of the threatening cues. One possible explanation for the differences could be due to the specificity of the images. Fashler and Katz [20] used images for which both individuals with, and without pain could perceive as threatening (e.g., an open wound, needle inserted into the skin etc.). In contrast, our study used images that were specific to back pain and were not deemed threatening for the control group. Todd et al. [5] propose that initial vigilance occurs when participants interpret the stimuli as threatening. The specificity of the image, and using a homogenous pain group, may, therefore, have influenced the attentional bias to pain related stimuli. Furthermore, the differences between the studies could be due to the image presentation time and type of probe stimulus. In the current study, the images were presented for 500 ms and the dot probe was either.. or : and each probe could appear on either side. In contrast, Fashler and Katz [20] presented the images for 2000 ms and participants were shown a single dot, the response required participants to press one of two buttons to indicate the side of the screen the dot was on. The significant differences in the methods between the studies may explain the differences in the reaction time data. In contrast to Fashler and Katz [20], Yang et al. [30] found that chronic pain participants had an early attentional bias towards catastrophe-based words, followed by avoidance of pain words. Due to the short stimuli presentation time within our study, we were only able to assess initial vigilance, consistent with previous research in pain populations [18]. This bottom up process is considered to be automatic in anxious individuals. In contrast to other studies identifying a vigilance-avoidance pattern [18,30], this study used images of physical activity (rather than words) associated with pain. Images with implied movement provide elements of action understanding. They may give more personal meaning, agency, ownership and motor response [31] for the viewed activity for chronic back pain participants compared to words, pain faces or images of an individual experiencing pain (e.g., someone grimacing while they are completing an activity). Future studies should present pain-related images for a longer duration to identify whether chronic back pain participants maintain vigilance or attend then avoid threatening images. Using images that are specific to the pain condition may also provide researchers with the ability to alter biases to allow for top down processing of attending to goal directed information. This enhanced attention to goal related information may reduce avoidance of activity and disability levels. Although a greater understanding of attention in this context is needed, preliminary evidence has supported the therapeutic benefits of attentional bias modification in pain populations [32,33].

In this study, chronic pain participants showed a significantly larger pupil diameter to threatening images compared to controls. As well as for light intensity, the pupil dilates under conditions of high attentional allocation and also in response to emotionally-congruent information [34,35]. In this regard, it has been suggested that pupil dilation is a physiological response that can indicate brain mechanisms associated with the processing of emotional information [36]. When viewing threatening, emotional images pupil dilation has also been found to be mediated by increased sympathetic activity (e.g., increased heart rate and skin conductance) [34]. According to the biopsychosocial model of pain [37], there is both a psychological and physiological response to pain. If individuals attend to their physiological reaction to emotional information, it increases their worry-based anxiety, based on schemas, causing them to associate the increased arousal with the pain and lead to active avoidance behaviors. The results from this study suggest that not only are individuals with chronic pain attending to pain-related images more than controls, but they are also allocating greater visual attention to them indicating that the stimuli having greater emotional congruence and meaning. This study suggests that investigating pupil diameter could be a useful addition to the study of chronic pain.

The eye gaze data from this study provides support for current models of attention and extends the current chronic pain literature. Models of attentional bias within chronic pain attribute slightly different roles to the process of attention. In general, they propose that individuals in pain are fearful of, and threatened by, pain [2,3,38], which causes them to over attend to pain-related information. Pain is prioritized over other demands for attention [39], which interferes with movement, leads to higher levels of anxiety, catastrophizing and ultimately exacerbation of levels of disability [40]. Understanding the mechanisms of attention to information which is perceived as threatening, is essential to better understand approaches to effective intervention.

The longer duration of attention to pain-related images in this study may be a function of the schemas associated with the movements. During experimental debriefs, some of the chronic pain participants commented that the images they viewed reminded them of activities in which they would expect to experience pain. Beck [41] proposed that maladaptive schemas cause individuals to have a preoccupation with threatening information and subsequently catastrophize due to a negative interpretive and attentional bias. Pincus and Morley [4] proposed the schema enmeshment model of pain (SEMP) in an attempt to explain recall bias in chronic pain patients through the operation of schemas. Pain schemas contain sensory, intensity, spatial and temporal features of pain, while illness schemas contain information about the consequences of illness, and self-schemas contain information about the self. The chronic pain experience may have illness related schemas about the implications of self-future activity, which causes enmeshment with the pain sensory, self and illness schemas. The anxiety experienced by the pain participants with particular activities they perceive as pain threatening leads to different behavioral and cognitive reactions [1]. The misinterpretation of pain stimuli leads to excessive fear of physical activity and avoidance of physical activity. This may be due to their negative cognitions and increased somatic anxiety about completing the activity, which leads to physical avoidance behavior [42]. Current interventions in the UK tend to focus on reducing a patient's disability through improved education about their pain and the opportunity to discuss problems with particular activities [43]. Understanding the cognitive and emotional mechanisms behind a patient's initial activity avoidance behavior may allow for more specific interventions that modify the way chronic pain patients not only attend to activity-related information, but also the way they interpret the planned movement. The interaction of these two cognitive biases will affect the processing of information, lead to behavior change and, potentially, reduce the patient's disability.

There were some limitations in the study. First, the PHODA images used were not assessed for their affective content (valence and arousal) or whether the images were personally meaningful to the individual. The images have, however, been used successfully in previous dot probe studies and to assess perceived harmfulness of daily activities [44,45] suggesting they have good ecological validity. Although we did not ask chronic pain participants to rate the images directly, in follow up manipulation checks, pain participants reported that they could attribute the images to behaviors in their daily life and that the activities would be difficult and painful for them to complete at home. Similarly, verbal follow up checks with the control group demonstrated that the PHODA images represented a "neutral" image set and they showed no bias to either image type. Therefore, the biases predicted in the chronic pain group can be attributed to the pain-specific content of the image set. Future studies should assess the valence and arousal of the images in larger and more varied pain populations. Future research should also consider asking patients to rate their personal relevance to them; there may be different attentional biases towards images that are more personally-relevant, compared to those that are not (e.g., see Lang's meaning propositions within Bioinformational Theory [46]).

Due to the recruitment strategy, there may be some selection bias. It has been suggested that pain patients who take part in research are often highly motivated, have more severe pain and respond better to treatment [47]. This is a continuing issue for pain research. We were, however, interested in the patients' cognitive response to threatening stimuli and did not implement an intervention. Future research may wish to consider comparing the health status of patients who volunteer, compared to those who decline to take part in a study.

Although the power analysis indicated there was sufficient power for this study, the sample size was low in comparison to other studies investigating attentional biases. Therefore, future research should aim to include a larger sample size. It should be noted that although the use of eye gaze is regarded as a more direct assessment of attention, it does not reflect overt attentional engagement. For example, visual attention can occur in the absence of eye movements [48] and eye tracking technology does not measure peripheral vision, which can be used to complete the dot-probe task accurately [17].

Despite these limitations, the present study provides further support for attentional biases towards pain-related images in chronic back pain participants. This finding is supported by additional data from eye gaze measurement techniques that provide a richer and more detailed analysis of the attentional biases in this population. Future studies should be conducted which investigate whether images that involve movement are more reliable at identifying attentional biases in chronic pain patients compared to pain-related words within a dot probe paradigm. Future research should also investigate the relationship between attention and interpretation of pain to provide an updated model to explain the mechanisms associated with patient responses to chronic pain. If the cognitive mechanisms of attention cause individuals with chronic pain to attend and dwell on painful stimuli, interventions that focus on modifying a patient's attention to goal-related outcomes (e.g., attentional bias modification) may have important beneficial effects on future quality of life.

Author Contributions: Conceptualization, Z.C.F., P.S.H. and N.E.F.; Formal analysis, Z.C.F.; Investigation, Z.C.F.; Methodology, Z.C.F., P.S.H. and N.E.F.; Project administration, Z.C.F.; Supervision, P.S.H. and N.E.F.; Writing—original draft, Z.C.F., P.S.H. and N.E.F.; Writing—review & editing, Z.C.F. and P.S.H.

Acknowledgments: The authors would like to thank the physiotherapy and administration staff at Kingsgate House in Stockport for their support throughout this project and allowing us to conduct this study in the clinic.

Conflicts of Interest: The authors declare no conflict of interest.

References

1. Eysenck, M.W. *Anxiety and Cognition: A Unified Theory*; Psychology Press: Hove, UK, 1997.
2. Vlaeyen, J.W.; Linton, S.J. Fear-avoidance and its consequences in chronic musculoskeletal pain: A state of the art. *Pain* **2000**, *85*, 317–332. [CrossRef]
3. Van Damme, S.; Legrain, V.; Vogt, J.; Crombez, G. Keeping pain in mind: A motivational account of attention to pain. *Neurosci. Biobehav. Rev.* **2010**, *34*, 204–213. [CrossRef] [PubMed]
4. Pincus, T.; Morley, S. Cognitive-processing bias in chronic pain: A review and integration. *Psychol. Bull.* **2001**, *127*, 599–617. [CrossRef] [PubMed]
5. Todd, J.; Sharpe, L.; Johnson, A.; Perry, K.N.; Colagiuri, B.; Dear, B.F. Towards a new model of attentional biases in the development, maintenance, and management of pain. *Pain* **2015**, *156*, 1589–1600. [CrossRef] [PubMed]
6. Crombez, G.; Van Ryckeghem, D.M.L.; Eccleston, C.; Van Damme, S. Attentional bias to pain-related information: A meta-analysis. *Pain* **2013**, *154*, 497–510. [CrossRef]
7. Schoth, D.E.; Nunes, V.D.; Liossi, C. Attentional bias towards pain-related information in chronic pain; a meta-analysis of visual-probe investigations. *Clin. Psychol. Rev.* **2012**, *32*, 13–25. [CrossRef]
8. Todd, J.; van Ryckeghem, D.M.; Sharpe, L.; Crombez, G. Attentional bias to pain-related information: A meta-analysis of dot-probe studies. *Health Psychol. Rev.* **2018**, *12*, 419–436. [CrossRef]
9. Kourtzi, Z.; Kanwisher, N. Activation in human mt/mst by static images with implied motion. *J. Cogn. Neurosci.* **2000**, *12*, 48–55. [CrossRef]

10. MacLeod, C.; Mathews, A.; Tata, P. Attentional bias in emotional disorders. *J. Abnorm. Psychol.* **1986**, *95*, 15–20. [CrossRef]
11. Mogg, K.; Bradley, B.P. Attentional bias in generalized anxiety disorder versus depressive disorder. *Cogn. Ther. Res.* **2005**, *29*, 29–45. [CrossRef]
12. Derakshan, N.; Salt, M.; Koster, E.H.W. Attentional control in dysphoria: An investigation using the antisaccade task. *Biol. Psychol.* **2009**, *80*, 251–255. [CrossRef] [PubMed]
13. Sharpe, L.; Brookes, M.; Jones, E.; Gittins, C.; Wufong, E.; Nicholas, M. Threat and fear of pain induces attentional bias to pain words: An eye-tracking study. *Eur. J. Pain* **2017**, *21*, 385–396. [CrossRef] [PubMed]
14. Yang, Z.; Jackson, T.; Gao, X.; Chen, H. Identifying selective visual attention biases related to fear of pain by tracking eye movements within a dot-probe paradigm. *Pain* **2012**, *153*, 1742–1748. [CrossRef] [PubMed]
15. Priebe, J.; Messingschlager, M.; Lautenbacher, S. Gaze behaviour when monitoring pain faces: An eye-tracking study. *Eur. J. Pain* **2015**, *19*, 817–825. [CrossRef] [PubMed]
16. Todd, J.; Sharpe, L.; Colagiuri, B.; Khatibi, A. The effect of threat on cognitive biases and pain outcomes: An eye-tracking study. *Eur. J. Pain* **2016**, *20*, 1357–1368. [CrossRef] [PubMed]
17. Vervoort, T.; Trost, Z.; Prkachin, K.M.; Mueller, S.C. Attentional processing of other's facial display of pain: An eye tracking study. *Pain* **2013**, *154*, 836–844. [CrossRef]
18. Liossi, C.; Schoth, D.E.; Godwin, H.J.; Liversedge, S.P. Using eye movements to investigate selective attention in chronic daily headache. *Pain* **2014**, *155*, 503–510. [CrossRef]
19. Schoth, D.E.; Godwin, H.; Liversedge, S.P.; Liossi, C. Eye movements during visual search for emotional faces in individuals with chronic headache. *Eur. J. Pain* **2015**, *19*, 722–732. [CrossRef]
20. Fashler, S.R.; Katz, J. Keeping an eye on pain: Investigating visual attention biases in individuals with chronic pain using eye-tracking methodology. *J. Pain Res.* **2016**, *9*, 551–561. [CrossRef]
21. Kugler, K.; Wijn, J.; Geilen, M.; de Jong, J.; Vlaeyen, J. *The Photograph Series of Daily Activities (Phoda). Cd-Rom Version 1.0*; Institute for Rehabilitation Research and School for Physiotherapy: Heerlen, The Netherlands, 1999.
22. Lang, P.J.; Bradley, M.M.; Cuthbert, B.N. *International Affective Picture System (IAPS): Affective Ratings of Pictures and Instruction Manual*; Technical Report A-8l; University of Florida: Gainesville, FL, USA, 2008.
23. Mogg, K.; Bradley, B.P.; Field, M.; De Houwer, J. Eye movements to smoking-related pictures in smokers: Relationship between attentional biases and implicit and explicit measures of stimulus valence. *Addiction* **2003**, *98*, 825–836. [CrossRef]
24. Cohen, J. *Statistical Power Analysis for the Behavioral Sciences*, 2nd ed.; Lawrence Earlbaum Associates: Hillsdale, NJ, USA, 1988.
25. Roelofs, J.; Peters, M.L.; Fassaert, T.; Vlaeyen, J.W. The role of fear of movement and injury in selective attentional processing in patients with chronic low back pain: A dot-probe evaluation. *J. Pain* **2005**, *6*, 294–300. [CrossRef] [PubMed]
26. Dear, B.F.; Sharpe, L.; Nicholas, M.K.; Refshauge, K. Pain-related attentional biases: The importance of the personal relevance and ecological validity of stimuli. *J. Pain* **2011**, *12*, 625–632. [CrossRef] [PubMed]
27. Franklin, Z.C.; Holmes, P.S.; Smith, N.C.; Fowler, N.E. Personality type influences attentional bias in individuals with chronic back pain. *PLoS ONE* **2016**, *11*, e0147035. [CrossRef] [PubMed]
28. Peelen, M.V.; Wiggett, A.J.; Downing, P.E. Patterns of fmri activity dissociate overlapping functional brain areas that respond to biological motion. *Neuron* **2006**, *49*, 815–822. [CrossRef] [PubMed]
29. Açık, A.; Bartel, A.; Koenig, P. Real and implied motion at the center of gaze. *J. Vis.* **2014**, *14*, 2. [CrossRef] [PubMed]
30. Yang, Z.; Jackson, T.; Chen, H. Effects of chronic pain and pain-related fear on orienting and maintenance of attention: An eye movement study. *J. Pain* **2013**, *14*, 1148–1157. [CrossRef] [PubMed]
31. Riach, M.; Wright, D.J.; Franklin, Z.C.; Holmes, P.S. Screen Position Preference Offers a New Direction for Action Observation Research: Preliminary Findings Using TMS. *Front. Hum. Neurosci.* **2018**, *12*, 26. [CrossRef]
32. Schoth, D.E.; Georgallis, T.; Liossi, C. Attentional bias modification in people with chronic pain: A proof of concept study. *Cogn. Behav. Ther.* **2013**, *42*, 233–243. [CrossRef]
33. Sharpe, L.; Ianiello, M.; Dear, B.F.; Perry, K.N.; Refshauge, K.; Nicholas, M.K. Is there a potential role for attention bias modification in pain patients? Results of 2 randomised, controlled trials. *Pain* **2012**, *153*, 722–731. [CrossRef]

34. Bradley, M.M.; Miccoli, L.; Escrig, M.A.; Lang, P.J. The pupil as a measure of emotional arousal and autonomic activation. *Psychophysiology* **2008**, *45*, 602–607. [CrossRef]
35. Duque, A.; Sanchez, A.; Vazquez, C. Gaze-fixation and pupil dilation in the processing of emotional faces: The role of rumination. *Cogn. Emot.* **2014**, *28*, 1347–1366. [CrossRef] [PubMed]
36. Siegle, G.J.; Steinhauer, S.R.; Thase, M.E.; Stenger, V.A.; Carter, C.S. Can't shake that feeling: Event-related fmri assessment of sustained amygdala activity in response to emotional information in depressed individuals. *Biol. Psychiatry* **2002**, *51*, 693–707. [CrossRef]
37. Waddell, G. 1987 Volvo award in clinical sciences. A new clinical model for the treatment of low-back pain. *Spine* **1987**, *12*, 632–644. [CrossRef]
38. Vlaeyen, J.W.; Linton, S.J. Fear-avoidance model of chronic musculoskeletal pain: 12 years on. *Pain* **2012**, *153*, 1144–1147. [CrossRef] [PubMed]
39. Eccleston, C.; Crombez, G. Pain demands attention: A cognitive–affective model of the interruptive function of pain. *Psychol. Bull.* **1999**, *125*, 356. [CrossRef] [PubMed]
40. Franklin, Z.C.; Smith, N.C.; Fowler, N.E. Influence of defensiveness on disability in a chronic musculoskeletal pain population. *Pain Pract.* **2016**, *16*, 882–889. [CrossRef]
41. Beck, A.T. *Cognitive Therapy and the Emotional Disorders*; International Universities Press: New York, NY, USA, 1976.
42. Crombez, G.; Eccleston, C.; Van Damme, S.; Vlaeyen, J.W.S.; Karoly, P. Fear-avoidance model of chronic pain: The next generation. *Clin. J. Pain* **2012**, *28*, 475–483. [CrossRef]
43. British Pain Society. Guidance for Pain Management Programmes for Adults. Available online: http://www.britishpainsociety.org/book_pmp2013_main.pdf (accessed on 8 July 2015).
44. Leeuw, M.; Goossens, M.E.J.B.; van Breukelen, G.J.P.; Boersma, K.; Vlaeyen, J.W.S. Measuring perceived harmfulness of physical activities in patients with chronic low back pain: The photograph series of daily activities—Short electronic version. *J. Pain* **2007**, *8*, 840–849. [CrossRef]
45. Barke, A.; Baudewig, J.; Schmidt-Samoa, C.; Dechent, P.; Kröner-Herwig, B. Neural correlates of fear of movement in high and low fear-avoidant chronic low back pain patients: An event-related fmri study. *Pain* **2012**, *153*, 540–552. [CrossRef]
46. Lang, P.J. A bio-informational theory of emotional imagery. *Psychophysiology* **1979**, *16*, 495–512. [CrossRef]
47. Nijs, J.; Inghelbrecht, E.; Daenen, L.; Hachimi-Idrissi, S.; Hens, L.; Willems, B.; Roussel, N.; Cras, P.; Wouters, K.; Bernheim, J. Recruitment bias in chronic pain research: Whiplash as a model. *Clin. Rheumatol.* **2011**, *30*, 1481. [CrossRef] [PubMed]
48. Zhao, M.; Gersch, T.M.; Schnitzer, B.S.; Dosher, B.A.; Kowler, E. Eye movements and attention: The role of pre-saccadic shifts of attention in perception, memory and the control of saccades. *Vis. Res.* **2012**, *74*, 40–60. [CrossRef] [PubMed]

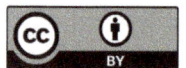

© 2018 by the authors. Licensee MDPI, Basel, Switzerland. This article is an open access article distributed under the terms and conditions of the Creative Commons Attribution (CC BY) license (http://creativecommons.org/licenses/by/4.0/).

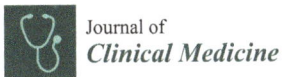

Article

A Meta-Epidemiological Appraisal of the Effects of Interdisciplinary Multimodal Pain Therapy Dosing for Chronic Low Back Pain

Elena Dragioti [1,*], Mathilda Björk [1,2], Britt Larsson [1] and Björn Gerdle [1]

[1] Pain and Rehabilitation Centre, and Department of Medical and Health Sciences, Linköping University, SE-581 85 Linköping, Sweden; mathilda.bjork@liu.se (M.B.); britt.larsson@liu.se (B.L.); bjorn.gerdle@liu.se (B.G.)
[2] Division of Occupational Therapy, Department of Social and Welfare Studies, Faculty of Health Sciences, Campus Norrkoping, Linköping University, SE-60174 Linköping, Sweden
* Correspondence: elena.dragioti@liu.se

Received: 21 May 2019; Accepted: 17 June 2019; Published: 18 June 2019

Abstract: Using a meta-analysis, meta-regression, and a meta-epidemiological approach, we conducted a systematic review to examine the influence of interdisciplinary multimodal pain therapy (IMPT) dosage on pain, disability, return to work, quality of life, depression, and anxiety in published randomised controlled trials (RCTs) in patients with non-specific chronic low back pain (CLBP). We considered all RCTs of IMPT from a Cochrane review and searched PubMed for additional RCTs through 30 September 2018. A subgroup random-effects meta-analysis by length, contact, and intensity of treatment was performed followed by a meta-regression analysis. Using random and fixed-effect models and a summary relative odds ratio (ROR), we compared the effect sizes (ES) from short-length, non-daily contact, and low-intensity RCTs with long-length, daily contact, and high-intensity RCTs. Heterogeneity was quantified with the I^2 metric. A total of 47 RCTs were selected. Subgroup meta-analysis showed that there were larger ES for pain and disability in RCTs with long-length, non-daily contact, and low intensity of treatment. Larger ES were also observed for quality of life in RCTs with short-length, non-daily contact, and low intensity treatment. However, these findings were not confirmed by the meta-regression analysis. Likewise, the summary RORs were not significant, indicating that the length, contact, and intensity of treatment did not have an overall effect on the investigated outcomes. For the outcomes investigated here, IMPT dosage is not generally associated with better ES, and an optimal dosage was not determined.

Keywords: programme dosage; interdisciplinary multimodal pain therapy; pain rehabilitation; low back pain; meta-analysis

1. Introduction

Currently, interdisciplinary multimodal pain therapy (IMPT) is used as a first-line therapy for chronic low back pain (CLBP) management [1–4]. IMPT, a long biopsychosocial treatment framework provided by a team of professionals, generally contains a synchronised combination of physical, educational, or psychological treatments in combination with measures for returning to work/studies [5,6]. Because IMPT can effectively treat patients with non-specific CLBP, it is strongly recommended [1–4]. Compared to usual care or physical treatment, IMPT has a consistent positive effect on disability and pain according to systematic reviews (SRs) [2,4]. In a new umbrella review, our team found suggestive evidence that IMPT might improve the likelihood of returning to work [5]. In addition, IMPT might decrease the personal and economic burden and increase the patients' treatment participation [2,7].

However, IMPT treatments are rather costly. The costs mainly depend on the treatment dosage, which includes the total duration, the contact (daily or non-daily), and intensity of treatment (number of contact hours per week) [8–10]. In addition, IMPT costs increase as the duration, contact, and intensity of treatment increase [8–10], and IMPT heavily depends on the involved professions. Typically, IMPT includes costs for physical therapists, psychologists, occupational therapists, physicians, and administration personnel [11]. Additionally, concerns include the costs of attending such treatments and the large societal costs of those patients who do not complete the treatments and do not return to work [11]. Therefore, the dosage of the treatment and the multidisciplinary nature of IMPT provide relatively high direct costs for both patients and the healthcare system [11]. Hence, variances in the IMPT dosage may lead to differences in both effectiveness and costs [8–10].

Presently, the optimal IMPT dosage and which dosage is efficacious for the patients with non-specific CLBP is unidentified [9], despite the need for a standardisation of such treatments [5,12]. A recent systematic review showed that IMPT dosage was never studied as a primary outcome, and its optimum dosage is currently unknown [10]. Our umbrella review also showed that a short duration of IMPT for CLBP patients with short-term and medium-term pain had the largest evidence of returning to work (highly suggestive evidence and suggestive evidence, respectively) [5]. A better understanding of how IMPT dosage is associated with outcome effects (e.g., pain, disability, and work status) should be considered when determining dosage. In turn, this could lead to better and more efficient patient care, which will benefit patients, rehabilitation facilities, insurers, and employers [8,11].

Here, we conducted a systematic review with meta-analysis and a meta-epidemiological appraisal to examine whether IMPT dosage is associated with better outcome effects in patients with non-specific CLBP.

2. Materials and Methods

This study was designed based on the Preferred Reporting Items for Systematic Reviews and Meta-Analyses (PRISMA) guidelines [13,14]. Because this meta-research project did not require patients to be directly involved, ethical approval was not required.

2.1. Literature Search and Study Selection

This study includes all randomised controlled trials (RCTs) included in Kamper et al.'s Cochrane systematic review [2]. We choose this review because it is the most recent and comprehensive review with the largest number of included RCTs. We also searched PubMed through 30 September 2018 for additional fully published RCTs in peer-reviewed journals investigating the effectiveness of IMPT on non-specific CLBP. The basic search strategy included the following key terms: chronic low back pain, interdisciplinary, multimodal pain therapy, multidisciplinary biopsychosocial rehabilitation, and randomised controlled trials (for details, see Box S1, Supplementary Materials).

We included only RCTs that (1) examined any IMPT versus any control (e.g., treatment as usual, and waiting list) or other treatment (e.g., physiotherapy and surgery), (2) included only adult men and women, (3) identified a diagnosis of a non-specific CLBP lasting more than three months, and (4) published in English expect for those included in the Kamper et al.'s review [2] as the provided data in this study were already translated into English.

We excluded studies if they (1) used a study design other than RCT, (2) compared different IMPTs with each other (i.e., head-to-head comparisons), (3) included participants with fewer than 50% diagnosed with non-specific CLBP, (4) included a diagnosis of LBP due to cancer, infection, inflammatory arthropathy, osteoporosis, high-velocity trauma, fracture, pregnancy, rheumatoid arthritis, or rheumatic pain, and (5) provided insufficient or inadequate data for quantitative synthesis.

2.2. Data Extraction

One investigator (E.D.) screened titles and abstracts, assessed the eligibility, extracted data, and rated the quality of the included RCTs. These were also checked by a second author (M.B.).

Any disagreements were resolved by consensus, or a third reviewer (B.G.) was consulted if disagreements persisted. The six primary outcomes of interest for this study were pain, disability, work status (return to work), quality of life, depression, and anxiety as reported by the original authors of the RCTs. We chose these outcomes because these were the most common outcomes in RCTs with adequate data for analysis. Other outcomes (e.g., fear avoidance and coping strategies) provided limited data for synthesis. Because of the same limitation (i.e., limited data for adequate synthesis), we also focused only on short-term outcomes (i.e., up to three months). The IMPT dosage was defined according to total duration (in weeks), daily contact or non-daily contact, and intensity of treatment (number of contact hours per week) [2,10].

2.3. Assessment of Bias

We used the updated Cochrane Back Review Group criteria [15] to rate the quality of the included RCTs, which include 12 criteria and assess the risk of bias (RoB). For each criterion, the quality of each RCT was classified as high (i.e., low RoB = 1), moderate (i.e., unclear RoB = 2), and low (i.e., high RoB = 3). Next, we evaluated an overall "risk of bias" assessment for each RCT by giving one point to each criterion when low RoB was indicated. Thus, RCTs satisfying at least six of the 12 criteria and having no having no serious flaws (e.g., 80% drop-out rate in one group) were considered as "low" risk of bias [15]. RCTs with serious flaws, or those in which fewer than six of the criteria are met were considered as having a "high" risk of bias [15]. It is important to note that the blinding is quite problematic in this field [2,10].

2.4. Data Synthesis and Analysis

We analysed data descriptively and conducted subgroup meta-analysis of all the outcomes of interest as listed above. Specifically, to explore the effects of IMPT dosage—i.e., the total duration (in weeks), the contact, and intensity of treatment (number of contact hours per week)—a series of random-effects meta-analyses [16] were conducted by clustering the RCTs according to the following variables: short length (in weeks; <5 weeks) vs. long length (≥5 weeks); non-daily contact vs. daily contact; and low intensity vs. high intensity (e.g., less than 30 h per week vs. more 30 h per week). Dichotomous outcomes were analysed by calculating the pooled odds ratio (OR), and continuous outcomes were analysed by calculating the standardised mean difference (SMD). Between-study heterogeneity was evaluated by Cochran's Q test [16] and quantified with the I^2 metric of inconsistency (low, moderate, large, and very large for values of <25, 25–49, 50–74, and >75%, respectively) [17,18]. We also calculated the 95% confidence intervals for the I^2. We used the regression asymmetry test and funnel plots to estimate publication bias for all outcomes of interest [19]. We also performed a random-effects meta-regression analysis [20] to examine the potential moderator effect of dosage aspects, mean age of the participants, gender (female), type of control (i.e., physical activity), and RoB assessment (i.e., RCTs with low risk as previously described) on treatment effects. The dosage aspects (duration and intensity) were included in the meta-regression analysis as continuous variables for a more accurate estimation [20]. The only exception was for contact since it was only in binary form.

To further systemically assess the potential influence of IMPT dosage on the outcomes of interest, we used a meta-epidemiological approach [21–23] comparing the magnitude of the effect size (ES) by the treatment dosage in terms of the total duration (in weeks), the contact, and intensity of treatment (number of contact hours per week) for each outcome. To match the outcome data and allow for the synthesis of the evidence, we transformed the SMD to a logOR for the continuous outcomes [22] based on a standardised formula [24].

From each outcome, we calculated a summary OR for the short-duration RCTs and long-duration RCTs, for the non-daily contact and daily contact, and for the low-intensity vs. high-intensity RCTs within the eligible RCTs using fixed-effect models [22,25]. This method is more proper for examining study design factors on treatment effects [21–23]. All comparisons were coined so that the experimental arm was always an IMPT vs. a control arm. Next, we obtained a relative OR (ROR) within all comparisons for each outcome [22]. A ROR that exceeds 1 equates to assessments providing a more favourable response to the experimental IMPT supported by an RCT with long duration, daily contact, and high intensity compared to RCTs with short duration, non-daily contact, and low intensity. To obtain a summary ROR (sROR) across all outcomes, we combined the natural logarithm estimates of the RORs for all comparisons [21] using fixed- and random-effects models [16,25].

The statistical analyses were made using STATA version 10.0 (STATA Corp, College Station, Texas, USA); a value of $p < 0.05$ (two-tailed) was set as the level of significance.

3. Results

We identified 41 RCTs from Kamper et al.'s study [2]. The electronic search yielded a total of 3799 potentially eligible titles. Following the search and screening and retrieval of 126 full text articles, six additional RCTs were determined to be eligible (Figure S1, Supplementary Materials). These articles were added to the 41 RCTs included in Kamper et al. [2] to make a total of 47 included RCTs (see Supplementary Materials for the list of refences of the included studies). The two independent investigators reached a very high level of agreement (43/47 RCTs). In the whole process, from screening to data extraction, any disagreement was discussed with a third researcher (B.G.) until a consensus was reached.

3.1. Characteristics of Included Studies

Table 1 presents the characteristics of studies. All the 47 included studies were RCTs published from 1990 to 2017. Most studies were conducted in Europe ($n = 34$; 74%). The number of participants ranged from 20 to 542 with a median number of 134 participants per study (interquartile range (IQR = 84–195), a median age of 44 years old (IQR = 41–47), a total treatment duration ranging from 1–16 weeks with a median of five weeks (IQR = 3–7), and a number of contact hours (per week) ranging from 1–100 h (median = 10; IQR = 3–30). Most RCTs provided a non-daily contact ($n = 26$; 56%). Although the definition of CLBP varied among studies, most studies defined CLBP as back pain lasting more than three months (Table 1). The number of datasets included in the meta-analysis per outcome varied from two (anxiety) to 28 (pain).

Table 1. Characteristics of included studies.

Author, Year *	Country	Sample Size	Female %	Mean Age (or Age Range)	Treatment	Control	Definition of Chronic LBP	Total Duration (Weeks)	Contact	Contact Duration (h/Week)	RoB Assessment
Abbassi, 2012	Iran	33	88	45	IMPT	TAU	LBP >6 months	7	Non-daily contact	4	Low risk
Alaranta, 1994	Finland	293	56	41	IMPT	Physical	LBP >6 months	6	Daily contact	100	High risk
Altmaier, 1992	USA	45	73	40	IMPT	Physical	LBP >3 months	3	Daily contact	20	High risk
Basler 1997	Germany	76	76	49	IMPT	TAU	LBP >6 months	12	Non-daily contact	2.5	High risk
Bendix, 1996/1998	Denmark	106	70	40	IMPT	TAU	LBP >6 months	3	Daily contact	49	High risk
Bendix, 1995/1998	Denmark	106	75	42	IMPT	Physical	LBP >6 months	4	Daily contact	45	High risk
Bendix, 2000	Denmark	138	65	41	IMPT	Physical	LBP >6 months	4	Daily contact	45	High risk
Coole, 2013	UK	51	53	44	IMPT	TAU	LBP >3 months	16	Non-daily contact	3	Low risk
Corey, 1996	Canada	138	NR	NR	IMPT	TAU	LBP >3 months	5	Daily contact	32.5	High risk
Fairbank, 2005	UK	349	51	18–55	IMPT	Surgery	LBP >1 year	3	Daily contact	75	Low risk
Harkapaa, 1989	Finland	309	37	45	IMPT	Physical	LBP for >2 years	3	Daily contact	100	High risk
Hellum, 2011	Norway	173	51	41	IMPT	Surgery	LBP >1 year	5	Non-daily contact	12	High risk
Henchoz, 2010	Switzerland	109	32	40	IMPT	Physical	LBP >3 months	3	Non-daily contact	30	High risk
Jackel, 1990	Germany	71	62	49	IMPT	WL	LBP >3 months	6	Daily contact	36	High risk
Jousset, 2004	France	84	33	40	IMPT	Physical	LBP >3 months	5	Daily contact	30	High risk
Kaapa, 2006	Finland	120	100	46	IMPT	Physical	LBP >1 year	7	Daily contact	100	Low risk
Kole-Snijders, 1999	Netherlands	148	64	40	IMPT	WL	LBP >6 months	8	Daily contact	13	High risk
Kool, 2007	Switzerland	174	21	42	IMPT	Physical	LBP >3 months	3	Non-daily contact	24	Low risk
Lambeek, 2010	Netherlands	134	42	18–65	IMPT	TAU	LBP >3 months	12	Non-daily contact	3	Low risk
Leeuw, 2008	Netherlands	85	48	45	IMPT	IMPT	LBP >3 months	16	Non-daily contact	2	Low risk
Linton, 2005	Sweden	185	83	49	IMPT	TAU	NR	6	Non-daily contact	2	High risk
Lukinmaa, 1989	Finland	158	53	44	IMPT	TAU	NR	1	Non-daily contact	2.5	High risk
Mangels, 2009	Germany	363	78	49	IMPT	Physical	ICD 10	4	Daily contact	100	Low risk
Meng, 2011	Germany	360	64	49	IMPT	TAU/IMPT	ICD 10	7	Non-daily contact	1	High risk
Mitchell, 1994	Canada	542	29	nr	IMPT	TAU	NR	8	Daily contact	35	High risk
Moix, 2003	Spain	30	53	54	IMPT	TAU	NR	11	Non-daily contact	1	High risk
Monticone, 2013	Italy	90	58	50	IMPT	TAU	LBP >3 months	5	Non-daily contact	3	Low risk
Monticone, 2014	Italy	20	NR	NR	IMPT	Physical	LBP >3 months	8	Non-daily contact	3	Low risk

Table 1. Cont.

Author, Year *	Country	Sample Size	Female %	Mean Age (or Age Range)	Treatment	Control	Definition of Chronic LBP	Total Duration (Weeks)	Contact	Contact Duration (h/Week)	RoB Assessment
Morone, 2011	Italy	73	64	60	IMPT	TAU	LBP >3 months	4	Non-daily contact	4	High risk
Morone, 2012	Italy	75	72	55	IMPT	TAU/Physical	LBP >3 months	4	Non-daily contact	4	High risk
Nicholas, 1991	Australia	58	52	41	IMPT	Physical	LBP >6 months	5	Non-daily contact	3.5	High risk
Nicholas, 1992	Australia	20	45	44	IMPT	Physical	LBP >6 months	5	Non-daily contact	3.5	High risk
Roche, 2007/2011	France	132	35	40	IMPT	Physical	LBP >3 months	5	Daily contact	30	Low risk
Smeets, 2006/2008	Netherlands	212	42	47	IMPT	WL	LBP >3 months	10	Non-daily contact	7.1	Low risk
Skouen, 2002	Norway	195	44	43	IMPT	TAU/IMPT	NR	4	Daily contact	30	High risk
Schweikert, 2006	Germany	409	17	47	IMPT	Physical	LBP >6 months	3	Daily contact	17.5	High risk
Strand, 2001	Norway	117	61	43	IMPT	TAU	ICPC diagnosis	5	Daily contact	30	High risk
Streibelt, 2009	Germany	222	17	46	IMPT	Physical	NR	3	Non-daily contact	20	High risk
Tavafian, 2008	Iran	102	100	43	IMPT	TAU	LBP >3 months	1	Non-daily contact	5	Low risk
Tavafian, 2011	Iran	197	22	45	IMPT	TAU	LBP >3 months	1	Non-daily contact	10	Low risk
Tavafian, 2014	Iran	178	75	44	IMPT	TAU	LBP >3 months	1	Daily contact	5	High risk
Tavafian, 2017	Iran	146	78	46	IMPT	TAU	LBP >3 months	1	Daily contact	5	Low risk
Tavafian, 2017	Iran	165	79	45	IMPT	TAU	LBP >3 months	1	Daily contact	5	Low risk
Turner, 1990	USA	96	49	44	IMPT	Physical/WL	LBP >6 months	8	Non-daily contact	2	High risk
Van den Hout, 2003	Netherlands	84	34	40	IMPT	IMPT	LBP >6 months	8	Non-daily contact	20	High risk
Vollenbroek-Hutten, 2004	Netherlands	163	NR	39	IMPT	TAU	LBP >6 months	7	Non-daily contact	9	Low risk
Von Korff, 2005	USA	240	63	50	IMPT	TAU	score >7/23 on RMDQ	1	Non-daily contact	3	High risk

* See references of included randomised controlled trials (RCTs) 1–47 in Supplementary Materials; ICD 10—International Statistical Classification of Diseases and Related Health Problems, Tenth Revision, ICPC—International Classification of Primary Care, LBP—lower back pain, IMPT—interdisciplinary multimodal pain therapy, NR—not reported, RMDQ—Roland Morris Disability Questionnaire, RoB—risk of bias, TAU—treatment as usual, UK—United Kingdom, USA—United States of America, WL—waiting list.

3.2. Risk of Bias in Included Studies

The results of the RoB assessment are presented in Table S1 (Supplementary Materials). Overall, 15 of the 47 studies (32%) were evaluated as low risk of bias. The most important methodological flaws were related to a lack of participant, clinician, and outcome assessment blinding; in particular, 46 out of 47 RCTs (almost 100%) had a high risk of bias in all three of these criteria (Figure 1). However, as in any psychotherapy [22], blinding is not possible, at least to participants or clinicians, in this type of treatment [2,10].

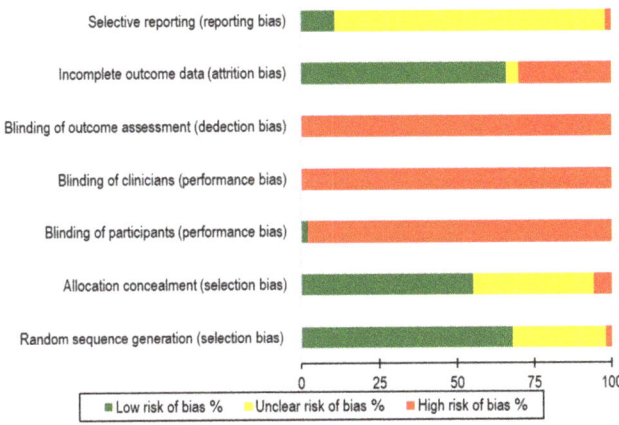

Figure 1. Risk of bias graph: assessments for seven risk of bias criteria presented as percentages across all included studies.

3.3. Publication Bias

Publication bias was observed for three outcomes (disability ($p = 0.018$), quality of life ($p = 0.060$), and depression ($p = 0.081$)), based on the funnel plots and Egger's regression test (see Figures S2–S6, Supplementary Materials). No publication bias remained for the outcome of pain ($p = 0.219$) after excluding the study of Monticone et al. (2013) (Reference 27 in Supplementary Materials) providing a large outlier as seen in Figure S2 (Supplementary Materials). Publication bias for anxiety outcome could not be estimated due to the inadequate number of included studies (only two RCTs).

3.4. Analyses for Outcomes of Interdisciplinary Multimodal Pain Therapy (IMPT) by Length, Contact, and Intensity

For each outcome, subgroup analysis was conducted for IMPT dosage by length, contact, and intensity (Table 2). There were larger ES for pain and disability in RCTs with long length, non-daily contact, and low intensity of treatment. Larger and significant ES were also observed for quality of life in RCTs with short length, non-daily contact, and low intensity of treatment. After excluding the study of Moticone et al. (2013/2014) (References 27,28 in Supplementary Materials), the ES were similar between the aspects of dosage for the outcomes of pain and disability (see Figures S7–S12, Supplementary Materials). The forest plots of the overall ES from all studies included for the six outcomes per RoB assessment, type of control, and aspects of dosage are provided in Figures S13–S18 (Supplementary Materials).

Table 2. Characteristics and subgroup meta-analysis for dose of IMPT by length, contact, and intensity of the six investigated outcomes.

Short-Term Outcomes	No. of RCTs	Average Total Duration (Median Weeks, IQR)	Average h/Week (Median, IQR)	Level of Daily/Non-Daily Contact (n)	Level of Active (i.e., Physical)/Non-Active Control (i.e., WL/TAU) (n)	Level of Low Risk/High Risk of Bias (n)	Overall ES (95% CI) Random-Effects Model	p-Value	I^2 (%; 95% CI) p-Value
Outcome 1: Pain									
Length									
Short length (<5 weeks)	12	3 (1–4)	7.5 (4–22)	8/4	6/6	3/9	SMD, −0.33 (−0.55 to −0.11)	0.003	81 (67–88) 0.000
Long length (≥5 weeks)	16	8 (5.5–10)	3.5 (2.7–10)	4/12	8/8	8/8	SMD, −0.45 (−0.73 to −0.17)	0.001	79 (64–85) 0.000
Contact									
Non-daily contact	16	7.5 (4.5–10)	3.3 (2.7–4)	0/16	7/9	6/10	SMD, −0.50 (−0.79 to −0.20)	0.001	80 (67–86) 0.000
Daily contact	12	3 (2–5.5)	22 (11.5–68)	12/0	7/5	5/7	SMD, −0.29 (−0.49 to −0.09)	0.005	78 (59–86) 0.000
Intensity									
<30 h per week	23	5 (3–8)	4 (3–7.1)	7/16	10/13	8/15	SMD, −0.42 (−0.62 to −0.20)	<0.000	81 (71–86) 0.000
>30 h per week	5	5 (4–6)	100 (36–100)	5/0	4/1	3/2	SMD, −0.32 (−0.63 to −0.05)	0.022	79 (31–89) 0.001
Outcome 2: Disability									
Length									
Short length (<5 weeks)	10	3 (1–4)	7.5 (4–30)	5/5	5/5	2/8	SMD, −0.27 (−0.48 to −0.07)	0.007	75 (47–85) 0.000
Long length (≥5 weeks)	17	7 (6–10)	3.5 (3–9)	4/13	9/8	9/8	SMD, −0.51 (−0.78 to −0.24)	<0.000	82 (73–88) 0.000
Contact									
Non-daily contact	18	7 (4–10)	3.5 (3–4)	0/18	8/10	7/11	SMD, −0.58 (−0.86 to −0.31)	<0.000	81 (70–87) 0.000
Daily contact	9	4 (1–3)	36 (18–100)	9/0	6/3	4/5	SMD, −0.16 (−0.33–0.01)	0.055	67 (16–82) 0.002
Intensity									
<30 h per week	20	6 (4–9)	3.8 (3–6)	3/17	8/12	8/12	SMD, −0.49 (−0.74 to −0.24)	<0.000	85 (78–89) 0.000
>30 h per week	7	5 (3–6)	100 (30–100)	6/1	6/1	3/4	SMD, −0.26 (−0.43 to −0.09)	0.003	54 (0–78) 0.043

Table 2. Cont.

Short-Term Outcomes	No. of RCTs	Average Total Duration (Median Weeks, IQR)	Average h/Week (Median, IQR)	Level of Daily/Non-Daily Contact (n)	Level of Active (i.e., Physical)/Non-Active Control (i.e., WL/TAU) (n)	Level of Low Risk/High Risk of Bias (n)	Overall ES (95% CI) Random-Effects Model	p-Value	I^2 (%; 95% CI) p-Value
Outcome 3: Return to work									
Length									
Short length (<5 weeks)	3	3 (1–4)	24 (3–30)	2/1	1/2	1/2	OR, 1.46 (0.82–2.62)	0.199	42 (0–83) 0.177
Long length (≥5 weeks)	2	5 (5–5)	30 (30–30)	2/0	2/0	1/1	OR, 1.10 (0.55–2.20)	0.786	0 (NA) # 0.938
Contact									
Non-daily contact	1	1 (1–1)	3 (3–3)	0/1	0/1	0/1	OR, 0.91 (0.31–2.68)	0.864	NA
Daily contact	4	4.5 (3.5–5)	30 (27–30)	4/0	1/3	2/2	OR, 1.46 (0.96–2.21)	0.075	12 (0–72) 0.332
Intensity									
<30 h per week	2	2 (1–3)	13.5 (3–24)	1/1	1/1	1/1	OR, 1.63 (0.65–4.09)	0.297	56 (NA) # 0.133
>30 h per week	3	5 (4–5)	30 (30–30)	3/0	2/1	1/2	OR, 1.12 (0.69–1.82)	0.645	0 (0–73) 0.994
Outcome 4: Quality of life									
Length									
Short length (<5 weeks)	8	1.5 (1–3.5)	7.5 (4–13.7)	5/3	3/5	2/6	SMD, 0.49 (0.14–0.84)	0.006	83 (65–90) 0.000
Long length (≥5 weeks)	1	10 (10–10)	7.1 (7.1–7.1)	0/1	1/0	1/0	SMD, 0.14 (−0.24–0.52)	0.470	NA
Contact									
Non-daily contact	4	4 (1–10)	4 (3–7.1)	0/4	2/2	2/2	SMD, 0.53 (0.09–0.98)	0.019	64 (0–86) 0.038
Daily contact	5	1.5 (1–3)	10 (5–18)	5/0	2/3	1/4	SMD, 0.38 (−0.06–0.81)	0.089	88 (70–93) 0.000
Intensity									
<30 h per week	8	2 (1–4))	6 (4–10)	4/4	3/5	2/6	SMD, 0.54 (0.25–0.83)	<0.000	75 (38–86) 0.000
>30 h per week	1	2 (2–2)	100 (100–100)	1/0	1/0	1/0	SMD, −0.38 (−0.74 to −0.02)	0.041 *	NA

Table 2. Cont.

Short-Term Outcomes	No. of RCTs	Average Total Duration (Median Weeks, IQR)	Average h/Week (Median, IQR)	Level of Daily/Non-Daily Contact (n)	Level of Active (i.e., Physical)/Non-Active Control (i.e., WL/TAU) (n)	Level of Low Risk/High Risk of Bias (n)	Overall ES (95% CI) Random-Effects Model	p-Value	I² (%; 95% CI) p-Value
Outcome 5: Depression									
Length									
Short length (<5 weeks)	2	3.5 (3–4)	58.8 (17.5–100)	2/0	2/0	1/1	SMD, 0.08 (−0.22–0.39)	0.584	71 (NA) # 0.063
Long length (≥5 weeks)	8	7.5 (5.5–9)	5.3 (2.8–21.5)	2/6	5/3	3/5	SMD, −0.09 (−0.29–0.11)	0.358	20 (0–64) 0.273
Contact									
Non-daily contact	6	8 (5–10)	3.5 (2–7.1)	0/6	4/2	2/4	SMD, 0.01 (−0.21–0.22)	0.959	0 (0–61) 0.562
Daily contact	4	5 (3.5–6.5)	68 (26.8–100)	4/0	3/1	2/2	SMD, −0.07 (−0.35–0.22)	0.653	72 (0–88) 0.013
Intensity									
<30 h per week	7	8 (5–10)	7.1 (2–17.5)	2/5	4/3	2/5	SMD, 0.12 (−0.03–0.27)	0.119	1 (0–59) 0.414
>30 h per week	3	5 (4–7)	100 (3.5–100)	2/1	3/0	2/1	SMD, −0.18 (−0.46–0.10)	0.202	46 (0–84) 0.155
Outcome 6: Anxiety									
Length									
Short length (<5 weeks)	1	3 (3–3)	17.5 (17.5–17.5)	1/0	1/0	0/1	SMD, 0.08 (−0.13–0.29)	0.455	NA
Long length (≥5 weeks)	1	5 (5–5)	3.5 (3.5–3.5)	0/1	1/0	0/1	SMD, −0.58 (−1.48–0.32)	0.209	NA
Contact									
Non-daily contact	1	5 (5–5)	3.5 (3.5–3.5)	0/1	1/0	0/1	SMD, −0.58 (−1.48–0.32)	0.209	NA
Daily contact	1	3 (3–3)	17.5 (17.5–17.5)	1/0	1/0	0/1	SMD, 0.08 (−0.13–0.29)	0.455	NA
Intensity									
<30 h per week	2	4 (3–5)	10.5 (3.5–17.5)	1/1	2/0	0/2	SMD, −0.10 (−0.67–0.48)	0.740	48 (NA) # 0.164
>30 h per week	0	0 (0–0)	0 (0–0)	0/0	0/0	0/0	NA	NA	NA

Notes: * favours control, # degrees of freedom (df n − 1) must be at least 2, CI—confidence interval, ES—effect size, OR—odds ratio, I²—I square metric of heterogeneity, IQR—interquartile range, TAU—treatment as usual, SMD—standardised mean difference, NA—not applicable, WL—waiting list.

3.5. Meta-Regression

In the meta-regression analyses, none of the examined variables displayed a moderating effect on the five examined outcomes (i.e., pain, disability, return to work, quality of life, and depression). For the anxiety outcome, there were insufficient observations to perform such analysis (Table S2, Supplementary Materials).

3.6. Comparison of Relative Odds Ratios

The comparison of RORs by length of treatment showed that, for pain and disability, the summary RORs were >1, demonstrating that the IMPT was more favourable in RCTs with long length of treatment (i.e., RCTs with duration of more than five weeks). However, the summary ROR was not significant (sROR = 1.48 (95% confidence interval (CI) 0.78–2.81, $p = 0.232$) using the random-effects model, showing that the length of treatment did not have an overall effect on the investigated outcomes (Figure 2). Very large heterogeneity was observed ($I^2 = 82\%$, 95% CI 55–90%). Under the fixed-effect models the sROR was, however, significant (Figure S19, Supplementary Materials).

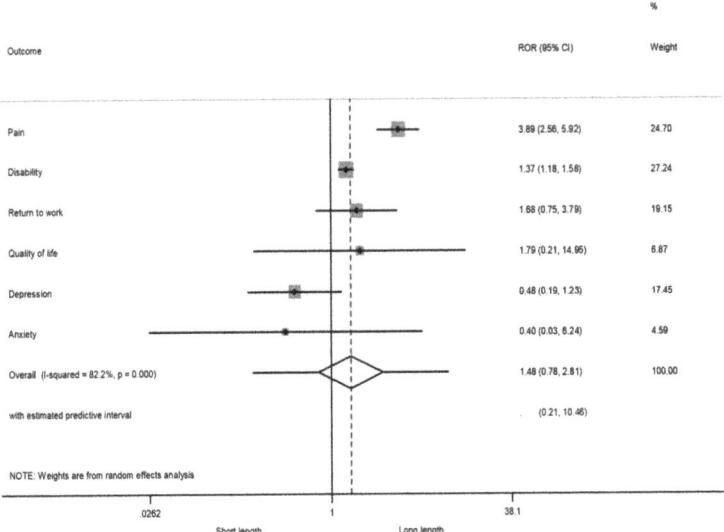

Figure 2. The relative odds ratios (RORs) and 95% confidence intervals (CIs) for each outcome, and the summary RORs and their 95% CIs at short term of a short-length treatment vs. long-length treatment. The RORs were calculated with a random-effects model. A ROR >1 favours long length; an ROR <1 favours short length.

The comparison of RORs by contact of treatment (i.e., non-daily contact vs. daily contact) showed that the summary ROR was <1 only for disability, a finding that indicates that the IMPT was more favourable in RCTs with non-daily contact of treatment (i.e., RCTs with at least 3 h per week). However, the summary ROR was not significant (sROR = 0.56; 95% CI 0.22–1.44; $p = 0.230$) according to the random-effects model (Figure 3), showing that the contact of treatment did not have an overall effect on the investigated outcomes, whereas the sROR was significant under the fixed-effect models (Figure S20, Supplementary Materials). Very large heterogeneity was also present ($I^2 = 93\%$, 95% CI 88–95%).

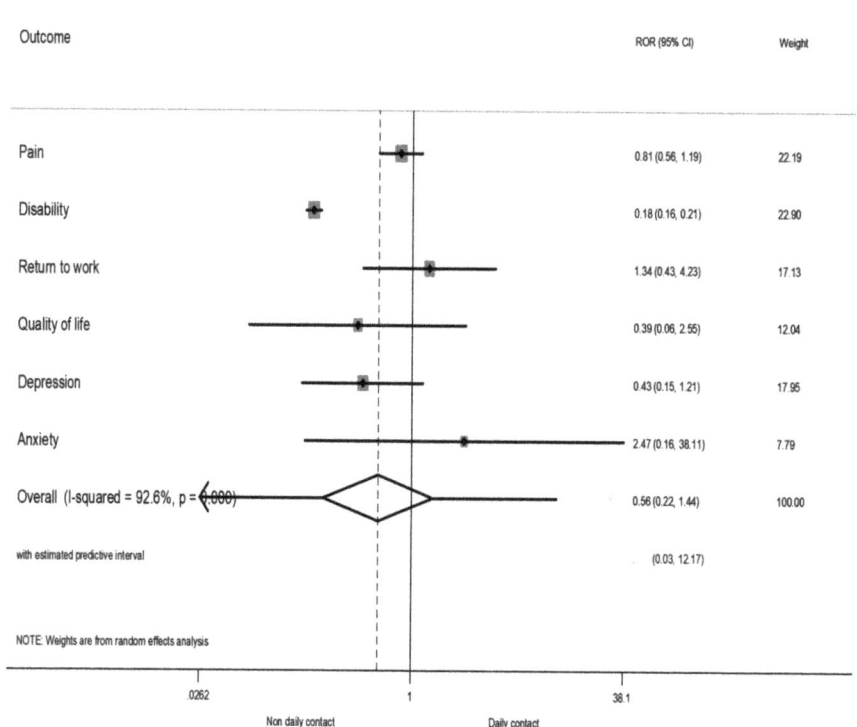

Figure 3. The relative odds ratios (RORs) and 95% confidence intervals (CIs) for each outcome, and the summary RORs and their 95% CIs at short term of non-daily contact vs. daily contact. The RORs were calculated with a random-effects model. A ROR >1 favours daily contact; an ROR <1 favours non-daily contact.

With respect to the intensity of treatment (i.e., low intensity vs. high intensity), the summary ROR was <1 only for disability, demonstrating that the IMPT was more favourable in RCTs with low intensity of treatment (i.e., RCTs with less than 30 h per week). The summary ROR was also not significant (sROR = 1.12; 95% CI 0.66–1.89; p = 0.672) using the random-effects model, showing that the intensity of treatment did not have an overall effect on the outcomes. Large heterogeneity was observed (I^2 = 70%, 95% CI 21–87%) (Figure 4). Similar results were evident when the fixed-effect models were used (Figure S21, Supplementary Materials). A sensitivity analysis excluding the study of Moticone et al. (2013/2014) (References 27,28 in Supplementary Materials) did not alter the overall effects between the comparison of RORs (Figures S22–S24, Supplementary Materials).

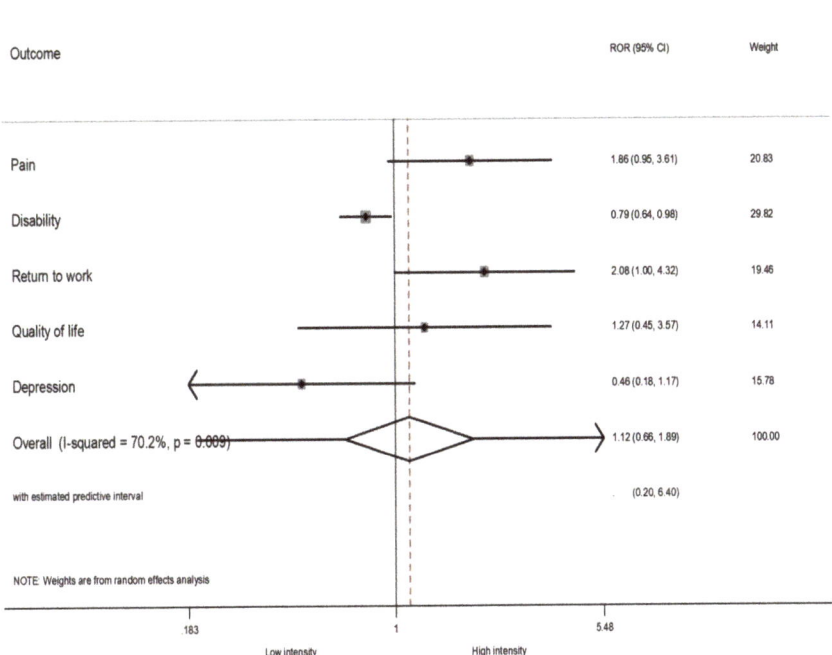

Figure 4. The relative odds ratios (RORs) and 95% confidence intervals (CIs) for each outcome, and the summary RORs and their 95% CIs at short term of low intensity vs. high intensity. The RORs were calculated with a random-effects model. A ROR >1 favours high intensity (i.e. >30 h per week); an ROR <1 favours low intensity (i.e. <30 h per week).

4. Discussion

When evaluating the 47 RCTs of IMPT by length, contact, and intensity, we found that IMPT dosage did not have an overall influence on the reported effects in patients with non-specific CLBP. Specifically, the summary RORs were not significant when we compared the effect estimates for the investigated outcomes from the short-length and the long-length treatments and the non-daily contact with the daily contact. There was no significant influence for either intensity of the treatment. Although we found large heterogeneity between RCTs, the meta-regression analysis revealed that none of the examined factors were potential factors for heterogeneity.

Yet, per individual outcome, some evidence exhibited that IMPT of more than five weeks may be related to more "favourable" effects for pain reduction, while a long treatment with non-daily contact and low intensity may be associated with more beneficial effects for disability. These results were supported by both subgroup meta-analyses and meta-analytical comparisons of RORs between the treatment effects. This study suggests that an optimal IMPT dosage from the published work is not possible to be standardised. This finding partly agrees with the idea that the published recommended IMPT dosages are somewhat arbitrary and primarily based on clinical expertise and experience [8]. Our study, however, did not confirm an overall IMPT dose–treatment–effect association in agreement with a recently published non-inferiority RCT [9].

To our knowledge, this is the first study to examine the influence of IMPT dosage in such a systematic appraisal followed by meta-analysis and meta-epidemiological approach across the largest dataset of published RCTs, calculating the magnitude of the observed effect. Our meta-epidemiological approach with comparison of RORs is suitable for examining study design factors and characteristics on treatment effects [21–23]. IMPT, a complex treatment, requires a broad set-up of outcome variables.

The present review had such a broad approach when evaluating IMPT dosage. Hence, we analysed dosage aspects for the individual outcomes and used a more comprehensive approach—the summary estimates of outcomes. Although IMPT dosing is rather essential in terms both of efficacy and healthcare costs [8,11], it was not systematically and thoroughly assessed in RCTs [9]. Few other studies that focused on IMPT dosage and these studies included a smaller number of RCTs or used different methodological methods and outcomes [4,10]. In a Cochrane review, Guzman et al. compared 12 IMPTs in 1964 patients with CLBP [4]. Their meta-analysis found that daily intensive IMPT (with more than 100 h per week) with respect to disability was more beneficial than monodisciplinary treatment. Evidence regarding other outcomes was either limited or ambivalent [4]. However, their review was not designed to directly study the influence of treatment dosage on outcome effects.

Waterschoot et al. conducted a systematic review analysing the influence of IMPT dosage on disability, work, and quality of life in patients with CLBP and included 18 studies [10]. As in our study, the studies included in that review varied in terms of dosage (total duration and contact hours) and outcome effects. Their linear mixed-effect modelling showed that duration in weeks was significantly associated with the aforesaid outcomes [10]. It was somewhat surprising that we did not find an association between duration of treatment (or any other dose aspect) and effects on pain, disability, return to work, quality of life, depression, or anxiety. An explanation could be that different components such as a professional's expertise or different types of professionals involved in an IMPT might have greater influence than the dosage variables. Waterschoot et al. also suggested that the content of such treatments is strongly related to dosage aspects; thus, the independent effect of dosage is not easily detectable [10]. A final explanation of the lack of association between and outcome effects is that there is also the possibility that the dosage does not actually influence the outcomes in this target group. The latter is supported by the subgroup analysis in Kamper et al. as they found that there was no pattern of smaller or larger effects for duration and contact with IMPT while the intensity of treatment slightly affected the treatment effects [2]. This finding is also supported by Reneman et al. who found that the dosage is not related to differences in disability [9].

One limitation of our study is that we did not explore the potential interaction of the role of professionals per RCT with length, contact, and intensity of treatment. Also, the individual components of IMPT may differ between RCTs without any difference in the overall dosage variables investigated here. Moreover, it is possible that some professionals might be unequally trained or have less clinical expertise for the application of the multidisciplinary treatment, and it might be hypothesised that these factors could affect the exact extent/dosage of a program. For example, well-trained professionals with extensive clinical expertise might require fewer contacts to help their patients. A related issue is the adherence to the treatment protocols within IMPT by the professionals. Many treatments require that the patients apply the achieved insights and knowledge in their home environments or jobs, and the time spent on this is usually not included in the stated doses. Furthermore, the severity of the clinical presentations of the patient groups, as well as the social context (e.g., with respect to the insurance situation) may differ substantially between RCTs; unfortunately, there are no established and standardised ways to compare chronic pain patient cohorts. It is also possible that the diversity of the professionals and the multidisciplinary nature of the treatment per se may lead to differences in treatment effects in relation to the variation of dosage [8,11]. However, there are no related data in the literature to either support or reject this hypothesis. Another limitation is that the dichotomisation between length was based on the median value of the total duration of the IMPT per week; thus, one may argue that this was somewhat subjective. However, in the literature, there is not a valid cut-off score to precisely define what is a short-length or long-length treatment, although the categorisation of contact and intensity was based on the available literature [4]. One may also argue that the overall dichotomisation of the dosage cannot accurately represent the wide spectrum of the total length in weeks, total number of hours, or the total number of contact hours per week. Indeed, our results confirm the wide variability in weeks, contact hours, and intensity as previously reported [10]. Nevertheless, the results of the meta-regression analysis using continuous variables of dosage were also not significant.

In addition, large heterogeneity was found, but it cannot be explained from the dosage choices, age, gender, low risk of bias, or type of control as presented in the published RCTs. This extensive heterogeneity contributed to different results from fixed and random-effects models with respect to the comparison between length and contact of treatment, and it can be better explained by the variation in professional teams and the contents of the IMPT. Finally, we based our research on studies from a Cochrane systematic review from 2014, and, despite the additional search on PubMed, we may have missed some information.

This study does not suggest that IMPT is not beneficial for patients with CLBP. On the contrary, our results found reliable but moderate effects on pain and disability following previous evidence [1–4]. In addition, even if IMPT dosage remains controversial, the lack of association between dosing and outcome effects may mean that the rehabilitation professionals should reconsider adopting lower dosages. We also assumed that an IMPT with duration of at least five weeks with non-daily contact and low intensity would reduce pain and disability and the costs of such treatments, and increase the rehab participation of patients suffering from chronic symptomatology, thereby avoiding exhaustive and long treatments. In turn, active participation could lead to more beneficial results. Undoubtedly, CLBP is a major cause of concern globally [7,26,27] and one of the leading causes of years lived with disability [28]; therefore, optimal treatments are needed [29].

5. Conclusions

In this study, we showed that the IMPT dosing in general is not associated with better effects on pain, disability, work status, quality of life, depression, and anxiety in patients with non-specific CLBP. Some evidence suggests the efficacy of a long program with non-daily contact and low intensity for only pain and disability per individual outcome level, but an overall optimal dosage was not likely to be identified. This knowledge will contribute to a better evaluation from pain rehabilitation professionals to obtain insight into dosage choices that may contribute to more efficacious treatments. Further research on this topic examining also long-term outcomes is warranted.

Supplementary Materials: The following are available online at http://www.mdpi.com/2077-0383/8/6/871/s1. Figure S1: Study flow diagram, Figure S2: Funnel plot for the pain outcome. Egger's test for publication bias was not significant ($p = 0.141$), Figure S3: Funnel plot for the disability outcome. Egger's test for publication bias was significant ($p = 0.018$), Figure S4: Funnel plot for the return to work outcome. Egger's test for publication bias was not significant ($p = 0.141$), Figure S5: Funnel plot for the quality of life outcome. Egger's test for publication bias was significant ($p = 0.060$), Figure S6: Funnel plot for the depression outcome. Egger's test for publication bias was significant ($p = 0.081$), Figure S7: Sensitivity analysis by length for the pain outcome, after excluding the study of Moticone et al. (2013/2014), Figure S8: Sensitivity analysis by contact for the pain outcome, after excluding the study of Moticone et al. (2013/2014), Figure S9: Sensitivity analysis by intensity for the pain outcome, after excluding the study of Moticone et al. (2013/2014), Figure S10: Sensitivity analysis by length for the disability outcome, after excluding the study of Moticone et al. (2013/2014), Figure S11: Sensitivity analysis by contact for the disability outcome, after excluding the study of Moticone et al. (2013/2014), Figure S12: Sensitivity analysis by intensity for the disability outcome, after excluding the study of Moticone et al. (2013/2014), Figure S13: Forest plot for the pain outcome all studies included, Figure S14: Forest plot for the disability outcome all studies included, Figure S15: Forest plot for the return to work outcome all studies included, Figure S16: Forest plot for the quality of life outcome all studies included, Figure S17: Forest plot for the depression outcome all studies included, Figure S18: Forest plot for the anxiety outcome all studies included, Figure S19: The relative odds ratios (RORs) and 95% confidence intervals (CIs) for each outcome at short term of a short-length treatment vs. long-length treatment. The RORs were calculated with a fixed-effect model. A ROR >1 favours long length; a ROR <1 favours short length, Figure S20: The relative odds ratios (RORs) and 95% confidence intervals (CIs) for each outcome at short term of a non-daily contact vs. daily contact. The RORs were calculated with a fixed-effect model. A ROR >1 favours daily contact; a ROR <1 favours non-daily contact, Figure S21: The relative odds ratios (RORs) and 95% confidence intervals (CIs) for each outcome at short term of a low intensity vs. high intensity. The RORs were calculated with a fixed-effect model. A ROR >1 favours high intensity (i.e., >30 h per week); a ROR <1 favours low intensity (i.e., <30 h per week), Figure S22: The relative odds ratios (RORs) and 95% confidence intervals (CIs) for each outcome at short term of a short-length treatment vs. long-length treatment, after excluding the study of Moticone et al. (2013/2014). The RORs were calculated with a random-effects model. A ROR >1 favours long length; a ROR <1 favours short length, Figure S23: The relative odds ratios (RORs) and 95% confidence intervals (CIs) for each outcome at short term of a non-daily contact vs. daily contact, after excluding the study of Moticone et al. (2013/2014). The RORs were calculated with a random-effects model. A ROR >1 favours daily contact; a

ROR <1 favours non-daily contact, Figure S24: The relative odds ratios (RORs) and 95% confidence intervals (CIs) for each outcome at short term of a low intensity vs. high intensity, after excluding the study of Moticone et al. (2013/2014). The RORs were calculated with a random-effects model. A ROR >1 favours high intensity (i.e., >30 h per week); a ROR <1 favours low intensity (i.e., <30 h per week), Table S1: Risk of bias (RoB) according to the Cochrane Back Review Group criteria, Table S2: Results of the meta-regression analyses of potential moderators of the six examined outcomes, Table S3: Checklist summarizing compliance with PRISMA guidelines, Box S1: Search details in PubMed, Box S2: References of included RCTs.

Author Contributions: E.D. and B.G. had the idea for the project, and E.D. primarily designed the study, which was discussed and finally approved by all authors. E.D. and M.B. extracted the data and E.D. ran the analysis. All authors wrote the first draft and commented on different versions of the paper. All authors approved the final version of the paper. The corresponding author had final responsibility for the decision to submit for publication.

Conflicts of Interest: The authors declare no conflicts of interest.

References

1. Saragiotto, B.T.; de Almeida, M.O.; Yamato, T.P.; Maher, C.G. Multidisciplinary biopsychosocial rehabilitation for nonspecific chronic low back pain. *Phys. Ther.* **2016**, *96*, 759–763. [CrossRef] [PubMed]
2. Kamper, S.J.; Apeldoorn, A.T.; Chiarotto, A.; Smeets, R.J.; Ostelo, R.W.; Guzman, J.; van Tulder, M.W. Multidisciplinary biopsychosocial rehabilitation for chronic low back pain. *Cochrane Database Syst. Rev.* **2014**, *9*, CD000963. [CrossRef] [PubMed]
3. Kamper, S.J.; Apeldoorn, A.T.; Chiarotto, A.; Smeets, R.J.; Ostelo, R.W.; Guzman, J.; van Tulder, M.W. Multidisciplinary biopsychosocial rehabilitation for chronic low back pain: Cochrane systematic review and meta-analysis. *BMJ* **2015**, *350*, h444. [CrossRef] [PubMed]
4. Guzman, J.; Esmail, R.; Karjalainen, K.; Malmivaara, A.; Irvin, E.; Bombardier, C. Multidisciplinary bio-psycho-social rehabilitation for chronic low back pain. *Cochrane Database Syst. Rev.* **2002**, *1*, CD000963.
5. Dragioti, E.; Evangelou, E.; Larsson, B.; Gerdle, B. Effectiveness of multidisciplinary programmes for clinical pain conditions: An umbrella review. *J. Rehabil. Med.* **2018**, *50*, 779–791. [CrossRef] [PubMed]
6. Scascighini, L.; Toma, V.; Dober-Spielmann, S.; Sprott, H. Multidisciplinary treatment for chronic pain: A systematic review of interventions and outcomes. *Rheumatology (Oxford)* **2008**, *47*, 670–678. [CrossRef]
7. Lambeek, L.C.; van Tulder, M.W.; Swinkels, I.C.; Koppes, L.L.; Anema, J.R.; van Mechelen, W. The trend in total cost of back pain in The Netherlands in the period 2002 to 2007. *Spine (Phila. Pa. 1976)* **2011**, *36*, 1050–1058. [CrossRef] [PubMed]
8. Reneman, M.F.; Waterschoot, F.P.C.; Bennen, E.; Schiphorst Preuper, H.R.; Dijkstra, P.U.; Geertzen, J.H.B. Dosage of pain rehabilitation programs: A qualitative study from patient and professionals' perspectives. *BMC Musculoskelet. Disord.* **2018**, *19*, 206. [CrossRef]
9. Reneman, M.F.; Waterschoot, F.P.C.; Burgerhof, J.G.M.; Geertzen, J.H.B.; Schiphorst Preuper, H.R.; Dijkstra, P.U. Dosage of pain rehabilitation programmes for patients with chronic musculoskeletal pain: A non-inferiority randomised controlled trial. *Disabil. Rehabil.* **2018**, *18*, 1–8. [CrossRef]
10. Waterschoot, F.P.; Dijkstra, P.U.; Geertzen, J.H.; Reneman, M.F. Dose or content? Effectiveness of pain rehabilitation programs for patients with chronic low back pain: A systematic review. Aurthor reply. *Pain* **2014**, *155*, 1902–1903. [CrossRef]
11. Chen, J.J. Outpatient pain rehabilitation programs. *Iowa Orthop. J.* **2006**, *26*, 102–106. [PubMed]
12. Kaiser, U.; Treede, R.D.; Sabatowski, R. Multimodal pain therapy in chronic noncancer pain-gold standard or need for further clarification? *Pain* **2017**, *158*, 1853–1859. [CrossRef]
13. Moher, D.; Liberati, A.; Tetzlaff, J.; Altman, D.G.; Group, P. Preferred reporting items for systematic reviews and meta-analyses: the PRISMA statement. *PLoS Med.* **2009**, *6*, e1000097. [CrossRef]
14. Liberati, A.; Altman, D.G.; Tetzlaff, J.; Mulrow, C.; Gotzsche, P.C.; Ioannidis, J.P.; Clarke, M.; Devereaux, P.J.; Kleijnen, J.; Moher, D. The PRISMA statement for reporting systematic reviews and meta-analyses of studies that evaluate health care interventions: Explanation and elaboration. *J. Clin. Epidemiol.* **2009**, *62*, e1–e34. [CrossRef] [PubMed]
15. Furlan, A.D.; Pennick, V.; Bombardier, C.; van Tulder, M.; Editorial Board, Cochrane Back Review Group. 2009 updated method guidelines for systematic reviews in the Cochrane Back Review Group. *Spine (Phila. Pa. 1976)* **2009**, *15*, 1929–1941. [CrossRef] [PubMed]
16. DerSimonian, R.; Laird, N. Meta-analysis in clinical trials. *Control Clin. Trials* **1986**, *7*, 177–188. [CrossRef]

17. Higgins, J.P.; Thompson, S.G.; Deeks, J.J.; Altman, D.G. Measuring inconsistency in meta-analyses. *BMJ* **2003**, *327*, 557–560. [CrossRef]
18. Higgins, J.P.; Thompson, S.G. Quantifying heterogeneity in a meta-analysis. *Stat. Med.* **2002**, *21*, 1539–1558. [CrossRef]
19. Egger, M.; Davey Smith, G.; Schneider, M.; Minder, C. Bias in meta-analysis detected by a simple, graphical test. *BMJ* **1997**, *315*, 629–634. [CrossRef]
20. Thompson, S.G.; Higgins, J.P. How should meta-regression analyses be undertaken and interpreted? *Stat. Med.* **2002**, *21*, 1559–1573. [CrossRef]
21. Sterne, J.A.; Juni, P.; Schulz, K.F.; Altman, D.G.; Bartlett, C.; Egger, M. Statistical methods for assessing the influence of study characteristics on treatment effects in 'meta-epidemiological' research. *Stat. Med.* **2002**, *21*, 1513–1524. [CrossRef]
22. Dragioti, E.; Dimoliatis, I.; Fountoulakis, K.N.; Evangelou, E. A systematic appraisal of allegiance effect in randomized controlled trials of psychotherapy. *Ann. Gen. Psychiatry* **2015**, *14*, 25. [CrossRef]
23. Evangelou, E.; Tsianos, G.; Ioannidis, J.P. Doctors' versus patients' global assessments of treatment effectiveness: Empirical survey of diverse treatments in clinical trials. *BMJ* **2008**, *336*, 1287–1290. [CrossRef] [PubMed]
24. Chinn, S. A simple method for converting an odds ratio to effect size for use in meta-analysis. *Stat. Med.* **2000**, *19*, 3127–3131. [CrossRef]
25. Altman, D.G.; Egger, M.; Smith, G.D. *Systematic Reviews in Health Care: Meta-Analysis in Context*, 2nd ed.; BMJ Publishing Group: London, UK, 2001.
26. Henschke, N.; Maher, C.G.; Refshauge, K.M.; Herbert, R.D.; Cumming, R.G.; Bleasel, J.; York, J.; Das, A.; McAuley, J.H. Prognosis in patients with recent onset low back pain in Australian primary care: Inception cohort study. *BMJ* **2008**, *337*, a171. [CrossRef] [PubMed]
27. Maetzel, A.; Li, L. The economic burden of low back pain: A review of studies published between 1996 and 2001. *Best Pract. Res. Clin. Rheumatol.* **2002**, *16*, 23–30. [CrossRef]
28. Vos, T.; Flaxman, A.D.; Naghavi, M.; Lozano, R.; Michaud, C.; Ezzati, M.; Shibuya, K.; Salomon, J.A.; Abdalla, S.; Aboyans, V.; et al. Years lived with disability (YLDs) for 1160 sequelae of 289 diseases and injuries 1990–2010: A systematic analysis for the Global Burden of Disease Study 2010. *Lancet* **2012**, *380*, 2163–2196. [CrossRef]
29. Oliveira, C.B.; Maher, C.G.; Pinto, R.Z.; Traeger, A.C.; Lin, C.C.; Chenot, J.F.; van Tulder, M.; Koes, B.W. Clinical practice guidelines for the management of non-specific low back pain in primary care: An updated overview. *Eur. Spine J.* **2018**, *27*, 2791–2803. [CrossRef]

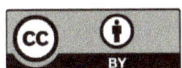

© 2019 by the authors. Licensee MDPI, Basel, Switzerland. This article is an open access article distributed under the terms and conditions of the Creative Commons Attribution (CC BY) license (http://creativecommons.org/licenses/by/4.0/).

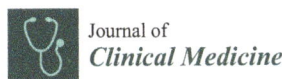

Review

The Evolving Case Supporting Individualised Physiotherapy for Low Back Pain

Jon Ford [1,2,*], Andrew Hahne [1], Luke Surkitt [2], Alexander Chan [2] and Matthew Richards [2]

1 School of Allied Health, La Trobe University, Kingsbury Drive, Bundoora 3086, Australia
2 Advance Healthcare, 157 Scoresby Road, Boronia 3155, Australia
* Correspondence: J.Ford@latrobe.edu.au

Received: 19 August 2019; Accepted: 22 August 2019; Published: 28 August 2019

Abstract: Low-back pain (LBP) is one of the most burdensome health problems in the world. Guidelines recommend simple treatments such as advice that may result in suboptimal outcomes, particularly when applied to people with complex biopsychosocial barriers to recovery. Individualised physiotherapy has the potential of being more effective for people with LBP; however, there is limited evidence supporting this approach. A series of studies supporting the mechanisms underpinning and effectiveness of the Specific Treatment of Problems of the Spine (STOPS) approach to individualised physiotherapy have been published. The clinical and research implications of these findings are presented and discussed. Treatment based on the STOPS approach should also be considered as an approach to individualised physiotherapy in people with LBP.

Keywords: low-back pain; physiotherapy; individualisation

1. Introduction

Low-back pain (LBP) is recognised as a common and costly problem in the Western world, with a global prevalence of 0.5 billion, the highest ranking cause of years lived with disability contributing 57·6 million years [1], and an increase in prevalence and disease burden of nearly 20% over the last 10 years [2]. People with LBP have historically been described as having a favourable natural history [3]; however, systematic reviews of primary care studies show that 28%–79% of people with acute LBP experience persistent or recurrent symptoms at 12 months [4,5]. Higher rates are supported by one large general population study which is likely to be a more accurate measure of persistency/recurrence than samples recruited from primary care settings [6].

Syntheses of clinical guidelines suggest international consensus in recommending initial exclusion of red flags and radiculopathy, and subsequent management of LBP as a "non-specific" condition on the basis that a nociceptive cause of symptoms cannot be identified [7–9]. Guideline-based treatment (Table 1) aims to minimise potential harm of treatments such as surgery or medication and maximise cost-effectiveness by utilising simple treatments such as advice [10,11]. However, the randomised controlled trials (RCTs) upon which guideline recommendations are based typically show small effect sizes of questionable clinical importance [8,9,12].

A potential reason for the limited effects demonstrated in RCTs on LBP is a false assumption that non-specific LBP is a homogeneous group. It has been postulated that multiple subgroups exist within the non-specific LBP population that are likely to respond differently to generic treatment [13]. In such circumstances, a false assumption of sample homogeneity in RCTs may lead to a treatment being inappropriately applied, resulting in either failure to respond or exacerbation of the condition. Based on this understanding, identifying valid subgroups for the purposes of an RCT has been described as a high research priority [14,15]. Meaningful subgroups enable treatment to be individualised to the patient presentation, potentially increasing the size of the effect [16]. An example of the value of individualised treatment is the management of inflammation in people with LBP. Guidelines suggest that non-steroidal anti-inflammatory drugs (NSAIDs) have small and short-term positive effects for LBP [8], yet these recommendations are based on RCTs selecting people with non-specific LBP. It is unlikely that every patient in this population has LBP with inflammatory processes as a contributing factor. It is, therefore, plausible that RCTs sampling populations with a greater likelihood of an inflammatory component to their LBP would show larger effects.

Table 1. Overview of interventions endorsed for non-specific low-back pain in evidence-based clinical practice guidelines (adapted from Foster et al. 2018) [9].

	Acute LBP (<6 weeks)	Persistent LBP (>12 weeks)
First line care	Advice Education	Advice Education Exercise CBT
Second line or adjunctive care	NSAIDs Superficial heat Manual therapy Massage Acupuncture	NSAIDs Selective norepinephrine reuptake inhibitors Manual therapy Acupuncture Yoga Mindfulness Interdisciplinary rehabilitation Discectomy or laminectomy for disc herniation with associated radiculopathy
Limited use in selected patients	Opioids Skeletal muscle relaxants Exercise CBT	Opioids Epidural injection
Not recommended	Paracetamol Systemic glucocorticoids Epidural injection	Paracetamol Systemic glucocorticoids
Insufficient evidence	Mindfulness Interdisciplinary rehabilitation Selective norepinephrine reuptake inhibitors Antiseizure medication Any surgery	Superficial heat Skeletal muscle relaxants

CBT = cognitive behavioural therapy, NSAIDs = non-steroidal anti-inflammatory drugs.

The argument for the importance of individualised treatment is further strengthened by considering the multi-dimensional nature of LBP. Clinical guidelines for LBP [9], the World Health Organisation's International Classification of Functioning, Disability and Health [17] and internationally accepted standards on clinical reasoning [18] all emphasise multiple factors that are relevant for the management of LBP including the pathoanatomical (e.g., nociceptive source of symptoms), psychosocial (e.g., fear avoidance), neurophysiological (e.g., central sensitisation and neuropathic pain) and genetic dimensions. The complexity of LBP is also reflected in the wide range of subgrouping approaches reported in systematic and narrative reviews [13,19–21]. Given the multidimensional and complex nature of LBP, it is almost axiomatic that a "one size fits all" approach to treatment provision in RCTs is likely to yield suboptimal results [13].

Based on the scale of the LBP problem, the limited data on treatment effectiveness, and the potential value of individualised treatment, the aim of this paper was to overview the evidence on individualised physiotherapy, including a contextualised presentation and discussion of a series of studies on the Specific Treatment of Problems of the Spine (STOPS) approach.

2. The Evidence on Individualised Physiotherapy for Low-Back Pain

A search on the evidence supporting individualised physiotherapy for LBP was conducted on PubMed using the Boolean term OR for individ*, subgroup*, classif* AND back pain AND "review" in the title. Reference lists of the retrieved papers, as well as recent clinical guidelines [7–9], were also checked for relevant evidence. A total of 546 citations were identified from PubMed, with 12 being deemed relevant for this overview.

Individualising treatment for LBP has been identified as a high research priority by a series of international expert panels [14,15] and a methodological framework for future research suggested [19,22]. However, research investigating the large number of heterogenous approaches for individualising treatment are of variable methodological quality [20,23–27]. Individualising physiotherapy based on movement is recommended in a professional guideline [28] but is not supported by recent clinical trials [29]. The STarT Back approach to individualising physiotherapy has been extensively researched in different contexts [30–42], and is recommended in clinical guidelines based on cost effectiveness [8,9]. However, the STarT Back approach only confers small clinical effects on activity limitation, and no long-term effects on pain compared to usual care [33].

Given the limited evidence supporting attempts to develop effective individualised physiotherapy approaches for LBP, exploration of alternative methods has merit.

3. A Series of Studies Supporting Individualised Physiotherapy for Low-Back Pain

The STOPS trial was a randomised controlled trial ($n = 300$) published in 2016 that concluded individualised physiotherapy was more effective than guideline-based advice for early persistent LBP [43]. This trial was part of a series of studies that will be overviewed to inform a discussion on the STOPS approach to individualised physiotherapy for LBP.

3.1. Prognosis in Identifying Potential Targets for Individualised Physiotherapy

Identification of prognostic factors can improve clinical decision making, understanding of disease processes, definitions of risk groups, and prediction of clinical outcomes [44]. Prognostic factors can also assist in identifying treatment targets to improve the effectiveness of individualised treatment [45,46]. Exploring and identifying gaps in the prognostic literature for LBP has been recommended as a research priority [47].

Prognostic studies and systematic reviews on LBP commonly evaluate specific prognostic factors [47,48] such as psychosocial distress [49–52], clinical features [53–56] and physical activity [57]. We are unaware of any high-quality studies evaluating a comprehensive range of biomedical (including pathoanatomical), psychological and social prognostic factors using multivariate methods in a large sample of people with LBP [46,58,59].

We, therefore, conducted a study that aimed to develop a multivariate prognostic model for back pain, leg pain and activity limitation in patients with LBP based on a comprehensive range of commonly used prognostic factors reflective of the biopsychosocial model of health [60]. Following univariate analyses of a range of variables from 300 participants in the STOPS trial, 58 variables progressed to multivariate analysis (Table A1). Five indicators of positive outcome (belonging to either the reducible discogenic pain or disc herniation with associated radiculopathy subgroups, below waist paraesthesia, walking as an easing factor and low transversus abdominis tone) and 10 indicators of negative outcome (both parents born overseas, deep leg symptoms, higher sick leave duration on the Örebro Musculoskeletal Pain Questionnaire [61], high multifidus tone, clinically determined inflammation [62,63], higher back and leg pain severity, lower Oswestry Disability Index [64] lifting capacity, lower capacity for light work (Örebro item) and higher Pain Drawing [65] scores based on percentage body chart coverage) were identified (Table 2).

Table 2. Back related healthcare utilization and costs per patient.

Resource	Resource Use: Units/Patient (SD), % of Patients Utilizing		Cost/Patient (SD) in US$		
	IP	Advice	IP	Advice	Between-Group Cost Difference (95% CI) *
Study physiotherapy	8.9 (2.1), 100%	1.8 (2.4), 99%	379.35 (87.10)	81.93 (18.46)	**297.72 (282.85 to 312.01)**
Medical consultations	1.7 (5.3), 32%	2.0 (4.2), 40%	86.95 (280.78)	110.55 (238.03)	−23.61 (−85.61 to 38.40)
Medical intervention Surgery (discectomy) Injections	0.01 (0.08), 0.7% 0.1 (0.3), 3.4%	0.02 (0.12), 1.5% 0.1 (0.5), 7.7	35.81 (434.18) 5.87 (36.32)	80.99 (650.40) 13.82 (56.10)	−45.18 (−174.68 to 84.32) −7.95 (−19.01 to 3.10)
Allied health consultations	3.3 (6.3), 38.8%	7.9 (12.3), 60.8%	152.38 (292.15)	324.47 (480.14)	**−172.09 (−264.94 to −79.25)**
Medication	57.0%	54.6%	59.87 (140.54)	85.60 (207.93)	−25.73 (−69.16 to 17.69)
Total Healthcare cost (95%CI)			782.82 (623.82 to 941.82)	755.79 (592.84 to 918.75)	27.03 (−200.29 to 254.35)
Work absence: Mean (95%CI), %	10.8 (4.6 to 17.1) days, 36%	20.5 (13.3 to 27.6) days, 44%	$1889.16 (680.86 to 3097.46)	$3884.67 (2497.22 to 5272.12)	**$ −1995.51 (−3847.03 to −143.98)**

IP = individualised physiotherapy; SD = standard deviation; *, Between-group comparisons analysed via linear mixed models, with positive values representing a higher cost in the individualised physiotherapy group relative to the advice group, significant between-group differences in bold.

Researchers and clinical practice guidelines [66] have suggested that biomedical factors are less relevant in the management of non-specific LBP and few studies have identified biomedical or physical factors of prognostic value [67]. However biomedical factors are commonly used by clinicians in decision making [68]. In our study, nine of the 15 prognostic factors related primarily to pathoanatomical mechanisms. In addition, previously reported psychosocial predictors such as depression, fear avoidance and recovery expectations were not prognostic when analysed in a multi-variate model of a comprehensive range of prognostic factors. These results provide support for the validity of the STOPS approach of individualised treatment based on a range of biomedical, psychological and social factors.

3.2. Development of an Individualised Physiotherapy Treatment Program

Identifying subgroups of different types of LBP is one way of individualising physiotherapy, and treatment targeting specific features or causal mechanisms underpinning the nature of the subgroup has the potential of being more effective in RCTs [13,16]. However, developing a LBP subgrouping system is challenging and the review literature shows that a wide array of approaches exist [13,19–21,25–27,29,69–72]. Historically, subgrouping systems have been developed by experts combining the best available evidence with their own clinical experience [73–77]. More recently, a standardised approach to subgroup development used in the medical domain [78] has been extrapolated to LBP [19,79] involving: initial evaluation of assessment methods of potential utility for subgrouping, hypothesis setting studies using a range of methodologies, a priori hypothesis testing studies and a series of further validation stages including analysis of impact of the subgrouping system on routine care (Figure 1). A key component of the hypothesis generation, hypothesis testing and subgroup validation studies is evaluation of treatment effect modifiers within a RCT. Treatment effect modifier studies aim to assess whether the effect of a treatment (relative to a comparison treatment) is different in people with certain characteristics (which are of potential use in defining a subgroup), compared to those without [80]. However, to be adequately powered treatment effect modifiers studies need to be around four times larger than studies investigating overall treatment effect [81,82]. Given the complexity of LBP, a relatively large number of variables require exploration for relevance to subgrouping, which further increases the necessary sample size in treatment effect modifier studies [83]. These issues mean that treatment effect modifier RCTs, with the associated high costs, are of questionable feasibility, particularly in certain research funding contexts such as Australia [71,84,85].

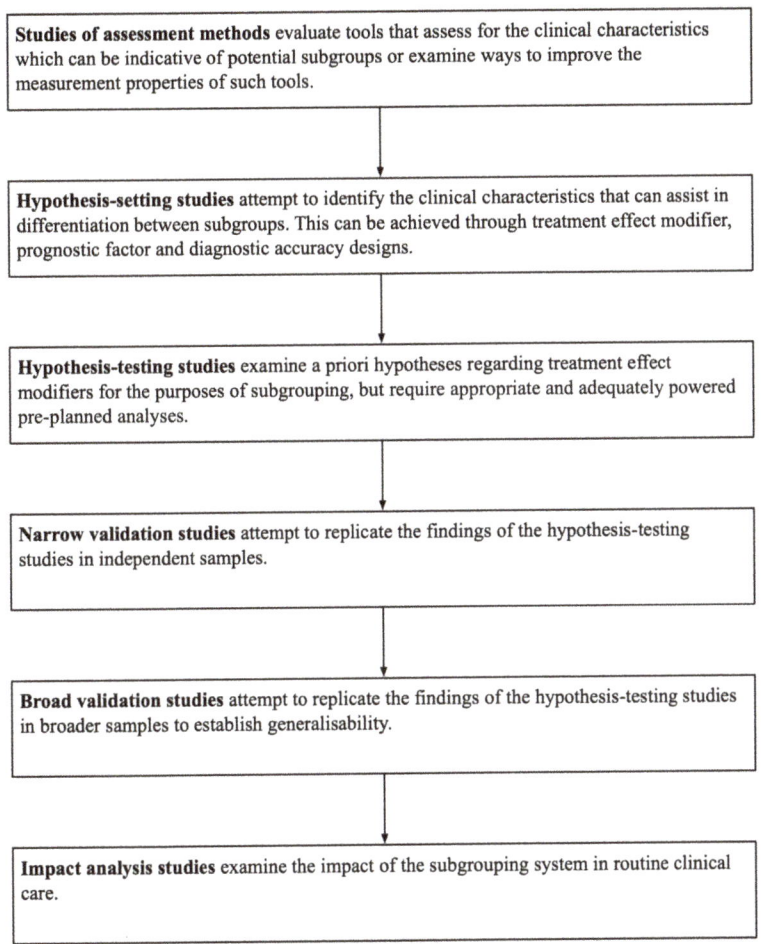

Figure 1. Conceptual phases of subgrouping research (adapted from Kent et al [19]).

A range of methodologies other than treatment effect modifiers can be used in the hypothesis setting stage of subgroup development, although each approach has significant limitations. Studies evaluating the diagnostic accuracy of different subgroup features/clinical measures are limited by the absence of suitable reference standards [7]. Commonly used reference standards such as imaging, discography and diagnostic blocks have all demonstrated significant false positives due, at least in part, to the complexity of LBP including psychosocial and neurophysiological influences [86]. Despite growing popularity [87] and defined methodological rigour, 'data driven' analyses for identifying and developing subgroups also have significant limitations. Statistical processes can result in artificial subgroups [88] of limited clinical use and/or meaningfulness [20,21,83] and a degree of judgement is required in undertaking the analyses with the potential for bias [20,88–90].

Contemporary methodologies for the development and validation of subgrouping systems work well in certain medical contexts to allow greater individualisation of treatment [78]. Yet, as described above, extrapolation of these principles to the complex domain of LBP has limited feasibility and methodological shortcomings. An alternative approach is the principle of "convergence of validity" described as when " ... evidence supporting or refuting the (subgrouping) system (is) gathered from different sources and from the use of different methods. In the best case scenario, these sources converge and indicate similar meanings of the underlying constructs being studied." [91] (p. 312). Implicit in this approach is an acceptance of the limitations of all research designs in relation to subgroup development.

As an alternative subgrouping strategy, convergence of validity is consistent with the original definitions of evidence-based practice that emphasise the constructive interaction between the research literature and clinical perspectives [92]. It also aligns with expert recommendations from the field of epidemiology [93] and mirrors the approach taken in other complex medical domains such as the classification of headache [94] and non-Hodgkin's lymphoma [95].

In essence, a convergence of validity approach is the equivalent to the hypothesis setting phase where a range of research methodologies are considered in developing a subgrouping system. In applying a convergence of validity approach, it is accepted that the complete validation of such a system, particularly through repeated treatment effect modifier studies, is not likely to be feasible. Yet this limitation in achieving full validation should not prohibit the use of the subgrouping system in other research designs, such as RCTs, provided the limitations of system validity are acknowledged.

Four papers [83,96–98] have been published in relation to the STOPS trial justifying and outlining detailed individualised treatment protocols on the basis of convergence of validity supporting five subgroups. This process has been further supported by two expert panels [99,100] and five systematic reviews [20,101–104]. Four of the subgroups were primarily based on clinical features indicative of a pathoanatomical diagnosis of the LBP and comprised: reducible discogenic pain, zygapophyseal joint pain, non-reducible discogenic pain, and disc herniation with associated radiculopathy. A fifth subgroup (multi-factorial persistent pain) captured people without a clear pathoanatomical classification along with likely psychosocial contributors to their delayed recovery as measured on the Örebro Musculoskeletal Pain Questionnaire [61].

Participants with reducible discogenic pain were prescribed a home program based on mechanical loading strategies that led to improvement or centralisation of symptoms. This included repeated/sustained movement exercises, a walking program, taping and postural advice [83]. Participants with zygapophysial joint dysfunction received targeted manual therapy comprising unilateral mobilisation ± manipulation applied with a rigorous clinical reasoning approach [96]. All participants apart from those in the MFP group received motor-control training targeting local muscles such as transversus abdominus leading into a pain contingent graded functional exercise program [96]. This was the primary treatment for participants with disc herniation with associated radiculopathy or non-reducible discogenic pain. Those with multifactorial persistent pain received physiotherapy focusing on psychosocial and neurophysiological rather than pathoanatomical mechanisms [98]. Progression of functional exercise in this subgroup was time-contingent, and cognitive restructuring/behavioural strategies were used targeting key barriers identified on the Örebro Musculoskeletal Pain Questionnaire.

Although subgroup membership determined the primary treatment approach, a range of other treatment components were also provided depending on identification of other pathoanatomical, psychosocial or neurophysiological barriers to recovery. All participants receiving individualised physiotherapy engaged in an explanation/discussion regarding: the nature/source of their symptoms, treatment options available outside of the RCT and timeframes for recovery. Participants also worked with the trial physiotherapists on goal setting, cognitive restructuring of counterproductive beliefs, behavioural strategies to support and reinforce the education program, as well as modifying unproductive behaviours and discharge planning. A range of optional treatment components were provided including: pain management strategies (pharmacological and non-pharmacological), management of inflammation in participants with a clinically determined inflammatory component to their pain, management of work issues, sleep strategies, relaxation and dealing with increases in pain (flare-ups). In participants failing to improve with a pathoanatomical approach initially, the trial physiotherapist determined whether transfer to the MFP treatment protocol was required. These treatment strategies were all applied in a manner individualised to the participant's presentation as determined by the trial physiotherapist.

3.3. Effectiveness of Individualised Physiotherapy

Based on the above-described research, the STOPS trial aimed to evaluate the effectiveness of individualised physiotherapy compared to guideline-based advice. Advice regarding prognosis and resuming normal activities is recommended in all clinical guidelines for people with LBP of over 6-weeks duration [8]. Prior to our clinical trials, there had been few published RCTs evaluating the effectiveness of individualised physiotherapy compared to guideline-based advice.

Other recent subgrouping approaches based on risk stratification such as STarT Back [33] and physical examination findings (i.e., movement patterns) do not address pathoanatomical factors despite this approach being common in clinical practice and the convergence of evidence that it may be important in clinical decision making for LBP [16,83,96–98].

Using the STOPS individualised physiotherapy protocol including manual therapy, directional preference management, postural re-education, motor control training, and graded functional exercise [83,96–98] we evaluated the effectiveness of individualised physiotherapy compared to guideline-based advice for 300 participants with early persistent LBP (6-weeks to 6-months duration) [43].

Results (Figure 2) showed that individualised physiotherapy was more effective than advice in improving activity limitation (at 10, 26 and 52-weeks) as well as back pain and leg pain (at 5, 10 and 26-weeks). Between-group mean differences were statistically significant in 71% of the primary and secondary outcomes measured in the trial. Participants receiving individualised physiotherapy took 5-8 weeks to achieve the same pain rating as those receiving advice at 12 months indicating a more rapid rate of recovery. Satisfaction with individualised treatment was high, and 92.3% of individualised physiotherapy participants completed the intervention. Based on contemporary definitions, these results are clinically important [105,106].

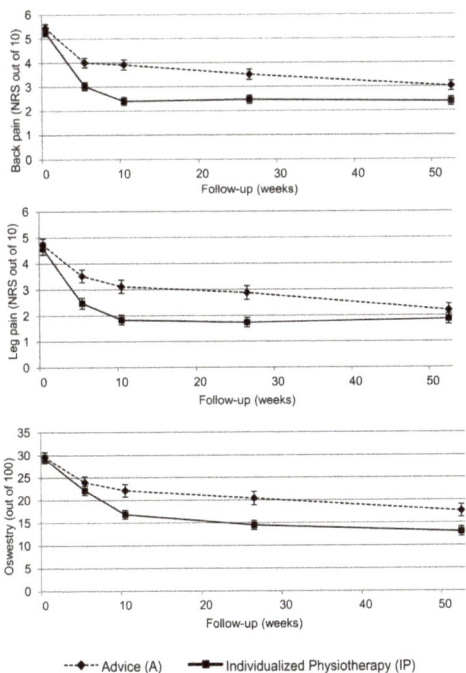

Figure 2. Group mean scores (error bars indicate standard errors) for primary outcomes at baseline and 5-, 10-, 26- and 52-week follow-up in the STOPS Trial (adapted from Ford et al. [43], permission admitted).

3.4. Cost-Effectiveness of Individualised Physiotherapy

Direct healthcare costs attributable to people with LBP in Western countries seeking healthcare is estimated at billions of dollars annually [107,108] and is predicted to rise [109,110]. Treatments that improve clinical outcomes such as pain and activity at a sustainable cost are urgently needed [111].

Guideline-based advice is a low-cost treatment that is commonly prescribed by medical practitioners [112] and physiotherapists [113]. However, low cost does not necessarily correspond to cost-effectiveness when treatment effects and all relevant costs (healthcare and other) are considered. There is insufficient evidence regarding the cost-effectiveness of advice for LBP according to one systematic review [111].

The STOPS trial showed that individualised physiotherapy was clinically more effective than guideline-based advice [43]. Given the treatment cost of delivering individualised physiotherapy (10 sessions) was higher than advice (2 sessions), consideration is required as to whether the larger effects were worth the additional cost. We therefore investigated the cost-effectiveness of individualised physiotherapy versus advice in people with LBP enrolled in the STOPS trial [114].

The results showed that total health care costs were similar for both groups despite individualised physiotherapy being more expensive than guideline-based advice (Table 2). This was due to 61% of participants receiving advice seeking further non-medical treatment outside the trial compared to 39% of participants receiving individualised physiotherapy (Table 2). Health benefits favoured individualised physiotherapy over advice (incremental Quality Adjusted Life Years = 0.06 (95%CI: 0.02 to 0.10)). Cost-effectiveness was established by the achievement of an Incremental Cost Effectiveness ratio of $US 422 per quality adjusted life year gained [114]. In addition, lower work absence across the 12-month follow-up resulted in income savings of $US 1995 (95%CI: 144 to 3847) per working participant in the individualised physiotherapy group compared to the advice group (Table 2).

3.5. Who Benefits Most from Individualised Physiotherapy Versus Advice?

Treatment effect modifier studies are helpful for determining characteristics of patients who respond best to a particular treatment relative to another in an RCT [19]. The STOPS treatment effect modifier study investigated several patient characteristics identified a priori and listed on the trial register [115] based on the hypothesis that participants with more severe, persistent or complex LBP would derive the largest benefits from individualised physiotherapy relative to advice. This hypothesis was supported by the results showing that participants with higher back pain intensity, higher Örebro scores (indicative of higher risk of persistent pain) or longer duration of symptoms derived the largest benefits from individualised physiotherapy relative to advice. These findings are of particular importance because the presence of these characteristics has been associated with a worse prognosis as well as higher treatment and societal costs [107,116,117]. Targeting individualised physiotherapy towards these higher risk groups may, therefore, result in even stronger treatment effectiveness and cost-effectiveness than those reported for the whole sample involved in the STOPS trial.

4. Discussion

Research into individualised physiotherapy is a high research priority that has, to date, yielded disappointing results in RCTs. The series of studies described in this paper support the development and validity of the STOPS subgrouping approach. In addition, three studies on the effectiveness, cost-effectiveness and treatment effect modifiers provide further support for the individualised treatment of LBP using the STOPS approach. We are unaware of any similar body of research on the utility of individualised physiotherapy based on a comprehensive biopsychosocial-based treatment model. There are a range of possible factors that may have contributed to the above-described results.

4.1. The Definition of Clinical Importance

Most RCTs on LBP demonstrating statistically significant results show small effects of questionable clinical importance [8,9]. However, the traditional definition of clinical importance based on the minimal clinically important difference (MCID) has been questioned given it was developed for use on individuals rather than group data and may not be appropriate for people with lower severity symptoms [105,118]. Authoritative contemporary guidelines recommend determining clinical importance using multiple methods of analysis including consistency of results across multiple primary and secondary outcome measures, risks/benefits of the treatments, consideration of the population being sampled, and the proportion of individual patients who demonstrate change in outcome measures in excess of the MCID *in addition* to between-group differences in mean scores [106,119,120].

The STOPS trial did not demonstrate clinically important between-group mean differences based on the MCID. However, in accordance with our a priori statistical plan [121], a primary outcome responder analysis was conducted. This analysis showed that participants receiving individualised physiotherapy had 1.8 and 1.6 times the chance of improving by at least 50% from baseline on back and leg pain, respectively, at the 10-week follow-up compared with those receiving advice alone. By 52 weeks, those having individualised physiotherapy also had 1.5 times the chance of improving by 50% from baseline on the Oswestry Disability Questionnaire compared with those receiving advice. All secondary outcomes favoured individualised physiotherapy, with the exception of work interference, but the cost-effectiveness study showed significantly lower work absence (and associated lost income) in the individualised physiotherapy group. In the secondary-outcomes responder analysis, participants receiving individualised physiotherapy had 1.3–4.1 times the chance of achieving a clinically important change compared with those receiving advice. Participant satisfaction was significantly greater and non-medical co-interventions significantly lower in the individualised physiotherapy group. All between-group comparisons should be interpreted in the context of large *within-group* improvements on all primary outcomes for both treatment groups [33]. Given the population sampled were ≥6-weeks post-injury where spontaneous recovery is limited [4,5], it is likely that both treatments were helpful, with individualised physiotherapy conferring additional benefits over and above advice. There were no serious adverse events in either group and with detailed published clinical protocols available, the STOPS approach to LBP is potentially accessible worldwide without extensive training common to other individualised physiotherapy approaches [33,122].

The clinical importance of the between-group differences as a measure of significance in the STOPS trial is further strengthened by the cost-effectiveness analysis. Results showed an incremental cost-effectiveness ratio (ICER) of US$422 per quality-adjusted life year (QALY), which compares favourably to other relevant RCTs in the field. Cognitive behavioural therapy is recommended in all clinical guidelines for LBP [8,9], but has an ICER of US$2773 per QALY gained for group cognitive behavioural therapy along with advice versus advice alone [123]. In another relevant RCT [124] five sessions of physiotherapy were not cost-effective compared with one session of advice as there were no significant differences in health outcomes. These data further support the clinical importance of the STOPS trial results by way of cost-effectiveness compared to guideline-based advice.

Another potential indicator of clinical importance from RCTs is the proportion of participants who complete the intervention. High drop-out rates in clinical trials may indicate that the intervention is not acceptable to participants on the basis of ineffectiveness, patient preferences, the required commitment to comply with treatment, or side-effects. Drop-out rates exceeding 15% have been reported for multiple LBP trials of graded activity [125], anticonvulsants [126], and in one trial of individualised physiotherapy [122]. The individualised physiotherapy group in the STOPS trial had a 7.7% drop-out rate, suggesting that the treatment was acceptable for most participants and giving further support to the clinical importance of the STOPS trial results.

4.2. Comparison Group Selection and Advice

When designing and interpreting RCTs, it is important for the researcher and consumer to carefully consider the comparison group. Common trial designs in LBP use no treatment, placebo treatment, advice, usual medical care or various types of physiotherapy interventions. There is no right or wrong approach to designing a comparison group in an RCT; it simply informs the hypothesis being tested. For example, a RCT comparing manual therapy to placebo manual therapy is designed to test the specific effect of manual therapy independent of any non-specific effects such as patient expectations, learning/conditioning effects and neurophysiological effects [127].

It is worth reflecting on the use of guideline-based advice in designing a RCT. Advice to stay active and reassurance regarding prognosis is recommended as first-line treatment in all clinical guidelines for acute and persistent LBP as described in Table 1 [9]. The evidence directly supporting the effectiveness and cost-effectiveness of guideline-based advice is sparse [111,128–130]. Nevertheless, it has been asserted that this treatment is just as effective as more costly and complex treatments [10,11]. Although not commonly used as the sole treatment approach by practitioners in the field [131], guideline-based advice is being advocated strongly as first line treatment ahead of other physiotherapeutic treatments such as manual therapy as well as medical treatments such as NSAIDs [8,9,131,132]. Given the low-quality evidence supporting guideline-based advice, it is possible that this approach is counterproductive, particularly if second-line treatments are more effective without being prohibitively more expensive. On this basis, guideline-based advice is an important comparison group in a RCT evaluating the effectiveness of commonly used second-line treatments (Table 1).

4.3. Use of a Pathoanatomical Approach

A major difference between the STOPS trial and the majority of the LBP research was the incorporation of pathoanatomical factors into the subgrouping approach and pathoanatomical-based decision making in the clinical protocol. Definitive criteria for pathoanatomical-based diagnosis and/or clinical decision making in LBP are not available [8]. It has been suggested that further research into and clinicians hypothesising about pathoanatomical barriers to recovery is likely to be at best, futile and, at worst, counterproductive to patient outcomes [66,133,134]. However, there is sparse evidence supporting this contention [16] and a pathoanatomical approach is common in clinical practice [68]. In addition, although there are likely to be benefits from addressing exercise/activity, lifestyle and psychosocial factors, the prognostic and treatment effects are small [134]. On this basis, it does not seem sensible to abandon clinical and research-based hypothesising on the role of pathoanatomy unless compelling evidence to do so is provided. Guideline-based advice is not informed by pathoanatomy and the mechanisms of effect are likely to be non-specific. As such, it is possible that a reason for the significant between-group differences in the STOPS trial was that assessment and treatment incorporated hypothesised pathoanatomical diagnoses and related clinical decision making. This premise was supported by the prevalence of pathoanatomical factors in the STOPS prognostic study and the convergence of results from a range of other research designs [83,96–98].

One example of this approach is the STOPS protocol, where treatment was individualised based on the hypothesised presence or absence of an inflammatory component to the LBP. The lumbar intervertebral disc is a biologically plausible contributor to LBP [135]. The mechanisms underpinning the symptoms of disc related pain and activity limitation are unclear, however substantial evidence exists supporting the role of inflammation in disc degeneration and disc herniation with associated radiculopathy (DHR) [136,137]. Studies investigating the composition and structure of lumbar discs have shown fibrosis, vascular invasion, inflammatory granulation tissue formation and extensive innervation along fissures in the posterior annulus fibrosis in painful degenerative discs and around symptomatic nerve roots. Such changes are not observed in non-painful degenerative or herniated discs [138,139].

Further evidence on the presence of and potential importance of inflammatory processes in degenerative discs and DHR [140] can be seen in disc tissue histologically [141–145], in the disc tissue using other inflammatory markers [146–151] and as measured by serum biomarkers in people with LBP [152]. A recent study showed that high serum tumour necrosis factor in acute LBP predicted poor recovery of pain and activity limitation at 6-months, providing further evidence of the relevance of inflammation [153].

Significant evidence suggests that inflammatory processes are a potential treatment target in clinical trials [136,137,154–156], particularly in people who may have discogenic pain [141–145]. Clinical features of inflammatory back pain such as spondyloarthropathy have been validated using practitioner surveys, expert panels and diagnostic accuracy studies [63,157–160]. These features include age <40 years, insidious onset, improvement with exercise, no improvement with rest and pain at night with improvement upon getting up from bed [161]. These results are similar to studies on the clinical features of disc related LBP and associated inflammation [144,145,147].

Although systematic reviews and guidelines suggest that NSAIDs are only a second-line treatment option for the management of LBP (Table 1), the literature above suggests that management of inflammatory processes might be more effective if targeted to individuals with clinical symptoms indicative of inflammation, particularly with a combination of pharmacological and other relevant management strategies. The clinical features suggestive of the presence of inflammation informed clinical decision making in the STOPS trial regarding when to implement anti-inflammatory treatment such as medication, taping, postural management and gentle walking. The identification of an inflammatory component was also important where inflammation may have hindered the effectiveness of mechanically based treatment approaches such as exercise, manual therapy or directional preference management [162,163]. The STOPS trial was unique in identifying clinically determined inflammation as a reason for exercising caution with mechanical treatment and simultaneously, treating inflammatory problems using anti-inflammatory treatment. The guideline-based advice comparison treatment gave no consideration to the role of inflammation. Therefore, clinical decision making based on the possible presence/absence of inflammation may have been a factor contributing to the significant between-group differences. This premise is further supported by the significance of clinically determined inflammation identified in the STOPS prognosis study.

4.4. Treatment Fidelity in Randomised Controlled Trials

Methods to maximise treatment fidelity in RCTs for physiotherapy interventions are highly variable and often poorly reported [164–169]. The STOPS trial employed a range of evidence-based methods [170] to enhance treatment fidelity including: specification regarding the treatment program design (140 page clinical manual with full detail on all aspects of individualised treatment); 16 hours of standardised practitioner training; review of practitioner treatment and practitioner feedback during the RCT (by way of study researchers reviewing the clinical notes followed by verbal feedback and group-based monthly case reviews); and evaluation of the participant's perspective/understanding of the treatment provided (qualitative exit interviews). Participants also completed exercise diaries that were checked by the physiotherapist at each visit. Similar methods were put in place with the advice treatment program. Given the relative complexity of the individualised physiotherapy, it is plausible that the treatment fidelity program would have had greater impact on patient outcomes in the individualised physiotherapy group. This could, therefore, have been an additional factor for the significant between-group differences observed in the STOPS trial.

4.5. The Importance of Motor Control

Motor control retraining focusing on posture, movement and muscle activation was a significant component of individualised physiotherapy for all participants apart from those in the multifactorial persistent pain (MFP) subgroup. The relevance and effectiveness of this approach is contentious [171] and there are significant inconsistencies in systematic review results [172–174]. Nevertheless, as the advice group did not receive motor control training this treatment component could have been responsible in part for the significant between-group effects. This premise is supported by the significance of suboptimal motor control identified in the STOPS prognosis study as well as the biological plausibility and potential pathoanatomical relevance of optimising motor control in people with LBP [175–178].

5. Clinical Implications

The clinical implications of the research presented in this paper are potentially substantial but need to be contextualised within an evidence-based framework. In order to make strong recommendations to practitioners, the findings need to be replicated in independent samples and/or systematic reviews updated to incorporate the relevant data into meta-analyses. However, the significance and consistency of the results are sufficient to challenge some of the common perceptions around evidence-based practice for LBP.

Guidelines routinely state that the vast majority of LBP patients should be considered as a non-specific condition where consideration of pathoanatomy is not possible or necessary [8,9]. Some guidelines go so far as to state that clinical decision making based on pathoanatomy may be harmful [66] despite sparse data to support this assertion. The results presented in this paper support the notion that hypothesising on and clinical decision making with regard to pathoanatomical considerations cannot be discounted and may lead to superior outcomes compared to a less targeted approach.

There is sparse data supporting the effectiveness of simple guideline-based advice. It is of interest that the RCT with the largest effect sizes in favour of advice incorporated a pathoanatomical explanation [179]. Despite this, advice in the absence of a pathoanatomical explanation is being recommended as first-line treatment for LBP of any duration [8,9]. The series of studies described in this paper suggest that further consideration and evaluation of guideline-based advice as a first-line treatment is required.

The generalisability of the STOPS trial results should be superior to most recent RCTs on individualised physiotherapy, where only a few experienced practitioners were used [122] and/or detailed clinical protocols were not published [33,122]. The treatment used in the STOPS trial was provided by physiotherapists with a range of experience, none of whom had a post-graduate qualification. It encompassed the most commonly used methods by physiotherapists [113,180,181] however the published treatment protocols have the potential to improve the quality of existing standards in clinical practice due to the detailed explanations and clinical decision making processes provided.

On the basis of the STOPS trial, practitioners can provide their patients with an average timeframe for expected treatment outcomes when receiving individualised physiotherapy. Patients are likely to experience rapid reductions in back/leg pain in the first 10 weeks of treatment, but optimal improvements in activity limitation are likely to take longer. Patients will also be reassured regarding the cost-effectiveness of the treatment, particularly with regards to minimising time off work.

6. Future Research

The results of this series of studies should be highly impactful on future research. Much of the research in LBP develop study designs, eligibility criteria, prognostic factors or treatment protocols that are relatively simplistic in nature. Whilst this approach renders research projects more feasible and potentially more methodologically rigorous, it does not reflect the real-world complexity of LBP and the associated treatment options that are likely to be most effective.

A pathoanatomical approach should be considered when planning future clinical research within the context of a truly biopsychosocial model for LBP.

More research is required on the relative importance of different components of individualised physiotherapy. Individualised physiotherapy also needs to be compared to other comparison groups and on different populations, particularly persistent LBP where more entrenched psychosocial and neurophysiological barriers to recovery are likely to be relevant.

Researchers should be encouraged by the clinical importance of the results in the STOPS trial and be emboldened to develop ambitious research hypotheses based on an in-depth understanding of both clinical and research perspectives.

Greater rigour should be applied to the development of clinical guidelines to ensure that low-quality evidence such as the sparse data and questionable cost-effectiveness supporting simple advice is acknowledged.

Researchers should follow the lead of the STOPS trial in providing detailed clinical protocols that are feely available in full-text. Such an approach would greatly accelerate the dissemination of evidence-based information to practitioners in the field and substantially improve external validity.

7. Conclusions

LBP is the most burdensome health problem in the world. Prior to the publication of the studies in this body of research, there was limited evidence for the effectiveness of individualised physiotherapy and a focus in clinical guidelines on advice as first-line treatment for LBP. Our series of studies challenge the role of advice alone in early persistent pain and suggests that the concept of non-specific LBP needs to be reconsidered. Furthermore, there are now detailed clinical protocols and quality evidence to support the STOPS approach to individualised physiotherapy in clinical practice and future research studies.

Author Contributions: Conceptualization, J.F. and A.H.; methodology, J.F., A.H., L.S., A.C. and M.R.; formal analysis, A.H. and J.F.; data curation, J.F., A.H., L.S., A.C. and M.R.; writing—original draft preparation, J.F. and A.H.; writing—review and editing, J.F., A.H., L.S., A.C. and M.R.; supervision, J.F.; project administration, J.F., A.H., L.S., A.C. and M.R.; funding acquisition, J.F.

Funding: Elements of the original research summarized in this review were supported by LifeCare Health, who provided facilities, personnel and resources to allow treatment of participants free of charge in the STOPS Trial.

Acknowledgments: We wish to acknowledge the physiotherapists who treated participants in the STOPS Trial free of charge.

Conflicts of Interest: The authors declare no conflict of interest LifeCare Health had no role in the design of the study; in the collection, analyses, or interpretation of data; in the writing of the manuscript, or in the decision to publish the results.

Appendix A

Table A1. Prognostic factors for Oswestry, back pain and leg pain obtained from the multivariate model.

Prognostic factor	Oswestry (0–100)			Back Pain (0–10)			Leg Pain (0–10)		
	N	B Coefficient (95% CI)	p-value	N	B Coefficient (95% CI)	p-value	N	B Coefficient (95% CI)	p-value
Intercept		−0.2 (−14.4 to 13.9)	0.975		0.0 (−1.962 to 2.019)	0.977		−2.0 (−4.3 to 0.4)	0.095
Subgroup									
Disc herniation/radiculopathy *	54	−1.3 (−5.0 to 2.3)	0.473 +	54	−0.6 (−1.2 to −0.1)	0.029 +	54	−0.3 (−0.9 to 0.3)	0.312 +
Reducible discogenic pain *	78	−3.2 (−5.9 to −0.6)	0.017 +	78	−0.9 (−1.3 to −0.4)	<0.001 +	70	−0.7 (−1.2 to −0.2)	0.005 +
Manual therapy group *	64	−2.6 (−5.5 to 0.3)	0.082 +	64	−0.5 (−1.0 to 0.0)	0.050 +	49	−0.2 (−0.7 to 0.4)	0.560 +
Multifactorial persistent pain *	8	−1.3 (−7.8 to 5.1)	0.683 +	8	0.2 (−0.5 to 0.8)	0.647	7	−0.2 (−1.4 to 0.9)	0.725 +
Parents born overseas									
Both born overseas #	165	3.4 (1.1 to 5.7)	0.004	165	0.6 (0.2 to 0.9)	0.003	141	0.5 (0.1 to 0.9)	0.026
One born overseas #	21	0.7 (−3.7 to 5.1)	0.761	21	0.2 (−0.4 to 0.8)	0.570	18	0.1 (−0.5 to 0.8)	0.723
Paresthesia below waist	134	−3.3 (−6.0 to −0.6)	0.016 +	134	−0.1 (−0.5 to 0.3)	0.607 +	125	−0.2 (−0.6 to 0.3)	0.498 +
Deep leg symptoms	145	2.5 (0.0 to 4.9)	0.053	145	0.2 (−0.2 to 0.6)	0.286	145	0.6 (0.2 to 1.0)	0.002
Walking eases symptoms	160	−2.0 (−4.2 to 0.2)	0.073 +	160	−0.5 (−0.9 to −0.2)	0.005 +	138	−0.2 (−0.6 to 0.2)	0.273 +
Lateral flexion limited by pain	116	1.0 (−1.3 to 3.4)	0.382	116	0.1 (−0.3 to 0.5)	0.536	106	0.4 (0.0 to 0.8)	0.055
Transversus abdominis low tone	109	−3.0 (−5.3 to −0.7)	0.012 +	109	−0.8 (−1.1 to −0.4)	<0.001 +	91	−0.4 (−0.9 to 0.0)	0.051
Multifidus high tone	60	2.0 (−1.2 to 5.1)	0.215	60	0.0 (−0.4 to 0.5)	0.918	47	0.7 (0.1 to 1.4)	0.019
Clinical inflammation	182	1.1 (−1.1 to 3.3)	0.342	182	0.4 (0.1 to 0.8)	0.020	165	−0.2 (−0.6 to −0.2)	0.311 +
Back pain severity	300	0.2 (−0.5 to 0.8)	0.556	300	0.3 (0.2 to 0.4)	<0.001	261	0.1 (0.0 to 0.2)	0.245
Leg pain severity	300	0.1 (−0.5 to 0.6)	0.764	300	0.0 (−0.1 to 0.1)	0.896	261	0.3 (0.2 to 0.4)	<0.001
Örebro sick leave duration (0–10)	300	1.1 (0.4 to 1.7)	0.002	300	0.1 (0.0 to 0.2)	0.112	261	0.1 (0.0 to 0.2)	0.219

*, relative to "non-reducible discogenic pain"; #, relative to "both parents born in Australia"; +, Positive prognostic indicator. Results are independent of time point, significant p-values in bold. Negative B-coefficients represent lower outcome scores and therefore a better outcome at follow-up in participants with the listed prognostic factor. Predicted outcome for a given patient can be calculated by applying the patient's score on each baseline factor to the B-coefficients, and adding the scores from each item together (including the intercept).

References

1. Global Burden of Disease 2016 Disease and Injury Incidence and Prevalence Collaborators. Global, regional, and national incidence, prevalence, and years lived with disability for 328 diseases and injuries for 195 countries, 1990–2016: A systematic analysis for the Global Burden of Disease Study 2016. *Lancet* **2017**, *390*, 1211–1259. [CrossRef]
2. Hurwitz, E.L.; Randhawa, K.; Yu, H.; Cote, P.; Haldeman, S. The Global Spine Care Initiative: a summary of the global burden of low back and neck pain studies. *Eur. Spine J.* **2018**, *27*, 796–801. [CrossRef] [PubMed]
3. Waddell, G. A new clinical model for the treatment of low back pain. *Spine* **1987**, *12*, 632–654. [CrossRef] [PubMed]
4. Itz, C.J.; Geurts, J.W.; van Kleef, M.; Nelemans, P. Clinical course of non-specific low back pain: a systematic review of prospective cohort studies set in primary care. *Eur. J. Pain* **2013**, *17*, 5–15. [CrossRef] [PubMed]
5. Costa, L.M.; Maher, C.G.; Hancock, M.J.; McAuley, J.H.; Herbert, R.D.; Costa, L.O. The prognosis of acute and persistent low-back pain: a meta-analysis. *CMAJ* **2012**, *184*, E613–E624. [CrossRef]
6. Vasseljen, O.; Woodhouse, A.; Bjorngaard, J.H.; Leivseth, L. Natural course of acute neck and low back pain in the general population: The HUNT study. *Pain* **2013**, *154*, 1237–1244. [CrossRef] [PubMed]
7. Hartvigsen, J.; Hancock, M.J.; Kongsted, A.; Louw, Q.; Ferreira, M.L.; Genevay, S.; Hoy, D.; Karppinen, J.; Pransky, G.; Sieper, J.; et al. What low back pain is and why we need to pay attention. *Lancet* **2018**, *391*, 2356–2367. [CrossRef]
8. Oliveira, C.B.; Maher, C.G.; Pinto, R.Z.; Traeger, A.C.; Lin, C.C.; Chenot, J.F.; van Tulder, M.; Koes, B.W. Clinical practice guidelines for the management of non-specific low back pain in primary care: An updated overview. *Eur. Spine J.* **2018**, *27*, 2791–2803. [CrossRef]
9. Foster, N.E.; Anema, J.R.; Cherkin, D.; Chou, R.; Cohen, S.P.; Gross, D.P.; Ferreira, P.H.; Fritz, J.M.; Koes, B.W.; Peul, W.; et al. Prevention and treatment of low back pain: Evidence, challenges, and promising directions. *Lancet* **2018**, *391*, 2368–2383. [CrossRef]
10. Michaleff, Z.A.; Maher, C.G.; Lin, C.W.; Rebbeck, T.; Jull, G.; Latimer, J.; Connelly, L.; Sterling, M. Comprehensive physiotherapy exercise programme or advice for chronic whiplash (PROMISE): A pragmatic randomised controlled trial. *Lancet* **2014**, *384*, 133–141. [CrossRef]
11. Machado, L.A.; Maher, C.G.; Herbert, R.D.; Clare, H.; McAuley, J.H. The effectiveness of the McKenzie method in addition to first-line care for acute low back pain: A randomized controlled trial. *BMC Med.* **2010**, *8*, 10. [CrossRef] [PubMed]
12. O'Keeffe, M.; Purtill, H.; Kennedy, N.; Conneely, M.; Hurley, J.; O'Sullivan, P.; Dankaerts, W.; O'Sullivan, K. Comparative Effectiveness of Conservative Interventions for Nonspecific Chronic Spinal Pain: Physical, Behavioral/Psychologically Informed, or Combined? A Systematic Review and Meta-Analysis. *J. Pain* **2016**, *17*, 755–774. [CrossRef] [PubMed]
13. Ford, J.J.; Hahne, A.J. Complexity in the physiotherapy management of low back disorders: Clinical and research implications. *Man. Ther.* **2013**, *18*, 438–442. [CrossRef] [PubMed]
14. Foster, N.E.; Dziedzic, K.S.; Windt, D.; Fritz, J.M.; Hay, E.M. Research priorities for non-pharmacological therapies for common musculoskeletal problems: Nationally and internationally agreed recommendations. *BMC Muscul. Disord.* **2009**, *10*, 3. [CrossRef] [PubMed]
15. Costa, L.; Koes, B.; Pransky, G.; Borkan, J.; Maher, C.; Smeets, R. Primary care research priorities in low back pain: An update. *Spine* **2013**, *38*, 148–156. [CrossRef] [PubMed]
16. Ford, J.J.; Hahne, A.J. Pathoanatomy and classification of low back disorders. *Man. Ther.* **2013**, *18*, 165–168. [CrossRef] [PubMed]
17. World Health Organization. *International Classification of Functioning, Disability and Health: ICF*; World Health Organization: Geneva, Switzerland, 2001.
18. Jones, M. Clinical reasoning: From the Maitland Concept and beyond. In *Maitland's Vertebral Manipulation. Management of Neuromusculoskeletal Disorders*, 8th ed.; Elsevier: Edinburgh, UK, 2014; pp. 14–54.
19. Kent, P.; Keating, J.L.; Leboeuf-Yde, C. Research methods for subgrouping low back pain. *BMC Med. Res. Methodol.* **2010**, *10*, 62. [CrossRef]
20. Ford, J.; Story, I.; O'Sullivan, P.; McMeeken, J. Classification systems for low back pain: A review of the methodology for development and validation. *Physical Therapy Rev.* **2007**, *12*, 33–42. [CrossRef]

21. Karayannis, N.; Jull, G.; Hodges, P. Physiotherapy movement based classification approaches to low back pain: comparison of subgroups through review and developer/expert survey. *BMC Muscull Disord.* **2012**, *13*, 24. [CrossRef]
22. Kent, P.; Hancock, M.; Petersen, D.H.; Mjosund, H.L. Clinimetrics corner: choosing appropriate study designs for particular questions about treatment subgroups. *J. Manipulative Physiol. Ther.* **2010**, *18*, 147–152. [CrossRef]
23. Fairbank, J.; Gwilym, S.E.; France, J.C.; Daffner, S.D.; Dettori, J.; Hermsmeyer, J.; Andersson, G. The role of classification of chronic low back pain. *Spine* **2011**, *36*, 19–42. [CrossRef] [PubMed]
24. Stynes, S.; Konstantinou, K.; Dunn, K.M. Classification of patients with low back-related leg pain: A systematic review. *BMC Muscul. Disord.* **2016**, *17*, 226. [CrossRef] [PubMed]
25. Saragiotto, B.T.; Maher, C.G.; Moseley, A.M.; Yamato, T.P.; Koes, B.W.; Sun, X.; Hancock, M.J. A systematic review reveals that the credibility of subgroup claims in low back pain trials was low. *J. Clin. Epidemiology* **2016**, *79*, 3–9. [CrossRef] [PubMed]
26. Kent, P.; Mjosund, H.L.; Petersen, D.H. Does targeting manual therapy and/or exercise improve patient outcomes in nonspecific low back pain? A systematic review. *BMC Med.* **2010**, *8*, 22. [CrossRef] [PubMed]
27. Kent, P.; Kjaer, P. The efficacy of targeted interventions for modifiable psychosocial risk factors of persistent nonspecific low back pain—A systematic review. *Man. Ther.* **2012**, *17*, 385–401. [CrossRef] [PubMed]
28. American Physical Therapy Association. Guide to physical therapy practice 3.0. In *Guide to Physical Therapist Practice 3.0*; APTA: Alexandria, Egypt, 2014.
29. Riley, S.P.; Swanson, B.T.; Dyer, E. Are movement-based classification systems more effective than therapeutic exercise or guideline based care in improving outcomes for patients with chronic low back pain? A systematic review. *J. Manual Manipulative Therapy* **2019**, *27*, 5–14. [CrossRef] [PubMed]
30. Hill, J.C.; Dunn, K.M.; Main, C.J.; Hay, E.M. Subgrouping low back pain: A comparison of the STarT Back Tool with the Orebro Musculoskeletal Pain Screening Questionnaire. *Eur. J. Pain* **2010**, *14*, 83–89. [CrossRef]
31. Hill, J.C.; Vohora, K.; Dunn, K.M.; Main, C.J.; Hay, E.M. Comparing the STarT back screening tool's subgroup allocation of individual patients with that of independent clinical experts. *Clin. J. Pain* **2010**, *26*, 783–787. [CrossRef]
32. Fritz, J.M.; Beneciuk, J.M.; George, S.Z. Relationship between categorization with the STarT Back Screening Tool and prognosis for people receiving physical therapy for low back pain. *Phys. Ther.* **2011**, *91*, 722–732. [CrossRef]
33. Hill, J.C.; Whitehurst, D.G.; Lewis, M.; Bryan, S.; Dunn, K.M.; Foster, N.E.; Konstantinou, K.; Main, C.J.; Mason, E.; Somerville, S.; et al. Comparison of stratified primary care management for low back pain with current best practice (STarT Back): A randomised controlled trial. *Lancet* **2011**, *378*, 1560–1571. [CrossRef]
34. Main, C.J.; Sowden, G.; Hill, J.C.; Watson, P.J.; Hay, E.M. Integrating physical and psychological approaches to treatment in low back pain: The development and content of the STarT Back trial's 'high-risk' intervention (STarT Back; ISRCTN 37113406). *Physiotherapy* **2012**, *98*, 110–116. [CrossRef] [PubMed]
35. Morso, L.; Kent, P.; Manniche, C.; Albert, H.B. The predictive ability of the STarT Back Screening Tool in a Danish secondary care setting. *Eur. Spine J.* **2013**, *23*, 120–128. [CrossRef] [PubMed]
36. Hill, J.C.; Afolabi, E.K.; Lewis, M.; Dunn, K.M.; Roddy, E.; van der Windt, D.A.; Foster, N.E. Does a modified STarT Back Tool predict outcome with a broader group of musculoskeletal patients than back pain? A secondary analysis of cohort data. *BMJ Open* **2016**, *6*, e012445. [CrossRef] [PubMed]
37. Mansell, G.; Hill, J.C.; Main, C.; Vowles, K.E.; van der Windt, D. Exploring what factors mediate treatment effect: Example of the STarT Back study high-risk intervention. *J. Pain* **2016**, *17*, 1237–1245. [CrossRef] [PubMed]
38. Morso, L.; Kongsted, A.; Hestbaek, L.; Kent, P. The prognostic ability of the STarT Back Tool was affected by episode duration. *Eur. Spine J.* **2016**, *25*, 936–944. [CrossRef] [PubMed]
39. Bier, J.D.; Sandee-Geurts, J.J.W.; Ostelo, R.; Koes, B.W.; Verhagen, A.P. Can primary care for back and/or neck pain in the Netherlands benefit from stratification for risk groups according to the STarT Back Tool-classification? *Arch. Phys. Med. Rehabil.* **2017**, *99*, 65–71. [CrossRef] [PubMed]
40. Magel, J.; Fritz, J.M.; Greene, T.; Kjaer, P.; Marcus, R.L.; Brennan, G.P. Outcomes of Patients With Acute Low Back Pain Stratified by the STarT Back Screening Tool: Secondary Analysis of a Randomized Trial. *Phys. Ther.* **2017**, *97*, 330–337. [CrossRef] [PubMed]

41. Suri, P.; Delaney, K.; Rundell, S.D.; Cherkin, D.C. Predictive Validity of the STarT Back Tool for Risk of Persistent Disabling Back Pain in a U.S. Primary Care Setting. *Arch. Phys. Med. Rehabil.* **2018**, *99*, 1533–1539. [CrossRef]
42. Rabey, M.; Kendell, M.; Godden, C.; Liburd, J.; Netley, H.; O'Shaughnessy, C.; O'Sullivan, P.; Smith, A.; Beales, D. STarT Back Tool risk stratification is associated with changes in movement profile and sensory discrimination in low back pain: A study of 290 patients. *Eur. J. Pain* **2019**, *23*, 823–834. [CrossRef]
43. Ford, J.J.; Hahne, A.J.; Surkitt, L.D.; Chan, A.Y.; Richards, M.C.; Slater, S.L.; Hinman, R.S.; Pizzari, T.; Davidson, M.; Taylor, N.F. Individualised physiotherapy as an adjunct to guideline-based advice for low back disorders in primary care: A randomised controlled trial. *Br. J. Sports Med.* **2016**, *50*, 237–245. [CrossRef]
44. Verkerk, K.; Luijsterburg, P.A.; Miedema, H.S.; Pool-Goudzwaard, A.; Koes, B.W. Prognostic factors for recovery in chronic nonspecific low back pain: A systematic review. *Phys. Ther.* **2012**, *92*, 1093–1108. [CrossRef] [PubMed]
45. Pincus, T.; Burton, A.K.; Vogel, S.; Field, A.P. A systematic review of psychological factors as predictors of chronicity/disability in prospective cohorts of low back pain. *Spine* **2002**, *5*, E109–E120. [CrossRef] [PubMed]
46. Ashworth, J.; Konstantinou, K.; Dunn, K.M. Prognostic factors in non-surgically treated sciatica: A systematic review. *BMC Muscul. Disord.* **2011**, *12*, 208. [CrossRef] [PubMed]
47. Hayden, J.A.; Chou, R.; Hogg-Johnson, S.; Bombardier, C. Systematic reviews of low back pain prognosis had variable methods and results: Guidance for future prognosis reviews. *J. Clin. Epidemiol.* **2009**, *62*, 781–796. [CrossRef] [PubMed]
48. Kent, P.; Keating, J. Can we predict poor recovery from recent-onset nonspecific low back pain? A systematic review. *Man. Ther.* **2008**, *13*, 12–28. [CrossRef] [PubMed]
49. Ramond, A.; Bouton, C.; Richard, I.; Roquelaure, Y.; Baufreton, C.; Legrand, E.; Huez, J.F. Psychosocial risk factors for chronic low back pain in primary care: A systematic review. *Fam. Pract.* **2011**, *28*, 12–21. [CrossRef] [PubMed]
50. Gray, H.; Adefolarin, A.T.; Howe, T.E. A systematic review of instruments for the assessment of work-related psychosocial factors (Blue Flags) in individuals with non-specific low back pain. *Man. Ther.* **2011**, *16*, 531–543. [CrossRef]
51. Iles, R.A.; Davidson, M.; Taylor, N.F. Psychosocial predictors of failure to return to work in non-chronic non-specific low back pain: A systematic review. *Occup. Environ. Med.* **2008**, *65*, 507–517. [CrossRef]
52. Hartvigsen, J.; Lings, S.; Leboeuf-Yde, C.; Bakketeig, L. Psychosocial factors at work in relation to low back pain and consequences of low back pain; a systematic, critical review of prospective cohort studies. *Occup. Environ. Med.* **2004**, *61*, e2.
53. Wong, A.Y.; Parent, E.C.; Funabashi, M.; Stanton, T.R.; Kawchuk, G.N. Do various baseline characteristics of transversus abdominis and lumbar multifidus predict clinical outcomes in non-specific low back pain? A systematic review. *Pain* **2013**, *154*, 2589–2602. [CrossRef]
54. Konstantinou, K.; Hider, S.L.; Jordan, J.L.; Lewis, M.; Dunn, K.M.; Hay, E.M. The Impact of Low Back-related Leg Pain on Outcomes as Compared With Low Back Pain Alone: A Systematic Review of the Literature. *Clin. J. Pain* **2013**, *29*, 644–654. [CrossRef] [PubMed]
55. Chorti, A.; Chortis, A.G.; Strimpakos, N.; McCarthy, C.J.; Lamb, S.E. The prognostic value of symptom responses in the conservative management of spinal pain: A systematic review. *Spine* **2009**, *34*, 2686–2699. [CrossRef] [PubMed]
56. Borge, J.; Leboeuf-Yde, C.; Lothe, J. Prognostic values of physical examination findings in patients with chronic low back pain treated conservatively: A systematic literature review. *J. Manipulative Physiol. Ther.* **2001**, *24*, 292–295. [CrossRef] [PubMed]
57. Hendrick, P.; Milosavljevic, S.; Hale, L.; Hurley, D.A.; McDonough, S.; Ryan, B.; Baxter, G.D. The relationship between physical activity and low back pain outcomes: A systematic review of observational studies. *Eur. Spine J.* **2011**, *20*, 464–474. [CrossRef] [PubMed]
58. Van Oort, L.; van den Berg, T.; Koes, B.W.; de Vet, R.H.; Anema, H.J.; Heymans, M.W.; Verhagen, A.P. Preliminary state of development of prediction models for primary care physical therapy: A systematic review. *J. Clin. Epidemiol.* **2012**, *65*, 1257–1266. [CrossRef]
59. Hilfiker, R.; Bachmann, L.M.; Heitz, C.A.; Lorenz, T.; Joronen, H.; Klipstein, A. Value of predictive instruments to determine persisting restriction of function in patients with subacute non-specific low back pain. Systematic review. *Eur. Spine J.* **2007**, *16*, 1755–1775. [CrossRef] [PubMed]

60. Ford, J.J.; Richards, M.C.; Surkitt, L.D.; Chan, A.Y.P.; Slater, S.L.; Taylor, N.F.; Hahne, A.J. Development of a Multivariate Prognostic Model for Pain and Activity Limitation in People With Low Back Disorders Receiving Physiotherapy. *Arch. Phys. Med. Rehabil.* **2018**, *99*, 2504–2512. [CrossRef]
61. Linton, S.; Boersma, K. Early identification of patients at risk of developing a persistent back problem: The predictive validity of the Örebro musculoskeletal pain questionnaire. *Clin. J. Pain* **2003**, *19*, 80–86. [CrossRef]
62. Walker, B.F.; Williamson, O.D. Mechanical or inflammatory low back pain. What are the potential signs and symptoms? *Man. Ther.* **2009**, *14*, 314–320. [CrossRef]
63. Keeling, S.O.; Majumdar, S.R.; Conner-Spady, B.; Battie, M.C.; Carroll, L.J.; Maksymowych, W.P. Preliminary validation of a self-reported screening questionnaire for inflammatory back pain. *J. Rheumatol.* **2012**, *39*, 822–829. [CrossRef]
64. Fairbank, J.C.; Pynsent, P.B. The Oswestry Disability Index. *Spine* **2000**, *25*, 2940–2952. [CrossRef] [PubMed]
65. Ransford, A.; Cairns, D.; Mooney, V. The pain drawing as an aid to the psychologic evaluation of patients with low-back pain. *Spine* **1976**, *1*, 127–134. [CrossRef]
66. Dagenais, S.; Tricco, A.C.; Haldeman, S. Synthesis of recommendations for the assessment and management of low back pain from recent clinical practice guidelines. *Spine J.* **2010**, *10*, 514–529. [CrossRef] [PubMed]
67. Hayden, J.A.; Dunn, K.M.; van der Windt, D.A.; Shaw, W.S. What is the prognosis of back pain? *Best Practice Res. Clin.l Rheumatol.* **2010**, *24*, 167–179. [CrossRef] [PubMed]
68. Kent, P.; Keating, J.L. Classification in non-specific low back pain: What methods do primary care clinicians currently use? *Spine* **2005**, *30*, 1433–1440. [CrossRef] [PubMed]
69. Haskins, R.; Rivett, D.A.; Osmotherly, P.G. Clinical prediction rules in the physiotherapy management of low back pain: A systematic review. *Man. Ther.* **2012**, *17*, 9–21. [CrossRef] [PubMed]
70. Patel, S.; Friede, T.; Froud, R.; Evans, D.W.; Underwood, M. Systematic review of randomized controlled trials of clinical prediction rules for physical therapy in low back pain. *Spine* **2013**, *38*, 762–769. [CrossRef]
71. Mistry, D.; Patel, S.; Hee, S.W.; Stallard, N.; Underwood, M. Evaluating the quality of subgroup analyses in randomized controlled trials of therapist-delivered interventions for nonspecific low back pain: A systematic review. *Spine* **2014**, *39*, 618–629. [CrossRef]
72. Haskins, R.; Osmotherly, P.G.; Rivett, D.A. Diagnostic clinical prediction rules for specific subtypes of low back pain: A systematic review. *J. Ortho. Sports Phys. Thera.* **2015**, *45*, 61–76. [CrossRef]
73. McKenzie, R.; May, S. *The Lumbar Spine: Mechanical Diagnosis and Therapy*, 2nd ed.; Orthopedic Physical Therapy Products: Waikanae, New Zealand, 2003.
74. Sahrmann, S. *Diagnosis and Treatment of Movement Impairment Syndromes*, 1st ed.; Mosby Inc: St Louis, MI, USA, 2002.
75. Petersen, T.; Laslett, M.; Thorsen, H.; Manniche, C.; Ekdahl, C.; Jacobsen, S. Diagnostic classification of non-specific low back pain. A new system integrating patho-anatomic and clinical categories. *Physiother. Theory Pract.* **2003**, *19*, 213–237. [CrossRef]
76. O'Sullivan, P. Lumbar segmental 'instability': Clinical presentation and specific stabilizing exercise management. *Man. Ther.* **2000**, *5*, 2–12. [CrossRef] [PubMed]
77. O'Sullivan, P. Diagnosis and classification of chronic low back pain disorders: Maladaptive movement and motor control impairments as underlying mechanism. *Man. Ther.* **2005**, *10*, 242–255. [CrossRef] [PubMed]
78. McGinn, T.; Guyatt, G.; Wyer, P.; Naylor, C.; Stiell, I.; Richardson, W. Users' guides to the medical literature XXII: How to use articles about clinical decision rules. *J. Am. Med. Assoc.* **2000**, *284*, 79–84. [CrossRef] [PubMed]
79. Kamper, S.J.; Maher, C.G.; Hancock, M.J.; Koes, B.W.; Croft, P.R.; Hay, E. Treatment-based subgroups of low back pain. A guide to appraisal of research studies and a summary of current evidence. *Best Practice Res. Clin. Rheumatology* **2010**, *24*, 181–191. [CrossRef] [PubMed]
80. Hancock, M.J.; Kjaer, P.; Korsholm, L.; Kent, P. Interpretation of subgroup effects in published trials. *Phys. Ther.* **2013**, *93*, 852–859. [CrossRef] [PubMed]
81. Hancock, M.; Herbert, R.D.; Maher, C.G. A guide to interpretation of studies investigating subgroups of responders to physical therapy interventions. *Phys. Ther.* **2009**, *89*, 698–704. [CrossRef] [PubMed]
82. Brookes, S.T.; Whitely, E.; Egger, M.; Smith, G.D.; Mulheran, P.A.; Peters, T.J. Subgroup analyses in randomized trials: Risks of subgroup-specific analyses; power and sample size for the interaction test. *J. Clin. Epidemiology* **2004**, *57*, 229–236. [CrossRef] [PubMed]

83. Ford, J.J.; Surkitt, L.D.; Hahne, A.J. A classification and treatment protocol for low back disorders. Part 2: directional preference management for reducible discogenic pain. *Physical Therapy Rev.* **2011**, *16*, 423–437. [CrossRef]
84. Gurung, T.; Ellard, D.R.; Mistry, D.; Patel, S.; Underwood, M. Identifying potential moderators for response to treatment in low back pain: A systematic review. *Physiotherapy* **2015**, *101*, 243–251. [CrossRef]
85. Maher, C.G. Natural course of acute neck and low back pain in the general population: The HUNT study. *Pain* **2013**, *154*, 1480–1481. [CrossRef]
86. Carragee, E.; Hannibal, M. Diagnostic evaluation of low back pain. *Orthop. Clin. North Am.* **2004**, *35*, 7–16. [CrossRef]
87. Stanton, T.; Hancock, M.; Maher, C.; Koes, B. Critical appraisal of clinical prediction rules that aim to optimize treatment selection for musculoskeletal conditions. *Phys. Ther.* **2010**, *90*, 843–854. [CrossRef] [PubMed]
88. Feinstein, A. Clinical biostatistics XIII: On homogeneity, taxonomy, and nosography. *Clin. Pharmacol. Ther.* **1972**, *13*, 114–129. [CrossRef] [PubMed]
89. Heinrich, I.; O'Hare, H.; Sweetman, B.; Anderson, J. Validation aspects of an empirically derived classification for "non-specific" low back pain. *Statistician* **1985**, *34*, 215–230. [CrossRef]
90. Klapow, J.; Slater, M.; Patterson, T.; Doctor, J.; Atkinson, J.; Garfin, S. An empirical evaluation of multidimensional clinical outcome in chronic low back pain patients. *Pain* **1993**, *55*, 107–118. [CrossRef]
91. George, S.; Delitto, A. Clinical examination variables discriminate among treatment-based classification groups: A study of construct validity in patients with acute low back pain. *Phys. Ther.* **2005**, *85*, 306–314.
92. Sackett, D.; Straus, S.; Richardson, W.; Rosenberg, W.; Haynes, R. *Evidence-Based Medicine*; Churchill Livingstone: London, UK, 2000.
93. Reitsma, J.B.; Rutjes, A.W.S.; Khan, K.S.; Coomarasamy, A.; Bossuyt, P.M. A review of solutions for diagnostic accuracy studies with an imperfect or missing reference standard. *J. Clin. Epidemiol.* **2009**, *62*, 797–806. [CrossRef] [PubMed]
94. International Headache Society. Headache Classification Committee of the International Headache Society (IHS) The International Classification of Headache Disorders, 3rd edition. *Cephalalgia* **2018**, *38*, 1–211. [CrossRef]
95. Swerdlow, S.H.; Campo, E.; Pileri, S.A.; Harris, N.L.; Stein, H.; Siebert, R.; Advani, R.; Ghielmini, M.; Salles, G.A.; Zelenetz, A.D.; et al. The 2016 revision of the World Health Organization classification of lymphoid neoplasms. *Blood* **2016**, *127*, 2375–2390. [CrossRef]
96. Ford, J.J.; Thompson, S.L.; Hahne, A.J. A classification and treatment protocol for low back disorders. Part 1: Specific manual therapy. *Physical Therapy Rev.* **2011**, *16*, 168–177. [CrossRef]
97. Ford, J.J.; Hahne, A.J.; Chan, A.Y.P.; Surkitt, L.D. A classification and treatment protocol for low back disorders. Part 3: functional restoration for intervertebral disc related disorders. *Physical Therapy Rev.* **2012**, *17*, 55–75. [CrossRef]
98. Ford, J.J.; Richards, M.J.; Hahne, A.J. A classification and treatment protocol for low back disorders. Part 4: Functional restoration for low back disorders associated with multifactorial persistent pain. *Physical Therapy Rev.* **2012**, *17*, 322–334. [CrossRef]
99. Wilde, V.; Ford, J.; McMeeken, J. Indicators of lumbar zygapophyseal joint pain: Survey of an expert panel with the Delphi Technique. *Phys. Ther.* **2007**, *87*, 1348–1361. [CrossRef] [PubMed]
100. Chan, A.Y.; Ford, J.J.; McMeeken, J.M.; Wilde, V.E. Preliminary evidence for the features of non-reducible discogenic low back pain: Survey of an international physiotherapy expert panel with the Delphi technique. *Physiotherapy* **2013**, *99*, 212–220. [CrossRef] [PubMed]
101. Hahne, A.J.; Ford, J.J.; McMeeken, J.M. Conservative management of lumbar disc herniation with associated radiculopathy: A systematic review. *Spine* **2010**, *35*, E488–E504. [CrossRef] [PubMed]
102. Richards, M.C.; Ford, J.J.; Slater, S.L.; Hahne, A.J.; Surkitt, L.D.; Davidson, M.; McMeeken, J.M. The effectiveness of physiotherapy functional restoration for post-acute low back pain: A systematic review. *Man. Ther.* **2012**, *18*, 4–25. [CrossRef] [PubMed]
103. Slater, S.L.; Ford, J.J.; Richards, M.C.; Taylor, N.F.; Surkitt, L.D.; Hahne, A.J. The effectiveness of sub-group specific manual therapy for low back pain: A systematic review. *Man. Ther.* **2012**, *17*, 201–212. [CrossRef] [PubMed]
104. Surkitt, L.D.; Ford, J.J.; Hahne, A.J.; Pizzari, T.; McMeeken, J.M. Efficacy of directional preference management for low back pain: a systematic review. *Phys. Ther.* **2012**, *92*, 652–665. [CrossRef] [PubMed]

105. Dworkin, R.H.; Turk, D.C.; McDermott, M.P.; Peirce-Sandner, S.; Burke, L.B.; Cowan, P.; Farrar, J.T.; Hertz, S.; Raja, S.N.; Rappaport, B.A.; et al. Interpreting the clinical importance of group differences in chronic pain clinical trials: IMMPACT recommendations. *Pain* **2009**, *146*, 238–244. [CrossRef] [PubMed]
106. Deyo, R.A.; Dworkin, S.F.; Amtmann, D.; Andersson, G.; Borenstein, D.; Carragee, E.; Carrino, J.; Chou, R.; Cook, K.; DeLitto, A.; et al. Report of the NIH Task Force on research standards for chronic low back pain. *J. Pain* **2014**, *15*, 569–585. [CrossRef] [PubMed]
107. Dagenais, S.; Caro, J.; Haldeman, S. A systematic review of low back pain cost of illness studies in the United States and internationally. *Spine J.* **2008**, *8*, 8–20. [CrossRef] [PubMed]
108. Maniadakis, N.; Gray, A. The economic burden of back pain in the UK. *Pain* **2000**, *84*, 95–103. [CrossRef]
109. Murray, C.J.; Vos, T.; Lozano, R.; Naghavi, M.; Flaxman, A.D.; Michaud, C.; Ezzati, M.; Shibuya, K.; Salomon, J.A.; Abdalla, S.; et al. Disability-adjusted life years (DALYs) for 291 diseases and injuries in 21 regions, 1990–2010: A systematic analysis for the Global Burden of Disease Study 2010. *Lancet* **2012**, *380*, 2197–2223. [CrossRef]
110. Hoy, D.; March, L.; Brooks, P.; Blyth, F.; Woolf, A.; Bain, C.; Williams, G.; Smith, E.; Vos, T.; Barendregt, J.; et al. The global burden of low back pain: estimates from the Global Burden of Disease 2010 study. *Ann. Rheum. Dis.* **2014**, *73*, 968–974. [CrossRef] [PubMed]
111. Lin, C.W.; Haas, M.; Maher, C.G.; Machado, L.A.; van Tulder, M.W. Cost-effectiveness of guideline-endorsed treatments for low back pain: A systematic review. *Eur. Spine J.* **2011**, *20*, 1024–1038. [CrossRef] [PubMed]
112. Britt, H.; Miller, G.C.; Henderson, J.; Bayram, C.; Valenti, L.; Harrison, C.; Charles, J.; Pan, Y.; Zhang, C.; Pollack, A.J.; et al. *General Practice Activity in Australia 2012–2013. General Practice Series No.33.*; Sydney University Press: Sydney, Austrilia, 2013.
113. Liddle, D.; Baxter, D.; Gracey, J. Physiotherapists' use of advice and exercise for the management of chronic low back pain: A national survey. *Man. Ther.* **2009**, *14*, 189–196. [CrossRef] [PubMed]
114. Hahne, A.J.; Ford, J.J.; Surkitt, L.D.; Richards, M.C.; Chan, A.Y.; Slater, S.L.; Taylor, N.F. Individualized Physical Therapy is Cost Effective Compared to Guideline-Based Advice for People with Low Back Disorders. *Spine* **2017**, *42*, E169–E176. [CrossRef] [PubMed]
115. Hahne, A.J.; Ford, J.J.; Richards, M.C.; Surkitt, L.D.; Chan, A.Y.P.; Slater, S.L.; Taylor, N.F. Who Benefits Most From Individualized Physiotherapy or Advice for Low Back Disorders? A Preplanned Effect Modifier Analysis of a Randomized Controlled Trial. *Spine* **2017**, *42*, E1215–E1224. [CrossRef]
116. Celestin, J.; Edwards, R.; Jamison, R. Pretreatment psychosocial variables as predictors of outcomes following lumbar surgery and spinal cord stimulation: A systematic review and literature synthesis. *Pain Med.* **2009**, *10*, 639–653. [CrossRef]
117. Hockings, R.L.; McAuley, J.H.; Maher, C.G. A systematic review of the predictive ability of the Orebro Musculoskeletal Pain Questionnaire. *Spine* **2008**, *33*, E494–E500. [CrossRef]
118. Ferreira, M.L.; Herbert, R.D. What does 'clinically important' really mean? *Aust. J. Physiother.* **2008**, *54*, 229–230. [CrossRef]
119. Guyatt, G.H.; Thorlund, K.; Oxman, A.D.; Walter, S.D.; Patrick, D.; Furukawa, T.A.; Johnston, B.C.; Karanicolas, P.; Akl, E.A.; Vist, G.; et al. GRADE guidelines: 13. Preparing summary of findings tables and evidence profiles-continuous outcomes. *J. Clin. Epidemiol.* **2013**, *66*, 173–183. [CrossRef] [PubMed]
120. Dworkin, R.H.; Turk, D.C.; Farrar, J.T.; Haythornthwaite, J.A.; Jensen, M.P.; Katz, N.P.; Kerns, R.D.; Stucki, G.; Allen, R.R.; Bellamy, N.; et al. Core outcome measures for chronic pain clinical trials: IMMPACT recommendations. *Pain* **2005**, *113*, 9–19. [CrossRef] [PubMed]
121. Hahne, A.J.; Ford, J.J.; Surkitt, L.D.; Richards, M.C.; Chan, A.Y.; Thompson, S.L.; Hinman, R.S.; Taylor, N.F. Specific treatment of problems of the spine (STOPS): Design of a randomised controlled trial comparing specific physiotherapy versus advice for people with subacute low back disorders. *BMC Muscul. Disord.* **2011**, *12*, 104. [CrossRef] [PubMed]
122. Vibe Fersum, K.; O'Sullivan, P.; Skouen, J.S.; Smith, A.; Kvale, A. Efficacy of classification-based cognitive functional therapy in patients with non-specific chronic low back pain: A randomized controlled trial. *Eur. J. Pain* **2013**, *17*, 916–928. [CrossRef] [PubMed]
123. Lamb, S.E.; Hansen, Z.; Lall, R.; Castelnuovo, E.; Withers, E.J.; Nichols, V.; Potter, R.; Underwood, M.R. Group cognitive behavioural treatment for low-back pain in primary care: A randomised controlled trial and cost-effectiveness analysis. *Lancet* **2010**, *375*, 916–923. [CrossRef]

124. Rivero-Arias, O.; Gray, A.; Frost, H. Cost-utility analysis of physiotherapy treatment compared with physiotherapy advice in low back pain. *Spine* **2006**, *31*, 1381–1387. [CrossRef]
125. Macedo, L.G.; Smeets, R.J.; Maher, C.G.; Latimer, J.; McAuley, J.H. Graded activity and graded exposure for persistent nonspecific low back pain: A systematic review. *Phys. Ther.* **2010**, *90*, 860–879. [CrossRef]
126. Enke, O.; New, H.A.; New, C.H.; Mathieson, S.; McLachlan, A.J.; Latimer, J.; Maher, C.G.; Lin, C.C. Anticonvulsants in the treatment of low back pain and lumbar radicular pain: A systematic review and meta-analysis. *Can. Med. Association J.* **2018**, *190*, E786–E793. [CrossRef]
127. Bialosky, J.E.; Bishop, M.D.; George, S.Z.; Robinson, M.E. Placebo response to manual therapy: Something out of nothing? *J. Manipulative Physiol. Ther.* **2011**, *19*, 11–19. [CrossRef]
128. Dahm, K.; Brurberg, K.G.; Jamtvedt, G.; Hagen, K.B. Advice to rest in bed versus advice to stay active for acute low-back pain and sciatica. *Cochrane. Database Syst. Rev.* **2010**, *6*, CD007612. [CrossRef] [PubMed]
129. Liddle, S.; Gracey, J.; Baxter, G. Advice for the management of low back pain: A systematic review of randomised controlled trials. *Man. Ther.* **2007**, *12*, 310–327. [CrossRef] [PubMed]
130. Abdel Shaheed, C.; Maher, C.G.; Williams, K.A.; McLachlan, A.J. Interventions available over the counter and advice for acute low back pain: Systematic review and meta-analysis. *J. Pain* **2014**, *15*, 2–15. [CrossRef] [PubMed]
131. Buchbinder, R.; van Tulder, M.; Öberg, B.; Costa, L.M.; Woolf, A.; Schoene, M.; Croft, P.; Buchbinder, R.; Hartvigsen, J.; Cherkin, D.; et al. Low back pain: A call for action. *Lancet* **2018**, *391*, 2384–2388. [CrossRef]
132. National Guideline Centre. National Guideline Centre. National Institute for Health and Care Excellence: Clinical Guidelines. In *Low Back Pain and Sciatica in Over 16s: Assessment and Management*; National Institute for Health and Care Excellence: London, UK, 2016.
133. O'Sullivan, P. It's time for change with the management of non-specific chronic low back pain. *Br. J. Sports Med.* **2012**, *46*, 224–227. [CrossRef] [PubMed]
134. O'Sullivan, K.; O'Sullivan, P.B.; O'Keeffe, M. The Lancet series on low back pain: reflections and clinical implications. *Br. J. Sports Med.* **2019**, *53*, 392–393. [CrossRef]
135. Bogduk, N. *Clinical and Radiological Anatomy of the Lumbar Spine*, 5th ed.; Churchill Livingstone: New York, NY, USA, 2012.
136. Peng, B.G. Pathophysiology, diagnosis, and treatment of discogenic low back pain. *World J. Orthopedics* **2013**, *4*, 42–52. [CrossRef] [PubMed]
137. Adams, M.A.; Stefanakis, M.; Dolan, P. Healing of a painful intervertebral disc should not be confused with reversing disc degeneration: Implications for physical therapies for discogenic back pain. *Clin. Biomech.* **2010**, *25*, 961–971. [CrossRef]
138. Peng, B.; Wu, W.; Hou, S.; Li, P.; Zhang, C.; Yang, Y. The pathogenesis of discogenic low back pain. *J. Bone Joint Surg. Br.* **2005**, *87*, 62–67. [CrossRef]
139. Peng, B.; Hao, J.; Hou, S.; Wu, W.; Jiang, D.; Fu, X.; Yang, Y. Possible pathogenesis of painful intervertebral disc degeneration. *Spine* **2006**, *31*, 560–566. [CrossRef]
140. Van den Berg, R.; Jongbloed, E.M.; de Schepper, E.I.T.; Bierma-Zeinstra, S.M.A.; Koes, B.W.; Luijsterburg, P.A.J. The association between pro-inflammatory biomarkers and nonspecific low back pain: A systematic review. *Spine J.* **2018**, *18*, 2140–2151. [CrossRef] [PubMed]
141. Gronblad, M.; Virri, J.; Tolonen, J.; Seitsalo, S.; Kaapa, E.; Kankare, J. A controlled immunohistochemical study of inflammatory cells in disc herniation tissue. *Spine* **1994**, *19*, 2744–2751. [CrossRef] [PubMed]
142. Habtemariam, A.; Gronglad, M.; Virri, J.; Seitsala, S.; Ruuskanen, M.; Karaharju, E. Immunocytochemical localization of immunoglobulins in disc herniations. *Spine* **1996**, *21*, 1864–1869. [CrossRef] [PubMed]
143. Habtemariam, A.; Gronglad, M.; Virri, J.; Seitsala, S.; Karaharju, E. A comparative immunohistochemical study of inflammatory cells in acute-stage and chronic-stage disc herniations. *Spine* **1998**, *23*, 2159–2166. [CrossRef] [PubMed]
144. Rothoerl, R.D.; Woertgen, C.; Holzschuh, M.; Rueschoff, J.; Brawanski, A. Is there a clinical correlate to the histologic evidence of inflammation in herniated lumbar disc tissue? *Spine* **1998**, *23*, 1197–1200. [CrossRef] [PubMed]
145. Virri, J.; Grönblad, M.; Seitsalo, S.; Habtemariam, A.; Kääpä, E.; Karaharju, E. Comparison of the prevalence of inflammatory cells in subtypes of disc herniations and associations with straight leg raising. *Spine* **2001**, *26*, 2311–2315. [CrossRef] [PubMed]

146. Miyamoto, H.; Saura, R.; Harada, T.; Doita, M.; Mizuno, K. The role of cyclooxygenase-2 and inflammatory cytokines in pain induction of herniated lumbar intervertebral disc. *Kobe J. Med. Sci.* **2000**, *46*, 13–28. [PubMed]
147. Piperno, M.; le Graverand, M.; Reboul, P.; Mathieu, P.; Tron, A. Phospholipase A2 activity in herniated lumbar discs: Clinical correlations and inhibition by piroxicam. *Spine* **1997**, *22*, 2061–2063. [CrossRef]
148. Jimbo, K.; Park, J.S.; Yokosuka, K.; Sato, K.; Nagata, K. Positive feedback loop of interleukin-1beta upregulating production of inflammatory mediators in human intervertebral disc cells in vitro. *J. Neurosurg. Spine* **2005**, *2*, 589–595. [CrossRef]
149. Brisby, H.; Byrod, G.; Olmarke, R.; Miller, V.; Aoki, Y.; Rydevik, B. Nitric oxide as a mediator of nucleus pulposus-induced effects on spinal nerve roots. *J. Orthop. Res.* **2000**, *18*, 815–820. [CrossRef]
150. Burke, J.; Watson, R.; McCormack, D.; Dowling, F.; Walsh, M.; Fitzpatrick, J. Intervertebral discs which cause low back pain secrete high levels of proinflammatory mediators. *J.f Bone Joint Surgery* **2002**, *84B*, 196–201.
151. Kang, J.; Georgescu, H.; McIntyre-Larkin, L.; Stefanovic-Racic, M.; Donaldson, W.r.; CH, E. Herniated lumbar intervertebral discs spontaneously produce matrix metalloproteinases, nitric oxide, interleukin-6, and prostaglandin E2. *Spine* **1996**, *21*, 271–277. [CrossRef] [PubMed]
152. Khan, A.N.; Jacobsen, H.E.; Khan, J.; Filippi, C.G.; Levine, M.; Lehman, R.A., Jr.; Riew, K.D.; Lenke, L.G.; Chahine, N.O. Inflammatory biomarkers of low back pain and disc degeneration: A review. *Ann. N. Y. Acad. Sci.* **2017**, *1410*, 68–84. [CrossRef] [PubMed]
153. Klyne, D.M.; Barbe, M.F.; van den Hoorn, W.; Hodges, P.W. ISSLS PRIZE IN CLINICAL SCIENCE 2018: longitudinal analysis of inflammatory, psychological, and sleep-related factors following an acute low back pain episode-the good, the bad, and the ugly. *Eur. Spine J.* **2018**, *27*, 763–777. [CrossRef] [PubMed]
154. Podichetty, V.K. The aging spine: The role of inflammatory mediators in intervertebral disc degeneration. *Cell. Mol. Biol.* **2007**, *53*, 4–18. [CrossRef] [PubMed]
155. Zhou, Y.; Abdi, S. Diagnosis and minimally invasive treatment of lumbar discogenic pain: A review of the literature. *Clin. J. Pain* **2006**, *22*, 468–481. [CrossRef]
156. Ross, J.S. Non-mechanical inflammatory causes of back pain: current concepts. *Skeletal Radiol.* **2006**, *35*, 485–487. [CrossRef]
157. Adizie, T.; Elamanchi, S.; Prabu, A.; Pace, A.V.; Laxminarayan, R.; Barkham, N. Knowledge of features of inflammatory back pain in primary care in the West Midlands: A cross-sectional survey in the United Kingdom. *Rheumatol. Int.* **2018**, *38*, 1859–1863. [CrossRef]
158. Sieper, J.; van der Heijde, D.; Landewe, R.; Brandt, J.; Burgos-Vagas, R.; Collantes-Estevez, E.; Dijkmans, B.; Dougados, M.; Khan, M.A.; Leirisalo-Repo, M.; et al. New criteria for inflammatory back pain in patients with chronic back pain: A real patient exercise by experts from the Assessment of SpondyloArthritis international Society (ASAS). *Ann. Rheum. Dis.* **2009**, *68*, 784–788. [CrossRef]
159. Calin, A.; Porta, J.; Fries, J.F.; Schurman, D.J. CLinical history as a screening test for ankylosing spondylitis. *JAMA* **1977**, *237*, 2613–2614. [CrossRef]
160. Underwood, M.R.; Dawes, P. Inflammatory back pain in primary care. *Br. J. Rheumatol.* **1995**, *34*, 1074–1077. [CrossRef] [PubMed]
161. Weisman, M.H. Inflammatory back pain: the United States perspective. *Rheum. Dis. Clin. North Am.* **2012**, *38*, 501–512. [CrossRef] [PubMed]
162. McKenzie, R. *The Lumbar Spine: Mechanical Diagnosis and Therapy*; Spinal Publication: Waikanae, New Zealand, 1981.
163. Maitland, G.D. *Vertebral Manipulation*, 5th ed.; Butterworth-Heinemann: Oxford, UK, 1986.
164. Van der Windt, D.; Hay, E.; Jellema, P.; Main, C. Psychosocial interventions for low back pain in primary care: lessons learned from recent trials. *Spine* **2008**, *33*, 81–89. [CrossRef] [PubMed]
165. Borrelli, B.; Sepinwall, D.; Ernst, D.; Bellg, A.J.; Czajkowski, S.; Breger, R.; DeFrancesco, C.; Levesque, C.; Sharp, D.L.; Ogedegbe, G.; et al. A new tool to assess treatment fidelity and evaluation of treatment fidelity across 10 years of health behavior research. *J. Consult. Clin. Psychol.* **2005**, *73*, 852–860. [CrossRef] [PubMed]
166. Perepletchikova, F.; Treat, T.A.; Kazdin, A.E. Treatment integrity in psychotherapy research: Analysis of the studies and examination of the associated factors. *J. Consulting Clin. Psychol.* **2007**, *75*, 829–841. [CrossRef] [PubMed]

167. Helmhout, P.; Staal, J.; Maher, C.; Petersen, T.; Rainville, J.; Shaw, W. Exercise therapy and low back pain: Insights and proposals to improve the design, conduct, and reporting of clinical trials. *Spine* **2008**, *33*, 1782–1788. [CrossRef] [PubMed]
168. Herbert, R.D.; Bo, K. Analysis of quality of interventions in systematic reviews. *Br. Med. J.* **2005**, *331*, 507–509. [CrossRef]
169. Karas, S.; Plankis, L. Consideration of treatment fidelity to improve manual therapy research. *J. Man. Manip. Ther.* **2016**, *24*, 233–237. [CrossRef]
170. Borrelli, B. The Assessment, Monitoring, and Enhancement of Treatment Fidelity In Public Health Clinical Trials. *J. Public Health Dent.* **2011**, *71*, S52–S63. [CrossRef]
171. Hodges, P.W.; van Dieen, J.H.; Cholewicki, J. Time to Reflect on the Role of Motor Control in Low Back Pain. *J. Orthop. Sports Phys. Ther.* **2019**, *49*, 367–369. [CrossRef]
172. Macedo, L.G.; Saragiotto, B.T.; Yamato, T.P.; Costa, L.O.; Menezes Costa, L.C.; Ostelo, R.W.; Maher, C.G. Motor control exercise for acute non-specific low back pain. *Cochrane Database Syst. Rev.* **2016**, *2*, cd012085. [CrossRef] [PubMed]
173. Saragiotto, B.T.; Maher, C.G.; Yamato, T.P.; Costa, L.O.; Menezes Costa, L.C.; Ostelo, R.W.; Macedo, L.G. Motor control exercise for chronic non-specific low-back pain. *Cochrane Database Syst. Rev.* **2016**, *1*, cd012004. [CrossRef] [PubMed]
174. Bystrom, M.G.; Rasmussen-Barr, E.; Grooten, W.J. Motor control exercises reduces pain and disability in chronic and recurrent low back pain: a meta-analysis. *Spine* **2013**, *38*, E350–E358. [CrossRef] [PubMed]
175. Hodges, P. *Spinal Control: The Rehabilitation of Back Pain*, 1st ed.; Hodges, P., Cholewicki, J., van Dieen, J., Eds.; Churchill Livingston: Edinburgh, UK, 2013.
176. Van Dieen, J.H.; Reeves, N.P.; Kawchuk, G.; van Dillen, L.; Hodges, P.W. Analysis of Motor Control in Low-Back Pain Patients: A Key to Personalized Care? *J. Orthop. Sports Phys. Ther.* **2018**, *49*, 1–24. [CrossRef] [PubMed]
177. Hodges, P.W.; Barbe, M.F.; Loggia, M.L.; Nijs, J.; Stone, L.S. Diverse Role of Biological Plasticity in Low Back Pain and Its Impact on Sensorimotor Control of the Spine. *J. Orthop. Sports Phys. Ther.* **2019**, *49*, 389–401. [CrossRef] [PubMed]
178. Van Dieen, J.H.; Reeves, N.P.; Kawchuk, G.; van Dillen, L.R.; Hodges, P.W. Motor Control Changes in Low Back Pain: Divergence in Presentations and Mechanisms. *J. Orthop. Sports Phys. Ther.* **2019**, *49*, 370–379. [CrossRef] [PubMed]
179. Indahl, A.; Velund, L.; Reikeraas, O. Good prognosis for low back pain when left untampered. *Spine* **1995**, *20*, 473–477. [CrossRef]
180. Li, L.; Bombardier, C. Physical Therapy Management of Low Back Pain: An Expolratory Survey of Therapist Approaches. *Phys. Ther.* **2001**, *81*, 1018–1028.
181. Gracey, J.; McDonough, S.M.; Baxter, D.G. Physiotherapy Management of Low Back Pain. A Survey of Current Practice in Northern Ireland. *Spine* **2002**, *27*, 406–411. [CrossRef]

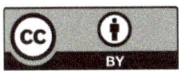 © 2019 by the authors. Licensee MDPI, Basel, Switzerland. This article is an open access article distributed under the terms and conditions of the Creative Commons Attribution (CC BY) license (http://creativecommons.org/licenses/by/4.0/).

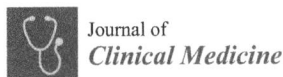

Review

Are Mindful Exercises Safe and Beneficial for Treating Chronic Lower Back Pain? A Systematic Review and Meta-Analysis of Randomized Controlled Trials

Liye Zou [1,†], Yanjie Zhang [2,†], Lin Yang [3,4], Paul D. Loprinzi [5], Albert S. Yeung [6], Jian Kong [6], Kevin W Chen [1], Wook Song [2,7], Tao Xiao [8,*] and Hong Li [9,10,*]

[1] Lifestyle (Mind-Body Movement) Research Center, College of Sports Science, Shenzhen University, Shenzhen 518060, China; liyezou123@gmail.com (L.Z.); Qigong4us@hotmail.com (K.W.C.)
[2] Health and Exercise Science Laboratory, Institute of Sports Science, Seoul National University, Seoul 08826, Korea; elite_zhangyj@163.com (Y.Z.); songw3@snu.ac.kr (W.S.)
[3] Cancer Epidemiology and Prevention Research, Alberta Health Services, Calgary, AB T2S 3C3, Canada; lin.yang@ahs.ca
[4] Departments of Oncology and Community Health Sciences, Cumming School of Medicine, University of Calgary, Calgary, AB T2N 4Z6, Canada
[5] Department of Health, Exercise Science and Recreation Management School of Applied Sciences, The University of Mississippi, Oxford, MS 36877, USA; pdloprin@olemiss.edu
[6] Department of Psychiatry, Massachusetts General Hospital, Harvard Medical School, Boston, MA 02114, USA; ayeung@mgh.harvard.edu (A.S.Y.); JKONG2@mgh.harvard.edu (J.K.)
[7] Institute on Aging, Seoul National University, Seoul 08826, Korea
[8] College of Mathematics and Statistics, Shenzhen University, Shenzhen 518060, China
[9] Shenzhen Key Laboratory of Affective and Social Cognitive Science, College of Psychology and Sociology, Shenzhen University, Shenzhen 518060, China
[10] Shenzhen Institute of Neuroscience, Shenzhen 518057, China
* Correspondence: taoxiao@szu.edu.cn (T.X.); lihongszu@szu.edu.cn (H.L.)
† These authors contributed equally to this work.

Received: 28 March 2019; Accepted: 6 May 2019; Published: 8 May 2019

Abstract: Background: Chronic low back pain (CLBP) is a common health issue worldwide. Tai Chi, Qigong, and Yoga, as the most widely practiced mindful exercises, have promising effects for CLBP-specific symptoms. Objective: We therefore conducted a comprehensive review investigating the effects of mindful exercises versus active and/or non-active controls while evaluating the safety and pain-related effects of mindful exercises in adults with CLBP. Methods: We searched five databases (MEDLINE, EMBASE, SCOPUS, Web of Science, and Cochrane Library) from inception to February 2019. Two investigators independently selected 17 eligible randomized controlled trials (RCT) against inclusion and exclusion criteria, followed by data extraction and study quality assessment. Standardized mean difference (SMD) was used to determine the magnitude of mindful exercises versus controls on pain- and disease-specific outcome measures. Results: As compared to control groups, we observed significantly favorable effects of mindful exercises on reducing pain intensity ($SMD = -0.37$, 95% CI -0.5 to -0.23, $p < 0.001$, $I^2 = 45.9\%$) and disability ($SMD = -0.39$, 95% CI -0.49 to -0.28, $p < 0.001$, $I^2 = 0\%$). When compared with active control alone, mindful exercises showed significantly reduced pain intensity ($SMD = -0.40$, $p < 0.001$). Furthermore, of the three mindful exercises, Tai Chi has a significantly superior effect on pain management ($SMD= -0.75$, 95% CI -1.05 to -0.46, $p < 0.001$), whereas Yoga-related adverse events were reported in five studies. Conclusion: Findings of our systematic review suggest that mindful exercises (Tai Chi and Qigong) may be beneficial for CLBP symptomatic management. In particular, Tai Chi appears to have a superior effect in reducing pain intensity irrespective of non-control comparison or active control comparison (conventional exercises, core training, and physical therapy programs). Importantly, training in these mindful exercises should be implemented with certified instructors to ensure quality of movement and injury prevention.

Keywords: Tai Chi; Yoga; Qigong; mind-body therapy; exercise; mind-body medicine; low back pain

1. Introduction

Low back pain is a common health issue worldwide, but notably, prevention and treatment of chronic low back pain (CLBP) is a major public health concern [1,2]. It has been widely recognized as the leading cause of disability, affecting work performance and general psychosomatic health and is associated with substantial economic and societal burden [2]. The estimated lifetime prevalence of CLBP is 12% to 33% in industrialized countries (period prevalence: 22% to 65% per year) [3]. The prevalence rate of CLBP is higher in adults than children and adolescents [4], particularly among the working population [5]. CLBP is widely treated with medications (e.g., nonsteroidal anti-inflammatory drug, analgesic, and muscle relaxant) to relieve pain, decrease inflammation, and reduce muscle tension [6]. However, these treatments may increase the likelihood of falls and drug-related side effects (e.g., mood disturbance, nausea, seizure, and/or tachycardia) among patients [6,7]. Furthermore, the long-term use of medications remains financially unaffordable in economically disadvantaged areas [7]. Other non-pharmacological treatments, such as physical therapy [8,9], spinal manipulation [10], and physical activity or exercise [11–13], have shown promising effects on improving CLBP-specific symptoms.

Tai Chi, Qigong (e.g., Baduanjin, Yijingjin, and Wuqinxi), and Yoga, also known as mindful exercises, are light-to-moderate intensity physical activities and have recently been popularized in both the fitness industry and clinical setting for disease prevention and symptomatic management [14–17]. Mindful exercises are typically performed at a slow pace, simultaneously integrated with mental focus on muscle and movement sense, rhythmic abdominal diaphragmatic breathing, and meditation [18–21]. These modalities may complement or act as an alternative practice to conventional rehabilitation programs [22–24]. Mindful exercises are beneficial for symptomatic management in a variety of diseases, such as multiple sclerosis [25,26], autism spectrum disorder [27], balance disorder [28,29], ankylosing spondylitis [30], mental illness [31,32], cerebrovascular disease [33], fibromyalgia [34], and knee osteoarthritis [35].

Recently, research has investigated the effects of mindful exercises in adults with CLBP. With the increasing number of experimental studies on this topic, two reviews were subsequently performed and published in 2013 [36,37]. Notably, these two systematic reviews only included eight to 10 randomized controlled trials (RCT) and focused on Yoga alone. Secondly, meta-analysis was only possible for the Yoga interventions versus non-active controls due to the small number of trials, lacking a direct comparison to active control conditions like conventional exercises or guideline-endorsed treatments. Thirdly, previous reviews simply evaluated the effectiveness of Yoga, but the safety of the broader mindful exercises in adults with CLBP still remains unknown. To fill these knowledge gaps, we therefore conducted an updated systematic review that includes all three most popular mindful exercises versus active and/or non-active controls while evaluating the safety and efficacy of mindful exercises in adults with CLBP.

2. Methods

2.1. Search Strategy

Two investigators independently searched five databases (MEDLINE, EMBASE, SCOPUS, Web of Science, and Cochrane library) from the inception to February 2019. We used two groups of keywords: (1) "Tai Chi" OR "Tai Chi Chuan" OR "Taiji" OR "Qigong" Or "Chi Kung" OR "Qi Gong" OR "Baduanjin" OR "Yijinjing" OR "Wuqinxi" OR "Yoga" OR "mind-body", OR "mindful exercise"; (2) "low back pain" OR "lower back pain" OR "back pain" OR "low back ache". Hand-searching was performed to identify relevant publications from the reference lists of eligible original articles and reviews. In addition to two separate investigators independently searching the five above-mentioned databases, these investigators also independently screened the titles and abstracts of the potentially eligible articles (described below). Full details on the search strategy and retrieval process are shown in Figure 1.

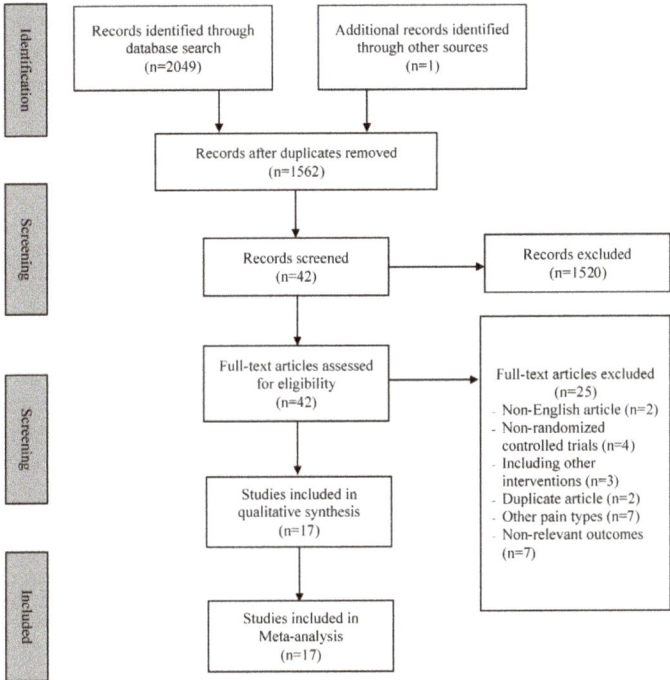

Figure 1. Flow chart of study searching.

2.2. Inclusion and Exclusion Criteria

In the present review, studies were only considered eligible if they: (1) were RCTs; (2) recruited adults diagnosed with CLBP (low back pain lasting or recurring for longer than 3 months [38]; (3) used at least one type of mindful exercise (e.g., Tai Chi, Qigong, and Yoga) or their combination as an intervention program; (4) included a control group using any form (e.g., aerobic exercise, self-care book, waitlist, or no treatment) other than mindful exercise; (5) reported at least one health outcome associated with disease-specific symptoms like pain, functional ability, or depression. Exclusion criteria were: (1) specific causes (e.g., spinal canal stenosis or herniated disc); (2) mindful exercise integrated with other treatments, like core training; (3) unobtainable data for calculating effect size (ES); (4) other types of publications, such as a case-study, observational study, or review articles.

2.3. Data Extraction and Quality Assessment

Detailed information of each included study were independently extracted by the two investigators and a third reviewer was consulted to reach consensus by discussion. Extracted information included the first author and year of publication, characteristics of participants (sample size and mean age), intervention protocol (mindful exercise, control type, and intervention duration), outcome measure (pain, disability, and/or depression), and reporting of an adverse event. In addition to descriptive information, the same investigators extracted the quantitative data for ES calculation.

Two investigators independently assessed methodological quality using the Physiotherapy Evidence Database (PEDro) scale. This scale consists of 11 items, including eligibility criteria, random allocation, allocation concealment, baseline equivalence, blinded assessor(s), blinded participants, blinded instructor, retention rate of ≥85%, intention-to-treat analysis (ITT), between group statistical comparisons, and point estimates of at least one set of outcome measures. One point is awarded for meeting each evaluation requirement. Since this review included all adults diagnosed with CLBP, the first eligibility criteria was not considered. Thus, each study could reach a maximum of 10 points: excellent (9–10 points), good (6–8 points), fair (4–5 points) and poor (less than 4 points) quality [39].

2.4. Statistical Analysis

The Comprehensive Meta-Analysis Software version 2.2 was employed to meta-analyze the extracted data. For each outcome, we used mean and standard deviations (SD) at baseline and post-intervention, along with the number of participants per group. If one study included two control groups, we halved the number of participants in the mindful exercise group with the two control groups, while mean and SD remained unchanged. We used random-effects model to calculate the pooled ES (standardized mean difference, SMD) to determine the magnitude of effect for mindful exercise intervention on two outcomes (pain and disability). Notably, we did not evaluate depression as an outcome variable, due to fewer than four studies evaluating this outcome [40]. Three levels of ES were adopted: small (0.2–0.49), moderate (0.50–0.79), and large (≥0.8) [40]. I^2 test was used to determine heterogeneity across included studies: $I^2 < 25\%$ (low), $I^2 < 50\%$ (moderate), and $I^2 > 75\%$ (high), respectively [40]. Furthermore, we performed sub-group analyses for categorical variables and meta-regression for continuous variables. The categorical variables included: (1) types of control condition (mindful exercise versus active control or non-active control), mindful exercise (Tai Chi, Yoga, and Qigong), and instrument; (2) use of allocation concealment. The continuous variables included mean age and total time spent over the entire intervention course (minutes). Finally, publication bias for each outcome was evaluated using the Egger's test and the visually-produced Funnel plot [40]. Subsequently, we removed studies that caused asymmetry.

3. Results

3.1. Search Results

Figure 1 describes the detailed search process of our meta-analysis. A total of 2049 potential studies were searched and 42 full-text publications were screened for further evaluation. After eliminating the irrelevant studies ($n = 25$), seventeen studies [41–57] were identified for data extraction and quality assessment.

3.2. Characteristics of Included Studies

Table 1 depicts the characteristics of the included studies, such as the sample size, age, intervention and control group details, and outcome measures. Seventeen studies [41–57] published in peer-review journals included a total of 2022 participants with CLBP. The mean age of participants ranged from 34 to 74 years. The sample size ranged from 20 to 320 per study. Intervention duration for the mindful exercise(s) lasted 1 to 24 weeks, with sessions occurring one to seven times per week (40 to 90 min per sessions). Control conditions varied greatly across the evaluated studies, including utilizing a self-care book, stretching exercise, and waitlist. Adverse events were reported in five Yoga intervention studies, including herniated discs (3.3% and 1.1%, respectively) [48,54,55], increased pain (2.6% and 14.1%, respectively) [53,54], and mild self-limited joint and back pain (7.1%) [56]. One study did not report an adverse event [57], while no adverse events were reported in the other mindful exercise intervention studies.

Table 1. Characteristics of randomized controlled trials in the meta-analysis.

Study	Participants		MA (years)	Mindful Exercise (Qualified Instructor)	Intervention Protocol		DR (wk)	Control Type	Outcome Measured		Safety
	Sample Size					Control			Pain and Disability		Adverse Events
Hall et al. (2011) [41]	160 CLBP; TC = 80; C = 80		44	2 × 40 min/wk, TC		Wait-list	10	Passive	Pain intensity (NRS), disability (RMDQ)		No adverse event
Blödt et al. (2015) [42]	127 CLBP; QG = 64; C = 63		47	1 × 90 min/wk, QG		1 × 60 min/wk Strengthening	12	Active	Pain intensity (VAS), disability (RMDQ)		No adverse event
Teut et al. (2016) [43]	176 CLBP; QG = 58; YG = 61; C = 57		73	1 × 90 min/wk, QG; 2 × 45 min/wk, YG		Waitlist	12	Passive	Pain intensity (VAS)		No adverse event
Phattharasupharerk et al. (2018) [44]	72 CLBP; QG = 36; C = 36		35	1 × 60 min/wk plus daily practice, YG		Waitlist	6	Passive	Pain intensity (VAS), disability (RMDQ)		No adverse event
Liu et al. (2019) [45]	43 CLBP; TC = 15; C1 = 15; C2 = 13		74	3 × 60 min/wk, TC		C1: Core training; C2: No intervention	12	C1: Active; C2: Passive	Pain intensity (VAS)		No adverse event
Galantino et al. (2004) [46]	22 CLBP		30–65	2 × 60 min/wk plus 7 × 60 min/wk (home), YG		No treatment	6	Passive	disability (ODI) Depression (BDI)		No adverse event
Sherman et al. (2005) [47]	101 CLBP; YG = 36; C1 = 35; C2 = 30		44	1 × 75 min/wk plus daily practice (home), YG		C1: 1 × 75min/wk + Daily practice, aerobic exercises and strength exercise; C2: Self-care book	12	C1: Active; C2: Passive	disability (RMDQ)		No adverse event
Williams et al. (2005) [48]	60 CLBP; YG = 30; C = 30		48	1 × 90 min/wk plus 5 × 30 min/wk (home), YG		Newsletters on back pain	16	Passive	Pain intensity (VAS), disability (ODI)		1 participant diagnosed with a herniated disc in YG
Tekur et al. (2008) [49]	80 CLBP; YG = 40; C = 40		48	7 × 120 min/wk, YG		Daily physical movements + education	1	Active	disability (ODI)		No adverse event
Williams et al. (2009) [50]	90 CLBP; YG = 43; C = 47		48	2 × 90 min/wk plus 7 × 30 min/wk (home), YG		Waitlist	24	Passive	Pain intensity (VAS), disability (ODI)		No adverse event
Saper et al. (2009) [51]	30 CLBP; YG = 15; C = 15		44	1 × 75 min/wk plus 7 × 30 min/wk (home), YG		Self-care book	12	Passive	Pain intensity (VAS), disability (RMDQ)		No adverse event
Cox et al. (2010) [52]	20 CLBP; YG = 10; C = 10		45	1 × 75 min/wk plus home practice, YG		Self-care book	12	Passive	Pain intensity (ABPS), disability (RMDQ)		No adverse event
Tilbrook et al. (2011) [53]	313 CLBP; YG = 156; C = 157		46	1 × 75min/wk plus 7 × 30 min/wk (home), YG		Self-care book	12	Passive	Pain intensity (ABPS), disability (RMDQ)		8 participants (increased pain) in YG
Sherman et al. (2011) [54]	228 CLBP; YG = 92; C1 = 91; C2 = 45		48	1 × 75 min/wk plus 6 × 20 min/wk (home), YG		C1: 1 × 75min/wk + 20 min/wk (home) Stretching exercise; C2: Self-care book	12	C1: Active; C2: Passive	Pain intensity (NRS) disability (RMDQ)		13 participants (increased pain) and 1 herniated disc in yoga
Nambi et al. (2014) [55]	60 CLBP; YG = 30; C = 30		44	1 × 60 min/wk plus 5 × 30 min/wk (home), YG		Exercise (strengthening and stretching) 35days/wk,	4	Active	Pain intensity (VAS)		1 herniated disc in YG
Saper et al. (2017) [56]	320 CLBP; YG = 127; C1 = 129; C2 = 64		46	1 × 75 min/wk plus 7 × 30 min/wk (home), YG		C1: 1 × 60min/wk, PT (stabilization and aerobic exercise); C2: Self-care book	12	C1: Active; C2: Passive	Pain intensity (NRS), disability (RMDQ)		9 and 14 participants (mild self-limited joint and back pain) in YG and PT, respectively
Kuvačić et al. (2018) [57]	30 CLBP; YG = 15; C = 15		34	2 × 75 min/wk, YG		Pamphlet program	8	Passive	Pain intensity (NRS), disability (ODI), depression (SDS)		Not reported

Note: TC = Tai Chi; YG = Yoga; QG = Qigong; PT = Physical therapy; C = control group; MA = mean age; wk = week; DR = duration; CLBP = Chronic lower back pain; VAS = Visual Analog Scale; NRS = Numeric Rating Scale; ABPS = Aberdeen Back Pain Scale; ODI = Oswestry Disability Index; RMDQ = Roland–Morris Disability Questionnaire; Self-care book refers to reading *The Back Pain Book*, which emphasizing self-care management strategies for low back pain such as the causes of back pain and advice on exercising, appropriate lifestyle modification, and guidelines for managing flare-up; Pamphlet program refers to knowledge about vertebral spine and its biomechanical aspects; BDI = Beck depression inventory; SDS = Zung self-rating depression scale.

3.3. Study Quality Assessment

Study quality for each evaluated experiment is summarized in Table 2. Overall, the included studies demonstrated good quality (6–8 points). Notably, no studies implemented subject blinding or therapist blinding, and only one study [56] adopted assessor blinding. Concealed allocation was conducted in 40% of the studies, and four studies did not use intention-to-treat analysis [48–50,55].

Table 2. Methodological quality of the included studies (PEDro assessment).

Study	Score	Methodological Quality	1	2	3	4	5	6	7	8	9	10	11
Hall et al., 2011 [41]	8	Good	✓	✓	✓	✓				✓	✓	✓	✓
Blödt et al., 2015 [42]	8	Good	✓	✓	✓	✓				✓	✓	✓	✓
Teut et al., 2016 [43]	8	Good	✓	✓	✓	✓				✓	✓	✓	✓
Phattharasuphaererk et al., 2018 [44]	7	Good	✓	✓		✓				✓	✓	✓	✓
Liu et al., 2019 [45]	7	Good	✓	✓		✓				✓	✓	✓	✓
Galantino et al., 2004 [46]	7	Good	✓	✓		✓				✓	✓	✓	✓
Sherman et al., 2005 [47]	8	Good	✓	✓	✓	✓				✓	✓	✓	✓
Williams et al., 2005 [48]	6	Good	✓	✓		✓				✓		✓	✓
Tekur et al., 2008 [49]	7	Good	✓	✓	✓	✓				✓		✓	✓
Williams et al., 2009 [50]	6	Good	✓	✓		✓				✓		✓	✓
Saper et al., 2009 [51]	8	Good	✓	✓	✓	✓				✓	✓	✓	✓
Cox et al., 2010 [52]	8	Good	✓	✓	✓	✓				✓	✓	✓	✓
Tilbrook et al., 2011 [53]	8	Good	✓	✓	✓	✓				✓	✓	✓	✓
Sherman et al., 2011 [54]	8	Good	✓	✓	✓	✓				✓	✓	✓	✓
Nambi et al., 2014 [55]	6	Good	✓	✓		✓				✓		✓	✓
Saper et al., 2017 [56]	9	Excellent	✓	✓	✓	✓			✓	✓	✓	✓	✓
Kuvačić et al., 2018 [57]	7	Good	✓	✓		✓				✓	✓	✓	✓

Studies were classified as having excellent (9–10), good (6–8), fair (4–5) or poor (<4)

Scale of item score: ✓, present. The PEDro scale criteria are (1) eligibility criteria; (2) random allocation; (3) concealed allocation; (4) similarity at baseline on key measures; (5) subject blinding; (6) therapist blinding; (7) assessor blinding; (8) more than 85% follow-up of at least one key outcome; (9) intention-to-treat analysis; (10) between-group statistical comparison for at least one key outcome; and (11) point estimates and measures of variability provided for at least one key outcome.

3.4. Meta-Analysis of Outcome Measured

3.4.1. Pain Intensity

There were 15 studies (18 pairs of intervention vs. control comparisons since three studies [43,54,56] included two control conditions) on pain intensity, measured by three different self-reported scales (Visual Analog Scale (VAS), Numeric Rating Scale (NRS), and Aberdeen Back Pain Scale (ABPS)). Based on the asymmetrical Funnel plot and the Egger's Regression test (Egger's regression intercept = −3.78, $p < 0.01$), we removed four comparisons [44,45,55,57] and the remaining studies showed a symmetrical Funnel plot (Figure 2) with Eggers test intercept = −1.54, $p = 0.16$. For the meta-analysis of 11 studies (14 comparisons), compared with the control groups, a significant benefit on reducing pain intensity was observed in favor of mindful exercises ($SMD = -0.37$, 95% CI −0.5 to −0.23, $p < 0.001$, $I^2 = 45.9\%$; Figure 3). Furthermore, we performed sub-group analyses and meta-regression for categorical variables (control type, type of mindful exercise, type of instrument, and use of allocation concealment) and continuous variables (mean age and total time). We observed significantly different effects on pain intensity across different types of mindful exercise ($Q = 8.46$, $p = 0.01$), with Tai Chi ($SMD = -0.75$, 95% CI −1.05 to −0.46, $p < 0.001$) and Yoga ($SMD = -0.33$, 95% CI −0.47 to −0.19, $p < 0.001$) showing significantly decreased pain intensity, but Qigong exercise did not demonstrate such an effect ($SMD = -0.21$, 95% CI −0.48 to 0.06, $p = 0.12$) (Table 3).

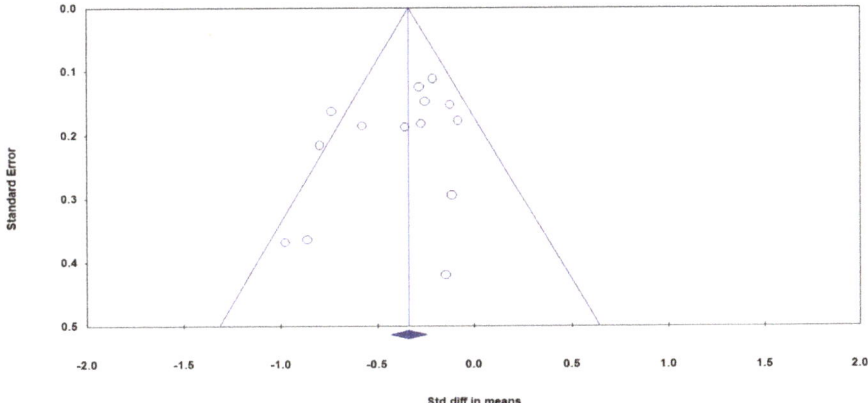

Figure 2. Funnel plot of publication bias for pain intensity.

Study name	Std diff in means	Standard error	Variance	Lower limit	Upper limit	Z-Value	p-Value
Teut 2016 YG vs WL	-0.27	0.18	0.03	-0.63	0.09	-1.49	0.14
Teut 2016 QG vs WL	-0.35	0.19	0.04	-0.72	0.01	-1.88	0.06
Liu 2019 TC vs CT	-0.86	0.36	0.13	-1.57	-0.15	-2.36	0.02
Saper 2009	-0.98	0.37	0.14	-1.70	-0.25	-2.65	0.01
Williams 2005	-0.11	0.30	0.09	-0.69	0.47	-0.38	0.70
Williams 2009	-0.80	0.22	0.05	-1.22	-0.37	-3.69	0.00
Hall 2011	-0.73	0.16	0.03	-1.05	-0.41	-4.51	0.00
Blodt 2015	-0.08	0.18	0.03	-0.43	0.27	-0.45	0.65
Saper 2017 YG vs PT	-0.28	0.12	0.02	-0.53	-0.04	-2.25	0.02
Saper 2017 YG vs SB	-0.12	0.15	0.02	-0.42	0.18	-0.79	0.43
Cox 2010	-0.15	0.42	0.18	-0.97	0.68	-0.35	0.73
Tilbrook 2011	-0.21	0.11	0.01	-0.43	0.01	-1.88	0.06
Sherman 2011 YG vs SB	-0.57	0.19	0.03	-0.94	-0.21	-3.10	0.00
Sherman 2011 YG vs SE	-0.25	0.15	0.02	-0.54	0.04	-1.70	0.09
	-0.37	0.07	0.00	-0.50	-0.23	-5.31	0.00

Figure 3. Effects of mindful exercises on pain intensity (YG = Yoga, WL = waitlist, TC = Tai Chi, CT = core training, QG = Qigong; PT = physical therapy, SB = self-care book; SE = stretching exercise). The red symbol represents the overall effect size in favor of mindful exercises.

3.4.2. Back-Specific Disability

Overall, there were 14 studies, including 17 pairs of mindful exercises vs. control comparisons (because three studies [47,54,56] included two control conditions, respectively), with disability measured by two different types of instruments (Roland–Morris Disability Questionnaire (RMDQ) and Oswestry Disability Index (ODI)). Based on the asymmetrical Funnel plot, we removed three outlying studies [47,49,51] and the remaining studies showed a symmetrical Funnel plot (Figure 4) with Eggers test intercept = −0.42, p = 0.53. For the meta-analysis in 12 studies (14 pairs of mindful exercises vs. control comparisons), compared with the control groups, the aggregated result showed a significant benefit in favor of mindful exercises on reducing disability (SMD = −0.39, 95% CI −0.49 to −0.28, $p < 0.001$, I^2 = 0%; Figure 5). We performed sub-group analyses and meta-regression for categorical variables (control type, type of mindful exercise, type of instrument, and use of allocation concealment) and continuous variables (mean age and total time) (Table 3). No significant differences were observed.

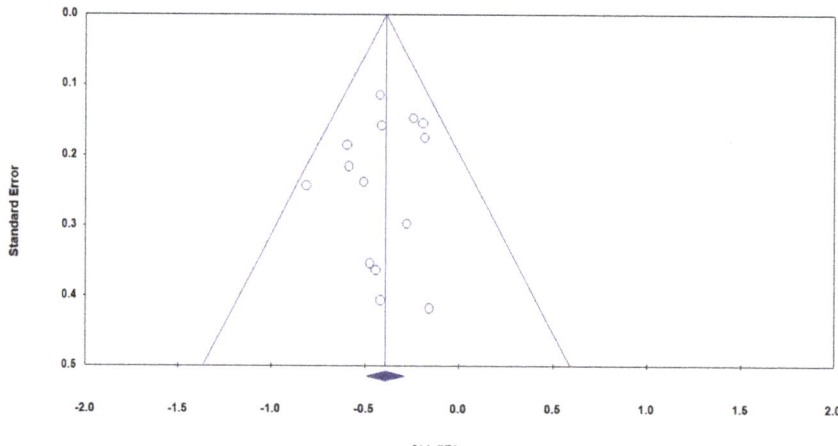

Figure 4. Funnel plot of publication bias for disability.

Study name	Std diff in means	Standard error	Variance	Lower limit	Upper limit	Z-Value	p-Value
Phattharasupharerk 2018	-0.81	0.24	0.06	-1.29	-0.33	-3.32	0.00
Hall 2011	-0.41	0.16	0.02	-0.72	-0.10	-2.61	0.01
Blodt 2015	-0.18	0.18	0.03	-0.52	0.16	-1.03	0.30
Cox 2010	-0.16	0.42	0.17	-0.97	0.66	-0.38	0.71
Sherman 2005 YG vs ASE	-0.51	0.24	0.06	-0.97	-0.04	-2.14	0.03
Tilbrook 2011	-0.42	0.11	0.01	-0.65	-0.20	-3.67	0.00
Saper 2009	-0.44	0.36	0.13	-1.15	0.27	-1.22	0.22
Saper 2017 YG vs SB	-0.19	0.16	0.02	-0.50	0.11	-1.23	0.22
Sherman 2011 YG vs SB	-0.24	0.15	0.02	-0.53	0.05	-1.64	0.10
Sherman 2011 YG vs SE	-0.60	0.19	0.03	-0.96	-0.23	-3.21	0.00
Galantino 2004	-0.42	0.41	0.16	-1.21	0.38	-1.02	0.31
Williams 2005	-0.27	0.30	0.09	-0.86	0.31	-0.92	0.36
Williams 2009	-0.59	0.22	0.05	-1.01	-0.16	-2.71	0.01
Kuvacic 2018	-0.47	0.35	0.13	-1.17	0.22	-1.34	0.18
	-0.39	0.05	0.00	-0.49	-0.28	-7.36	0.00

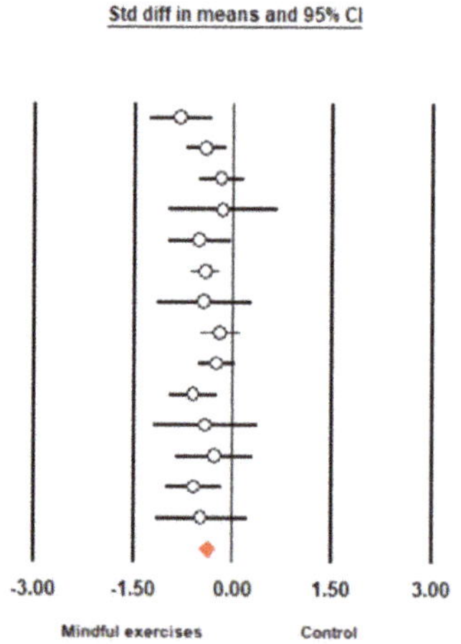

Figure 5. The effect of mindful exercises on disability (YG = Yoga, ASE = Aerobic and strength exercise, SB = self-care book, SE = stretching exercise).The red symbol below represents the overall effect size in favor of mindful exercises.

Table 3. The effect of mind-body exercise in moderator analysis.

Categorical Moderator	Outcome	Covariates	No. of Studies/Comparisons	SMD	95% Confidence Interval	I^2%	Test for Between-Group Hoterogeneity		
							Q-Value	df(Q)	p-Value
Control Type	Pain intensity	Active	7	−0.40	−0.48 to −0.20	53.2%	0.08	1	0.78
		Passive	7	−0.35	−0.46 to −0.21	46.5%			
	Disability	Active	4	−0.28	−0.47 to −0.09	0%	1.62	1	0.20
		Passive	10	−0.43	−0.55 to −0.31	0%			
Mindful Type	Pain intensity	Yoga	10	−0.33	−0.47 to −0.19	33.7%	8.46	2	0.01*
		TC	2	−0.75	−1.05 to −0.46	0%			
		Qigong	2	−0.21	−0.48 to 0.06	10.0%			
	Disability	Yoga	11	−0.38	−0.50 to −0.26	0%	0.16	2	0.92
		TC	1	−0.41	−0.72 to −0.10	0%			
		Qigong	2	−0.47	−1.09 to 0.14	77.2%			
		ABPS	2	−0.21	−0.42 to 0.01	0%			
Instruments	Pain intensity	VAS	7	−0.43	−0.68 to −0.18	50.5%	2.1	2	0.35
		NRS	5	−0.38	−0.59 to −0.17	60.1%			
	Disability	RMDQ	10	−0.38	−0.49 to −0.27	0%	0.36	1	0.55
		ODI	4	−0.47	−0.76 to −0.18	39.5%			
Allocation Concealment	Pain intensity	Yes	11	−0.33	−0.46 to −0.19	50.9%	1.19	1	0.28
		No	3	−0.59	1.05 to −0.13	0%			
	Disability	Yes	9	−0.35	−0.46 to −0.24	0%	2.27	1	0.13
		No	5	−0.56	−0.80 to −0.31				
Continuous moderator	Outcome	No. of studies/comparisons	β	95% Confidence Interval			Q-value	df(Q)	p-value
Age	Pain intensity	14	−0.00108	−0.01080 to 0.00865			0.05	1	0.83
	Disability	14	0.02454	−0.00706 to 0.05614			2.32	1	0.13
Total Time	Pain intensity	14	0.00002	−0.00007 to 0.00012			0.22	1	0.64
	Disability	14	−0.00002	−0.00012 to 0.00009			0.10	1	0.75

VAS = Visual Analog Scale; RMDQ = Roland-Morris Disability Questionnaire; SMD = Standardized Mean Difference; TC = Tai Chi; * $p < 0.01$.

4. Discussion

Mindful exercises are increasingly accepted by clinicians worldwide as an alternative therapy for chronic disease symptomatic management. To the best of our knowledge, this is the first systematic review to comprehensively evaluate the existing literature regarding the safety and pain- and disease-specific effects of three commonly practiced mindful exercises (Tai Chi, Qigong, and Yoga) among adults with CLBP. Our findings indicated that mindful exercises may be effective in reducing pain intensity and disability among CLBP patients. More importantly, the beneficial effects of mindful exercises were observed comparing to both non-active and active controls. Notably, several Yoga interventions induced varied adverse events (e.g., injury).

4.1. Pain Intensity

Overall, mindful exercises may be effective in reducing pain intensity level, with a small intervention effect ($SMD = -0.37$). However, we observed non-significant effects on this outcome in five comparisons [42,43,48,51,52] and marginally significant effects in three comparisons [43,47,53]. Such results may be attributed to inadequacy of weekly instructor-led training time (75 to 90 min) [42,43,47,53], relatively small sample size [48,51,52] (20 to 60 participants), and/or direct comparison to active controls (strengthening or stretching exercise) [42,47]. When compared with an active control alone, mindful exercises showed significantly reduced pain intensity ($SMD = -0.40$, $p < 0.001$). This suggests that mindful exercise may be more beneficial for pain management than conventional exercise (strengthening and/or stretching exercise) and guideline-endorsed (core training or physical therapy) programs. Furthermore, results from the sub-group analyses indicated that, when compared to Yoga and Qigong, Tai Chi appeared to have a superior effect on pain relief. Such positive intervention effects reached a moderate level ($SMD = -0.75$). Tai Chi emphasizes neutral spine or standing with upright posture during performance, providing an opportunity to strengthen core muscles (similar to a guideline-endorsed core training program) to reduce pain intensity. Additionally, a previous RCT by Hall [58] indicated that Tai Chi can reduce pain-catastrophizing, which partially mediates the effect of Tai Chi on pain intensity among adults with CLBP. Conversely, adverse events (increased pain, reduced range of motion at joints, and/or herniated disc) were reported in several Yoga intervention studies but not in Tai Chi studies. This is likely due to the Yoga routine, which involves movements of bending forward and backwards at the low back, which may initiate or exacerbate pain intensity. Taken together, Tai Chi may be a more suitable mindful exercise in rehabilitation programs for CLBP rather than Yoga.

4.2. Back-Specific Disability

In this meta-analysis, we observed a small overall positive effect (SMD = -0.39) of mindful exercise on disability. Of the 12 studies (including 14 comparisons), six comparisons (Qigong vs. waitlist, Tai Chi vs. waitlist, Yoga vs. aerobic plus strength exercises, Yoga vs. Waitlist, Yoga vs. self-care book, Yoga vs. stretching exercise, and Yoga vs. waitlist) [41,44,47,50,53,54] showed significant effects on CLBP-specific disability, whereas the other eight [42,46,48,51,52,54,56,57] demonstrated positive effects. Throughout the 12-week intervention period, weekly instructor-based training length ranged from 75 to 90 min in Qigong [42] and Yoga [54,56], which may not be sufficient to achieve significant reductions in disability risk. Notably, Neiyanggong, as one type of Qigong exercise, is not as popular as Baduanjin and Wuqinxi Qigong. Thus, it presumably takes beginners much longer to understand the principle and movement concepts, particularly during the initial stage of motor learning (cognitive stage) [59]. A 90-min session per week during a 12-week Neiyanggong intervention may not be sufficient to maximize the potential benefits of this modality of exercise. Likewise, movements in Yoga routine are relatively complex and require a certified instructor, and self-practice at home may lead to incorrect movement patterns, which may have contributed to the deterioration in disability or caused the observed adverse events (increased pain, herniated disc, and/or reduced range of motion at joints) reported in the five Yoga intervention studies [48,53–56]. Second, three studies included relatively small sample sizes of 20 [52], 30 [51] and 60 participants [48], which may have affected the power of detecting significant differences on disability risk.

4.3. Strengths and Limitations for Future Research

Strengths of this systematic review are as follows: (1) we provide a comprehensive review regarding the effectiveness of mindful exercises on CLBP disease-specific symptoms; (2) we were the first to include three popular mindful exercises; (3) we compared mindful exercises with active controls (conventional exercises and guideline-endorsed physical therapy); and (4) we evaluated the safety of mindful exercises in adults with CLBP [60,61]. Several limitations should be considered: (1) this review only included English-language studies, which possibly excluded Chinese-language journals that may be more likely to publish Tai Chi and Qigong studies; (2) we limited our meta-analysis to pain intensity and disability. We were not able to meta-analyze data on depressive symptomology (and other related outcomes) due to fewer than four studies reporting data on this outcome. Thus, future studies should include psychological outcome measures; (3) blinding of assessors was only used in one study (blinding of instructor and participants are, however, unrealistic), and it remains unclear whether greater expectations were associated with reduced pain intensity and disability in the mindful exercise groups; (4) some studies did not use "intention to treat analysis" and "allocation concealment", which possibly overestimated the pooled effect size; (5) none of studies used follow-up assessments, so it is difficult to determine how long the beneficial effects of mindful exercise interventions lasted in adults with CLBP; (6) previous studies suggest that different brain mechanisms are associated with different mindful exercises, thus, future studies should comparatively investigate different mind-body exercises as well as their underlying mechanisms [62,63].

5. Conclusions

Findings of our systematic review suggest that mindful exercises (Yoga, Tai Chi, and Qigong) may be beneficial for CLBP symptomatic management, irrespective of non-control comparison or active control comparison (conventional exercises, core training, and physical therapy programs). The potential of Tai Chi as a routine non-pharmacological approach for CLBP needs to be rigorously evaluated in future studies. Importantly, training in these mindful exercises should be implemented with certified instructors, to ensure quality of movement and injury prevention. Before definitive conclusions can be drawn, future work is needed that employs more robust study designs and implements long-term follow-up assessments.

Author Contributions: L.Z., Y.J.Z., A.Y., K.W.C., L.Y., P.D.L., T.X., and H.L. contributed to the conception and design of the review. Y.J.Z. and L.Z. applied the search strategy. L.Z. and Y.J.Z. applied the selection criteria. L.Z., Y.J.Z. and H.L. completed assessment of risk of bias. All authors analyzed and interpreted the data. All authors wrote this manuscript. All authors edited this manuscript. L.Z., Y.J.Z., T.X., and H.K. are responsible for the overall project.

Acknowledgments: The leading author would like to thank his family members (wife, son, daughter, and parents) for their consistent support.

Conflicts of Interest: The authors declare no conflict of interest.

References

1. Shmagel, A.; Foley, R.; Ibrahim, H. Epidemiology of chronic low back pain in US adults: Data from the 2009–2010 national health and nutrition examination survey. *Arthritis Care Res.* **2016**, *68*, 1688–1694. [CrossRef]
2. Murray, C.J.; Atkinson, C.; Bhalla, K.; Birbeck, G.; Burstein, R. The state of US health, 1990–2010: Burden of diseases, injuries, and risk factors. *JAMA* **2013**, *310*, 591–608. [CrossRef]

3. Taimela, S.; Kujala, U.M.; Salminen, J.J.; Viljanen, T. The prevalence of low back pain among children and adolescents: A nationwide, cohort-based questionnaire survey in Finland. *Spine* **1997**, *22*, 1132–1136. [CrossRef] [PubMed]
4. Balague, F.; Troussier, B.; Salminen, J.J. Non-specific low back pain in children and adolescents: Risk factors. *Eur. Spine J.* **1999**, *8*, 429–438. [CrossRef]
5. Richard, G.; David, W. The Adult Spine: Principles and Practice-Second Edition. *Neurosurgery* **1997**, *41*, 1208–1209. [CrossRef]
6. Enthoven, W.; Roelofs, P.; Deyo, R. Non-steroidal anti-inflammatory drugs for chronic low back pain. *Cochrane Database Syst. Rev.* **2016**, *2*, 012087. [CrossRef] [PubMed]
7. Marquardt, K.A.; Alsop, J.A.; Albertson, T.E. Tramadol exposures reported to statewide poison control system. *Ann. Pharmacother.* **2005**, *39*, 1039–1044. [CrossRef] [PubMed]
8. Shipton, E.A. Physical Therapy Approaches in the Treatment of Low Back Pain. *Pain Ther.* **2018**, *7*, 127–137. [CrossRef] [PubMed]
9. Burns, S.A.; Cleland, J.A.; Rivett, D.A.; Snodgrass, S.J. Effectiveness of physical therapy interventions for low back pain targeting the low back only or low back plus hips: A randomized controlled trial protocol. *Braz. J. Phys. Ther.* **2018**, *22*, 424–430. [CrossRef]
10. Cuenca-Martínez, F.; Cortés-Amador, S.; Espí-López, G.V. Effectiveness of classic physical therapy proposals for chronic non-specific low back pain: A literature review. *Phys. Ther. Res.* **2018**, *21*, 16–22. [CrossRef]
11. Searle, A.; Spink, M.; Ho, A.; Chuter, V. Exercise interventions for the treatment of chronic low back pain: A systematic review and meta-analysis of randomised controlled trials. *Clin. Rehabil.* **2015**, *29*, 1155–1167. [CrossRef] [PubMed]
12. Gordon, R.; Bloxham, S. A Systematic Review of the Effects of Exercise and Physical Activity on Non-Specific Chronic Low Back Pain. *Healthcare* **2016**, *4*, 22. [CrossRef]
13. Miyamoto, G.C.; Lin, C.C.; Cabral, C.M.; Van-Dongen, J.M.; Van-Tulder, M.W. Costeffectiveness of exercise therapy in the treatment of non-specific neck pain and low back pain: A systematic review with meta-analysis. *Br. J. Sports Med.* **2019**, *53*, 172–181. [CrossRef] [PubMed]
14. Zhou, S.; Zhang, Y.; Kong, Z.; Loprinzi, P.D.; Hu, Y.; Ye, J.; Liu, S.; Yu, J.J.; Zou, L. The Effects of tai chi on markers of atherosclerosis, lower-limb physical function, and cognitive ability in adults aged over 60: A randomized controlled trial. *Int. J. Environ. Res. Public Health* **2019**, *16*, 753. [CrossRef] [PubMed]
15. Zou, L.; Zeng, N.; Huang, T.; Yeung, A.S.; Wei, G.X.; Liu, S.J.; Zhou, J.; Hu, R.; Hui, S.S. The Beneficial Effects of Mind-body Exercises for People with Mild Cognitive Impairment: A Systematic Review with Meta-Analysis. *Arch. Phys. Med. Rehabil.* **2019**, in press. [CrossRef] [PubMed]
16. Zou, L.; Sasaki, J.E.; Wei, G.-X.; Huang, T.; Yeung, A.S.; Neto, O.B.; Chen, K.W.; Hui, S.C. Effects of mind–body exercises (Tai Chi/Yoga) on heart rate variability parameters and perceived stress: A systematic review with meta-analysis of randomized controlled trials. *J. Clin. Med.* **2018**, *7*, 404. [CrossRef] [PubMed]
17. Zou, L.; Yeung, A.; Li, C.; Wei, G.; Chen, K.; Kinser, P.; Chan, J.; Ren, Z. Effects of meditative movements on major depressive disorder: A systematic Review and meta-analysis of randomized controlled trials. *J. Clin. Med.* **2018**, *7*, 195. [CrossRef] [PubMed]
18. Zou, L.; Han, J.; Tsang, W.; Yeung, A. Effects of Tai Chi on lower limb proprioception in adults aged over 55: A systematic review ad meta-analysis. *Arch. Phys. Med. Rehabil.* **2018**, in press. [CrossRef]
19. Zou, L.; Sasaki, J.; Zeng, N.; Wang, C.; Sun, L.A. Systematic Review with Meta-Analysis of Mindful Exercises on Rehabilitative Outcomes among post-stroke patients. *Arch. Phys. Med. Rehabil.* **2018**, *9*, 2355–2364. [CrossRef] [PubMed]
20. Zou, L.; Yeung, A.; Li, C.; Chiou, S.; Zeng, N.; Tzeng, H. Effects of mind-body movement on balance function in stroke survivors: A meta-analysis of randomized controlled trials. *Int. J. Environ. Res. Public Health* **2018**, *15*, 1292. [CrossRef]
21. Zou, L.; Yeung, A.; Zeng, N.; Wang, C.; Sun, L.; Thomas, G.; Wang, H. Effects of Mind-Body Exercises for Mood and Functional Capabilities in Post-Stroke Patients: An Analytical Review of Randomized Controlled Trials. *Int. J. Environ. Res. Public Health* **2018**, *15*, 721. [CrossRef]
22. Zou, L.; Wang, C.; Tian, Z.; Wang, H.; Shu, Y. Effect of Yang-Style Tai Chi on Gait Parameters and Musculoskeletal Flexibility in Healthy Chinese Older Women. *Sports* **2017**, *5*, 52. [CrossRef]

23. Zhang, Y.; Loprinzi, P.D.; Yang, L.; Liu, J.; Liu, S.; Zou, L. The Beneficial Effects of Traditional Chinese Exercises for Adults with Low Back Pain: A Meta-Analysis of Randomized Controlled Trials. *Medicina* **2019**, *55*, 118. [CrossRef] [PubMed]
24. Zou, L.; Albert, Y.; Quan, X.; Wang, H. A Systematic review and meta-analysis of mindfulness-based (Baduanjin) exercise for alleviating musculoskeletal pain and improving sleep quality in people with chronic diseases. *Int. J. Environ. Res. Public Health* **2018**, *15*, 206. [CrossRef] [PubMed]
25. Zou, L.; SasaKi, J.; Wang, H.; Xiao, Z.; Fang, Q.; Zhang, M. A Systematic Review and Meta-Analysis Baduanjin Qigong for Health Benefits: Randomized Controlled Trials. *Evid. Based Complement. Altern. Med.* **2017**, *2017*. [CrossRef] [PubMed]
26. Zou, L.; Wang, H.; Xiao, Z.; Fang, Q.; Zhang, M.; Li, T. Tai chi for health benefits in patients with multiple sclerosis: A systematic review. *PLoS ONE* **2017**, *12*, e0170212. [CrossRef] [PubMed]
27. Zou, L.; Xiao, Z.; Wang, H.; Wang, C.; Hu, X.; Shu, Y. Asian martial arts for Children with Autism Spectrum Disorder: A Systematic Review. *Arch. Budo* **2017**, *13*, 79–92.
28. Zou, L.; Wang, H.; Yu, D. Effect of a long-term modified Tai Chi-based intervention in attenuating bone mineral density in postmenopausal women in southeast China: Study protocol for a randomized controlled trial. *Clin. Trials Degener. Dis.* **2017**, *2*, 46–52.
29. Zou, L.; Wang, C.; Chen, K.; Shu, Y.; Chen, X.; Luo, L.; Zhao, X. The effect of Taichi practice on attenuating bone mineral density loss: A systematic review and meta-analysis of randomized controlled trials. *Int. J. Environ. Res. Public Health* **2017**, *14*, 1000. [CrossRef]
30. Zou, L.; Wang, H.; Li, T.; Lu, L. Effect of traditional Chinese mind-body exercise on disease activity, spinal mobility, and quality of life in patients with ankylosing spondylitis. *Trav. Hum.* **2017**, *80*, 1585–1597.
31. Zou, L.; Wang, C.; Yeung, A.; Liu, Y.; Pan, Z. A Review Study on the beneficial effects of baduanjin. *J. Altern. Complement. Med.* **2018**, *24*, 324–335. [CrossRef] [PubMed]
32. Zou, L.; Yeung, A.; Quan, X. Mindfulness-based baduanjin exercise for depression and anxiety in people with physical or mental illnesses: A systematic review and meta-analysis of randomized controlled trials. *Int. J. Environ. Res. Public Health* **2018**, *15*, 321. [CrossRef]
33. Zou, L.; Wang, C.; Chen, X.; Wang, H. Baduanjin Exercise for Stroke Rehabilitation: A Systematic Review with Meta-Analysis of Randomized Controlled Trials. *Int. J. Environ. Res. Public Health* **2018**, *15*, 600. [CrossRef] [PubMed]
34. Theadom, A.; Cropley, M.; Smith, H.E.; Feigin, V.L.; Mcpherson, K. Mind and body therapy for fibromyalgia. *Cocrane Database Syst. Rev.* **2015**, *9*, CD001980. [CrossRef] [PubMed]
35. Selfe, T.K.; Innes, K.E. Mind-body therapies and osteoarthritis of the knee. *Curr. Rheumatol. Rev.* **2009**, *5*, 204–211. [CrossRef]
36. Holtzman, S.; Beggs, R.T. Yoga for chronic low back pain: A meta-analysis of randomized controlled trials. *Pain Res. Manag.* **2013**, *18*, 267–272. [CrossRef]
37. Cramer, H.; Lauche, R.; Haller, H.; Dobos, G. A systematic review and meta-analysis of yoga for low back pain. *Clin. J. Pain* **2013**, *29*, 450–460. [CrossRef]
38. Treede, R.D.; Rief, W.; Barke, A.; Aziz, Q.; Bennett, M.; Benoliel, R.; Wang, S.J. Chronic pain as a symptom or a disease: The IASP classification of chronic pain for the international classification of disease (ICD-11). *Pain* **2019**, *160*, 19–27. [CrossRef]
39. Maher, C.; Sherrington, C.; Herbert, R.; Moseley, A.; Elkins, M. Reliability of the PEDro scale for rating quality of randomized controlled trials. *Phys. Ther.* **2003**, *83*, 713–721. [CrossRef] [PubMed]
40. Higgins, J.P.; Green, S. *Cochrane Handbook for Systematic Reviews of Interventions*; John Wiley & Sons: New York, NY, USA, 2011; ISBN 9780470057964.
41. Hall, A.M.; Maher, C.G.; Lam, P.; Ferreira, M.; Latimer, J. Tai chi exercise for treatment of pain and disability in people with persistent low back pain: A randomized controlled trial. *Arthritis Care Res.* **2011**, *63*, 1576–1583. [CrossRef]
42. Blödt, S.; Pach, D.; Kaster, T.; Lüdtke, R.; Icke, K.; Reisshauer, A.; Witt, C.M. Qigong versus exercise therapy for chronic low back pain in adults—A randomized controlled non-inferiority trial. *Eur. J. Pain (UK)* **2015**, *19*, 123–131. [CrossRef]
43. Teut, M.; Knilli, J.; Daus, D.; Roll, S.; Witt, C.M. Qigong or Yoga Versus No Intervention in Older Adults with Chronic Low Back Pain—A Randomized Controlled Trial. *J. Pain* **2016**, *17*, 796–805. [CrossRef]

44. Phattharasupharerk, S.; Purepong, N.; Eksakulkla, S.; Siriphorn, A. Effects of Qigong practice in office workers with chronic non-specific low back pain: A randomized control trial. *J. Bodyw. Mov. Ther.* **2018**. [CrossRef]
45. Liu, J.; Yeung, A.; Xiao, T.; Tian, X.; Kong, Z.; Zou, L.; Wang, X. Chen-Style Tai Chi for Individuals (Aged 50 Years Old or Above) with Chronic Non-Specific Low Back Pain: A Randomized Controlled Trial. *Int. J. Environ. Res. Public Health* **2019**, *16*, 517. [CrossRef]
46. Galantino, M.L.; Bzdewka, T.M.; Eissler-Russo, J.L.; Holbrook, M.L.; Mogck, E.P.; Geigle, P.; Farrar, J.T. The impact of modified hatha yoga on chronic low back pain: A pilot study. *Altern. Ther. Health Med.* **2004**, *10*, 56–59. [CrossRef]
47. Sherman, K.J.; Cherkin, D.C.; Erro, J.; Miglioretti, D.L.; Deyo, R.A. Comparing yoga, exercise, and a self-care book for chronic low back pain: A randomized, controlled trial. *Ann. Intern. Med.* **2005**, *143*, 849–856. [CrossRef] [PubMed]
48. Williams, K.A.; Petronis, J.; Smith, D.; Goodrich, D.; Wu, J.; Ravi, N.; Doyle, E.J.; Juckett, R.G.; Kolar, M.M.; Gross, R. Effect of Iyengar yoga therapy for chronic low back pain. *Pain* **2005**, *115*, 107–117. [CrossRef]
49. Tekur, P.; Singphow, C.; Nagendra, H.R.; Raghuram, N. Effect of Short-Term Intensive Yoga Program on Pain, Functional Disability and Spinal Flexibility in Chronic Low Back Pain: A Randomized Control Study. *J. Altern. Complement. Med.* **2008**, *14*, 637–644. [CrossRef]
50. Williams, K.; Ph, D.; Abildso, C.; Ph, D.; Steinberg, L.; Ph, D.; Doyle, E.; Epstein, B.; Pt, M.D.; Smith, D. Evaluation of the effectiveness and efficacy of Iyengar Yoga Therapy on Chronic Low Back Pain. *Spine* **2009**, *34*, 2066–2076. [CrossRef] [PubMed]
51. Saper, R.B.; Sherman, K.J.; Cullum-Dugan, D.; Davis, R.B.; Phillips, R.S.; Culpepper, L. Yoga for chronic low back pain in a predominantly minority population: A pilot randomized controlled trial. *Altern. Ther. Health Med.* **2009**, *15*, 18–27. [CrossRef]
52. Cox, H.; Torgerson, D.; Semlyen, A.; Tilbrook, H.; Watt, I.; Aplin, J.; Trewhela, A. A randomised controlled trial of yoga for the treatment of chronic low back pain: Results of a pilot study. *Complement. Ther. Clin. Pract.* **2010**, *16*, 187–193. [CrossRef]
53. Tilbrook, H.E.; Cox, H.; Hewitt, C.E.; Kangombe, A.R.; Chuang, L.H.; Jayakody, S.; Aplin, J.D. Yoga for Chronic Low Back Pain. *Ann. Intern. Med.* **2011**, *155*, 569–578. [CrossRef]
54. Sherman, K.J.; Cherkin, D.C.; Wellman, R.D.; Cook, A.J.; Hawkes, R.J.; Delaney, K.; Deyo, R.A. A randomized trial comparing yoga, stretching, and a self-care book for chronic low back pain. *Arch. Intern. Med.* **2011**, *171*, 2019–2026. [CrossRef] [PubMed]
55. Nambi, G.S.; Inbasekaran, D.; Khuman, R.; Devi, S. Changes in pain intensity and health related quality of life with Iyengar yoga in nonspecific chronic low back pain: A randomized controlled study. *Int. J. Yoga* **2014**, *7*, 48–53. [CrossRef] [PubMed]
56. Saper, R.B.; Lemaster, C.; Delitto, A.; Sherman, K.J.; Herman, P.M.; Sadikova, E.; Stevans, J.; Keosaian, J.E.; Cerrada, C.J.; Femia, A.L. Yoga, Physical Therapy, or Education for Chronic Low Back Pain. *Ann. Intern. Med.* **2017**, *167*, 85. [CrossRef] [PubMed]
57. Kuvačić, G.; Fratini, P.; Padulo, J.; Antonio, D.I.; De Giorgio, A. Effectiveness of yoga and educational intervention on disability, anxiety, depression, and pain in people with CLBP: A randomized controlled trial. *Complement. Ther. Clin. Pract.* **2018**, *31*, 262–267. [CrossRef]
58. Hall, A.M.; Kamper, S.J.; Emsley, R.; Maher, C.G. Does pain-catestrophising mediate the effects of tai Chi on treatment outcomes ofr people with low back pain? *Complement. Ther. Med.* **2016**, *25*, 61–66. [CrossRef] [PubMed]
59. Enghauser, R. Motor learning and the dance technique class: Science, tradition and pedagogy. *J. Dance Educ.* **2003**, *3*, 87–95. [CrossRef]
60. Wayne, P.M.; Berkowitz, D.L.; Litrownik, D.E.; Buring, J.E.; Yeh, G.Y. What do we really know about the safety of tai chi? A systematic review of adverse event reports in randomized trials. *Arch. Phys. Med. Rehabil.* **2014**, *95*, 2470–2483. [CrossRef]
61. Zou, L.; Zhang, Y.; Liu, Y.; Tian, X.; Xiao, T.; Liu, X.; Yeung, A.S.; Liu, J.; Wang, X. The effects of tai chi chuan versus core stability training on lower-limb neuromuscular function in aging individuals with non-specific chronic lower back pain. *Medicina* **2019**, *55*, 60. [CrossRef] [PubMed]

62. Liu, J.; Tao, J.; Liu, W.; Huang, J.; Xue, X.; Li, M.; Yang, M.; Zhu, J.; Lang, C.; Park, J.; et al. Different modulation effects of tai chi chuan and baduanjin on resting state functional connectivity of the default mode network in older adults. *Soc. Cogn. Affect. Neurosci.* **2019**, *14*, 217–224. [CrossRef] [PubMed]
63. Tao, J.; Chen, X.; Liu, J.; Egorova, N.; Xue, X.; Liu, W.; Zheng, G.; Li, M.; Wu, J.; Hu, K.; et al. Tai Chi Chuan and Baduanjin mind-body training changes resting-state low-frequency fluctuations in the frontal lobe of older adults: A resting-state fmri study. *Front. Hum. Neurosci.* **2017**, *11*, 514. [CrossRef] [PubMed]

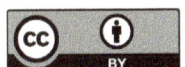

© 2019 by the authors. Licensee MDPI, Basel, Switzerland. This article is an open access article distributed under the terms and conditions of the Creative Commons Attribution (CC BY) license (http://creativecommons.org/licenses/by/4.0/).

MDPI
St. Alban-Anlage 66
4052 Basel
Switzerland
Tel. +41 61 683 77 34
Fax +41 61 302 89 18
www.mdpi.com

Journal of Clinical Medicine Editorial Office
E-mail: jcm@mdpi.com
www.mdpi.com/journal/jcm